SURVIVAL GUIDE TO
MIDWIFERY

Diane M. Fraser

BEd MPhil PhD MTD RN RM
Emeritus Professor of Midwifery and Former Head of the Academic Division
of Midwifery, School of Nursing, Midwifery and Physiotherapy, Faculty of
Medicine and Health Sciences, University of Nottingham, Nottingham, UK

Margaret A. Cooper

BA MTD RGN RM
Former Director of Pre-Registration Midwifery Programmes and Associate
Professor, School of Nursing, Midwifery and Physiotherapy, Faculty of Medicine
and Health Sciences, University of Nottingham, Nottingham, UK

SECOND EDITION

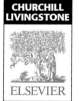

CHURCHILL
LIVINGSTONE

ELSEVIER

EDINBURGH   LONDON   NEW YORK   OXFORD   PHILADELPHIA
ST LOUIS   SYDNEY   TORONTO 2012

CHURCHILL
LIVINGSTONE
ELSEVIER

First edition 2008
Second edition 2012

ISBN 9780702045868

British Library Cataloguing in Publication Data
A catalogue record for this book is available from the British Library

Library of Congress Cataloging in Publication Data
A catalog record for this book is available from the Library of Congress

ELSEVIER your source for books,
journals and multimedia
in the health sciences

www.elsevierhealth.com

Working together to grow
libraries in developing countries

www.elsevier.com | www.bookaid.org | www.sabre.org

ELSEVIER   BOOK AID International   Sabre Foundation

The
Publisher's
policy is to use
**paper manufactured
from sustainable forests**

Printed in China

MIDWIFERY

Commissioning Editor: Mairi McCubbin
Development Editor: Carole McMurray
Project Manager: Vinod Kumar
Designer/Design Direction: Miles Hitchen
Illustration Manager: Jennifer Rose

Contents

Preface

This revised *Survival Guide* was developed in response to requests from midwives and student midwives. Whilst there are excellent textbooks for midwives, size precludes them from being carried around in clinical practice. This pocket-sized reference text enables students and midwives to draw upon and advance knowledge and understanding during practice, as well as providing a useful revision text for examinations and assessments.

No attempt has been made to replace full textbooks, as more detail, especially on psycho-social issues, and evidence sources continue to be essential and can only be provided in a larger and more comprehensive book. To allow easy reading, no references have been included in this *Survival Guide* and readers are directed to textbooks for this purpose and to explore wider practice issues.

The strategy when this *Survival Guide* was developed was to summarise information considered to be key for quick reference during practice. A list of common abbreviations, medications, drug calculations, terms and normal values have been included in this revised edition as an easily accessible source of information.

Nottingham, 2011

Diane M. Fraser
Margaret A. Cooper

Acknowledgements

These must be given to the *Myles Textbook for Midwives* authors on whose chapters this *Survival Guide* has been based. They are: Jean Bain, Diane Barrowclough, Terri Coates, Helen Crafter, Susan and Victor Dapaah, Margie Davies, Soo Downe, Jean Duerden, Carole England, Phil Farrell, Alison Gibbs, Claire Greig, Adela Hamilton, Jenny Hassall, Sally Inch, Judith Lee, Carmel Lloyd, Sally Marchant, Carol McCormick, Sue McDonald, Irene Murray, Margaret Oates, Patricia Percival, Maureen Raynor, Annie Rimmer, Jane Rutherford, Judith Simpson, Norma Sittlington, Amanda Sullivan, Ian Symonds, Ros Thomas, Denise Tiran, Tom Turner, Anne Viccars and Stephen Wardle.

In addition, thanks are extended to consultant obstetrician Margaret Ramsay and midwife teachers at the University of Nottingham for sharing their expertise.

Common Abbreviations

Use with caution, as some may have more than one meaning.

ACTH	Adrenocorticotrophic hormone
AFP	Alpha fetoprotein
AID	Artificial insemination by donor
AIH	Artificial insemination by husband
AIMS	Association for Improvements in the Maternity Services
ALT	Alanine transaminase
ANC	Antenatal clinic
APH	Antepartum haemorrhage
ARM	Artificial rupture of membranes
BBA	Born before arrival
BFI	Baby-Friendly Initiative
BMI	Body mass index
BMR	Basal metabolic rate
BP	Blood pressure
BPD	Biparietal diameter
BPM	Beats per minute
BTS	Blood Transfusion Service
CCT	Controlled cord traction
CDH	Congenital dislocation of hips
CEMACH	Confidential Enquiry into Maternal and Child Health
CF	Cystic fibrosis
CMV	Cytomegalovirus
CNS	Central nervous system
CNST	Clinical negligence scheme for trusts
CPAP	Continuous positive airways pressure
CPR	Cardiopulmonary resuscitation
CQC	Care Quality Commission
CSF	Cerebrospinal fluid
CTG	Cardiotocograph
CVP	Central venous pressure
CVS	Chorionic villus sampling
D&C	Dilatation and curettage
DIC	Disseminated intravascular coagulation
DVT	Deep vein thrombosis

EBM	Expressed breast milk
ECG	Electrocardiogram
ECV	External cephalic version
EDD	Expected date of delivery
EEG	Electroencephalogram
EFM	Electronic fetal monitoring
EUA	Examination under anaesthetic
FACH	Forceps to aftercoming head
FAS	Fetal alcohol syndrome
FBC	Full blood count
FBS	Fetal blood sampling
FDPs	Fibrin degradation products
FGM	Female genital mutilation
FH	Fetal heart
FHH	Fetal heart heard
FIGO	International Federation of Gynaecologists and Obstetricians
FSE	Fetal scalp electrode
FSH	Follicle-stimulating hormone
GA	General anaesthetic
GBS	Group B haemolytic streptococcus
GI	Gastrointestinal
GIFT	Gamete intrafallopian transfer
G6PD	Glucose 6-phosphate dehydrogenase
G&S	Group and save serum
GTT	Glucose tolerance test
GU	Genitourinary
Hb	Haemoglobin
HBV	Hepatitis B virus
HCG	Human chorionic gonadotrophin
HDN	Haemolytic disease of the newborn
HDU	High-dependency unit
HELLP	Haemolysis, elevated liver enzymes, low platelets
HIV	Human immunodeficiency virus
HPL	Human placental lactogen
HPV	Human papillomavirus
HVS	High vaginal swab
ICM	International Confederation of Midwives
ICSI	Intracytoplasmic sperm injection
ICU	Intensive care unit
IG	Immunoglobulin
IM	Intramuscular
IOL	Induction of labour
IUCD	Intrauterine contraceptive device
IU(F)D	Intrauterine (fetal) death
IUGR	Intrauterine growth restriction

IV	Intravenous
LAM	Lactational amenorrhoea method
LFT	Liver function tests
LGA	Large for gestational age
LH	Luteinising hormone
LMP	Last menstrual period
L:S	Lecithin:sphyngomyelin
LSA	Local Supervising Authority
LSCS	Lower segment caesarean section
MAP	Mean arterial pressure
MSU	Midstream specimen of urine
NEC	Necrotising enterocolitis
NICE	National Institute for Health and Clinical Excellence
NICU	Neonatal intensive care unit
NMC	Nursing and Midwifery Council
NND	Neonatal death
NSF	National Service Framework
NT	Nuchal translucency
NTD	Neural tube defect
PE	Pulmonary embolism (care – may also be used for pre-eclampsia)
PGD	Patient group direction
PIH	Pregnancy-induced hypertension
PKU	Phenylketonuria
PPH	Postpartum haemorrhage
PROM	Premature rupture of membranes
PV	Per vaginam
RBC	Red blood cell
RCM	Royal College of Midwives
RCOG	Royal College of Obstetricians and Gynaecologists
RCT	Randomised controlled trial
RDS	Respiratory distress syndrome
Rh	Rhesus
SB	Stillbirth
SCBU	Special care baby unit
SGA	Small for gestational age
SIDS	Sudden infant death syndrome
SLE	Systemic lupus erythematosus
SPD	Symphysis pubis dysfunction
SROM	Spontaneous rupture of membranes
STI	Sexually transmitted infection
TIA	Transient ischaemic attack
TOP	Termination of pregnancy
TPN	Total parenteral nutrition
TSH	Thyroid-stimulating hormone

U&E	Urea and electrolytes
UNICEF	United Nations Children's Fund
USS	Ultrasound scan
UTI	Urinary tract infection
VBAC	Vaginal birth after caesarean
VDRL	Venereal Disease Research Laboratory
VE	Vaginal examination
WHO	World Health Organisation
ZIFT	Zygote intrafallopian transfer

Section 1

Anatomy and Reproduction

CHAPTER 1

The Female Pelvis and the Reproductive Organs

THE FEMALE PELVIS

The normal pelvis is comprised of four pelvic bones:
- two innominate bones
- one sacrum
- one coccyx.

The innominate bones (Fig. 1.1)
Each innominate bone is composed of three parts:
- the ilium
- the ischium
- the pubic bone.

The ilium
- At the front of the iliac crest is a bony prominence known as the *anterior superior iliac spine*; below it is the *anterior inferior iliac spine*.
- Two similar points at the other end of the iliac crest are called the *posterior superior* and the *posterior inferior iliac spines*.
- The concave anterior surface of the ilium is the *iliac fossa*.

The ischium
The ischium is the thick lower part.
- The *ischial tuberosity* is the prominence on which the body rests when sitting.
- Behind and a little above the tuberosity is an inward projection, the *ischial spine*.

In labour the station of the fetal head is estimated in relation to the ischial spines.

The pubic bone
- This has a body and two oar-like projections: the *superior ramus* and the *inferior ramus*.
- The two pubic bones meet at the symphysis pubis and the two inferior rami form the *pubic arch*, merging into a similar ramus on the ischium.

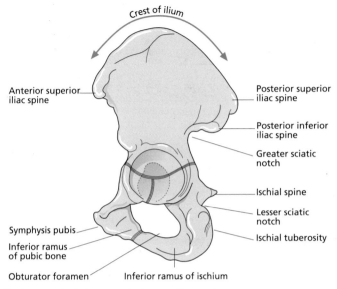

Fig. 1.1: Innominate bone showing important landmarks.

- The space enclosed by the body of the pubic bone, the rami and the ischium is called the *obturator foramen*.
- The innominate bone contains a deep cup, the *acetabulum*, which receives the head of the femur.
  On the lower border of the innominate bone are found two curves:
- One extends from the posterior inferior iliac spine up to the ischial spine and is called the *greater sciatic notch*. It is wide and rounded.
- The other lies between the ischial spine and the ischial tuberosity and is the *lesser sciatic notch*.

The sacrum
This is a wedge-shaped bone consisting of five fused vertebrae. The first sacral vertebra juts forward and is called the *sacral promontory*.

The coccyx
The coccyx consists of four fused vertebrae, forming a small triangular bone.

The pelvic joints
There are four pelvic joints:
- The *symphysis pubis* is formed at the junction of the two pubic bones, which are united by a pad of cartilage.
- Two *sacroiliac joints* join the sacrum to the ilium and thus connect the spine to the pelvis.

- The *sacrococcygeal joint* is formed where the base of the coccyx articulates with the tip of the sacrum.

In the non-pregnant state there is very little movement in these joints, but during pregnancy endocrine activity causes the ligaments to soften, which allows the joints to give.

The pelvic ligaments
Each of the pelvic joints is held together by ligaments:
- *interpubic* ligaments at the symphysis pubis
- *sacroiliac* ligaments
- *sacrococcygeal* ligaments.

Two other ligaments are important in midwifery:
- the sacrotuberous ligament
- the sacrospinous ligament.

The sacrotuberous ligament runs from the sacrum to the ischial tuberosity, and the sacrospinous ligament from the sacrum to the ischial spine. These two ligaments cross the sciatic notch and form the posterior wall of the pelvic outlet.

THE TRUE PELVIS

The true pelvis is the bony canal through which the fetus must pass during birth. It has a brim, a cavity and an outlet.

The pelvic brim
The fixed points on the pelvic brim are known as its landmarks (see Fig. 1.2 and Box 1.1).

Diameters of the brim
Three diameters are measured (Figs 1.3 and 1.4):
- anteroposterior
- oblique
- transverse.

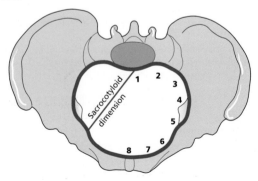

Fig. 1.2: Brim or inlet of female pelvis (see Box 1.1).

Box 1.1 Landmarks of the pelvic brim (commencing posteriorly)

See Figure 1.2 for numbers
- Sacral promontory (1)
- Sacral ala or wing (2)
- Sacroiliac joint (3)
- Iliopectineal line: the edge formed at the inward aspect of the ilium (4)
- Iliopectineal eminence: a roughened area formed where the superior ramus of the pubic bone meets the ilium (5)
- Superior ramus of the pubic bone (6)
- Upper inner border of the body of the pubic bone (7)
- Upper inner border of the symphysis pubis (8)

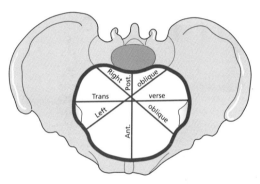

Fig. 1.3: View of pelvic inlet showing diameters.

The anteroposterior diameter

This is a line from the sacral promontory to the upper border of the symphysis pubis.
- When the line is taken to the uppermost point of the symphysis pubis, it is called the *anatomical conjugate* (12 cm).
- When it is taken to the posterior border of the upper surface, it is called the *obstetrical conjugate* (11 cm).
- The *diagonal conjugate* is also measured anteroposteriorly from the lower border of the symphysis to the sacral promontory. It may be estimated on vaginal examination as part of a pelvic assessment and should measure 12–13 cm.

The oblique diameter

This is a line from one sacroiliac joint to the iliopectineal eminence on the opposite side of the pelvis (12 cm).

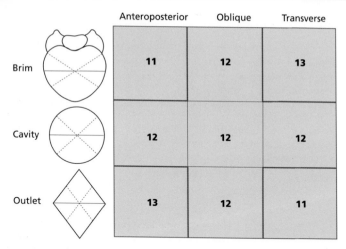

Fig. 1.4: Measurements of the pelvic canal in centimetres.

The transverse diameter
This is a line between the points furthest apart on the iliopectineal lines (13 cm).

Another dimension is described, the *sacrocotyloid* (see Fig. 1.2). It passes from the sacral promontory to the iliopectineal eminence on each side and measures 9–9.5 cm.

The pelvic cavity
This extends from the brim above to the outlet below.
- The anterior wall is formed by the pubic bones and symphysis pubis and its depth is 4 cm.
- The posterior wall is formed by the curve of the sacrum, which is 12 cm in length.

The cavity forms a curved canal; its lateral walls are the sides of the pelvis, which are mainly covered by the obturator internus muscle.

The cavity is circular in shape and its diameters are all considered to be 12 cm (see Fig. 1.4).

The pelvic outlet
Two outlets are described: the *anatomical* and the *obstetrical*. The obstetrical outlet includes the narrow pelvic strait, through which the fetus must pass. This outlet is diamond shaped. Its three diameters are as follows (see Fig. 1.4):
- The *anteroposterior diameter* is a line from the lower border of the symphysis pubis to the sacrococcygeal joint.
- The *oblique diameter* is said to be between the obturator foramen and the sacrospinous ligament, although there are no fixed points.
- The *transverse diameter* is a line between the two ischial spines.

THE FALSE PELVIS

The false pelvis is the part of the pelvis situated above the pelvic brim. It is of no significance in obstetrics.

PELVIC INCLINATION

When a woman is standing in the upright position, her pelvis is on an incline; as can be seen in Figure 1.5, the brim is tilted and forms an angle of 60° with the horizontal floor. The angles are important to understand when women are in different positions for an abdominal examination.

The pelvic planes

These are imaginary flat surfaces at the brim, cavity and outlet of the pelvic canal at the levels of the lines described above.

The axis of the pelvic canal

A line drawn exactly half-way between the anterior wall and the posterior wall of the pelvic canal would trace a curve known as the *curve of Carus*. An understanding of this is necessary when assessing progress in labour.

THE FOUR TYPES OF PELVIS (TABLE 1.1)

Classically, the pelvis has been described according to the shape of the brim. If one of the important measurements is reduced by 1 cm or more from the

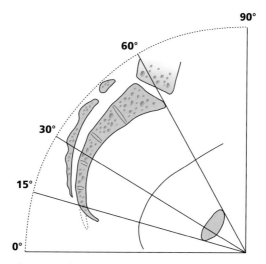

Fig. 1.5: Median section of the pelvis showing the inclination of the planes and the axis of the pelvic canal.

Table 1.1 Features of the four types of pelvis

Features	Gynaecoid	Android	Anthropoid	Platypelloid
Brim	Rounded	Heart shaped	Long oval	Kidney shaped
Forepelvis	Generous	Narrow	Narrowed	Wide
Side walls	Straight	Convergent	Divergent	Divergent
Ischial spines	Blunt	Prominent	Blunt	Blunt
Sciatic notch	Rounded	Narrow	Wide	Wide
Subpubic angle	90°	<90°	>90°	>90°
Incidence	50%	20%	25%	5%

normal, the pelvis is said to be contracted; this may give rise to difficulty in labour or necessitate caesarean section.

The *gynaecoid pelvis* is the ideal pelvis for childbearing. Its main features are:
- a rounded brim
- generous forepelvis (the part in front of the transverse diameter)
- straight side walls
- a shallow cavity with a broad, well-curved sacrum, blunt ischial spines, a rounded sciatic notch and a subpubic angle of 90°.

It is found in women of average build and height with a shoe size of 4 or larger.

THE PELVIC FLOOR

The pelvic floor is formed by the soft tissues that fill the outlet of the pelvis. The most important of these is the strong diaphragm of muscle slung like a hammock from the walls of the pelvis. Through it pass the urethra, the vagina and the anal canal. The pelvic floor comprises two muscle layers:
- the superficial layer (Fig. 1.6)
- the deep layer (Fig. 1.7).

THE VULVA

The term 'vulva' applies to the external female genital organs (Fig. 1.8).

THE VAGINA

The vagina is a canal running from the vestibule to the cervix, passing upwards and backwards into the pelvis along a line approximately parallel to the plane of the pelvic brim.

A knowledge of the relations of the vagina to other organs is essential for the accurate examination of the pregnant woman and the safe birth of her baby (see Figs 1.9 and 1.10)

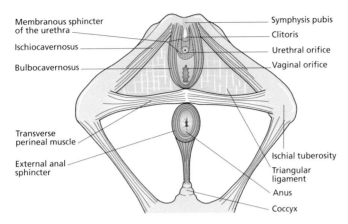

Fig. 1.6: Superficial muscle layer of the pelvic floor.

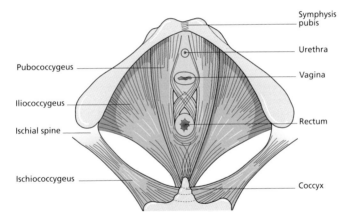

Fig. 1.7: Deep muscle layer of the pelvic floor.

THE UTERUS

The uterus is situated in the cavity of the true pelvis.

Relations
See Figures 1.9 and 1.10.

Supports
The uterus is supported by the pelvic floor and maintained in position by several ligaments.

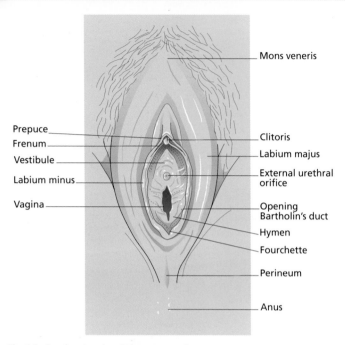

Fig. 1.8: Female external genital organs, or vulva.

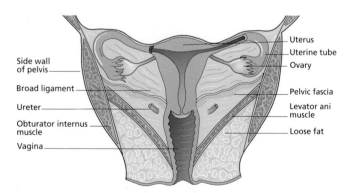

Fig. 1.9: Coronal section through the pelvis.

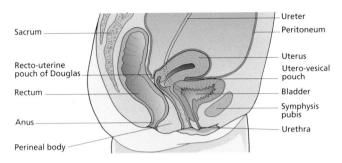

Fig. 1.10: Sagittal section of the pelvis.

Structure

The non-pregnant uterus is a hollow, muscular, pear-shaped organ. It is 7.5 cm long, 5 cm wide and 2.5 cm in depth, each wall being 1.25 cm thick. The cervix forms the lower third of the uterus and measures 2.5 cm in each direction. The uterus consists of the following parts:

The body or corpus
This forms the upper two-thirds of the uterus.

The fundus
The fundus is the domed upper wall between the insertions of the uterine tubes.

The cornua
These are the upper outer angles of the uterus where the uterine tubes join.

The uterine tubes extend laterally from the cornua of the uterus towards the side walls of the pelvis. They arch over the ovaries, the fringed ends hovering near the ovaries in order to receive the oocyte. Each tube is 10 cm long. The lumen of the tube provides an open pathway from the outside to the peritoneal cavity. The uterine tube has four portions:
- the interstitial portion
- the isthmus
- the ampulla
- the infundibulum (Fig. 1.11).

The cavity
The cavity is a potential space between the anterior and posterior walls. It is triangular in shape, the base of the triangle being uppermost.

The isthmus
The isthmus is a narrow area between the cavity and the cervix, which is 7 mm long. It enlarges during pregnancy to form the lower uterine segment.

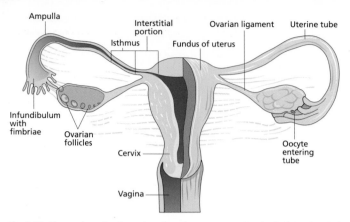

Fig. 1.11: The uterine tubes in section. Note the oocyte entering the fimbriated end of one tube.

The cervix
This protrudes into the vagina.
- The *internal os* is the narrow opening between the isthmus and the cervix.
- The *external os* is a small round opening at the lower end of the cervix. After childbirth it becomes a transverse slit.
- The *cervical canal* lies between these two ora and is a continuation of the uterine cavity.

Layers
The layers of the uterus are called:
- the endometrium
- the myometrium
- the perimetrium.

The endometrium
This forms a lining of ciliated epithelium on a base of connective tissue or stroma.

In the uterine cavity this endometrium is constantly changing in thickness throughout the menstrual cycle. The basal layer does not alter, but provides the foundation from which the upper layers regenerate. The epithelial cells are cubical in shape and dip down to form glands that secrete an alkaline mucus.

The cervical endometrium does not respond to the hormonal stimuli of the menstrual cycle to the same extent. Here the epithelial cells are tall and columnar in shape and the mucus-secreting glands are branching racemose glands. The cervical endometrium is thinner than that of the body and is folded into a pattern known as the 'arbor vitae'. The portion of the cervix that protrudes into the vagina is covered with squamous epithelium similar to that lining the vagina. The point where the epithelium changes, at the external os, is termed the squamocolumnar junction.

The myometrium

This layer is thick in the upper part of the uterus but sparser in the isthmus and cervix. Its fibres run in all directions and interlace to surround the blood vessels and lymphatics that pass to and from the endometrium. The outer layer is formed of longitudinal fibres that are continuous with those of the uterine tube, the uterine ligaments and the vagina.

In the cervix the muscle fibres are embedded in collagen fibres, which enable it to stretch in labour.

The perimetrium

This is a double serous membrane, an extension of the peritoneum, which is draped over the uterus, covering all but a narrow strip on either side and the anterior wall of the supravaginal cervix, from where it is reflected up over the bladder.

Blood supply

The uterine artery arrives at the level of the cervix and is a branch of the internal iliac artery. It sends a small branch to the upper vagina, and then runs upwards in a twisted fashion to meet the ovarian artery and form an anastomosis with it near the cornu. The ovarian artery is a branch of the abdominal aorta. It supplies the ovary and uterine tube before joining the uterine artery. The blood drains through corresponding veins.

Lymphatic drainage

Lymph is drained from the uterine body to the internal iliac glands and also from the cervical area to many other pelvic lymph glands.

Nerve supply

This is mainly from the autonomic nervous system, sympathetic and parasympathetic, via the inferior hypogastric or pelvic plexus.

THE OVARIES

The ovaries are situated within the peritoneal cavity. They are attached to the back of the broad ligaments but are supported from above by the ovarian ligament medially and the infundibulopelvic ligament laterally. Each ovary is composed of a medulla and cortex, covered with germinal epithelium. (See Ch. 3 for changes associated with the menstrual cycle.)

CHAPTER 2

The Female Urinary Tract

The urinary system has important functions in connection with the control of water and electrolyte balance and of blood pressure.

THE KIDNEYS

The kidneys are two bean-shaped glands that have both endocrine and exocrine secretions.

Functions
Functions of the kidneys are shown in Box 2.1.

Position and appearance
The kidneys are positioned at the back of the abdominal cavity, high up under the diaphragm. Each kidney is about 10 cm long, 6.5 cm wide and 3 cm thick. It weighs around 120 g and is covered with a tough, fibrous capsule.

The inner border of the organ is indented at the hilum; here the large vessels enter and leave, and the ureter is attached by its funnel-shaped upper end to channel the urine away.

Inner structure
- The glandular tissue is formed of *cortex* on the outside and *medulla* within. The cortex is dark with a rich blood supply, whereas the medulla is paler.
- A collecting area for urine merges with the upper ureter and is called the *pelvis*. It is divided into branches or calyces.
- Each calyx forms a cup over a projection of the medulla known as a *pyramid*. There are some 12 pyramids in all and they contain bundles of tubules leading from the cortex.
- The tubules create a lined appearance and these are the *medullary rays*.
- The base of each pyramid is curved and the cortex arches over it and projects downwards between the pyramids, forming columns of tissue (*columns of Bertini*).

The nephrons (Fig. 2.1)
The tissue of the kidney is made up of about 1 million nephrons, which are its functional units.
- Each nephron starts at a knot of capillaries called a *glomerulus*.
- It is fed by a branch of the renal artery, the *afferent arteriole*. (Afferent means 'carrying towards'.)

Box 2.1 Functions of the kidneys

- Elimination of waste, particularly the breakdown products of protein, such as urea, urates, uric acid, creatinine, ammonia and sulphates
- Elimination of toxins
- Regulation of the water content of the blood and indirectly of the tissues
- Regulation of the pH of the blood
- Regulation of the osmotic pressure of the blood
- Secretion of the hormones renin and erythropoietin

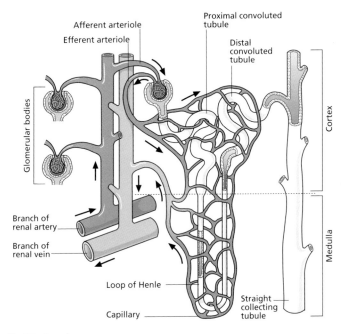

Fig. 2.1: A nephron.

- The blood is collected up again into the *efferent arteriole*. (Efferent means 'carrying away'.)
- Surrounding the glomerulus is a cup known as the *glomerular capsule*, into which fluid and solutes are exuded from the blood.
- The glomerulus and capsule together comprise the *glomerular body*. The pressure within the glomerulus is raised because the afferent arteriole is

of a wider bore than the efferent arteriole; this factor forces the filtrate out of the capillaries and into the capsule. At this stage there is no selection; any substance with a small molecular size will filter out.

- The cup of the capsule is attached to a tubule, as a wine glass is to its stem. The tubule initially winds and twists, then forms a straight loop which dips into the medulla, rising up into the cortex again to wind and turn before joining a *straight collecting tubule*, which receives urine from several nephrons.
- The first twisting portion of the nephron is the *proximal convoluted tubule*, the loop is termed the *loop of Henle* and the second twisting portion is the *distal convoluted tubule*.

The whole nephron is about 3 cm in length. The straight collecting tubule runs from the cortex to a medullary pyramid; it forms a medullary ray and receives urine from over 4000 nephrons along its length.

Juxtaglomerular apparatus

The distal convoluted tubule returns to pass alongside granular cells of the afferent arteriole, and this part of the tubule is called the *macula densa*. The two are known as the *juxtaglomerular apparatus*. The granular cells secrete renin, whereas the macula densa cells monitor the sodium chloride concentration of fluid passing through.

Blood supply

The renal arteries are early branches of the descending abdominal aorta and divert about a quarter of the cardiac output into the kidneys. Blood is collected up and returned via the renal vein.

THE MAKING OF URINE

This takes place in three stages:

- filtration
- reabsorption
- secretion.

Filtration

Water and the substances dissolved in it are passed from the glomerulus into the glomerular capsule as a result of the raised intracapillary pressure. Blood components such as corpuscles and platelets, as well as plasma proteins, which are large molecules, are kept in the blood vessel; water, salts and glucose escape through the filter as the *filtrate*. Fluid passes out at about 2 ml per second or 120 ml per minute. Ninety-nine per cent of this must be recovered. Filtration is increased in pregnancy, as it helps to eliminate the additional waste substances created by maternal and fetal metabolism.

Reabsorption

The body selects from the filtrate those substances that it needs: water, salts and glucose.

Normally, all the glucose is reabsorbed; only if there is already more than sufficient in the blood will any be excreted in the urine. The level of blood glucose at which this happens is the *renal threshold* for glucose:

- In the non-pregnant woman, the threshold is 10 mmol/l.
- In the pregnant woman, the threshold is 8.3 mmol/l.

It is more likely, therefore, that glucose will appear in the urine during pregnancy.

The water is almost all reabsorbed. The posterior pituitary gland controls the reabsorption of water by producing antidiuretic hormone (ADH). Minerals are selected according to the body's needs. The reabsorption of sodium is controlled by aldosterone, which is produced in the cortex of the adrenal gland. The interaction of aldosterone and ADH maintains water and sodium balance. The pH of the blood must be controlled and if it is tending towards acidity then acids will be excreted. However, if the opposite pertains, alkaline urine will be produced.

Secretion

Certain substances, such as creatinine and toxins, are added directly to the urine in the ascending arm of the loop of Henle.

ENDOCRINE ACTIVITY

The kidney secretes two hormones:

- *Renin* is produced in the afferent arteriole and is secreted when the blood supply to the kidneys is reduced and in response to lowered sodium levels. It acts on angiotensinogen, which is present in the blood, to form angiotensin, which raises blood pressure and encourages sodium reabsorption.
- *Erythropoietin* stimulates the production of red blood cells.

THE URINE

An adult passes between 1 and 2 litres of urine daily, depending on fluid intake. Pregnant women secrete large amounts of urine because of the increased glomerular filtration rate. In the first day or two postpartum a major diuresis occurs and urine output is copious. The specific gravity of urine is 1.010–1.030. It is composed of:

- 96% water
- 2% urea
- 2% other solutes.

Urea and uric acid clearance are increased in pregnancy. Urine is usually acid and contains no glucose or ketones; nor should it carry blood cells or bacteria. Women are susceptible to urinary tract infection (UTI) but this is usually an ascending infection acquired via the urethra. A low count, less than 100 000 per ml, of bacteria in the urine (bacteriuria) is treated as insignificant.

THE URETERS

The ureters convey urine from the kidneys to the bladder. They assist the passage of urine by the muscular peristaltic action of their walls. The upper end is funnel shaped and merges into the pelvis of the kidney, where the urine is received from the renal tubules.

Each tube is about 25–30 cm long and runs from the renal hilum to the posterior wall of the bladder. In the abdomen the ureters pass down the posterior wall, remaining outside the peritoneal cavity. On reaching the pelvic brim, they descend along the side walls of the pelvis to the level of the ischial spines and then turn forwards to pass beside the uterine cervix and enter the bladder from behind. They pass through the bladder wall at an angle, so that when the bladder contracts to expel urine the ureters are closed off and reflux is prevented.

The hormones of pregnancy, particularly progesterone, relax the walls of the ureters and allow dilatation and kinking. In some women this is quite marked and it tends to result in a slowing down or stasis of urinary flow, making infection a greater possibility.

THE BLADDER

The bladder is the urinary reservoir, storing the urine until it is convenient for it to be voided. It is described as being pyramidal and its base is triangular. When it is full, however, it becomes more globular in shape as its walls are distended. Although it is a pelvic organ, it may rise into the abdomen when full.

Structure

- The base of the bladder is termed the *trigone*. It is situated at the back of the bladder, resting against the vagina. Its three angles are formed by the exit of the urethra below and the two slit-like openings of the ureters above. The apex of the trigone is thus at its lowest point, which is also termed the neck.
- The anterior part of the bladder lies close to the pubic symphysis and is termed the *apex* of the bladder. From it the urachus runs up the anterior abdominal wall to the umbilicus. The empty bladder is of similar size to the uterus; when full of urine, its capacity is around 600 ml but it is capable of holding more, particularly under the influence of pregnancy hormones.

THE URETHRA

The urethra is 4 cm long in the female and consists of a narrow tube buried in the outer layers of the anterior vaginal wall. It runs from the neck of the bladder and opens into the vestibule of the vulva as the urethral meatus. During labour the urethra becomes elongated, as the bladder is drawn up into the abdomen, and may become several centimetres longer.

MICTURITION

The urge to pass urine is felt when the bladder contains about 200–300 ml of urine; psychological and other external stimuli may also trigger a desire to empty the bladder. The sphincters relax, the detrusor muscle contracts and urine is passed. In summary, the bladder fills and then contracts as a reflex response. The internal sphincter opens by the action of Bell's muscles. If the urge is not resisted, the external sphincter relaxes and the bladder empties. The act of emptying may be speeded by raising intra-abdominal pressure either to initiate the process or throughout voiding. The act of micturition can be temporarily postponed.

Key points for practice are summarised in Box 2.2.

Box 2.2 Key points for practice

- Pregnant and postnatal women produce large amounts of urine
- Glucose in the urine might be due to a temporary reduced reabsorption threshold or diabetes (pre-existing or gestational)
- Protein in the urine might be due to contamination, UTI, pre-eclampsia or renal dysfunction
- A full bladder can impede progress in labour and prevent contraction of the uterus following birth

CHAPTER 3

Hormonal Cycles: Fertilisation and Early Development

The hypothalamus is the ultimate source of control, governing the anterior pituitary gland by hormonal pathways. The anterior pituitary gland in turn governs the ovary via hormones. Finally, the ovary produces hormones that control changes in the uterus. All these changes occur simultaneously and in harmony. A woman's moods may change along with the cycle, and emotional influences can alter the cycle because of the close relationship between the hypothalamus and the cerebral cortex.

THE OVARIAN CYCLE

- Under the influence of follicle-stimulating hormone (FSH) and, later, luteinising hormone (LH) the Graafian follicle matures and moves to the surface of the ovary. At the same time it swells and becomes tense, finally rupturing to release the secondary oocyte into the fimbriated end of the uterine tube; this is *ovulation*.
- The empty follicle, known as the *corpus luteum*, collapses, the granulosa cells enlarge and proliferate over the next 14 days, and the whole structure becomes irregular in outline and yellow in colour.
- Unless pregnancy occurs, the corpus luteum atrophies and becomes the *corpus albicans*.

Ovarian hormones
Oestrogen
This is produced under the influence of FSH by the granulosa cells and the theca in increasing amounts until the degeneration of the corpus luteum, when the level falls. The effects of oestrogen are as follows:
- It is responsible for the secondary female sex characteristics.
- It influences the production of cervical mucus and the structure of the vaginal epithelium.
- During the cycle, it causes the proliferation of the uterine endometrium.
- It inhibits FSH and encourages fluid retention.

Progesterone
This, with related compounds, is produced by the corpus luteum under the influence of LH. They act only on tissues that have previously been affected by oestrogen.

The effects of progesterone are mainly evident during the second half of the cycle:

- It causes secretory changes in the lining of the uterus, when the endometrium develops tortuous glands and an enriched blood supply in readiness for the possible arrival of a fertilised oocyte.
- It causes the body temperature to rise by 0.5°C after ovulation and gives rise to tingling and a sense of fullness in the breasts prior to menstruation.

Relaxin

This hormone is at its maximum level between weeks 38 and 42 of pregnancy. It originates in the corpus luteum.

Relaxin is thought to relax the pelvic girdle, to soften the cervix and to suppress uterine contractions.

PITUITARY CONTROL

Under the influence of the hypothalamus, which produces gonadotrophin-releasing hormone (GnRH), the anterior pituitary gland secretes two gonadotrophins: FSH and LH. The gonadotrophic activity of the hypothalamus and the pituitary is influenced by positive and negative feedback mechanisms from ovarian hormones.

FSH

This hormone causes several Graafian follicles to develop and enlarge, one of them more prominently than all the others. FSH stimulates the secretion of oestrogen. The level of FSH rises during the first half of the cycle and when the oestrogen level reaches a certain point its production is stopped.

LH

This is first produced a few days after the anterior pituitary starts producing FSH. Rising oestrogen causes a surge in both FSH and LH levels, the ripened follicle ruptures and ovulation occurs. Levels of both gonadotrophins then fall rapidly. Progesterone inhibits any new rise in LH in spite of high oestrogen levels, but if no pregnancy occurs, the corpus luteum degenerates after 14 days. The negative feedback effect of progesterone ceases and FSH and LH levels rise again to begin a new cycle.

Prolactin

This is also produced in the anterior pituitary gland, but it does not play a part in the control of the ovary. If produced in excessive amounts, however, it will inhibit ovulation.

THE UTERINE CYCLE OR MENSTRUAL CYCLE

The average cycle is taken to be 28 days long. The first day of the cycle is the day on which menstruation begins (Fig. 3.1). There are three main phases and they affect the tissue structure of the endometrium, controlled by the ovarian hormones.

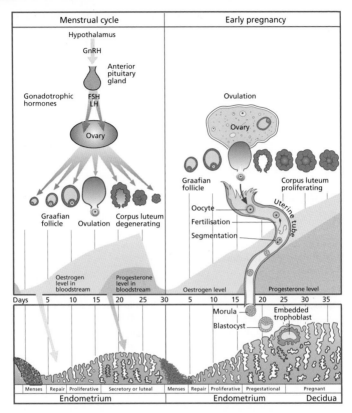

Fig. 3.1: The menstrual cycle and early pregnancy. Left: action of the gonadotrophic hormones on the ovary and of the ovarian hormones on the endometrium. Right: ovulation, fertilisation, decidual reaction and embedding of the fertilised oocyte.

FERTILISATION

Following ovulation, the oocyte passes into the uterine tube and is moved along towards the uterus. At this time the cervix, under the influence of oestrogen, secretes a flow of alkaline mucus that attracts the spermatozoa. Sperm that reach the loose cervical mucus survive to propel themselves towards the uterine tubes, while the remainder are destroyed by the acid medium of the vagina. More will die en route. Those that reach the uterine tube meet the oocyte, usually in the ampulla. During this journey the sperm finally become mature and capable of releasing the enzyme hyaluronidase, which allows penetration of the zona pellucida and the cell membrane surrounding the oocyte. Only one sperm will enter the oocyte. The sperm and the oocyte each contribute half the complement of chromosomes to make a total of 46.

● The sperm and oocyte are known as the male and female *gametes*.
● The fertilised oocyte is known as the *zygote*.

Fertilisation is most likely to occur when intercourse takes place not more than 48 hours before or 24 hours after ovulation.

DEVELOPMENT OF THE ZYGOTE

When the oocyte has been fertilised, it continues its passage through the uterine tube and reaches the uterus 3 or 4 days later.

● During this time the zygote divides and subdivides to form a cluster of cells known as the *morula*.
● Next, a fluid-filled cavity appears in the morula, which now becomes known as the *blastocyst*.
● Around the outside of the blastocyst there is a single layer of cells known as the *trophoblast*.
● The remaining cells are clumped together at one end forming the *inner cell mass*.

The trophoblast will form the placenta and chorion, while the inner cell mass will become the fetus, amnion and umbilical cord.

See Chapter 9 for calculation of the expected date of delivery based on menstrual history.

The decidua

This is the name given to the endometrium during pregnancy. From the time of conception the increased secretion of oestrogens causes the endometrium to grow to four times its non-pregnant thickness. The corpus luteum also produces large amounts of progesterone, which stimulate the secretory activity of the endometrial glands and increase the size of the blood vessels. This accounts for the soft, vascular, spongy bed in which the blastocyst implants. The three layers of the decidua are:

● the basal layer
● the functional layer
● the compact layer.

The trophoblast

Small projections begin to appear all over the surface of the blastocyst, becoming most prolific at the area of contact. These trophoblastic cells differentiate into layers:

● the outer syncytiotrophoblast (syncytium)
● the inner cytotrophoblast.

The inner cell mass

While the trophoblast is developing into the placenta, the inner cell mass is forming the fetus itself. The cells differentiate into three layers, each of which will form particular parts of the fetus:

- The *ectoderm* mainly forms the skin and nervous system.
- The *mesoderm* forms bones and muscles and also the heart and blood vessels, including those in the placenta. Certain internal organs also originate in the mesoderm.
- The *endoderm* forms mucous membranes and glands.

Two cavities appear in the inner cell mass:

- The *amniotic cavity* is filled with fluid, and gradually enlarges and folds around the embryo to enclose it.
- *The yolk sac* provides nourishment for the embryo until the trophoblast is sufficiently developed to take over.

The embryo

This name is applied to the developing offspring after implantation and until 8 weeks after conception.

Problems of development are summarised in Box 3.1.

Box 3.1 Problems of development

- Implantation bleeding – lighter than a period, not usually significant
- Ectopic pregnancy – suspect when there is abdominal pain and amenorrhoea
- Hydatidiform mole – gross malformation of the trophoblast
- Miscarriage/abortion – threatened, inevitable, missed

See also Chapter 11

CHAPTER 4

The Placenta

Originating from the trophoblastic layer of the fertilised oocyte, the placenta links closely with the mother's circulation to carry out functions that the fetus is unable to perform for itself during intrauterine life.

DEVELOPMENT

Initially, the zygote appears to be covered with a fine, downy hair, which consists of the projections from the trophoblastic layer. These proliferate and branch from about 3 weeks after fertilisation, forming the *chorionic villi*. The villi become most profuse in the area where the blood supply is richest – that is, in the basal decidua.

- This part of the trophoblast is known as the *chorion frondosum* and it will eventually develop into the placenta.
- The villi under the capsular decidua, being less well nourished, gradually degenerate and form the *chorion laeve*, which is the origin of the chorionic membrane.

The villi erode the walls of maternal blood vessels as they penetrate the decidua, opening them up to form a lake of maternal blood in which they float. The maternal blood circulates slowly, enabling the villi to absorb food and oxygen and excrete waste. Each chorionic villus is a branching structure arising from one stem (Fig. 4.1). The placenta is completely formed and functioning from 10 weeks after fertilisation.

Circulation through the placenta

- Fetal blood, low in oxygen, is pumped by the fetal heart towards the placenta along the umbilical arteries and transported along their branches to the capillaries of the chorionic villi.
- Having yielded up carbon dioxide and absorbed oxygen, the blood is returned to the fetus via the umbilical vein.
- The maternal blood is delivered to the placental bed in the decidua by spiral arteries and flows into the blood spaces surrounding the villi. It is thought that the direction of flow is similar to a fountain; the blood passes upwards and bathes the villus as it circulates around it and drains back into a branch of the uterine vein.

It is impossible for the maternal and fetal circulations to mix unless any villi are damaged.

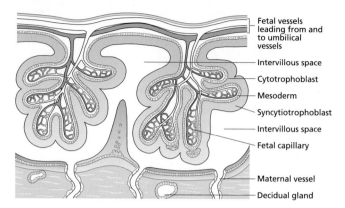

Fig. 4.1: Chorionic villi.

THE MATURE PLACENTA

Functions

The 'Green B' mnemonic (Box 4.1) can be helpful.

Appearance of the placenta at term

The placenta is a round, flat mass about 20 cm in diameter and 2.5 cm thick at its centre.

- *The maternal surface*. The surface is arranged in about 20 cotyledons (lobes), which are separated by sulci. The cotyledons are made up of lobules, each of which contains a single villus with its branches.

Box 4.1 Functions of the mature placenta

- **G**lycogen storage plus iron and fat-soluble vitamins
- **R**espiration
- **E**xcretion
- **E**ndocrine:
  - *Human chorionic gonadotrophin* (HCG) – is produced by the cytotrophoblastic layer of the chorionic villi
  - *Oestrogens* – as the activity of the corpus luteum declines, the placenta takes over the production of oestrogens
  - *Progesterone* – is made in the syncytial layer of the placenta
  - *Human placental lactogen* (HPL) – has a role in glucose metabolism in pregnancy
- **N**utrition
- **B**arrier to some but not all infections

- *The fetal surface.* The amnion covering the fetal surface of the placenta gives it a white, shiny appearance. Branches of the umbilical vein and arteries are visible, spreading out from the insertion of the umbilical cord, which is normally in the centre. The amnion can be peeled off the surface, leaving the chorionic plate from which the placenta has developed and which is continuous with the chorion.
- *The fetal sac.* The fetal sac consists of a double membrane. The outer membrane is the chorion; this is a thick, opaque, friable membrane. The inner, smooth, tough, translucent membrane is the amnion, which contains the amniotic fluid.

AMNIOTIC FLUID

Functions
These are listed in Box 4.2.

Volume
- The total amount of amniotic fluid increases throughout pregnancy until 38 weeks' gestation, when there is about 1 litre.
- It then diminishes slightly until term, when approximately 800 ml remains.
- If the total amount exceeds 1500 ml, the condition is known as *polyhydramnios*.
- If there is less than 300 ml, the term *oligohydramnios* is applied.

Constituents
Amniotic fluid is a clear, pale, straw-coloured fluid consisting of 99% water. The remaining 1% is dissolved solid matter, including food substances and waste products. In addition, the fetus sheds skin cells, vernix caseosa and lanugo into the fluid. Abnormal constituents of the liquor, such as meconium in the case of fetal distress, may give valuable diagnostic information about the condition of the fetus.

Box 4.2 Functions of the amniotic fluid

- Distends the amniotic sac and allows for the growth and movement of the fetus
- Equalises pressure and protects the fetus from jarring and injury
- Maintains a constant temperature for the fetus
- Provides small amounts of nutrients
- Protects the placenta and umbilical cord from the pressure of uterine contractions in labour, as long as the membranes remain intact, Also aids effacement of the cervix and dilatation of the uterine os, particularly where the presenting part is poorly applied

THE UMBILICAL CORD

The umbilical cord extends from the fetus to the placenta and transmits the umbilical blood vessels: two arteries and one vein. These are enclosed and protected by *Wharton's jelly*. The whole cord is covered in a layer of amnion continuous with that covering the placenta. The length of the average cord is about 50 cm.

True knots should be noted on examination of the cord, but they must be distinguished from false knots, which are lumps of Wharton's jelly on the side of the cord and are not significant.

ANATOMICAL VARIATIONS OF THE PLACENTA AND THE CORD

These are listed in Box 4.3. Except for the dangers noted, these varieties of conformation have no clinical significance.

See Chapter 19 for inspection after birth.

Box 4.3 Anatomical variations of the placenta and the cord

Succenturiate lobe of placenta

- A small extra lobe is present, separate from the main placenta but joined to it by blood vessels that run through the membranes to reach it
- A hole in the membranes with vessels running to it is likely to indicate a retained lobe

Circumvallate placenta

- An opaque ring is seen on the fetal surface of the placenta
- It is formed by a doubling back of the chorion and amnion and may result in the membranes leaving the placenta nearer the centre instead of at the edge as is usual

Battledore insertion of the cord

- The cord is attached at the very edge of the placenta in the manner of a table-tennis bat

Velamentous insertion of the cord

- The cord is inserted into the membranes some distance from the edge of the placenta
- The umbilical vessels run through the membranes from the cord to the placenta
- If the placenta is normally situated, no harm will result to the fetus, but the cord is likely to become detached upon applying traction during active management of the third stage of labour
- If the placenta is low lying, the vessels may pass across the uterine os. The term applied to the vessels lying in this position is vasa praevia. In this

Box 4.3 Anatomical variations of the placenta and the cord—cont'd

case there is great danger to the fetus when the membranes rupture and even more so during artificial rupture, as the vessels may be torn, leading to rapid exsanguination of the fetus

Bipartite placenta

- Two complete and separate parts are present, each with a cord leaving it
- The bipartite cord joins a short distance from the two parts of the placenta

Tripartite placenta

- This is similar to bipartite, but with three distinct parts

CHAPTER 5

The Fetus

Knowledge of fetal development is needed to estimate the approximate age of a baby born before term and appreciate the ways in which developmental abnormalities arise.

TIME SCALE OF DEVELOPMENT

- For the first 3 weeks following conception the term *zygote* is used.
- From 3–8 weeks after conception it is known as the *embryo*.
- Following this it is called the *fetus* until birth. Development within the uterus is summarised in Box 5.1.

FETAL ORGANS

Blood

The fetal haemoglobin is termed HbF. It has a much greater affinity for oxygen and is found in greater concentration (18–20 g/dl at term). Towards the end of pregnancy the fetus begins to make adult-type haemoglobin (HbA).

In utero, the red blood cells have a shorter lifespan, this being about 90 days by the time the baby is born.

The renal tract

The kidneys begin to function and the fetus passes dilute urine from 10 weeks' gestation.

The adrenal glands

The fetal adrenal glands produce the precursors for placental formation of oestriols. They are also thought to play a part in the initiation of labour.

The liver

The fetal liver is comparatively large in size. From the third to the sixth month of intrauterine life, it is responsible for the formation of red blood cells, after which they are mainly produced in the red bone marrow and the spleen.

Towards the end of pregnancy, iron stores are laid down in the liver.

The alimentary tract

The digestive tract is mainly non-functional before birth. Sucking and swallowing of amniotic fluid containing shed skin cells and other debris begin about 12 weeks after conception. Digestive juices are present before birth and they act on the swallowed substances and discarded intestinal cells to form meconium. This is normally retained in the gut until after birth, when it is passed as the first stool of the newborn.

Box 5.1 Summary of development

0–4 weeks after conception

- Rapid growth
- Formation of the embryonic plate
- Primitive central nervous system forms
- Heart develops and begins to beat
- Limb buds form

4–8 weeks

- Very rapid cell division
- Head and facial features develop
- All major organs laid down in primitive form
- External genitalia present but sex not distinguishable
- Early movements
- Visible on ultrasound from 6 weeks

8–12 weeks

- Eyelids fuse
- Kidneys begin to function and fetus passes urine from 10 weeks
- Fetal circulation functioning properly
- Sucking and swallowing begin
- Sex apparent
- Moves freely (not felt by mother)
- Some primitive reflexes present

12–16 weeks

- Rapid skeletal development
- Meconium present in gut
- Lanugo appears
- Nasal septum and palate fuse

16–20 weeks

- 'Quickening' – mother feels fetal movements
- Fetal heart heard on auscultation
- Vernix caseosa appears
- Fingernails can be seen
- Skin cells begin to be renewed

20–24 weeks

- Most organs become capable of functioning
- Periods of sleep and activity
- Responds to sound
- Skin red and wrinkled

24–28 weeks

- Survival may be expected if born
- Eyelids reopen
- Respiratory movements

Continued

Box 5.1 Summary of development—cont'd

28–32 weeks

- Begins to store fat and iron
- Testes descend into scrotum
- Lanugo disappears from face
- Skin becomes paler and less wrinkled

32–36 weeks

- Increased fat makes body more rounded
- Lanugo disappears from body
- Head hair lengthens
- Nails reach tips of fingers
- Ear cartilage soft
- Plantar creases visible

36–40 weeks after conception (38–42 weeks after last menstrual period, LMP)

- Term is reached and birth is due
- Contours rounded
- Skull firm

The lungs

It is mainly the immaturity of the lungs that reduces the chance of survival of infants born before 24 weeks' gestation, owing to the limited alveolar surface area, the immaturity of the capillary system in the lungs and the lack of adequate surfactant. Surfactant is a lipoprotein that reduces the surface tension in the alveoli and assists gaseous exchange. It is first produced from about 20 weeks' gestation and the amount increases until the lungs are mature at about 30–34 weeks. At term the lungs contain about 100 ml of lung fluid. This is expelled during birth but mostly absorbed and carried away by the lymphatics and blood vessels.

There is some movement of the thorax from the third month of fetal life and more definite diaphragmatic movements from the sixth month.

The central nervous system

The fetus is able to perceive strong light and to hear external sounds. Periods of wakefulness and sleep occur.

The skin

- From 18 weeks after conception the fetus is covered with a white, protective, creamy substance called *vernix caseosa*.
- At 20 weeks the fetus will be covered with a fine downy hair called *lanugo*; at the same time the head hair and eyebrows begin to form.
- Lanugo is shed from 36 weeks and a full-term infant has little left.
- Fingernails develop from about 10 weeks but the toenails do not form until about 18 weeks.

THE FETAL CIRCULATION

The key to understanding the fetal circulation (Fig. 5.1) is the fact that oxygen is derived from the placenta. At birth there is a dramatic alteration in this situation and an almost instantaneous change must occur. Several temporary structures, in addition to the placenta itself and the umbilical cord, enable the fetal circulation to function while allowing for the changes at birth (Box 5.2).

THE FETAL SKULL

The fetal skull (Fig. 5.2) contains the delicate brain, which may be subjected to great pressure as the head passes through the birth canal.

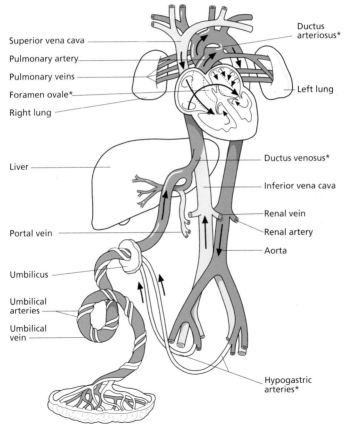

Superior vena cava
Pulmonary artery
Pulmonary veins
Foramen ovale*
Right lung

Ductus arteriosus*
Left lung

Liver

Ductus venosus*
Inferior vena cava
Renal vein
Renal artery
Aorta

Portal vein

Umbilicus
Umbilical arteries
Umbilical vein

Hypogastric arteries*

Fig. 5.1: Fetal circulation. The arrows show the course taken by the blood. The temporary structures are asterisked.

Box 5.2 Temporary structures within the fetal circulation

- Umbilical vein
- Ductus venosus
- Foramen ovale
- Ductus arteriosus
- Hypogastric arteries

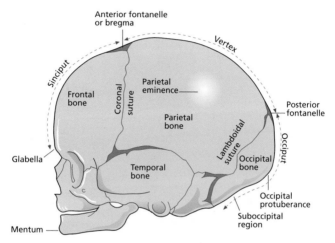

Fig. 5.2: Fetal skull showing regions and landmarks of obstetrical importance.

Ossification

The bones of the fetal head originate in two different ways:

- The face is laid down in cartilage and is almost completely ossified at birth, the bones being fused together and firm.
- The bones of the vault are laid down in membrane and are much flatter and more pliable. They ossify from the centre outwards and this process is incomplete at birth, leaving small gaps which form the sutures and fontanelles. The ossification centre on each bone appears as a boss or protuberance.

Bones of the vault (Fig. 5.3)

There are five main bones in the vault of the fetal skull:

- the *occipital bone*
- the two *parietal bones*
- the two *frontal bones*.

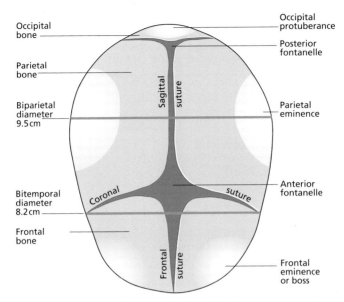

Fig. 5.3: View of fetal head from above (head partly flexed), showing bones, sutures and fontanelles.

In addition to these five, the upper part of the *temporal bone* forms a small part of the vault.

Sutures and fontanelles

Sutures are cranial joints and are formed where two bones adjoin. Where two or more sutures meet, a fontanelle is formed. There are several sutures and fontanelles in the fetal skull. Those of greatest obstetrical significance are shown in Box 5.3.

The sutures and fontanelles, because they consist of membranous spaces, allow for a degree of overlapping of the skull bones during labour and birth.

Box 5.3 Sutures and fontanelles of significance in the fetal skull

- Lambdoidal suture
- Sagittal suture
- Coronal suture
- Frontal suture
- Posterior fontanelle or lambda
- Anterior fontanelle or bregma

Regions and landmarks of the fetal skull

The skull is divided into the vault, the base and the face:

- The *vault* is the large, dome-shaped part above an imaginary line drawn between the orbital ridges and the nape of the neck.
- The *base* is composed of bones that are firmly united to protect the vital centres in the medulla.
- *The face* is composed of 14 small bones, which are also firmly united and non-compressible.

The regions of the skull are described as in Box 5.4.

Diameters of the fetal skull

The measurements of the skull are important to understand the relationship between the fetal head and the mother's pelvis (Table 5.1 and Fig. 5.4). Some diameters are more favourable than others for easy passage through the pelvic canal.

Attitude of the fetal head

This term is used to describe the degree of flexion or extension of the head on the neck. The attitude of the head determines which diameters will present in labour and therefore influences the outcome.

Presenting diameters

The diameters of the head, which are called the presenting diameters, are those that are at right angles to the curve of Carus. There are always two:

- an anteroposterior or longitudinal diameter
- a transverse diameter.

The diameters presenting in the individual cephalic or head presentations are as described below.

Box 5.4 Regions of the fetal skull

Occiput
- Lies between the foramen magnum and the posterior fontanelle
- The part below the occipital protuberance is known as the suboccipital region

Vertex
- Bounded by the posterior fontanelle, the two parietal eminences and the anterior fontanelle

Sinciput or brow
- Extends from the anterior fontanelle and the coronal suture to the orbital ridges

Face
- Small in the newborn baby
- Extends from the orbital ridges and the root of the nose to the junction of the chin and the neck
- The point between the eyebrows is known as the glabella
- The chin is termed the mentum and is an important landmark

Table 5.1 Diameters of the fetal skull	
Name of diameter	**Measurement**
Transverse diameters (Fig. 5.3)	
Biparietal	9.5 cm
Bitemporal	8.2 cm
Anteroposterior or longitudinal (Fig. 5.4)	
Suboccipitobregmatic (SOB)	9.5 cm
Suboccipitofrontal (SOF)	10 cm
Occipitofrontal (OF)	11.5 cm
Mentovertical (MV)	13.5 cm
Submentovertical (SMV)	11.5 cm
Submentobregmatic (SMB)	9.5 cm

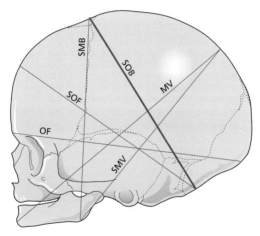

Fig. 5.4: Anteroposterior diameters of the fetal skull (see Table 5.1).

Vertex presentation

When the head is well flexed, the suboccipitobregmatic diameter and the biparietal diameter present. As these two diameters are the same length, 9.5 cm, the presenting area is circular, which is the most favourable shape for dilating the cervix. The diameter that distends the vaginal orifice is the suboccipitofrontal diameter, 10 cm (see Ch. 18).

When the head is not flexed but erect, the presenting diameters are the occipitofrontal, 11.5 cm, and the biparietal, 9.5 cm. This situation often arises when the occiput is in a posterior position. If it remains so, the diameter distending the vaginal orifice will be the occipitofrontal, 11.5 cm.

Brow presentation

When the head is partially extended, the mentovertical diameter, 13.5 cm, and the bitemporal diameter, 8.2 cm, present. If this presentation persists, vaginal birth is extremely unlikely.

Face presentation

When the head is completely extended, the presenting diameters are the submentobregmatic, 9.5 cm, and the bitemporal, 8.2 cm.

The submentovertical diameter, 11.5 cm, will distend the vaginal orifice (see Ch. 21 for mechanisms in labour.)

Moulding

This is the term applied to the change in shape of the fetal head that takes place during its passage through the birth canal. Alteration in shape is possible because the bones of the vault allow a slight degree of bending and the skull bones are able to override at the sutures. This overriding allows a considerable reduction in the size of the presenting diameters while the diameter at right angles to them is able to lengthen owing to the give of the skull bones.

In a normal vertex presentation, with the fetal head in a fully flexed attitude, the suboccipitobregmatic and the biparietal diameters will be reduced and the mentovertical will be lengthened. The shortening may amount to as much as 1.25 cm.

The intracranial membranes and sinuses (Fig. 5.5)

The skull contains delicate structures, some of which may be damaged if the head is subjected to abnormal moulding during delivery. Among the most important are the folds of dura mater and the venous sinuses associated with them (Box 5.5).

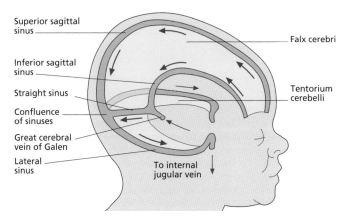

Fig. 5.5: Intracranial membranes and venous sinuses. Arrows show direction of blood flow.

Box 5.5 Intracranial membranes and sinuses

- Falx cerebri
- Tentorium cerebelli
- Superior sagittal sinus
- Inferior sagittal sinus
- Great cerebral vein of Galen
- Straight sinus
- Two lateral sinuses

Section 2

Pregnancy

CHAPTER 6

Preparing for Pregnancy

Preparing for pregnancy is a positive step towards enhancing pregnancy outcome and provides prospective parents with options that may not be available once a pregnancy is confirmed.

PRECONCEPTION CARE

The aims of preconception care are:
- to ensure that the woman and her partner are in an optimal state of physical and emotional health at the onset of pregnancy
- to provide prospective parents with a series of options that may not be available once a pregnancy is confirmed.

The preconception period refers to a timespan of anything from 3 months to 1 year before conception.

Box 6.1 outlines the information and investigations that may be required.

GENERAL HEALTH AND FERTILITY

Body weight

Fertility and obesity are closely linked, with subfertility-related problems occurring in women below and above the desirable range of body weight.
- The Quetelet or body mass index (BMI) is calculated by dividing the weight in kilograms by the height in metres squared.
- The desirable or healthy range is between 18.5 and 24.9.

Substantial evidence is accumulating that corroborates the relationship between an increased risk of pregnancy complications/adverse pregnancy outcomes and excess weight and obesity in women. Overweight women should be encouraged to lose weight before conception; however, some caution is required, as consuming an energy-deficient diet immediately prior to conception may result in nutritional deficiencies that could disadvantage the fetus. Dietary changes and weight loss should occur at least 3–4 months before attempting conception.

Principles of a healthy diet

A simple and easy guide is to advise women to eat:
- more starchy foods, such as cereals and bread
- at least five portions of fruit and vegetables daily
- fewer fatty foods.

Box 6.1 Information and investigations in a preconception programme

History
- Family history
- Medical history
- Menstrual history
- Obstetric history
- Method of contraception
- Medication
- Occupation
- Diet
- Smoking
- Alcohol

Observations/investigations
- Height and weight
- Blood pressure
- Urinalysis
- Stool sample
- Blood tests:
  - Haemoglobin
  - Folic acid and vitamin levels
  - Rubella immunity
  - Venereal disease research laboratory (VDRL)
  - Haemoglobinopathies
  - Lead and trace elements
- Hair analysis (controversial)
- Male – semen analysis
- Female – cervical smear, high vaginal swab (HVS)

Folate, folic acid and neural tube defects

Folic acid is a water-soluble vitamin belonging to the B complex.

- The term 'folates' is used to describe the folic acid derivatives that are found naturally in food.
- The term 'folic acid' is used to refer to the synthetic form found in vitamin supplements and fortified foods.

The main sources of folate in the UK diet are listed in Box 6.2.

Folates are vulnerable to heat and readily dissolve in water; therefore considerable losses can occur as a result of cooking or prolonged storage. Folic acid is more stable and better absorbed than folate and is added to many brands of bread and breakfast cereal in the UK.

- To reduce the risk of first occurrence of neural tube defects (NTDs), all women should increase their daily folate and folic acid intake by an additional 400 µg prior to conception and during the first 12 weeks of pregnancy.

Box 6.2 Principal sources of dietary folate

- Dark green vegetables
- Potatoes
- Fruit and fruit juices
- Beans
- Yeast extract

- Women with a history of a previous child with NTD should take a daily dose of 5 mg of folic acid to reduce the risk of recurrence.
- This dose is also recommended in women with diabetes, those taking antiepileptic medication, and those who have malabsorption syndrome.

Vitamin A

Vitamin A is essential for embryogenesis, growth and epithelial differentiation, but a high intake of the retinol form of vitamin A is known to be teratogenic.

Women who are pregnant or planning a pregnancy should avoid eating liver and liver products such as pâté or liver sausage, as these contain large amounts of retinol.

PRE-EXISTING MEDICAL CONDITIONS AND DRUGS

Diabetes

Infants of insulin-dependent diabetic mothers have ten times the general population risk of congenital malformation and five times the risk of stillbirth. Diabetic complications, such as retinopathy and nephropathy, may worsen during pregnancy, particularly if associated with hypertension. Women who have severe neuropathy or cardiovascular disease may be advised against pregnancy.

- The aim of preconception care is to achieve normoglycaemia both pre- and periconception, as many of the problems seen in the insulin-dependent diabetic mother are a direct result of hyperglycaemia.
- The safety of currently available oral hypoglycaemic agents in pregnancy is not well established.

Epilepsy

The major anticonvulsant drugs used to treat epilepsy are known to have teratogenic effects, and the newer antiepileptic drugs have not yet been sufficiently evaluated. Pregnancy is also known to alter the metabolism of antiepileptic drugs, with approximately one-third of women experiencing an increase in the number of seizures.

- The aim of preconception care is to help the woman plan her pregnancies carefully and to keep her seizure free on the lowest possible dose of anticonvulsants. For some women this may mean withdrawal of therapy and for others a reduction from polytherapy to monotherapy.
- Some anticonvulsant drugs are folate antagonists; therefore folic acid supplements are needed.

Phenylketonuria

Phenylketonuria (PKU) is an inborn error of metabolism. Some women with PKU discontinue treatment during middle childhood. However, unless they resume careful dietary control around the time of conception, the toxic effect of phenylalanine (Phe) on the developing embryo/fetus results in a high rate of fetal abnormality.

Oral contraception

Oral contraception should be stopped at least 3 months, and preferably 6 months, prior to planning a pregnancy to allow for the resumption of natural hormone regulation and ovulation. Also, the oral contraceptive pill is associated with vitamin and mineral imbalances that may need correcting.

Drug abuse

Disruption of the menstrual cycle is common among women using drugs like ecstasy, amfetamines, opiates and anabolic steroids, and heavy drug use during pregnancy is associated with miscarriage, preterm labour, low birth weight, stillbirth and abnormalities. A poor socioeconomic environment is a compounding factor. Some women may be trying to come off tranquillisers and this process can take many weeks.

ENVIRONMENTAL FACTORS

Smoking

Fertility and pregnancy are adversely affected by smoking. In women, smoking can induce early menopause and menstrual problems; in men it can cause abnormalities in sperm morphology and motility. During pregnancy, there is an increased risk of spontaneous abortion, preterm delivery, low birth weight and perinatal mortality because of antepartum haemorrhage and placental abruption. Nutritional status tends to be compromised in smokers.

- The aim of preconception care is to help the woman stop smoking, and partner involvement is known to enhance success.
- Health professionals should ask about smoking at every opportunity that advice and assistance for smoking cessation can be given.

Alcohol

Alcohol is a teratogen. Fetal alcohol syndrome (FAS) is the term used to describe the congenital malformations associated with excessive maternal alcohol intake during pregnancy. High alcohol intakes in women have been associated with menstrual disorders and decreased fertility.

- Women should ideally abstain from alcohol or limit alcohol consumption in pregnancy to no more than one standard unit of alcohol twice in a week.
- Women with a drink problem will need specialist referral for treatment and support.

Exercise

Moderate exercise is known to be beneficial for health and the benefits of regular exercise for the healthy pregnant woman appear to outweigh the risks. However, exercise intensity should be modified according to maternal symptoms and should not continue to fatigue or exhaustion.

Workplace hazards and noxious substances

Employees are protected by the Control of Substances Hazardous to Health (COSHH) regulations. Exposure to solvents, ionising radiation and anaesthetic gases is known to be toxic and associated with central nervous system defects, microcephaly and an increased risk of miscarriage. Heavy metals are also known to be toxic.

There has been concern about working with visual display units (VDUs) during pregnancy and there are reports of an increased risk of miscarriages or birth defects. However, taken as a whole, the scientific studies that have been carried out to date do not show any link.

GENETIC COUNSELLING

A family history of genetic disorders, a previous baby affected with a congenital abnormality and childbearing left until later years all increase the risk of giving birth to an abnormal child. For such couples, referral for genetic counselling will help them to decide what is best.

Mendelian inheritance

Genetic disorders can occur as a result of Mendelian inheritance and are termed either dominant or recessive (see Ch. 34).

Chromosome abnormalities

- Chromosome aberrations include the *trisomies*, of which trisomy 21 (Down syndrome) is the most common; trisomy 13 and 18 are more rare. Age factors are significant, particularly in Down syndrome, for which the risk is 1% for a woman around 40 years of age.
- *Monosomies* are usually lethal and non-viable autosomal trisomies are extremely common in spontaneous abortions. Sex chromosome abnormalities, such as Turner syndrome (XO) and Klinefelter syndrome (XXY), have a rare recurrence rate in families.
- In *translocation*, extra chromosome material is translocated onto another chromosome; it is regarded as balanced when the total amount of chromosome material is normal but only 45 chromosomes are present. Reciprocal translocations can also occur, in which there is an exchange of chromosome material but no change in chromosome number. The recurrence risk is low if neither parent is a balanced carrier for the translocation.

Non-Mendelian disorders

The more common congenital abnormalities, such as NTDs and congenital heart disease, do not follow the Mendelian inheritance pattern, as there is no identified genetic locus; they are therefore referred to as *multifactorial*. These conditions arise as a result of a combination or interaction of environmental and genetic factors. The recurrence risk of such conditions depends upon the incidence of the disorder but is increased among close relatives.

Prenatal diagnosis

Ultimately, the goal of genetic counselling is to prevent or avoid a genetic disorder. Preconception care, involving a multidisciplinary team, is the way to achieve this.

INFERTILITY

Infertility is categorised as *primary* if there has been no prior conception and *secondary* if there has been a previous pregnancy, irrespective of the outcome.

Approximately one-third of cases of infertility involve problems with both partners, and in one-third of couples the causes of infertility remain unexplained. The most common causes are:

- ovulation failure
- sperm disorders.

Much of the initial management of the infertile couple is via primary care. The investigative process is aimed at achieving:

- an accurate diagnosis and definition of any cause
- an accurate estimation of the chance of conceiving without treatment
- a full appraisal of treatment options.

Specialised investigations may need to be undertaken in a dedicated, specialist infertility clinic where there is access to appropriately trained staff and a multiprofessional team.

ASSISTED REPRODUCTION TECHNIQUES

A range of assisted reproduction techniques (Box 6.3) is available to treat the infertile couple and it is important for the appropriate treatment option to be offered.

Box 6.3 Some assisted reproduction techniques

- Ovulation induction
- Intrauterine insemination (IUI)
- Donor insemination (DI) or artificial insemination by donor (AID)
- In-vitro fertilisation/embryo transfer (IVF/ET)
- Gamete intrafallopian transfer (GIFT)
- Zygote intrafallopian transfer (ZIFT)
- Intracytoplasmic sperm injection (ICSI)

CHAPTER 7

Change and Adaptation in Pregnancy

PHYSIOLOGICAL CHANGES IN THE REPRODUCTIVE SYSTEM

THE BODY OF THE UTERUS

After conception, the uterus develops to provide a nutritive and protective environment in which the fetus will develop and grow.

Decidua

After embedding of the blastocyst there is thickening and increased vascularity of the lining of the uterus, or decidua. Decidualisation, influenced by progesterone and oestradiol, is most marked in the fundus and upper body of the uterus.

- The decidua is believed to maintain functional quiescence of the uterus during pregnancy; spontaneous labour is thought to result from the activation of the decidua with resultant prostaglandin release following withdrawal of placental hormones.
- The decidua and trophoblast also produce relaxin, which appears to promote myometrial relaxation, and may have a role to play in cervical ripening and rupture of fetal membranes.

Myometrium

Uterine growth is due to *hyperplasia* (increase in number due to division) and *hypertrophy* (increase in size) of myometrial cells under the influence of oestrogen (Table 7.1). The dimensions of the uterus vary considerably, however, depending on the age and parity of the woman.

The three layers of the myometrium become more clearly defined during pregnancy.

Table 7.1 Uterine growth during pregnancy		
	Prior to pregnancy	At term
Weight of uterus	60–80 g	1000 g
Size of uterus	7.5 × 5 × 2.5 cm	30 × 22.5 × 20 cm

Muscle layers

- The outer longitudinal layer of muscle fibres is thin. It consists of a network of bundles of smooth muscles. These pass longitudinally from the front of the isthmus anteriorly over the fundus and into the vault of the vagina posteriorly, and extend into the round and transverse ligaments.
- The thicker middle layer comprises interlocked spiral myometrial fibres that are perforated in all directions by blood vessels. Each cell in this layer has a double curve so that the interlacing of any two gives the approximate form of a figure of eight. Due to this arrangement, contraction of these cells after birth causes constriction of the blood vessels, providing 'living ligatures'.
- The inner circular layer is arranged concentrically around the longitudinal axis of the uterus and bundle formation is diffuse. It forms sphincters around the openings of the uterine tubes and around the internal cervical os.

Uterine activity in pregnancy

The myometrium is both contractile (can lengthen and shorten) and elastic (can enlarge and stretch) to accommodate the growing fetus and allow involution following the birth.

- The contractile ability of the myometrium is dependent on the interaction between two contractile proteins, actin and myosin.
- The interaction of actin and myosin brings about contraction, whereas their separation brings about relaxation under the influence of intracellular free calcium.
- The coordination of synchronous contractions across the whole organ is due to the presence of gap junctions that connect myometrial cells and provide connections for electrical activity. Gap junctions are absent for most of the pregnancy but appear in significant numbers near term, manifesting themselves as *Braxton Hicks contractions*.
- The formation of gap junctions is promoted by oestrogens and prostaglandins.
- Progesterone, prostacyclin and relaxin, however, are all involved in inhibiting the formation of gap junctions by reducing cell excitability and cell connections and so limiting myometrial activity to small clumps of cells, thus maintaining uterine quiescence during pregnancy.

Uterine activity can be measured as early as 7 weeks' gestation, when Braxton Hicks contractions can occur every 20–30 minutes and may reach a pressure of up to 10 mmHg. These contractions facilitate uterine blood flow through the intervillous spaces of the placenta, promoting oxygen delivery to the fetus. Braxton Hicks contractions are usually painless but may cause some discomfort when their intensity exceeds 15 mmHg.

In the last few weeks of pregnancy, *prelabour* occurs:

- Further increases in myometrial contractions cause the muscle fibres of the fundus to be drawn up.
- The actively contracting upper uterine segment becomes thicker and shorter in length and exerts a slow, steady pull on the relatively fixed cervix.
- This causes the beginning of cervical stretching and ripening known as effacement, and thinning and stretching of the passive lower uterine segment.

There is little rebound between contractions, however; hence there is no cervical dilatation at this time.

Perimetrium

The perimetrium is a thin layer of peritoneum that protects the uterus. It is deflected over the bladder anteriorly to form the uterovesical pouch, and over the rectum posteriorly to form the pouch of Douglas.

- The double folds of perimetrium (broad ligaments), hanging from the uterine tubes and extending to the lateral walls of the pelvis, become longer and wider with increasing tension exerted on them as the uterus enlarges and rises out of the pelvis.
- The anterior and posterior folds open out so that they are no longer in apposition and can therefore accommodate the greatly enlarged uterine and ovarian arteries and veins.
- The round ligaments (contained within the hanging folds of perimetrium) provide some anterior support for the enlarging uterus and undergo considerable hypertrophy and stretching during pregnancy, which may cause discomfort.

Blood supply

The uterine blood flow progressively increases from approximately 50 ml/min at 10 weeks' gestation to 450–750 ml/min at term.

CHANGES IN UTERINE SHAPE AND SIZE

For the first few weeks the uterus maintains its original pear shape, but as pregnancy advances the corpus and fundus assume a more globular form (Box 7.1).

THE CERVIX

The cervix is composed of only about 10% muscular tissue, the remainder being collagenous tissue. During pregnancy the cervix remains firmly closed, providing a seal against external contamination and holding in the contents of the uterus. It remains 2.5 cm long throughout pregnancy but becomes softer

Box 7.1 Changes in the pregnant uterus

10 weeks

- The uterus is about the size of an orange

12 weeks

- The uterus is about the size of a grapefruit
- It is no longer anteverted and anteflexed and has risen out of the pelvis and become upright
- The fundus may be palpated abdominally above the symphysis pubis
- The globular upper segment is sitting on an elongated stalk formed from the isthmus, which softens and which will treble in length from 7 to 25 mm between the 12th and 36th weeks

20 weeks

- The fundus of the uterus can be palpated at the level of the umbilicus
- As the uterus continues to rise in the abdomen, the uterine tubes become progressively more vertical, which causes increasing tension on the broad and round ligaments

30 weeks

- The fundus may be palpated midway between the umbilicus and the xiphisternum

38 weeks

- The uterus reaches the level of the xiphisternum
- As the upper segment muscle contractions increase in frequency and strength, the lower uterine segment develops more rapidly and is stretched radially; along with cervical effacement and softening of the tissues of the pelvic floor, this permits the fetal presentation to begin its descent into the upper pelvis
- This leads to a reduction in fundal height known as *lightening*, relieving pressure on the upper part of the abdomen but increasing pressure in the pelvis. In the majority of multiparous women, however, engagement rarely occurs prior to labour

and swollen under the influence of oestradiol and progesterone. Its increased vascularity makes it look bluish in colour. Under the influence of progesterone the mucous glands become distended and increase in complexity, resulting in the secretion of a thick, viscous, mucoid discharge. It forms a cervical plug called the *operculum*, which provides protection from ascending infection.

As uterine activity builds up during pregnancy, the cervix gradually softens, or *ripens*, and the canal dilates. *Effacement* or *taking up of the cervix* normally occurs in the primigravida during the last 2 weeks of pregnancy but does not usually take place in the multigravida until labour begins. Effacement of the cervix is a mechanism whereby the following occur:

- The connective tissue of the long firm cervix is progressively softened by prostaglandins and shortened from the top downwards.

- The softened muscular fibres at the level of the internal cervical os are pulled upwards or 'taken up' into the lower uterine segment and around the fetal presenting part and the forewaters.
- The canal that was about 2.5 cm long becomes a mere circular orifice with paper-thin edges.
- The mucus plug is expelled as effacement progresses.

THE VAGINA

During pregnancy the muscle layer hypertrophies and oestrogen causes the vaginal epithelium to become thicker and more vascular. The altered composition of the surrounding connective tissue increases the elasticity of the vagina, making dilatation easier during the birth of the baby.

In pregnancy there is an increased rate of desquamation of the superficial vaginal mucosa cells. These epithelial cells release more glycogen, which is acted on by *Döderlein's bacilli*, a normal commensal of the vagina, producing lactic acid and hydrogen peroxide. This leads to the increased and more acidic (pH 3.5–6.0) white vaginal discharge known as *leucorrhoea*.

CHANGES IN THE CARDIOVASCULAR SYSTEM

Understanding changes in the cardiovascular system is important in the care of women with normal pregnancies, as well as for the management of women with pre-existing cardiovascular disease.

THE HEART

- The heart enlarges by about 12% between early and late pregnancy.
- The growing uterus elevates the diaphragm, the great vessels are unfolded and the heart is correspondingly displaced upwards, with the apex moved laterally to the left by about 15°.
- By mid-pregnancy more than 90% of women develop an ejection systolic murmur, which lasts until the first week postpartum. If unaccompanied by any other abnormalities, it reflects the increased stroke output.
- Twenty per cent develop a transient diastolic murmur and 10% develop continuous murmurs, heard over the base of the heart, owing to increased mammary blood flow.
- Rotational and axis changes during pregnancy cause an inverted T wave to be apparent on the electrocardiogram (ECG) – essential to note if resuscitation is required.

Cardiac output

- The increase in cardiac output ranges from 35 to 50% in pregnancy, from an average of 5 L/min before pregnancy to approximately 7 L/min by the 20th week; thereafter the changes are less dramatic.
- The increased cardiac output is due to rises in both stroke volume and heart rate.

- The increase in heart rate begins in the 7th week and by the third trimester it has increased by 10–20%.
- Heart rates are typically 10–15 beats per minute faster than those of the non-pregnant woman.
- The stroke volume increases by 10% during the first half of pregnancy, and reaches a peak at 20 weeks' gestation that is maintained until term.

BLOOD

Blood pressure

- Early pregnancy is associated with a marked decrease in diastolic blood pressure but little change in systolic pressure. With reduced peripheral vascular resistance the systolic blood pressure falls an average of 5–10 mmHg below baseline levels and the diastolic pressure falls 10–15 mmHg by 24 weeks' gestation.
- Thereafter blood pressure gradually rises, returning to prepregnant levels at term. Posture can have a major effect on blood pressure. The supine position can decrease cardiac output by as much as 25%.
- Compression of the inferior vena cava by the enlarging uterus during the late second and third trimesters results in reduced venous return, which in turn decreases stroke volume and cardiac output.

The pregnant woman may suffer from *supine hypotensive syndrome*, which consists of hypotension, bradycardia, dizziness, light-headedness, nausea and even syncope if she remains in the supine position too long. By rolling the woman onto her left side the cardiac output can be instantly restored.

Blood volume

The total maternal blood volume increases 30–50% in singleton pregnancies.

The plasma volume, which corresponds with the increase in blood volume, increases by 50% over the course of the pregnancy. In a normal first pregnancy it may increase by about 1250 ml above non-pregnant levels and in subsequent pregnancies it may increase by about 1500 ml. The increase starts in the first trimester, expands rapidly up until 32–34 weeks' gestation, and then in the last few weeks of pregnancy it plateaus with very little change. The increase in plasma volume reduces the viscosity of the blood and improves capillary flow.

Red cell mass increases during pregnancy in response to the extra oxygen requirements of maternal and placental tissue. Approximately 10–15% of women will have an increase in and reactivation of maternal fetal haemoglobin. The increase in red cell mass appears to be constant throughout pregnancy but it is most marked from about 20 weeks. In spite of the increased production of red blood cells, the marked increase in plasma volume causes dilution of many circulating factors. As a result, the red cell count, haematocrit and haemoglobin concentration all decrease (Table 7.2).

Table 7.2 Falling haemoglobin and haematocrit in pregnancy despite rising blood volume and red cell mass

	Week of pregnancy			
	Non-pregnant	20	30	40
Plasma volume (ml)	2600	3150	3750	3850
Red cell mass (ml)	1400	1450	1550	1650
Total blood volume (ml)	4000	4600	5300	5500
Haematocrit (packed cell volume, PCV) (%)	35.0	32.0	29.0	30.0
Haemoglobin (g/dl)	13.3	11.0	10.5	11.0

In healthy women with iron stores, the mean haemoglobin concentration:

- falls from 13.3 g/dl in the non-pregnant state to 11 g/dl in early pregnancy
- is at its lowest at around 32 weeks' gestation when plasma volume expansion is maximal
- after this time rises by approximately 0.5 g/dl, returning to 11 g/dl around the 36th week of pregnancy.

Anaemia in pregnancy has been defined as a haemoglobin of less than 11 g/dl in the first and third trimesters and less than 10.5 g/dl in the second trimester. Iron therapy is unnecessary unless:

- serial estimations show that the haemoglobin has fallen below 10 g/dl, *or*
- there is a progressive reduction in mean cell volume and low serum ferritin levels.

Iron metabolism

The increased red cell mass and the needs of the developing fetus and placenta lead to increased iron requirements in pregnancy. Iron demand increases from 2 to 4 mg daily. A healthy diet containing 10–14 mg of iron per day, 1–2 mg (5–10%) of which is absorbed, provides sufficient iron for the majority of pregnant women. Caffeine interferes with iron absorption.

Plasma protein

The total serum protein content falls within the first trimester and remains reduced throughout pregnancy. Albumin plays an important role:

- as a carrier protein for some hormones, drugs, free fatty acids and unconjugated bilirubin
- because of its influence in decreasing colloid osmotic pressure, causing physiological oedema.

Clotting factors

Major changes in the coagulation system lead to the *hypercoagulable state* of normal pregnancy. The increased tendency to clot is caused by:

- reduced plasma fibrinolytic activity
- an increase in circulating fibrin degradation products in the plasma.

White blood cells (leucocytes)

From 2 months the total white cell count rises in pregnancy and reaches a peak at 30 weeks, mainly because of the increase in numbers of neutrophil polymorphonuclear leucocytes. This enhances the blood's phagocytic and bactericidal properties.

Table 7.3 is a summary of changes in blood values in pregnancy.

Immunity

Human chorionic gonadotrophin (HCG) and prolactin are known to suppress the immune response of pregnant women. Lymphocyte function is depressed. There is also decreased resistance to certain viral infections. Serum levels of immunoglobulins IgA, IgG and IgM decrease steadily from the 10th week of pregnancy, reaching their lowest level at 30 weeks and remaining at this level until term.

Table 7.3 Summary of common blood values and their changes			
	Normal range (non-pregnant)	**Change in pregnancy**	**Timing**
Protein (total)	65–85 g/L	↓10 g/L	By 20 weeks then stable
Albumin	30–48 g/L	↓10 g/L	Most by 20 weeks then gradual
Fibrinogen	1.7–4.1 g/L	↑2 g/L	Progressively from third month
Platelets	$150–400 \times 10^9$ L	Slight decrease	No significant change until 3–5 days postpartum
Clotting time	6–12 min approx.	Little change	
White cell count	$4–11 \times 10^9$ L	9×10^9 L	Peaks at 30 weeks then plateaus
Red cell count	4.5×10^{12} L	3.8×10^{12} L	Declines progressively to 30–34 weeks

CHANGES IN THE RESPIRATORY SYSTEM

- Increased cardiac output in pregnancy leads to a substantial increase in pulmonary blood flow.
- The blood volume expansion and vasodilatation of pregnancy result in hyperaemia and oedema of the upper respiratory mucosa, which predispose the pregnant woman to nasal congestion, epistaxis and even changes in voice.
- As the uterus enlarges, the diaphragm is elevated by as much as 4 cm, and the ribcage is displaced upwards. Expansion of the ribcage causes the *tidal volume* to be increased by 30–40%. Although the respiratory rate is little changed in pregnancy from the normal 14 or 15 breaths per minute, breathing is deeper even at rest.
- Both the alveolar oxygen partial pressure and the arterial oxygen partial pressure (PaO_2) are increased from non-pregnant values of 98–100 mmHg to pregnant values of 101–104 mmHg.
- The rise in tidal volume and decrease in residual volume facilitates a 15–20% increase in oxygen consumption, which supports the additional metabolic requirements of mother and fetus.
- The 'hyperventilation of pregnancy' causes a 15–20% decrease in maternal arterial carbon dioxide partial pressure ($PaCO_2$) from an average of 5 kPa (35–40 mmHg) in the non-pregnant woman to 4 kPa (30 mmHg) or lower in late pregnancy. The fall in $PaCO_2$ is matched by an equivalent fall in plasma bicarbonate concentration from the non-pregnant values, resulting in mild alkalaemia.

CHANGES IN THE URINARY SYSTEM

- The kidneys increase in weight and lengthen by 1 cm.
- Under the influence of progesterone the calyces and renal pelves dilate.
- The ureters also dilate and lengthen and are thrown into curves of varying sizes. The right ureter is usually more dilated than the left, owing to the dextrorotation of the uterus, and as pregnancy advances the supine or upright posture may cause partial ureteric obstruction as the enlarged uterus compresses both ureters at the pelvic brim.
- All these factors can lead to urinary stasis and an increased risk of urinary tract infection in pregnancy.
- After the 4th month of pregnancy the bladder trigone is lifted and there is thickening of its intraureteric margin; this process continues until term, resulting in a deepened and widened trigone. Bladder pressure increases and may result in reduced bladder capacity. To compensate for this, the urethra lengthens and intraurethral pressure increases.
- The muscles of the internal urethral sphincter relax, which, along with pressure from the pregnant uterus on the bladder, causes a significant number of women to experience some degree of stress incontinence.

Antenatal teaching of pelvic floor exercises is important for helping to resolve this troublesome feature of pregnancy.

- Urgency of micturition and urge incontinence also increase in pregnancy, partly because of the effects of progesterone on the detrusor muscle. These all usually resolve spontaneously during the puerperium.
- Numerous factors affect renal function in pregnancy, including:
  - increased plasma volume
  - increased glomerular filtration rate (GFR)
  - increased renal plasma flow
  - alterations in hormones such as adrenocorticotrophic hormone (ACTH), antidiuretic hormone (ADH), aldosterone, cortisol, thyroid hormone and HCG.

Studies have shown:

- a 45% increase in creatinine clearance by 9 weeks' gestation
- a peak at about 32 weeks' gestation of about 50% above non-pregnant levels
- a significant decrease towards non-pregnant levels prior to birth.

Plasma levels of urea and creatinine decrease in proportion with the increase in GFR during normal pregnancy. Many women with proteinuria before pregnancy experience a progressive increase in the amount of protein spilled during pregnancy; however, the upper limit of normal is considered to be 300 mg over 24 hours. The increased GFR coupled with impaired tubular reabsorption capacity for filtered glucose results in excretion of glucose (*glycosuria*) at some time during pregnancy in 50% of women.

The urine is more alkaline owing to the presence of glucose and to the increased renal loss of bicarbonate caused by the alkalaemia of pregnancy. Renin rises early in pregnancy and continues to increase until term. It acts on angiotensinogen to form increased amounts of angiotensin I and subsequently II (Fig. 7.1). Increased production of angiotensin II stimulates the release of increased levels of aldosterone. Aldosterone prevents the increased loss of sodium that could occur as a result of the increased GFR and the natriuretic effects of progesterone. Despite elevated aldosterone levels, potassium excretion is decreased, possibly because of the effects of progesterone.

CHANGES IN THE GASTROINTESTINAL SYSTEM

- The gums become oedematous, soft and spongy during pregnancy, probably owing to the effect of oestrogen, which can lead to bleeding when the gums are mildly traumatised, as with a toothbrush. Occasionally a focal, highly vascular swelling known as *epulis* (or gingivitis) develops; it is caused by growth of the gum capillaries. It usually regresses spontaneously after delivery.
- Profuse salivation, or ptyalism, is an occasional complaint in pregnancy.
- Dietary changes in pregnancy, such as aversion to coffee, alcohol and fried foods, are very common, as are cravings for salted and spiced foods.

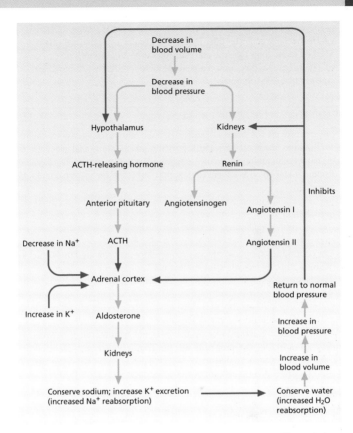

Fig. 7.1: The renin–angiotensin system. (From Wallace 2005 p. 232, with permission of Elsevier, London.)

Pica, the term given to the bizarre craving for and compulsive, secret chewing of food or ingestion of non-food substances (e.g. ice, coal, disinfectants), is also reasonably common.

- Although in early pregnancy many women experience nausea, an increase in appetite may also be noticed, with the daily food intake increasing by up to 200 kcal.
- Many women notice an increase in thirst in pregnancy because of the resetting of osmotic thresholds for thirst and vasopressin.
- As pregnancy progresses, the enlarging uterus displaces the stomach and intestines. At term the stomach attains a vertical position rather than its normal horizontal one. These mechanical forces lead

to increased intragastric pressure and a change in the angle of the gastro-oesophageal junction, leading to greater oesophageal reflux.

- Marked reduction of gastric and intestinal tone and motility plus relaxation of the lower oesophageal sphincter predispose to heartburn, constipation and haemorrhoids.

CHANGES IN METABOLISM

In order to provide for increased basal metabolic rate and oxygen consumption, as well as the needs of the rapidly growing uterus, fetus and placenta, the pregnant woman undergoes many metabolic changes.

- Protein metabolism is enhanced to supply substrate for maternal and fetal growth.
- Fat metabolism increases, as evidenced by elevation of all lipid fractions in the blood.
- Carbohydrate metabolism, however, demonstrates the most dramatic changes.

The continuous supply of glucose required by the growing fetus is met by:

- the intake of glucose when the mother eats
- the enhanced secretion of insulin in response to glucose.

HPL or other growth-related hormones may contribute to the process by reducing peripheral insulin sensitivity and there may be alterations in the characteristics of insulin binding to its receptor.

Optimal blood glucose levels in the pregnant woman range between 4.4 and 5.5 mmol/L. In the pregnant woman hypoglycaemia is defined as a concentration below 3.3 mmol/L.

It is recommended that pregnant women do not:

- fast
- skip meals
- restrict carbohydrate intake.

Maternal blood glucose levels are of critical importance for fetal wellbeing and prolonged fasting in pregnancy produces a more intense ketonaemia, which is dangerous to fetal health.

Muslim women are exempt from fasting while pregnant.

MATERNAL WEIGHT

Weight gain during pregnancy comprises:

- the products of conception (fetus, placenta and amniotic fluid)
- hypertrophy of several maternal tissues (uterus, breasts, blood, fat stores and extracellular and extravascular fluid) (Table 7.4).

An optimal weight gain for an average pregnancy is 12.5 kg, 9 kg of which is gained in the last 20 weeks. Appropriate weight gain for each individual woman is now based on the prepregnancy BMI, which reflects the mother's weight-to-height ratio.

Table 7.4 Distribution of average increase in weight		
	Weight gain (kg)	Percentage of total weight
Maternal		
Uterus	0.9	7.2
Breasts	0.4	3.2
Fat	4.0	32
Blood	1.2	9.6
Extracellular fluid	1.2	9.6
Total	7.7	61.6
Fetal		
Fetus	3.3	26.4
Placenta	0.7	5.6
Amniotic fluid	0.8	6.4
Total	4.8	38.4
Grand total	12.5	100

SKELETAL CHANGES

- During pregnancy, relaxation of the pelvic joints results from hormonal changes. Oestrogen, progesterone and relaxin all appear to be implicated.
- This allows some expansion of the pelvic cavity during descent of the fetal head in labour. The increase in width of the symphysis pubis, which has been associated with severe pelvic pain, occurs more in multiparous than in primigravid women, and returns to normal soon after birth.
- Posture usually alters to compensate for the enlarging uterus, particularly if abdominal muscle tone is poor. A progressive lordosis shifts the woman's centre of gravity back over her legs.
- There is also increased mobility of the sacroiliac and sacrococcygeal joints, which may contribute to the alteration in maternal posture, leading to low back pain in late pregnancy, particularly in the multiparous woman.

SKIN CHANGES

Pigmentation

From the 3rd month until term, some degree of skin darkening is observed in 90% of all pregnant women:

- The pigmented linea alba, now called the *linea nigra*, runs from the os pubis to above the umbilicus.
- Pigmentation of the face, which affects at least half of all pregnant women, is called *chloasma* or *melasma*, or 'mask of pregnancy'.

Melasma is caused by melanin deposition into epidermal or dermal macrophages. Epidermal melanosis usually regresses postpartum but dermal melanosis may persist for up to 10 years in one-third of women. Chloasma can be minimised or prevented by avoiding sun exposure and using high-protection factor sun creams.

Stretch marks

As maternal size increases, stretching occurs in the collagen layer of the skin, particularly over the breasts, abdomen and thighs. In some women the areas of maximum stretch become thin and stretch marks, *striae gravidarum*, appear as red stripes changing to glistening, silvery white lines approximately 6 months after the birth.

Itching

Although not common, itching of the skin in pregnancy (not due to liver disease) can be distressing. Obstetric cholestasis (see Ch. 12) must be excluded before assuming itching is a problem in pregnancy.

Hair

The proportion of growing hairs to resting hairs is increased in pregnancy so the woman reaches the end of pregnancy with many over-aged hairs. This ratio is reversed after delivery so that sometimes alarming amounts of hair are shed during brushing or washing. Normal hair growth is usually restored by 6–12 months. Mild hirsutism is common during pregnancy, particularly on the face.

Other skin changes

A rise in temperature by 0.2–0.4°C occurs as a result of the effects of progesterone and the increased basal metabolic rate (BMR). Angiomas or *vascular spiders* (minute red elevations on the skin of the face, neck, arms and chest) and *palmar erythema* (reddening of the palms) frequently occur, possibly as a result of the high levels of oestrogen. They are of no clinical significance and disappear after pregnancy.

CHANGES IN THE BREASTS

Major changes take place in the breasts during pregnancy owing to the increased blood supply; these changes are stimulated by secretion of oestrogen and progesterone from both corpus luteum and placenta. Among these changes is the formation of new ducts and acini cells (Box 7.2).

Box 7.2 Breast changes in chronological order

3–4 weeks

- There may be a prickling, tingling sensation due to increased blood supply, particularly around the nipple

6–8 weeks

- Breasts increase in size, becoming painful, tense and nodular due to hypertrophy of the alveoli
- Delicate bluish surface veins become visible just beneath the skin

8–12 weeks

- Montgomery's tubercles become more prominent on the areola; these hypertrophic sebaceous glands secrete sebum, which keeps the nipple soft and supple
- Pigmented areas around the nipple (the primary areola) darken, and may enlarge and become more erectile

16 weeks

- Colostrum can be expressed
- The secondary areola develops, with further extension of the pigmented areas that is often mottled in appearance

Late pregnancy

- Colostrum may leak from the breasts
- Progesterone causes the nipple to become more prominent and mobile

CHANGES IN THE ENDOCRINE SYSTEM

During pregnancy the intrauterine tissues can produce many of the peptide and steroid hormones that are produced by the endocrine glands in the non-pregnant state. Many hormones exert their actions indirectly by interacting with cytokines and chemokines. Early effects of placental hormones are described in Chapter 3. Later physiological effects caused by hormones have been highlighted throughout this chapter as they impact on the various systems, and are now summarised.

Placental hormones

These are listed in Box 7.3.

Pituitary gland and its hormones

- The pituitary gland enlarges during pregnancy owing to hypertrophy of the anterior lobe. Secretion of FSH and LH is greatly inhibited during pregnancy by the negative feedback of progesterone and oestrogen.
- In contrast there is increased secretion of hormones by the pituitary gland. The anterior lobe secretes:
- thyroid-stimulating hormone (TSH)
- ACTH

Box 7.3 Placental hormones

HCG

- Produced by the trophoblast
- Maintains the corpus luteum
- Forms the basis for the pregnancy test
- Suppresses the immune response

HPL

- Detected in the trophoblast
- Participates in important metabolic processes

Oestrogens

- Stimulate the liver to produce serum cortisol, testosterone and thyroid-binding proteins
- Cause proliferation of the ductal system of the breasts, secretion of prolactin, growth of the uterus and onset of contractions

Progesterone

- Synthesised within the syncytiotrophoblast
- Maintains uterine quiescence
- Relaxes smooth muscle

- prolactin
- melanocyte-stimulating hormone (MSH).

The posterior lobe of the pituitary gland secretes:

- oxytocin
- antidiuretic hormone (ADH, vasopressin).

Prolactin is essential for lactation and levels rise up to 10-fold during pregnancy and lactation. Its effect of producing milk is suppressed during pregnancy by high levels of oestrogen and progesterone. There is also intrauterine production of prolactin from cells within the decidua.

The posterior pituitary gland releases oxytocin throughout pregnancy. Concentrations of oxytocin in the maternal circulation do not change significantly during pregnancy or prior to the onset of labour, but do rise late in the second stage of labour. There is, however, an increased uterine sensitivity to oxytocin during labour that is influenced by the ratio of oestrogen to progesterone. The pulsatile release produces more effective uterine contractions. Oxytocin is also important for successful lactation.

Thyroid function

Alterations in the structure and function of the thyroid gland cause many thyroid symptoms to be mimicked in pregnancy, resulting in diagnostic confusion in the interpretation of thyroid function tests. Overall control of the thyroid gland, however, is unaltered during normal pregnancy.

- There is a moderate increase in size early in pregnancy.

- There is a marked increase in thyroid-binding globulin, and the bound forms of thyroxine (T_4) and tri-iodothyronine (T_3) peak at about 12 weeks' gestation.

Circulating concentrations of unbound (inactive) T_3 and T_4 are essentially unaltered. Similarly, TSH shows no change in pregnancy.

Adrenal glands

- In early pregnancy the levels of ACTH are reduced, but from 3 months until term there is a significant rise, along with an increase in serum concentrations of circulating free cortisol.
- The placenta and the trophoblast cells also produce corticotrophin-releasing factor and ACTH. These hormones are important in relation to the priming of myometrial activity and may also influence the fetal adrenals.
- The raised levels of unbound cortisol are reflected in the excretion of double the amount of urinary cortisol.
- From 15 weeks' gestation until the third trimester there is a 10-fold increase in the secretion of aldosterone and deoxycorticosterone by the maternal adrenal glands and also by fetal intrauterine tissues, which is stimulated to a certain extent by the acute rise in ACTH. Its main means of control is via the renin–angiotensin system (see Fig. 7.1) with involvement of factors such as atrial natriuretic peptide and angiotensins.

DIAGNOSIS OF PREGNANCY

- Amenorrhoea, breast changes, nausea, changes in food and drink preference, overwhelming tiredness, frequency of micturition and backache often convince women that they are pregnant (Table 7.5).
- The fluttering movements of the fetus felt by the mother, known as *quickening*, are normally felt by a primigravid woman at 18–20 weeks, and a multigravid woman at 16–18 weeks.
- Using transvaginal ultrasound, the gestational sac can be visualised at 4.5 weeks and heart pulsation can be seen at 5 weeks.
- Using transabdominal ultrasound, visualisation of the gestational sac and heart pulsation is possible 1 week later.
- Doppler can detect the fetal heart at 11–12 weeks' gestation.
- The palpation of fetal parts and fetal movements from about 22 weeks are good positive signs of pregnancy.
- Biochemical pregnancy tests depend on the detection of HCG, produced by the trophoblast. HCG can be detected in blood as early as 6 days after conception, and in urine 26 days after conception. Many different pregnancy tests are available, but the most popular over-the-counter home pregnancy test is the *enzyme-linked immunosorbent assay* (ELISA).

Table 7.5 Signs of pregnancy

Sign	Time of occurrence (gestational age)	Differential diagnosis
Possible (presumptive) signs		
Early breast changes (unreliable in multigravida)	3–4 weeks +	Contraceptive pill
Amenorrhoea	4 weeks +	Hormonal imbalance Emotional stress Illness
Morning sickness	4–14 weeks	Gastrointestinal disorders Pyrexial illness Cerebral irritation, etc.
Bladder irritability	6–12 weeks	Urinary tract infections Pelvic tumour
Quickening	16–20 weeks +	Intestinal movement, 'wind'
Probable signs		
Presence of HCG in: Blood Urine	9–10 days 14 days	Hydatidiform mole Choriocarcinoma
Softened isthmus (Hegar's sign)	6–12 weeks	
Blueing of vagina (Chadwick's sign)	8 weeks +	
Pulsation of fornices (Osiander's sign)	8 weeks +	Pelvic congestion
Uterine growth	8 weeks +	Tumours
Changes in skin pigmentations	8 weeks +	
Uterine soufflé	12–16 weeks	Increased blood flow to uterus, as in large uterine myomas or ovarian tumours
Braxton Hicks contractions	16 weeks	
Ballottement of fetus	16–28 weeks	

Table 7.5 Signs of pregnancy—cont'd

Sign	Time of occurrence (gestational age)	Differential diagnosis
Positive signs		
Visualisation of gestational sac by:		
Transvaginal ultrasound	4.5 weeks	
Transabdominal ultrasound	5.5 weeks	
Visualisation of heart pulsation by:		
Transvaginal ultrasound	5 weeks	
Transabdominal ultrasound	6 weeks	
Fetal heart sounds by:		
Doppler	11–12 weeks	
Fetal stethoscope	20 weeks +	
Fetal movements:		
Palpable	22 weeks +	
Visible	Late pregnancy	
Fetal parts palpated	24 weeks +	
Visualisation of fetus by:		
X-ray	16 weeks +	

CHAPTER 8

Common Disorders of and Exercises for Pregnancy

Common disorders experienced by some women as a consequence of the physiological changes occurring in their body are listed in Box 8.1.

RELIEF OF ACHES AND PAINS

Back and pelvic pain

- Backache can be eased by good posture and practice of the transversus and pelvic-tilting exercises in standing, sitting and lying positions.
- Women complaining of severe pain involving more than one area of the pelvis (*pelvic arthropathy*) should be referred to a women's health physiotherapist for assessment, advice and possible manipulation.
- Sciatica-like pain may be relieved by lying on the side away from the discomfort so that the affected leg is uppermost. Pillows should be placed strategically to support the whole limb.
- Symphysis pubis dysfunction (SPD), formerly known as diastasis of the symphysis pubis, is covered in Chapter 12.

Midwives should be aware of necessary precautions and correct positions in relation to labour.

Cramp

Women can help prevent cramp in pregnancy by practising foot and leg exercises.

- To relieve sudden cramp in the calf muscles while in the sitting position, the woman should hold the knee straight and stretch the calf muscles by pulling the foot upwards (dorsiflexing) at the same time.
- Alternatively, standing firmly on the affected leg and striding forwards with the other leg will stretch the calf muscles and solve the problem.

Rib stitch or discomfort

Discomfort around the ribcage can often be relieved by:

- adopting a good posture
- specifically stretching one or both arms upwards, depending on which side the pain affects.

Box 8.1 Common disorders of pregnancy

- Nausea and vomiting
- Breast discomfort
- Backache and ligament pain
- Leg cramp
- Headaches
- Fatigue
- Constipation
- Emotional lability

ANTENATAL EXERCISES

Exercises must be adapted for different circumstances. The positions that pregnant women adopt for exercises should be carefully considered:

- Women should not lie flat in the later second and third trimesters because of the danger of supine hypotension.
- Instead, a half-lying position with the back raised to an angle of approximately 35° can be used.
- Foot and leg exercises and pelvic tilting can be performed in sitting or half-lying positions, whereas transversus and pelvic floor exercises can be carried out in any position.

Muscles of good tone are more elastic and will regain their former length more efficiently and more quickly after being stretched than muscles of poor tone. Exercising the abdominal muscles antenatally will ensure a speedy postnatal return to normal, effective pushing in labour and the lessening of backache in pregnancy. An important function of the abdominal muscles is the control of pelvic tilt. As the ligaments around the pelvis stretch and no longer give such firm support to the joints, the muscles become the second line of defence, helping to prevent an exaggerated pelvic tilt and unnecessary strain on the pelvic ligaments. Overstretched ligaments and weakened abdominal muscles during pregnancy can lead to chronic skeletal problems postnatally as well as backache antenatally. Exercises for the transversus muscles (transversus exercise) and rectus muscles (pelvic tilting) help to prevent this and maintain good abdominal tone.

Exercises that involve the oblique abdominal muscles should be avoided in later pregnancy as they may cause diastasis recti.

Transversus exercise

To tone the deep transverse abdominal muscles and to help prevent backache:

- Sit comfortably or kneel on all fours with a level spine.
- Breathe in and out, then gently pull in the lower part of the abdomen below the umbilicus, keeping the spine still and breathing normally.

- Hold for up to 10 seconds then relax gently.
- Repeat up to 10 times.

Pelvic tilting or rocking

To encourage good posture and ease backache:

- Adopt a half-lying position, well supported with pillows, and the knees bent and feet flat.
- One hand should be placed under the small of the back and the other on top of the abdomen.
- Tighten the abdominals and buttocks, and press the small of the back down on to the hand underneath.
- Breathe normally; hold for up to 10 seconds then relax.
- Repeat up to 10 times.
  Pelvic tilting can also be performed sitting, standing or kneeling.

Pelvic floor exercise

To maintain the tone of the muscles so they retain their functions and to help the muscles to relax during parturition and regain their former strength quickly during the puerperium:

- Sit, stand or half-lie with legs slightly apart.
- Close and draw up around the back passage as though preventing a bowel action then repeat around the front two passages as though preventing the flow of urine.
- Draw up inside and hold for as long as possible, up to 10 seconds, breathing normally, then relax.
- Repeat up to 10 times.

This simple exercise can be practised anywhere and at any time. It will build up the endurance of the postural slow-twitch fibres in the pelvic floor but can also be performed quickly up to 10 times without holding the contraction. This works the fast-twitch fibres, which need to work quickly to prevent leakage (e.g. when coughing). All women should practise this exercise very regularly antenatally, particularly after emptying the bladder. For those with diminished pelvic floor awareness, attempting to 'stop midstream' occasionally or 'gripping' on to an imaginary tampon that is slipping out may assist the ability to contract the correct muscles.

Foot and leg exercises

To improve the circulation and prevent or alleviate cramp, oedema and varicose veins, each of the following should be repeated several times per day:

- Bend and stretch the ankles.
- Circle feet at the ankles.
- Brace the knees and let go.

Additional information

- Advise pregnant women to avoid long periods of standing, which may increase oedema, but encourage walking.
- Discourage sitting or lying with legs crossed, which can impede the circulation.

- Describe how to relieve cramp.
- Advise on correct use of support tights.
- Stress the importance of supporting footwear of sensible height.
- Advise sitting with feet elevated whenever possible and with heels higher than hips if oedema is present.

STRESS, RELAXATION AND RESPIRATION

Tension manifests itself with muscle tightening and shows in the ways listed in Box 8.2.

When tension increases, breathing often becomes shallow and rapid; when severe, breath holding may feature. The higher the stress level, the greater is the degree of postural change that will be evident. Mental tension often leads to physical tension and a vicious circle is established. Muscles can work singly but usually they work in groups and when any group of muscles is working, the opposite group relaxes. This is a physiological fact and is known as *reciprocal inhibition* or *reciprocal relaxation*.

Reciprocal relaxation ensures that, when following a series of instructions for the whole body, one will be able to bring release of tension and relaxation to all areas.

Respiration

Respiration is affected by stress and adapted breathing is one of the easiest ways of assisting relaxation. Breathing can be used to increase the depth of relaxation by varying its speed; slower breathing leads to deeper relaxation. Natural rhythmic breathing must not be confused with specific unnatural levels or rates of breathing. Women in labour frequently breathe very rapidly at the peak of a contraction but should be encouraged not to do so. Persistent rapid breathing or breath holding is usually a sign of panic.

Very slow deep breathing can cause hyperventilation, which produces tingling in the fingers and may proceed to carpopedal spasm and even tetany. Rapid shallow breathing or panting is only tracheal and can lead to hypoventilation with subsequent oxygen deprivation. During pregnancy, labour and birth, emphasis should be placed on easy, rhythmic breathing and on avoiding very deep breathing, shallow panting or long periods of breath holding.

Box 8.2 Signs of tension

- Frowning face
- Tense jaw
- Hunched shoulders
- Elbows bent and close to sides
- Fingers gripping or tapping
- Trunk bent forward
- Crossed legs
- Feet pulled up or tapping

CHAPTER 9

Antenatal Care

AIM OF ANTENATAL CARE

The aim is to monitor the progress of pregnancy in order to support maternal health and normal fetal development. The midwife critically evaluates the physical, psychological and sociological effects of pregnancy on the woman and her family by:

- developing a partnership with the woman
- providing a holistic approach to the woman's care that meets her individual needs
- promoting an awareness of the public health issues for the woman and her family
- exchanging information with the woman and her family and enabling them to make informed choices about pregnancy and birth
- being an advocate for the woman and her family during her pregnancy, supporting her right to choose care that is appropriate for her own needs and those of her family
- recognising complications of pregnancy and appropriately referring women within the multidisciplinary team
- assisting the woman and her family in their preparations to meet the demands of birth, and making a birth plan
- assisting the woman in making an informed choice about methods of infant feeding and giving appropriate and sensitive advice to support her decision
- offering education for parenthood within a planned programme or on an individual basis
- working in partnership with other pertinent organisations.

THE INITIAL ASSESSMENT (BOOKING VISIT)

The purpose of this visit is to:

- introduce the woman to the maternity service
- share information in order to discuss, plan and implement care for the duration of the pregnancy, the birth and postnatally.

The earlier the first contact is made with the midwife, the more appropriate and valuable the advice given relating to nutrition and care of the developing fetal organs. Medical conditions, infections, smoking, alcohol and drug taking may all have a profound and detrimental effect on the fetus during this time.

Models of midwifery care

Options for place of birth include:

- the home
- a birth centre
- a peripheral unit
- a tertiary hospital.

The majority of women receive antenatal care in the community, either in their own home or at a local clinic. Hospital-based clinics are available for women who receive care from an obstetrician or physician in addition to their midwife.

INTRODUCTION TO THE MIDWIFERY SERVICE

The woman's introduction to midwifery care is crucial in forming her initial impressions of the maternity service. The midwife can promote communication with the woman by:

- using gentle questioning
- good listening skills
- making open-ended statements
- reflecting back key words used during the discussion to encourage and facilitate exploration of what is being said.

Communication encompasses the writing of accurate, comprehensive and contemporaneous records of information given and received and the plan of care that has been agreed.

Observations

Observation of physical characteristics is also important. Posture and gait can indicate back problems or previous trauma to the pelvis. The woman may be lethargic, which could be an indication of extreme tiredness, anaemia, malnutrition or depression.

Social history

It is important to assess the response of the whole family to the pregnancy and to aim to improve health and reduce health inequalities in pregnant women and their young children. The midwife may, in partnership with the woman, advocate referral to a social worker, or to other multiprofessional agencies. Questioning about domestic abuse is important but requires discretion.

General health

General health should be discussed and advice given when required. The woman, her partner and other family members should be informed about the direct and passive effects of smoking on the baby. Alcohol abuse is less common but can affect the baby. It is recommended that women limit alcohol consumption to no more than one standard unit twice in a week.

Menstrual history

The midwife needs to know how to determine the expected date of birth (still referred to as EDD). Mothers expect this estimation while waiting for an ultrasound scan or if a scan is declined or not available. Abdominal assessment of uterine size can be made in conjunction with gestational age during the antenatal consultation. The midwife has a role in helping the woman to understand that an EDD is 1 day within a 5-week time frame during which her baby reaches term and may be born.

The EDD is calculated by adding 9 calendar months and 7 days to the date of the first day of the woman's last menstrual period (LMP). This method assumes that:

- the woman takes regular note of regularity and length of time between periods
- conception occurred 14 days after the first day of the last period; this is true only if the woman has a regular 28-day cycle
- the last period of bleeding was true menstruation; implantation of the zygote may cause slight bleeding.

Naegele's rule suggests that the duration of a pregnancy is 280 days. However, controversy exists over the suitability of applying Naegele's rule to determine EDD; therefore ultrasound scanning has become the more accurate and commonly used method for predicting the EDD. This depends on an experienced ultrasonographer being both available and accessible, and also requires the woman's consent. Ultrasound before 14 weeks confirms the EDD; the 18–20 week scan identifies abnormalities.

If the woman has taken oral contraceptives within the previous 3 months, this may also confuse estimation of dates because breakthrough bleeding and anovular cycles lead to inaccuracies. Some women become pregnant with an intrauterine contraceptive device (IUCD) still in place. Although the pregnancy is likely to continue normally, the position of the IUCD may be determined using ultrasound techniques.

Obstetric history

In order to give a summary of a woman's childbearing history, the descriptive terms -gravida and -para are used:

- 'Gravid' means 'pregnant', 'gravida' means 'a pregnant woman' and a subsequent number indicates the number of times she has been pregnant regardless of outcome.
- 'Para' means 'having given birth'; a woman's parity refers to the number of times that she has given birth to a child, live or stillborn, excluding miscarriages and abortions.

A *grande multigravida* is a woman who has been pregnant five times or more irrespective of outcome. A *grande multipara* is a woman who has given birth five times or more.

Any form of abortion occurring in a Rhesus negative woman requires prophylactic administration of anti-D immunoglobulin to reduce the risk of Rhesus incompatibility in a subsequent pregnancy (see Ch. 35).

Confidential information may be recorded in a clinic-held summary of the pregnancy and not in the woman's hand-held record if she requests this.

Repeated spontaneous abortion (miscarriage) may indicate conditions such as genetic abnormality, hormonal imbalance or incompetent cervix. The woman may be more anxious about this pregnancy, minor disturbances in pregnancy may be exacerbated and preoccupation with the pregnancy may lead to other psychological, social or physical problems.

A risk assessment should be carried out based on the woman's obstetric and medical history and current pregnancy. This will enable the midwife and woman to:

- discuss the progress of the pregnancy
- determine the frequency of antenatal visits and the location of antenatal care
- identify appropriate screening techniques and other health professionals who may need to be involved.

Place of birth will also be influenced by the risk assessment but in all cases the ultimate decision is taken by the mother, who should make an informed choice (Box 9.1).

Box 9.1 Factors that may require additional antenatal surveillance or advice

Initial assessment
- Age less than 18 years or 40 years and over
- Grande multiparity (more than five previous births)
- Vaginal bleeding at any time during pregnancy
- Unknown or uncertain EDD
- Late booking

Past obstetric history
- Stillbirth or neonatal death
- Baby small or large for gestational age
- Congenital abnormality
- Rhesus isoimmunisation
- Pregnancy-induced hypertension
- Two or more terminations of pregnancy
- Three or more spontaneous miscarriages
- Previous preterm labour
- Cervical cerclage in past or present pregnancy
- Previous caesarean section or uterine surgery
- Ante- or postpartum haemorrhage
- Precipitate labour
- Multiple pregnancy

Maternal health
- Previous history of deep vein thrombosis or pulmonary embolism
- Chronic illness, blood disorders

Continued

Box 9.1 Factors that may require additional antenatal surveillance or advice—cont'd

- Hypertension, cardiac disease
- History of infertility
- Uterine anomaly, including fibroids
- Substance abuse (drugs, alcohol, smoking)
- Family history of diabetes or genetic disorder
- Psychological or psychiatric disorders

Examination at the initial assessment

- Blood pressure 140/90 mmHg or above
- Maternal obesity or underweight according to body mass index (BMI)

Medical history

During pregnancy both the mother and the fetus may be affected by a medical condition, or a medical condition may be altered by the pregnancy; if untreated, there may be serious consequences for the woman's health.

Family history

Certain conditions are genetic in origin, others are familial or related to ethnicity, and some are associated with the physical or social environment in which the family lives.

PHYSICAL EXAMINATION

Prior to the physical examination of a pregnant woman, her consent and comfort are primary considerations. Sophisticated biochemical assessments and ultrasound investigations can enhance clinical observations.

Weight

- All women should be weighed or asked for a prepregnant weight at booking; if it is within the normal body mass index (BMI) range, repeated weighing is not recommended.
- Women with a BMI of 30 or above or 18 or under should be carefully monitored and offered nutritional counselling.

Blood pressure

Blood pressure is taken in order to ascertain normality and provide a baseline reading for comparison throughout pregnancy.

- The systolic recording may be falsely elevated if a woman is nervous or anxious; long waiting times can cause additional stress. A full bladder can also cause an increase in blood pressure.
- The woman should be comfortably seated or resting in a lateral position on the couch when the blood pressure is taken. Brachial artery pressure is highest when sitting and lower when in the recumbent position.

- A systolic blood pressure of 140 mmHg or diastolic pressure of 90 mmHg at booking is indicative of hypertension and will need careful monitoring during pregnancy with both midwife and obstetrician support.

Urinalysis

- At the first visit a midstream specimen should be sent to the laboratory for culture to exclude asymptomatic bacteriuria.
- Urinalysis for proteinuria is performed at every visit.

Blood tests in pregnancy

The midwife should explain why blood tests are carried out to enable women to make informed choices. The midwife should be fully aware of the difference between screening and diagnostic tests, and of their accuracy, and should discuss these options with the women. Blood tests taken at the initial assessment include the ones listed in Box 9.2.

Rhesus negative women who have threatened miscarriage, amniocentesis or any other uterine trauma should be given anti-D gamma-globulin within a few days of the event. If the titration demonstrates a rising antibody response, then more frequent assessment will be made in order to plan management by a specialist in Rhesus disease.

THE MIDWIFE'S EXAMINATION AND ADVICE

The midwife's general examination of the woman is holistic and should encompass her physical, social and psychological wellbeing and provide advice on the alleviation of common disorders.

Nausea and vomiting

These are said to affect over 50% of pregnancies. The cause is thought to be a combination of:

- hormonal changes
- psychological adjustments
- neurological factors.

Box 9.2 Blood tests performed at initial assessment

- ABO blood group and Rhesus (Rh) factor
- Full blood count
- Venereal Disease Research Laboratory (VDRL) test
- HIV antibodies
- Rubella immune status
- Hepatitis B screening
- Investigations for other blood disorders (in women and their partners of some ethnic groups – for example, sickle-cell disease or thalassaemia)

The midwife may suggest remedies such as:

- eating a dry biscuit or cracker with a drink before rising in the morning
- avoiding spicy or pungent odours
- eating little and often (helps to maintain the body's blood sugar levels; drinking small amounts of fluid between meals will help to maintain hydration).

Other suggested remedies have included:

- the use of neurological devices, which transmit electrical stimulation via the wrist and are thought to trigger sensory and neurological impulses that control vomiting
- complementary therapies, such as acupuncture and homeopathic and herbal remedies, which may be of benefit in minimising discomfort.

Nausea and vomiting generally improve around the 16th week of pregnancy. A small proportion of affected women will develop a more serious condition known as hyperemesis gravidarum, which requires urgent referral to a doctor.

Bladder and bowel function

Bladder and bowel function may be discussed. Dietary advice may be necessary at this visit or later in the pregnancy, with reference to how hormonal changes may alter normal bowel and kidney function. The midwife should be able to advise women on how to avoid constipation, for example, by taking a high-fibre diet and maintaining an adequate fluid intake. If constipation persists, then haemorrhoids may develop, caused by straining at defaecation.

Vaginal discharge

Vaginal discharge increases in pregnancy; the woman may discuss any increase or changes with the midwife. Once the woman has identified what is normal she will then be able to report any changes to the midwife during subsequent visits.

- If the discharge is itchy, causes soreness, is any colour other than creamy-white or has an offensive odour, then infection is likely and should be investigated further.
- Later in pregnancy the woman may report a change from leucorrhoea to a heavier mucous discharge. Mucoid loss is evidence of cervical changes, and if it occurs before the 37th week, may be an early sign of preterm labour.
- The obstetrician will investigate vaginal bleeding during pregnancy; however, in early pregnancy spotting may occur at the time when menstruation would have been due.
- Early bleeding is not uncommon; the midwife should advise the woman to rest at this time and to avoid sexual intercourse until the pregnancy is more stable.

Abdominal examination

This should be performed at each antenatal visit (see below). At the initial assessment the midwife will observe for signs of pregnancy. It is unlikely that the uterus will be palpable abdominally before the 12th week of gestation. If it has previously been retroverted, it may not be palpable until the 16th week.

Oedema

This is not likely to be in evidence during the initial assessment but may occur as the pregnancy progresses. Physiological oedema occurs after rising in the morning and worsens during the day; it is often associated with daily activities or hot weather. At visits later in pregnancy the midwife should observe for oedema and ask the woman about symptoms.

Varicosities

These are more likely to occur during pregnancy and are a predisposing cause of deep vein thrombosis. The woman should be asked to report any tenderness that she feels either during the examination or at any time during the pregnancy. Advice about support tights can be offered.

ABDOMINAL EXAMINATION

The abdominal examination is carried out to establish and affirm that fetal growth is consistent with gestational age during the progression of pregnancy.

PREPARATION

The bladder should be emptied. Privacy is essential. The woman should be lying comfortably with her arms by her sides to relax the abdominal muscles. She should then sit up to discuss the findings with the midwife.

METHOD

Inspection

- The size of the uterus is assessed approximately by observation.
- The shape of the uterus is longer than it is broad when the lie of the fetus is longitudinal. If the lie is transverse, the uterus is low and broad.
- The multiparous uterus may lack the snug ovoid shape of the primigravid uterus. Often it is possible to see the shape of the fetal back or limbs.
- If the fetus is in an occipitoposterior position, a saucer-like depression may be seen at or below the umbilicus.
- The midwife may observe fetal movements or they may be felt by the mother; this can help the midwife determine the position of the fetus.
- Lax abdominal muscles in the multiparous woman may allow the uterus to sag forwards; this is known as *pendulous abdomen* or anterior obliquity of the uterus. In the primigravida it is a serious sign, as it may be due to pelvic contraction.

Skin changes

- Stretch marks known as *striae gravidarum* from previous pregnancies appear silvery and recent ones appear pink.
- A *linea nigra* may be seen; this is a normal dark line of pigmentation running longitudinally in the centre of the abdomen below and sometimes above the umbilicus.
- Scars may indicate previous obstetric or abdominal surgery.

Palpation

- To determine the height of the fundus the midwife places her hand just below the xiphisternum.
- Pressing gently, she moves her hand down the abdomen until she feels the curved upper border of the fundus, noting the number of fingerbreadths that can be accommodated between the two.
- Alternatively, the distance between the fundus and the symphysis pubis can be determined with a tape measure.

The height of the fundus correlates well with gestational age, especially during the earlier weeks of pregnancy (Fig. 9.1).

- If the uterus is unduly big, the fetus may be large, but multiple pregnancy or polyhydramnios may be suspected.
- When the uterus is smaller than expected, the LMP date may be incorrect, or the fetus may be small for gestational age.

Fundal palpation

This determines the presence of the breech or the head. This information will help to diagnose the lie and presentation of the fetus.

- Watching the woman's reaction to the procedure, the midwife lays both hands on the sides of the fundus, fingers held close together and curving round the upper border of the uterus.

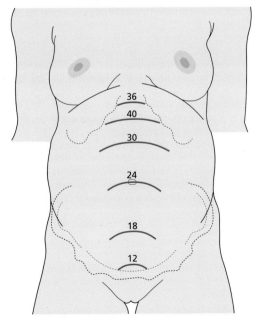

Fig. 9.1: Growth of the uterus, showing the fundal heights at various weeks of pregnancy.

- Gentle yet deliberate pressure is applied using the palmar surfaces of the fingers to determine the soft consistency and indefinite outline that denotes the breech. Sometimes the buttocks feel rather firm but they are not as hard, smooth or well defined as the head.
- With a gliding movement the fingertips are separated slightly in order to grasp the fetal mass, which may be in the centre or deflected to one side, to assess its size and mobility. The breech cannot be moved independently of the body, as the head can.
- The head is much more distinctive in outline than the breech, being hard and round; it can be balloted (moved from one hand to the other) between the fingertips of the two hands because of the free movement of the neck.

Lateral palpation

This is used to locate the fetal back in order to determine position.

- The hands are placed on either side of the uterus at the level of the umbilicus.
- Gentle pressure is applied with alternate hands in order to detect which side of the uterus offers the greater resistance.
- More detailed information is obtained by feeling along the length of each side with the fingers. This can be done by sliding the hands down the abdomen while feeling the sides of the uterus alternately.
- Some midwives prefer to steady the uterus with one hand and, using a rotary movement of the opposite hand, to map out the back as a continuous smooth resistant mass from the breech down to the neck; on the other side the same movement reveals the limbs as small parts that slip about under the examining fingers.
- 'Walking' the fingertips of both hands over the abdomen from one side to the other is an excellent method of locating the back. The fingers should be dipped deeply into the abdominal wall. The firm back can be distinguished from the fluctuating amniotic fluid and the receding knobbly small parts. To make the back more prominent, fundal pressure can be applied with one hand and the other used to 'walk' over the abdomen. Palpating from the neck upwards and inwards can locate the anterior shoulder.

Pelvic palpation

Pelvic palpation will identify the fetal presentation; however, as this can cause discomfort to the woman it is not recommended before 36 weeks.

- Ask the woman to bend her knees slightly in order to relax the abdominal muscles.
- Suggest that she breathe steadily; relaxation may be helped if she sighs out slowly.
- The sides of the uterus just below umbilical level are grasped snugly between the palms of the hands with the fingers held close together, and pointing downwards and inwards.
- If the head is presenting, a hard mass with a distinctive round, smooth surface will be felt. The midwife should also estimate how much of the

fetal head is palpable above the pelvic brim to determine engagement. The two-handed technique appears to be the more comfortable for the woman and gives the most information. Pawlik's manoeuvre is sometimes used to judge the size, flexion and mobility of the head but the midwife must be careful not to apply undue pressure. It should be used only if absolutely necessary. The midwife grasps the lower pole of the uterus between her fingers and thumb, which should be spread wide enough apart to accommodate the fetal head.

Auscultation

Routine auscultation of the fetal heart is not recommended; however, when requested by the mother it may provide some reassurance.

- A Pinard's stethoscope is placed on the mother's abdomen, at right angles to it over the fetal back (Fig. 9.2).
- The ear must be in close, firm contact with the stethoscope but the hand should not touch it while listening.
- The stethoscope should be moved about until the point of maximum intensity is located where the fetal heart is heard most clearly.
- The midwife should count the beats per minute, which should be in the range of 110–160.
- The midwife should take the woman's pulse at the same time as listening to the fetal heart to enable her to distinguish between the two.

In addition, ultrasound equipment (e.g. a Sonicaid or Doppler) can be used for this purpose, so that the woman may also hear the fetal heartbeat.

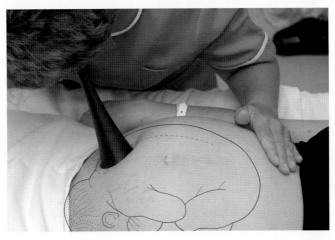

Fig. 9.2: Auscultation of the fetal heart.

FINDINGS

The midwife assesses all the information which she has gathered and critically evaluates the wellbeing of the mother and the fetus. Deviation from the expected growth and development should be referred to the obstetrician.

Gestational age

During pregnancy the uterus is expected to grow at a predicted rate and in early pregnancy uterine size will usually equate with the gestation estimated by dates. Later in pregnancy, increasing uterine size gives evidence of continuing fetal growth but is less reliable as an indicator of gestational age.

Multiple pregnancy increases the overall uterine size and should be diagnosed by 24 weeks' gestation. In a singleton pregnancy the fundus reaches the umbilicus at 22–24 weeks and the xiphisternum at 36 weeks. In the last month of pregnancy lightening occurs as the fetus sinks down into the lower pole of the uterus. The uterus becomes broader and the fundus lower. In the primigravida, strong, supportive abdominal muscles encourage the fetal head to enter the brim of the pelvis.

Lie

The lie of the fetus is the relationship between the long axis of the fetus and the long axis of the uterus. In the majority of cases the lie is *longitudinal* owing to the ovoid shape of the uterus; the remainder are oblique or transverse.

Attitude

Attitude is the relationship of the fetal head and limbs to its trunk. The attitude should be one of flexion.

Presentation

Presentation refers to the part of the fetus that lies at the pelvic brim or in the lower pole of the uterus. Presentations can be:

- vertex
- breech
- shoulder
- face
- brow.

Vertex, face and brow are all head or cephalic presentations.

Denominator

The denominator is the name of the part of the presentation, which is used when referring to fetal position. Each presentation has a different denominator and these are as follows:

- In the vertex presentation it is the occiput.
- In the breech presentation it is the sacrum.
- In the face presentation it is the mentum.

Although the shoulder presentation is said to have the acromion process as its denominator, in practice the dorsum is used to describe the position. In the brow presentation no denominator is used.

Position

The position is the relationship between the denominator of the presentation and six points on the pelvic brim. In addition, the denominator may be found in the midline either anteriorly or posteriorly, especially late in labour. This position is often transient and is described as *direct anterior* or *direct posterior*.

Anterior positions are more favourable than posterior positions because, when the fetal back is in front, it conforms to the concavity of the mother's abdominal wall and can therefore flex more easily. When the back is flexed, the head also tends to flex and a smaller diameter presents to the pelvic brim. There is also more room in the anterior part of the pelvic brim for the broad biparietal diameter of the head.

The positions in a vertex presentation are summarised in Box 9.3 and Figures 9.3–9.8.

Box 9.3 Positions in a vertex presentation

Left occipitoanterior (LOA)
- The occiput points to the left iliopectineal eminence
- The sagittal suture is in the right oblique diameter of the pelvis (Fig. 9.3)

Right occipitoanterior (ROA)
- The occiput points to the right iliopectineal eminence
- The sagittal suture is in the left oblique diameter of the pelvis (Fig. 9.4)

Left occipitolateral (LOL)
- The occiput points to the left iliopectineal line midway between the iliopectineal eminence and the sacroiliac joint
- The sagittal suture is in the transverse diameter of the pelvis (Fig. 9.5)

Right occipitolateral (ROL)
- The occiput points to the right iliopectineal line midway between the iliopectineal eminence and the sacroiliac joint
- The sagittal suture is in the transverse diameter of the pelvis (Fig. 9.6)

Left occipitoposterior (LOP)
- The occiput points to the left sacroiliac joint; the sagittal suture is in the left oblique diameter of the pelvis (Fig. 9.7)

Right occipitoposterior (ROP)
- The occiput points to the right sacroiliac joint; the sagittal suture is in the right oblique diameter of the pelvis (Fig. 9.8)

Direct occipitoanterior (DOA)
- The occiput points to the symphysis pubis; the sagittal suture is in the anteroposterior diameter of the pelvis

Direct occipitoposterior (DOP)
- The occiput points to the sacrum; the sagittal suture is in the anteroposterior diameter of the pelvis

In breech and face presentations the positions are described in a similar way using the appropriate denominator.

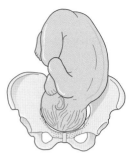

Fig. 9.3: Left occipitoanterior.

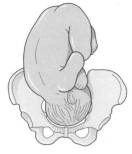

Fig. 9.4: Right occipitoanterior.

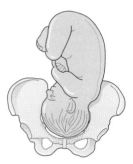

Fig. 9.5: Left occipitolateral.

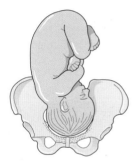

Fig. 9.6: Right occipitolateral.

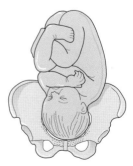

Fig. 9.7: Left occipitoposterior.

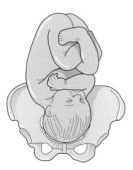

Fig. 9.8: Right occipitoposterior.

Engagement

Engagement is said to have occurred when the widest presenting transverse diameter has passed through the brim of the pelvis. In cephalic presentations this is the biparietal diameter, and in breech presentations the bitrochanteric diameter. Engagement in a cephalic presentation demonstrates that the maternal pelvis is likely to be adequate for the size of the fetus and that the baby will birth vaginally.

In a primigravid woman the head normally engages at any time from about 36 weeks of pregnancy, but in a multipara this may not occur until after the onset of labour. When the vertex presents and the head is engaged the following will be evident on clinical examination:

- Only two-fifths to three-fifths of the fetal head is palpable above the pelvic brim (Fig. 9.9).
- The head is not mobile.
- On rare occasions the head is not palpable abdominally because it has descended deeply into the pelvis.

If the head is not engaged, the findings are as follows:

- More than half of the head is palpable above the brim.
- The head may be high and freely movable (ballotable) or partly settled in the pelvic brim and consequently immobile.

If the head does not engage in a primigravid woman at term, there is a possibility of a malposition or cephalopelvic disproportion. Referral to an obstetrician should be made.

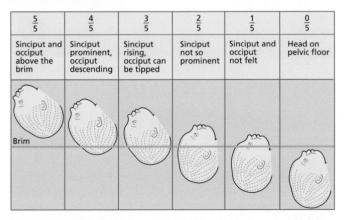

$\frac{5}{5}$	$\frac{4}{5}$	$\frac{3}{5}$	$\frac{2}{5}$	$\frac{1}{5}$	$\frac{0}{5}$
Sinciput and occiput above the brim	Sinciput prominent, occiput descending	Sinciput rising, occiput can be tipped	Sinciput not so prominent	Sinciput and occiput not felt	Head on pelvic floor

Fig. 9.9: Descent of the fetal head estimated in fifths palpable above the pelvic brim.

ONGOING ANTENATAL CARE

The information gathered during the antenatal visits will enable the midwife and pregnant woman to determine the appropriate pattern of antenatal care. The following schedule is based on guidelines from the UK's National Institute for Health and Clinical Excellence (NICE).

16 weeks
- Review, discuss and document results of screening tests undertaken at initial assessment.
- Investigate a haemoglobin level below 11 g/dl and consider iron supplementation.
- Measure blood pressure.
- Urinalysis for proteinuria.
- Information exchange and review of care plan.

18–20 weeks
- Ultrasound scan to detect fetal anomalies.

25 weeks
- Measure fundal height.
- Measure blood pressure.
- Urinalysis for proteinuria.
- Information exchange and review of care plan.

28 weeks
- Offer repeat screening for anaemia and atypical red-cell alloantibodies.
- Investigate a haemoglobin level below 10.5 g/dl and consider iron supplementation.
- Offer anti-D to Rhesus negative women.
- Measure fundal height.
- Measure blood pressure.
- Urinalysis for proteinuria.
- Information exchange and review of care plan.

31 weeks (nulliparous women)
- Measure fundal height.
- Measure blood pressure.
- Urinalysis for proteinuria.
- Review, discuss and document results of screening tests undertaken at 28-week assessment.
- Information exchange and review of care plan.

34 weeks
- Offer a second dose of anti-D to Rhesus negative women.
- Measure fundal height.
- Measure blood pressure.
- Urinalysis for proteinuria.
- *Multiparous women* – review, discuss and document results of screening tests undertaken at 28-week assessment.
- Information exchange and review of care plan.

36 weeks
- Measure blood pressure.
- Urinalysis for proteinuria.
- Measure fundal height.

- Check presentation of fetus; refer to obstetrician if breech.
- Information exchange and review of care plan.

38 weeks
- Measure blood pressure.
- Urinalysis for proteinuria.
- Measure fundal height.
- Information exchange and review of care plan.

40 weeks (nulliparous women)
- Measure blood pressure.
- Urinalysis for proteinuria.
- Measure fundal height.
- Information exchange and review of care plan.

41 weeks
- Measure blood pressure.
- Urinalysis for proteinuria.
- Measure fundal height.
- Information exchange and review of care plan.
- Offer a membrane sweep.
- Offer induction of labour.

CHAPTER 10

Specialised Fetal Investigations

Advances in technology mean that assessment of the fetus during pregnancy has become increasingly sophisticated and more widespread. Biochemical tests on maternal serum are commonly performed in order to identify which pregnancies carry a high risk of Down syndrome (trisomy 21) and ultrasound scanning is continually being refined.

PSYCHOLOGICAL ASPECTS OF PRENATAL TESTING

Prenatal testing is a two-edged sword. It enables midwives and doctors to give people choices. However, they may increase the amount of anxiety and psychological trauma experienced in pregnancy.

Anxiety caused by consideration of possible fetal abnormality may be accompanied by moral or religious dilemmas. For instance, tests that can diagnose chromosomal or genetic abnormalities also carry a risk of procedure-induced miscarriage. Many parents agonise about whether to subject a potentially normal fetus to this risk in order to obtain this information. Parents may then need to consider whether they wish to terminate or continue with an affected pregnancy. Informed consent must be given (Box 10.1).

TESTS FOR FETAL ABNORMALITY

Broadly speaking, there are two types of test for fetal anomaly:
- screening tests
- diagnostic tests.

Screening for fetal abnormality
Screening tests aim to identify a proportion of individuals (often around 5% of a population) who have the highest chances of a named disorder. This makes it possible to target further investigations towards those with the best indication. Mothers who undergo screening tests will be classified as above or below an action limit, whereby they are recalled and offered follow-up procedures.

The performance of a screening test is defined in a number of ways (Box 10.2).

Diagnosis of fetal abnormality
Diagnostic tests are performed in order to confirm or disprove the presence of a particular abnormality.

Box 10.1 Information required for obtaining informed consent

- Purpose of the procedure
- All risks and benefits to be reasonably expected
- Details of all possible future treatments that could arise as a consequence of testing
- Disclosure of all appropriate techniques that may be advantageous
- The option of refusing any tests
- The offer to answer any queries

Box 10.2 Performance criteria for screening tests

Detection rate/sensitivity
- The proportion of affected pregnancies that would be identified as high risk

False-positive rate
- The proportion of unaffected pregnancies with a high-risk classification
- The higher the specificity, the fewer the false positives

False-negative rate
- The proportion of affected pregnancies that would not be identified as high risk
- The higher the sensitivity, the fewer the false negatives

THE USE OF ULTRASOUND IN OBSTETRICS

Most mothers undergo at least one ultrasound scan during pregnancy. This procedure can enable assessment and monitoring of many aspects of the pregnancy and is often presented as 'routine'. It can be used in order to screen for and to diagnose fetal abnormalities. Ultrasound works by transmitting sound at a very high pitch, via a probe, in a narrow beam. When the sound waves enter the body and encounter a structure, some of that sound is reflected back. The amount of sound reflected varies according to the type of tissue encountered. Generally, pictures are transmitted in 'real time', which enables fetal movements to be seen.

FIRST TRIMESTER PREGNANCY SCANS

Many areas offer mothers a scan in early pregnancy. The purpose of this is to establish:
- that the pregnancy is viable and intrauterine
- gestational age
- fetal number (and chorionicity or amnionicity in multiple pregnancies)
- detection of gross fetal abnormalities, such as anencephaly.

There is evidence to suggest that at least one scan is beneficial, mainly in reducing the need to induce labour for postmaturity. A gestation sac can usually be visualised from 5 weeks' gestation and a small embryo from 6 weeks. Until 13 weeks, gestational age can be accurately assessed by crown–rump length (CRL) measurement. Mothers are asked to attend with a full bladder, since this aids visualisation of the uterus at an early gestation.

Measurement of nuchal translucency at 10–14 weeks as a screen for Down syndrome

Information about the fetus can be gained by observation of the nuchal translucency (NT) at 10–14 weeks' gestation. This involves measuring the thickness of the subcutaneous collection of fluid at the back of the neck. Increased NT is used as a basis upon which to screen for Down syndrome. The main advantage of this test is that it offers an early way of assessing the mother's risk for Down syndrome. Increased NT is also associated with other structural (mainly cardiac) and genetic syndromes, and this enables increased pregnancy surveillance to be arranged. However, a disadvantage of this knowledge is that parents may suffer considerable anxiety until later scans offer some degree of reassurance.

SECOND TRIMESTER ULTRASOUND SCANS

After 13 weeks of pregnancy, gestational age is primarily assessed using the biparietal diameter (BPD). It is a very useful measurement during the second trimester, but becomes less accurate towards the end of pregnancy because the shape of the head may alter. Limbs are also measured, most notably the femur.

The detailed fetal anomaly scan

This scan is usually performed at 18–22 weeks of pregnancy. Visualisation of fetal anatomy is more difficult before that time, although some ultrasound departments have very sophisticated equipment which can identify anomalies much earlier. The purpose of this scan is to reassure the mother that the fetus has no obvious structural abnormalities. Detection rates vary considerably, but it is thought that around 50% of significant abnormalities are identified at this time.

Some structural problems do not have associated sonographic signs and some fetal abnormalities may not appear until later in pregnancy. Diagnosis may therefore be missed.

Markers for chromosomal abnormality

Markers are minor sonographic clue signs that increase the chance that the fetus has a chromosomal abnormality. (Most are associated with Down syndrome.) The strength of association between each individual marker and Down syndrome varies considerably. When markers are identified, it is important to consider whether there are other risk factors, such as advancing maternal age or increased NT measurement at 10–14 weeks. The mother's aggregate risk for Down syndrome can then be calculated, taking all these factors into account.

THIRD TRIMESTER PREGNANCY SCANS

In general, late pregnancy scans are performed in response to a specific clinical need and not as a screen of the low-risk pregnant population. However, fetal abnormalities may come to light or be reassessed at this time. Many late scans are performed as a means of monitoring fetal wellbeing, growth and development.

Fetal growth

Many scans are performed in order to detect instances when growth deviates from normal.

- Fetuses with excessive growth (*macrosomia*) have increased perinatal mortality and morbidity.
- Fetuses may be small because they are preterm or because they are small for gestational age.
- Sometimes, these two problems overlap.

In general, growth-restricted babies can be divided into two groups:

- Those with symmetrical growth restriction.
- Those with asymmetrical growth restriction.

Most symmetrically small fetuses are entirely normal and may be genetically predetermined to be small. However, in some instances this may be caused by chromosomal abnormalities, infection or environmental factors such as maternal substance misuse.

Asymmetrical growth restriction

These fetuses have a head size appropriate for gestational age, but thin bodies. This is generally caused by placental insufficiency. Glycogen stores in the liver are reduced, so there are fewer energy reserves for the fetus during labour. Asymmetrically growth-restricted fetuses are therefore more likely to suffer antenatal or perinatal asphyxia, or both. Other potential problems include hypoglycaemia, hypothermia and premature birth.

In order to assess fetal growth, the gestational age must be accurately assessed on scan before 24 weeks. Women at high risk of having an abnormally grown fetus should have serial scans – often at 28, 32 and 36 weeks. Where there is a particular concern, growth may be measured every 2 weeks. The most important measurements are head circumference and abdominal circumference. In this way, trends in fetal growth can be assessed.

DOPPLER ULTRASONOGRAPHY

In recent years, there have been major developments in the use of Doppler ultrasound techniques for the study of maternal and fetal circulation. Abnormalities in Doppler measurements may be detected before growth becomes impaired and can be used as a prognostic indicator.

BIOPHYSICAL PROFILING

Another ultrasound measure of fetal wellbeing is the fetal biophysical profile. This is used to determine whether there are signs of fetal hypoxia or compromised placental function, or both. A score is calculated on the basis of five criteria (Box 10.3).

Findings from growth scans, biophysical profile scores and cardiotocography (CTG) recordings should be considered collectively, taking into account the full clinical picture and obstetric history.

SCREENING FOR FETAL ABNORMALITY FROM MATERNAL SERUM

Neural tube defect screening

Alpha fetoprotein (AFP) is present in fetal serum and amniotic fluid by 6 weeks' gestation. Thereafter, the levels alter according to gestation. When the fetus has an open neural tube defect, AFP can escape in increased amounts, causing levels to be raised in maternal serum. A blood sample from the mother at 15–18 weeks' gestation has a detection rate of 98%. Since the AFP level varies according to gestational age, it is important to assess the gestation accurately before results can be reliably interpreted.

Down syndrome screening from maternal serum

A variety of biochemical markers in maternal serum have been used, in order to assess the risk of Down syndrome. The most common ones are:

- AFP (reduced in many affected pregnancies)
- human chorionic gonadotrophin (HCG) (which is usually raised)
- unconjugated oestriol (uE_3, which is usually low).

If all three markers are used, this is called the *triple test*. If only AFP and HCG are used, this is called the *double test*. Maternal blood is sampled at 15–18 weeks' gestation.

The levels of biochemical markers are considered in conjunction with maternal age. A combined risk is then calculated. If this risk is greater than a specified limit (often 1 in 250), the mother is considered to be in a high-risk group and is offered further diagnostic tests.

Box 10.3 Criteria used in biophysical profiling

- Fetal breathing movements
- Fetal movements
- Fetal tone
- Fetal reactivity
- Qualitative amniotic fluid volume

INVASIVE DIAGNOSTIC TESTS

If mothers are found to have an increased risk of chromosomal or genetic problems, they may wish to undergo a diagnostic procedure. The two most frequently used tests are:

- chorionic villus sampling (CVS)
- amniocentesis.

These tests provide the opportunity to examine the fetal karyotype (the number and structure of chromosomes, visible through a microscope during mitotic metaphase) or for DNA analysis for particular gene mutations, or both.

Chorionic villus sampling

CVS is the acquisition of chorionic villi (placental tissue) under continuous ultrasound guidance. This may be performed at any stage after 10 weeks of pregnancy.

Access may be achieved transcervically (until 13 weeks' gestation) or via the transabdominal route.

The main advantage of CVS is that this is the earliest way mothers can obtain definitive information about the chromosomal/genetic status of the fetus. The main disadvantage with CVS is the procedure-induced risk of miscarriage, which is 0.5–2%.

Amniocentesis

This is usually performed after 15 weeks' gestation, as early amniocentesis has a higher loss rate than early CVS. The procedure involves transabdominal insertion of a fine needle into the amniotic fluid cavity, under continuous ultrasound guidance; 15 ml of amniotic fluid are aspirated. Cytogenetic, molecular (DNA) and biochemical analyses are possible. Amniocytes are often examined. These comprise cells that have been shed from several fetal sites, including skin, lungs and renal tract. The risk of procedure-induced miscarriage is 1%.

Recent advances in cytogenetic techniques mean that mothers can obtain an initial set of results (usually for Down syndrome) and then a full culture result after 2–3 weeks. This involves the use of fluorescent in-situ hybridisation (FISH), whereby a specific probe 'paints' the chromosomes to be examined. Cells are examined to determine whether there are two or three signals for this chromosome. Two is the normal count, whereas three indicates Down syndrome.

Fetal blood sampling

The use of this technique has declined in recent years because improved molecular and cytogenetic techniques allow more diagnoses to be made from chorionic villi or amniotic fluid. However, fetal blood may be advantageous when there are ambiguous findings from placental tissue. Also, when there is Rhesus isoimmunisation, it may be necessary to determine the fetal haemoglobin. When this is low, an intrauterine transfusion may be performed. Blood can be sampled from the umbilical cord or intrahepatic umbilical vein; the latter is less risky. The loss rate also depends upon the gestation and condition of the fetus. In uncomplicated procedures after 20 weeks, the loss rate is around 1%.

CHAPTER 11

Abnormalities of Early Pregnancy

BLEEDING IN PREGNANCY

Vaginal bleeding during pregnancy is abnormal. If the woman presents with a history of bleeding in the current pregnancy, it is important to establish when it occurred. How much blood was lost, the colour of the loss and whether it was associated with any pain should be noted. If the symptoms have subsided, it is important to advise the mother to report any recurrence.

Assessment of fetal condition will depend on gestation. Ultrasound scanning can confirm viability of the pregnancy before heart sounds are audible or movements felt. In the second trimester the use of ultrasound equipment can elicit the heart sounds, and note of fetal movements may also be made.

IMPLANTATION BLEEDING

As the trophoblast erodes the endometrial epithelium and the blastocyst implants, a small vaginal blood loss may be apparent to the woman. It occurs around the time of expected menstruation and may be mistaken for a period, although lighter. It is of significance if the estimated date of delivery is to be calculated from menstrual history.

CERVICAL ECTROPION

This condition is commonly and erroneously known as a cervical erosion. High levels of oestrogen cause proliferation of columnar epithelial cells, found in the cervical canal. These occupy a wider area, including the vaginal aspect of the cervix, encroaching on the squamous epithelial cells (metaplasia). The junction between is everted into the vagina. This ectropion is a physiological response to the hormonal changes in pregnancy. As the cells are vascular it may cause intermittent blood-stained loss, or spontaneous bleeding particularly following sexual intercourse. Normally, treatment is not required in pregnancy and the ectropion will usually disappear during the puerperium.

CERVICAL POLYPS

Small, vascular pedunculated growths attached to the cervix may bleed during pregnancy. They can be visualised on speculum examination and no treatment is required during pregnancy, unless bleeding is profuse or a cervical smear suggests malignancy.

CARCINOMA OF THE CERVIX

Carcinoma of the cervix is the most frequently diagnosed cancer in pregnancy. It is a treatable condition if detected early.

Cervical intraepithelial neoplasia (CIN) is the precursor to invasive cancer of the cervix. If the condition is detected at this stage, treatment can be given and the cytology reverts to normal. The principal screening test used is the Papanicolaou smear (Pap smear).

Types

There are two main types of cervical cancer:

- squamous cell carcinoma
- adenocarcinoma.

The latter is less common.

Clinical presentation

- Bleeding is the most common symptom.
- Vaginal discharge is the next most common.

As symptoms may be mistakenly diagnosed as symptoms of pregnancy, there may be delay in diagnosis.

Investigation

- A Papanicolaou smear test will detect atypical cells on the surface of the cervix, or within the endocervix.
- When changes are detected, a repeat smear test, followed by colposcopy, is indicated.
- Biopsies can be taken to reveal the extent of the lesion.

The mother and her partner should be fully informed about any tests and treatments that are offered and when and from whom results will be available. A positive test result following a smear test will cause anxiety to the mother and her family and it is important that accurate information is available, along with supportive counselling.

Treatment

Treatment depends on the stage of the disease and gestation. Laser treatment or cryotherapy following colposcopy can be carried out on an outpatient basis and will result in the destruction of the abnormal area of cells.

Cone biopsy under general anaesthesia involves excision of cervical tissue and is both a diagnostic tool and a treatment, but it may increase the risk to the mother. The cervix is highly vascular in pregnancy and the risk of haemorrhage is high, as is the possibility of causing the mother to miscarry. Delaying treatment until the end of pregnancy is an option for women who are found to have early changes in cervical cytology.

If the changes to the cervix are advanced and diagnosis is made in the first or second trimester, the mother may have to make a choice as to whether to terminate the pregnancy in order to undergo treatment. If diagnosis is made later in pregnancy, a decision to deliver the fetus may be taken to allow the mother to commence treatment.

SPONTANEOUS MISCARRIAGE

Spontaneous miscarriage is defined as the involuntary loss of the products of conception prior to 24 weeks' gestation.

Incidence

Fifteen per cent of all confirmed pregnancies are said to result in miscarriages, the majority of which happen in the first trimester. The different outcomes of potential miscarriage (abortion) have varying signs and symptoms (Fig. 11.1 and Table 11.1).

Sequelae to early pregnancy loss

- Language should be appropriate, avoiding terms such as 'products' or 'scrape', recognising that most women will be grieving for the lost baby.
- Regardless of gestation, the parents may want to see and hold the baby. Some parents may want to see the loss when there is no body.
- Creation of memories is important for the grieving process, and midwives can assist by taking photographs of the baby for the parents, and by providing a letter or certificate to confirm the loss.
- Parents need information on how the remains will be disposed of. Under 24 weeks' gestation the baby is not registrable in the UK; it is therefore not a legal requirement for the baby to be buried or cremated but nevertheless respectful disposal is paramount. At no time should any fetal remains be included with hospital clinical waste. Parents may wish to take the remains home; burial in a garden is not precluded in this instance. If cremation is considered, then midwives should be aware that the size of the fetus may result in few ashes, if any.
- Full written consent must be given by the mother for postmortem or any other investigations involving fetal tissue. Follow-up after miscarriage is needed, with parents being given the opportunity to receive further information about their loss and be offered advice regarding future pregnancies.

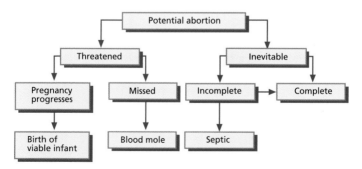

Fig. 11.1: Possible outcomes of potential miscarriage (abortion).

Table 11.1 Signs of miscarriage

Signs and symptoms	Threatened miscarriage	Inevitable miscarriage	Incomplete miscarriage	Complete miscarriage	Delayed miscarriage	Septic miscarriage
Pain	Variable	Severe/rhythmical	Severe	Diminishing/none	None	Severe/variable
Bleeding	Scanty	Heavy/clots	Heavy profuse	Minimal/none	Some spotting possible Brown loss	Variable May smell offensive
Cervical os	Closed	Open	Open	Closed	Closed	Open
Uterus (if palpable)	Soft, no tenderness	Tender, may be smaller than expected	Tender/painful	Firm, contracted	Smaller than expected	Bulky/tender/painful
Additional signs and symptoms			Tissue present in cervix Shock			

INDUCED ABORTION

Termination of pregnancy before 24 weeks' gestation is legal in the UK within the terms of current legislation.

Methods

- Abortion can be carried out in the first trimester, using vacuum aspiration, dilatation and evacuation under general anaesthetic. Medical methods using mifepristone and prostaglandin are licensed for use up to the 63rd day from the first day of a woman's last menstrual period.
- In the second trimester, medical methods are used. Extrauterine prostaglandin, accompanied by large doses of oxytocin, produces uterine contractions. The mother experiences labour pains and the process may be protracted.
- Prophylactic antibiotics may be given following termination, and for non-sensitised Rhesus negative women, anti-D immunoglobulin is recommended.

RECURRENT MISCARRIAGE

Recurrent miscarriage is defined as the loss of three or more consecutive pregnancies. The incidence of recurrent miscarriage suggests that there are significant underlying causes and the loss of the pregnancy is not chance. Factors associated with recurrent miscarriage are listed in Box 11.1. In many cases no causative factor is identified. Women should be referred to specialist clinics where a screening service is available.

CERVICAL INCOMPETENCE

Cervical incompetence describes painless dilatation of the cervix in the second or early third trimester, allowing bulging membranes through the cervical os into the vagina. Miscarriage or preterm birth may occur if the membranes rupture. Cervical incompetence recurs in subsequent pregnancies.

Causes

- Trauma to the cervix during dilatation and curettage or induced abortion.
- Cone biopsy or congenital weakness of the cervix.

Box 11.1 Some factors associated with recurrent miscarriage

- Genetic causes
- Immunological factors
- Hypersecretion of LH
- Infection
- Structural anomalies

Treatment

Treatment for subsequent pregnancies by cervical cerclage remains controversial. If undertaken, it is carried out after the risk of early miscarriage is thought to be past. At 14 weeks' gestation a non-absorbable suture may be inserted at the level of the internal os. This remains in situ until 38 weeks or the onset of labour, when it is removed.

The use of the term 'cervical incompetence' is now questioned because of the negative context it engenders.

ECTOPIC PREGNANCY

An ectopic pregnancy is one where implantation occurs at a site other than the uterine cavity. Sites can include:

- the uterine tube
- an ovary
- the cervix
- the abdomen.

Women require prompt, appropriate treatment for this life-threatening condition. Midwives need to consider the possibility of ectopic pregnancy being responsible for unexplained abdominal pain and bleeding in early pregnancy.

Risk factors for ectopic pregnancy

Any of the alterations of the normal function of the uterine tube in transporting the gametes listed in Box 11.2 contributes to the risk of ectopic pregnancy.

Clinical presentation (Box 11.3)

Tubal pregnancy rarely remains asymptomatic beyond 8 weeks.

- Pelvic pain can be severe.
- Acute symptoms are the result of tubal rupture and relate to the degree of haemorrhage there has been.
- Ultrasound enables an accurate diagnosis of tubal pregnancy, making management more proactive.

Box 11.2 Risk factors for ectopic pregnancy

- Previous ectopic pregnancy
- Previous surgery on the uterine tube
- Exposure to diethylstilboestrol in utero
- Congenital abnormalities of the tube
- Previous infection including chlamydia, gonorrhoea and pelvic inflammatory disease
- Use of intrauterine contraceptive devices
- Assisted reproductive techniques

Box 11.3 Signs of ectopic pregnancy

Typical signs
- Localised/abdominal pain
- Amenorrhoea
- Vaginal bleeding or spotting

Atypical signs
- Shoulder pain
- Abdominal distension
- Nausea, vomiting
- Dizziness, fainting

- Vaginal ultrasound, combined with the use of sensitive blood and urine tests which detect the presence of human chorionic gonadotrophin (HCG), helps to ensure diagnosis is made earlier.
- If the tube ruptures, shock may ensue; therefore resuscitation, followed by laparotomy, is needed.
- The mother should be offered follow-up support and information regarding subsequent pregnancies.

GESTATIONAL TROPHOBLASTIC DISEASE

Gestational trophoblastic disease is a general term covering:
- hydatidiform mole (benign)
- choriocarcinoma (malignant).

HYDATIDIFORM MOLE

Hydatidiform mole applies to a gross malformation of the trophoblast in which the chorionic villi proliferate and become avascular. They are found in the cavity of the uterus and, very rarely, within the uterine tube. As this condition can lead to the development of cancer, accurate diagnosis, treatment and follow-up are essential. Two forms of mole have been identified:
- complete hydatidiform mole
- partial mole.

The complete form carries an increased risk of choriocarcinoma.

Clinical presentation

See Box 11.4. Diagnosis is confirmed by ultrasound scan and serum HCG levels.

Treatment

The aim of treatment is to remove all trophoblast tissue. In some cases the hydatidiform mole aborts spontaneously. Where this does not occur, vacuum aspiration or dilatation and curettage is necessary. Spontaneous expulsion of the mole carries less risk of malignant change.

Box 11.4 Clinical presentation of hydatidiform mole

- Exaggerated signs of pregnancy, appearing by 6–8 weeks due to high levels of HCG
- Bleeding or a blood-stained vaginal discharge after a period of amenorrhoea
- Ruptured vesicles, resulting in a light pink or brown vaginal discharge, or detached vesicles, which may be passed vaginally
- Anaemia as a result of the gradual loss of blood
- Early-onset pre-eclampsia
- On examination, uterine size exceeding that expected for gestation; on palpation, a uterus that feels 'doughy' or elastic

All women who have been treated for hydatidiform mole in the UK are recorded on a central register. Women confirmed as having a complete mole require follow-up over a 2-year period. Pregnancy should be avoided during the follow-up period. Intrauterine contraceptive devices are contraindicated and hormonal methods of contraception should not be used until levels of HCG have returned to normal.

ADMINISTRATION OF ANTI-D IMMUNOGLOBULIN IN EARLY PREGNANCY

Significant fetomaternal haemorrhage can occur following early pregnancy loss; therefore anti-D immunoglobulin should be administered to reduce the risk of isoimmunisation in Rhesus negative women.

RETROVERSION OF THE UTERUS

When the long axis of the uterus is directed backwards during pregnancy, the uterus is said to be retroverted. In most cases it corrects spontaneously, the uterus rising out of the pelvis into the abdomen as pregnancy progresses, and there are no further problems. If the retroverted uterus fails to rise out of the pelvic cavity by the 14th week, it is said to be incarcerated.

FIBROIDS (LEIOMYOMAS)

These are firm, benign tumours of muscular and fibrous tissue, ranging in size from very small to very large.

Effect of pregnancy on fibroids

Fibroids do not significantly increase in size during pregnancy; however, they may become more vascular and oedematous, making them softer and more difficult to detect on palpation.

Effect of fibroids on pregnancy

- Early pregnancy loss is associated with submucosal fibroids. Outcome of pregnancy is dependent on the position of the fibroid.
- Lesser effects include mild abdominal pain.

- Fibroids located in the lower segment or on the cervix can prevent descent of the fetal head, causing malpresentation and obstructed labour and resulting in the need for caesarean section.
- Severe postpartum haemorrhage may be caused if the fibroids prevent the complete separation of the placenta or contraction of the uterus. In anticipation of this, blood should be available for urgent cross-matching.

Removal of fibroids during caesarean section should be avoided because of the risk of profuse haemorrhage.

Red degeneration of fibroids

Degeneration of a fibroid occurs if a rapidly growing fibroid exceeds the available blood supply.

HYPEREMESIS GRAVIDARUM

Excessive nausea and vomiting that start between 4 and 10 weeks' gestation, resolve before 20 weeks, and require intervention are known as hyperemesis gravidarum. The aetiology of hyperemesis is uncertain, with multifactorial causes such as endocrine, gastrointestinal and psychological factors proposed. Rising levels of oestrogen and HCG appear to be significant.

Diagnosis is made where there is a history of persistent, severe nausea and vomiting in early pregnancy; causes of vomiting not due to pregnancy need to be excluded. A mother suspected of suffering from hyperemesis presents as being unable to retain food or fluids. She may have lost weight, and be distressed and debilitated by her symptoms. The impact of nausea and vomiting on the woman and her daily life should not be underestimated. The woman requires admission to hospital for assessment and for management of symptoms.

Clinical presentation

- A history of the frequency and severity of the bouts of vomiting is taken.
- The mother's appearance is noted, including any dryness or inelasticity of the skin. In severe cases jaundice may be apparent.
- Additional signs of dehydration, such as rapid pulse, low blood pressure and dry furred tongue, may be seen.
- The mother's breath may smell of acetone, a sign of ketosis.
- Elevated haematocrit, alterations in electrolyte levels and ketonuria are associated with dehydration.

Management

- Hypovolaemia and electrolyte imbalance are corrected by intravenous infusion.
- Vitamin supplements can be given parenterally, particularly where hyperemesis has been prolonged.
- Initially nothing is given by mouth, to allow time for the vomiting to be controlled.
- Fluids and diet are gradually reintroduced as the woman's condition improves, but this is closely monitored.
- Antiemetics may be prescribed.

CHAPTER 12

Problems of Pregnancy

ABDOMINAL PAIN IN PREGNANCY

Abdominal pain is a common complaint in pregnancy. It is probably suffered by all women at some stage, and therefore presents a problem for the midwife of how to distinguish between:

- the physiologically normal (e.g. mild indigestion or muscle stretching)
- the pathological but not dangerous (e.g. degeneration of a fibroid)
- the dangerously pathological requiring immediate referral to the appropriate medical practitioner for urgent treatment (e.g. ectopic pregnancy or appendicitis).

The midwife should take a detailed history and perform a physical examination in order to reach a decision about whether to refer the woman. Treatment will depend on the cause (Box 12.1) and the maternal and fetal conditions.

UTERINE FIBROID DEGENERATION

Uterine fibroid degeneration may cause recurrent acute pain during pregnancy and is due to a diminished blood supply that may cause central core necrosis of a fibroid or fibroids.

Management
- Rest and analgesia are required.
- Be aware that enlargement of the fibroid may occasionally impede the progress of labour and lead to rupture of the uterus.

SEVERE UTERINE TORSION

Severe uterine torsion refers to rotation of the uterus by more than 90°, which may cause pain in the latter half of pregnancy.

Management
- Bed rest is necessary, altering the maternal position to correct the torsion spontaneously
- Analgesia is required.
- In severe cases a laparotomy will need to be performed in order for a clear diagnosis to be made.
- Delivery by caesarean section may be performed, either preceded or followed by manipulation of the uterus.

Box 12.1 Causes of abdominal pain in pregnancy

Pregnancy-specific causes

Physiological

- Heartburn, excessive vomiting, constipation
- Round ligament pain
- Severe uterine torsion
- Braxton Hicks contractions
- Miscellaneous discomfort in late pregnancy

Pathological

- Ectopic pregnancy
- Miscarriage
- Uterine fibroids
- Placental abruption
- Preterm labour
- Severe pre-eclampsia
- Uterine rupture

Incidental causes (consider domestic abuse)

Common pathology

- Appendicitis
- Intestinal obstruction
- Cholecystitis
- Inflammatory bowel disease
- Peptic ulcer
- Renal disease
- Ovarian pathology, e.g. torsion
- Acute pancreatitis
- Urinary tract infection
- Malaria
- Tuberculosis (may be associated with HIV infection)

Rare pathology

- Rectus haematoma
- Sickle-cell crisis
- Porphyria
- Arteriovenous haemorrhage
- Malignant disease

SYMPHYSIS PUBIS DYSFUNCTION (PELVIC GIRDLE PAIN [PGP])

This refers to abnormal relaxation of ligaments, causing increased mobility of the pubic joint. The woman may complain of pain at any time from the 28th week of pregnancy.

Management
- Reduce non-essential weight-bearing activities and avoid straddle movements that abduct the hips, e.g. squatting.
- A supportive panty girdle or 'tubigrip' and comfortable shoes may help when the woman is up and about.
- Refer to an obstetric physiotherapist for advice and treatment.
- In severe cases, bed rest on a firm mattress may be necessary.
- Postnatal physiotherapy will aid the strengthening and stabilisation of the joint.

ANTEPARTUM HAEMORRHAGE (APH)

Antepartum haemorrhage is bleeding from the genital tract after the 24th week of gestation and before the onset of labour.

Effect on the fetus
Fetal mortality and morbidity are increased as a result of severe vaginal bleeding in pregnancy. Stillbirth or neonatal death may occur. Premature placental separation and consequent hypoxia may result in severe neurological damage in the baby.

Effect on the mother
If bleeding is severe, it may be accompanied by shock and disseminated intravascular coagulation (DIC). The mother may die or be left with permanent ill health.

Types of APH (Table 12.1)
- Bleeding from local lesions of the genital tract (*incidental causes*).
- Placental separation due to *placenta praevia* or *placental abruption*.

INITIAL APPRAISAL OF A WOMAN WITH APH

APH is unpredictable and the woman's condition can deteriorate rapidly at any time. A rapid decision about the urgency of need for a medical or paramedic presence, or both, must be made, often at the same time as observing and talking to the woman and her partner.

Assessment of physical condition
Maternal condition
- Take a history from the woman.
- Observe pulse rate, respiratory rate, blood pressure and temperature.
- Look for any pallor or breathlessness.
- Assess the amount of blood lost.
- Perform a gentle abdominal examination, observing for signs that the woman is going into labour.
- *On no account must any vaginal or rectal examination be done; nor may an enema or suppository be given to a woman suffering from an APH.*

Table 12.1 Causes of bleeding in late pregnancy

Cause	Incidence (%)
Placenta praevia	31.0
Placental abruption	22.0
'Unclassified bleeding', e.g.:	47.0
Marginal	
Show	
Cervicitis	
Trauma	
Vulvovaginal varicosities	
Genital tumours	
Genital infections	
Haematuria	
Vasa praevia	
Other	

Fetal condition

- The mother should be asked if the baby has been moving as much as normal.
- Attempt to auscultate the fetal heart; ultrasound apparatus may be used in order to obtain information.

Factors to aid differential diagnosis

The location of the placenta is perhaps the most critical piece of information that will be needed in order to make a correct diagnosis; initially, the midwife may not have this fact at her disposal. However, if she is able to elicit the information listed in Box 12.2 from her observations and from talking to the woman and her partner, then this will help her to arrive at a provisional diagnosis.

Supportive treatment

- Provide emotional reassurance.
- Give rapid fluid replacement (warmed) with a plasma expander, and later with whole blood if necessary.
- Give analgesia.
- If at home, arrange transfer to hospital.
- Subsequent management depends on the definite diagnosis.

PLACENTA PRAEVIA

In this condition the placenta is partially or wholly implanted in the lower uterine segment on either the anterior or posterior wall.

Box 12.2 Diagnosis of antepartum haemorrhage

Pain
- Did the pain precede bleeding and is it continuous or intermittent?

Onset of bleeding
- Was this associated with any event such as abdominal trauma or sex?

Amount of visible blood loss
- Is there any reason to suspect that some blood has been retained in utero?

Colour of the blood
- Is it bright red or darker in colour?

Degree of shock
- Is this commensurate with the amount of blood visible or more severe?

Consistency of the abdomen
- Is it soft or tense and board-like?

Tenderness of the abdomen
- Does the mother tense on abdominal palpation?

Lie, presentation and engagement
- Are any of these abnormal when account is taken of parity and gestation?

Audibility of the fetal heart
- Is the fetal heart heard?

Ultrasound scan
- Does a scan suggest that the placenta is in the lower uterine segment?

The lower uterine segment grows and stretches progressively after the 12th week of pregnancy. In later weeks this may cause the placenta to separate and severe bleeding can occur.

Degrees of placenta praevia

See Box 12.3 and Figs 12.1–12.8.

Box 12.3 Degrees of placenta praevia

Type 1 placenta praevia
- The majority of the placenta is in the upper uterine segment
- Blood loss is usually mild and the mother and fetus remain in good condition
- Vaginal birth is possible

Type 2 placenta praevia
- The placenta is partially located in the lower segment near the internal cervical os
- Blood loss is usually moderate, although the conditions of the mother and fetus can vary
- Vaginal birth is possible, particularly if the placenta is anterior

Box 12.3 Degrees of placenta praevia—cont'd

Type 3 placenta praevia
- The placenta is located over the internal cervical os but not centrally
- Bleeding is likely to be severe
- Vaginal birth is inappropriate

Type 4 placenta praevia
- The placenta is located centrally over the internal cervical os
- Torrential haemorrhage is very likely
- Caesarean section is essential

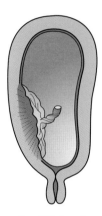

Fig. 12.1: Type 1.

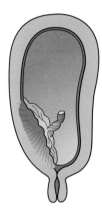

Fig. 12.2: Type 2.

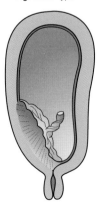

Fig. 12.3: Type 3.

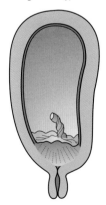

Fig. 12.4: Type 4.

Fig. 12.1–12.4: Types of placenta praevia.

Fig. 12.5: Type 1.

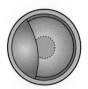

Fig. 12.6: Type 2.

Fig. 12.7: Type 3.

Fig. 12.8: Type 4.

Fig. 12.5–12.8: Relation of placenta praevia to cervical os.

Indications of placenta praevia

Bleeding from the vagina is the only sign and it is painless. The uterus is not tender or tense. The presence of placenta praevia should be considered when:

- the fetal head is not engaged in a primigravida (after 36 weeks)
- there is a malpresentation, especially breech
- the lie is oblique or transverse
- the lie is unstable, usually in a multigravida.

Localisation of the placenta using ultrasonic scanning will confirm the existence of placenta praevia and establish its degree.

Management of placenta praevia

The management of placenta praevia depends on:

- the amount of bleeding
- the condition of mother and fetus
- the location of the placenta
- the stage of the pregnancy.

PLACENTAL ABRUPTION

Premature separation of a normally situated placenta occurring after the 24th week of pregnancy is referred to as *placental abruption*. The aetiology is not always clear; some predisposing factors are listed in Box 12.4.

Blood loss may be:

- revealed
- concealed
- mixed.

Box 12.4 Predisposing factors in placental abruption

- Pregnancy-induced hypertension
- A sudden reduction in uterine size: e.g. when the membranes rupture or after the birth of a first twin
- Direct trauma to the abdomen
- High parity
- Previous caesarean section
- Cigarette smoking

Management of different degrees of placental abruption

Mild separation of the placenta

In this case the placental separation and the haemorrhage are slight. Mother and fetus are in a stable condition. There is no indication of maternal shock and the fetus is alive with normal heart sounds. The consistency of the uterus is normal and there is no tenderness on abdominal palpation.

- An ultrasound scan can determine the placental location and identify any degree of concealed bleeding.
- Fetal condition should be assessed while bleeding persists by frequent or continuous monitoring of the fetal heart rate. Subsequently, cardiotocography (CTG) should be carried out once or twice daily.
- If the woman is not in labour and the gestation is less than 37 weeks, she may be cared for in an antenatal ward for a few days. She may then go home if there is no further bleeding and the placenta has been found to be in the upper uterine segment.
- Women who have passed the 37th week of pregnancy may be offered induction of labour, especially if there has been more than one episode of mild bleeding.
- Further heavy bleeding or evidence of fetal distress may indicate that a caesarean section is necessary.

Moderate separation of the placenta

This describes placental separation of about one-quarter. A considerable amount of blood may be lost, some of which will escape from the vagina and some of which will be retained as a retroplacental clot or an extravasation into the uterine muscle. The mother will be shocked, with a raised pulse rate and a lowered blood pressure. There will be a degree of uterine tenderness and abdominal guarding. The fetus may be alive, although hypoxic; intrauterine death is also a possibility.

The immediate aims of care are to reduce shock and to replace blood loss:

- Fluid replacement should be monitored with the aid of a central venous pressure line.
- The fetal condition should be assessed with continuous CTG if the fetus is alive, in which case immediate caesarean section may be indicated once the woman's condition is stabilised.

If the fetus is in good condition or has already died, vaginal birth may be contemplated. Such a birth is advantageous because it enables the uterus to contract and control the bleeding. The spontaneous onset of labour frequently accompanies moderately severe placental abruption, but if it does not, then amniotomy is usually sufficient to induce labour. Oxytocin may be used with great care, if necessary. Delivery is often quite sudden after a short labour. The use of drugs to attempt to stop labour is usually inappropriate.

Severe separation of the placenta

This is an acute obstetric emergency; at least two-thirds of the placenta has become detached and 2000 ml of blood or more are lost from the circulation. Most or all of the blood can be concealed behind the placenta. The woman will be severely shocked, perhaps to a degree far beyond what might be expected from the amount of visible blood loss. The blood pressure will be lowered; the reading may lie within the normal range owing to a preceding hypertension. The fetus will almost certainly be dead. The woman will have very severe abdominal pain with excruciating tenderness; the uterus has a board-like consistency. Features associated with severe haemorrhage are:

- coagulation defects
- renal failure
- pituitary failure.

Treatment is the same as for moderate haemorrhage.

- Whole blood should be transfused rapidly and subsequent amounts calculated in accordance with the woman's central venous pressure.
- Labour may begin spontaneously in advance of amniotomy and the midwife should be alert for signs of uterine contraction causing periodic intensifying of the abdominal pain.
- However, if bleeding continues or a compromised fetal heart rate is present, caesarean section may be required as soon as the woman's condition has been adequately stabilised.
- The woman requires constant explanation and psychological support, despite the fact that, because of her shocked condition, she may not be fully conscious.
- Pain relief must also be considered.
- The woman's partner will also be very concerned, and should not be forgotten in the rush to stabilise the woman's condition.

Complications

See Box 12.5.

Box 12.5 Complications of placental abruption

- Disseminated intravascular coagulation
- Postpartum haemorrhage
- Renal failure
- Pituitary necrosis

BLOOD COAGULATION FAILURE

DISSEMINATED INTRAVASCULAR COAGULATION (DIC)

This is a situation of inappropriate coagulation within the blood vessels, which leads to the consumption of clotting factors. As a result, clotting fails to occur at the bleeding site. DIC is rare when the fetus is alive and it usually starts to resolve when the baby is born. DIC is never a primary disease – it always occurs as a response to another disease process.

Events that trigger DIC include:

- placental abruption
- intrauterine fetal death, including delayed miscarriage
- amniotic fluid embolism
- intrauterine infection, including septic abortion
- pre-eclampsia and eclampsia.

Management

The midwife should be alert for signs that clotting is abnormal, and the assessment of the nature of the clot should be part of her routine observation during the third stage of labour. Oozing from a venepuncture site or bleeding from the mucous membrane of the mother's mouth and nose must be noted and reported. Blood tests should include full blood count and blood grouping, clotting studies and the levels of platelets, fibrinogen and fibrin degradation products (FDPs).

Treatment involves the replacement of blood cells and clotting factors in order to restore equilibrium. This is usually done by the administration of fresh frozen plasma and platelet concentrates. Banked red cells will be transfused subsequently.

HEPATIC DISORDERS AND JAUNDICE IN PREGNANCY

Some liver disorders are specific to pregnant women, and some pre-existing or coexisting disorders may complicate the pregnancy (Box 12.6).

Box 12.6 Hepatic disorders of pregnancy

Specific to pregnancy

- Intrahepatic cholestasis of pregnancy
- Acute fatty liver in pregnancy
- Pre-eclampsia and eclampsia (see Ch.14)
- Severe hyperemesis gravidarum (see Ch. 11)

Pre-existing or coexisting in pregnancy

- Gall bladder disease
- Hepatitis

INTRAHEPATIC CHOLESTASIS OF PREGNANCY (ICP)

This is an idiopathic condition that begins in pregnancy, usually in the third trimester but occasionally as early as the first trimester. It resolves spontaneously following birth, but has a 60–80% recurrence rate in subsequent pregnancies. It is not a life-threatening condition for the mother, but she is at increased risk of preterm labour, fetal compromise and meconium staining and her stillbirth risk is increased by 15% unless there is active management of her pregnancy.

Clinical presentation
- There is pruritus at night.
- Fifty per cent of women affected will develop mild jaundice.
- Fever, abdominal discomfort and nausea and vomiting may occur.
- Urine may be darker and stools paler than usual.

Investigation
- Blood tests for an increase in bile acids, serum alkaline phosphatase, bilirubin and transaminases.
- Differential diagnosis: hepatic viral studies, an ultrasound scan of the hepatobiliary tract, an autoantibody screen.

Management
- Apply local antipruritic agents.
- Give vitamin K supplements for the mother.
- Monitor fetal wellbeing.
- Consider elective delivery when the fetus is mature, or earlier if the fetal condition appears to be compromised by the intrauterine environment.
- Give sensitive psychological care.
- Monitor the mother if she uses oral contraception in the future.

GALL BLADDER DISEASE

Pregnancy appears to increase the likelihood of gallstone formation but not the risk of developing acute cholecystitis.

Diagnosis
- Previous history.
- An ultrasound scan of the hepatobiliary tract.

Treatment
- Provide symptomatic relief of biliary colic by analgesia, hydration, nasogastric suction and antibiotics.
- Surgery should be avoided, if possible.

VIRAL HEPATITIS (B)

Viral hepatitis is the most common cause of jaundice in pregnancy. Acute infection affects approximately 1 in 1000 pregnancies and has an incubation period of 1–6 months.

Clinical presentation

- Nausea, vomiting, anorexia.
- Pain over the liver.
- Mild diarrhoea.
- Jaundice lasting several weeks.
- Malaise.

The main means of spread is via blood, blood products and sexual activity. The virus can also be transmitted across the placenta. In healthy adults 90% of cases resolve completely within 6 months. In the remaining 10%, hepatitis B surface antigen (HBsAg) remains in the serum and the woman is considered to be a chronic carrier.

Diagnosis

- The woman's history of her symptoms and lifestyle.
- Serological studies.

Management

- Provide relief of symptoms.
- Implement infection control measures if the woman is considered to be infectious.
- Provide information about the disease, nutrition and sexual health.
- Monitor liver function/fetal wellbeing.
- Assess fetal wellbeing.
- Offer immunisation to household contacts once their HBsAg seronegativity is established.
- Sexual partners should be traced and offered testing and vaccination.
- Postnatally, the mother should be encouraged to accept vaccination for the baby.
- Advice about breastfeeding remains controversial.

SKIN DISORDERS

Many women suffer from physiological pruritus in pregnancy, especially over the abdomen.

Management

- Give reassurance and apply calamine lotion over the affected area.
- If pruritus is generalised, exclude other causes, e.g. intrahepatic cholestasis.

DISORDERS OF THE AMNIOTIC FLUID

There are two chief abnormalities of amniotic fluid: polyhydramnios (or hydramnios) and oligohydramnios.

POLYHYDRAMNIOS

The amount of liquor present in a pregnancy is estimated by measuring 'pools' of liquor around the fetus with ultrasound scanning. The single deepest pool is measured to calculate the amniotic fluid volume (AFV). However, where possible, a more accurate diagnosis may be gained by measuring the liquor in each of four quadrants around the fetus in order to establish an amniotic fluid index (AFI).

Polyhydramnios is said to be present when the AFV exceeds 8 cm, or the calculated AFI is more than 24 cm.

Causes
These include:
- oesophageal atresia
- open neural tube defect, anencephaly
- multiple pregnancy, especially in the case of monozygotic twins
- maternal diabetes mellitus
- rarely, an association with Rhesus isoimmunisation
- chorioangioma, a rare tumour of the placenta
- in many cases, an unknown cause.

Types
Chronic polyhydramnios
This is gradual in onset, usually starting from about the 30th week of pregnancy. It is the most common type.

Acute polyhydramnios
This is very rare. It usually occurs at about 20 weeks and comes on very suddenly. The uterus reaches the xiphisternum in about 3 or 4 days. It is frequently associated with monozygotic twins or severe fetal abnormality.

Diagnosis
The mother may complain of breathlessness and discomfort. If the polyhydramnios is acute in onset, she may have severe abdominal pain. The condition may cause exacerbation of symptoms associated with pregnancy, such as indigestion, heartburn and constipation. Oedema and varicosities of the vulva and lower limbs may be present.

Abdominal examination
- On inspection the uterus is larger than expected for the period of gestation and is globular in shape. The abdominal skin appears stretched and shiny with marked striae gravidarum and obvious superficial blood vessels.
- On palpation the uterus feels tense and it is difficult to feel the fetal parts, but the fetus may be balloted between the two hands. A fluid thrill may be elicited by placing a hand on one side of the abdomen and tapping the other side with the fingers.
- Ultrasonic scanning is used to confirm the diagnosis of polyhydramnios and may also reveal a multiple pregnancy or fetal abnormality.

Complications
These include:
- maternal ureteric obstruction
- increased fetal mobility leading to unstable lie and malpresentation

- cord presentation and prolapse
- prelabour (and often preterm) rupture of the membranes
- placental abruption when the membranes rupture
- preterm labour
- increased incidence of caesarean section
- postpartum haemorrhage
- raised perinatal mortality rate.

Management

Care will depend on the condition of the woman and fetus, the cause and degree of the polyhydramnios and the stage of pregnancy. The presence of fetal abnormality will be taken into consideration in choosing the mode and timing of delivery. If gross abnormality is present, labour may be induced; if the fetus is suffering from an operable condition such as oesophageal atresia, it may be appropriate to arrange transfer to a neonatal surgical unit.

Mild asymptomatic polyhydramnios is managed expectantly.

For a woman with symptomatic polyhydramnios:

- An upright position will help to relieve any dyspnoea and she may be given antacids to relieve heartburn and nausea.
- If the discomfort from the swollen abdomen is severe, then therapeutic amniocentesis, or amnioreduction, may be considered. However, this is not without risk, as infection may be introduced or the onset of labour provoked. No more than 500 ml should be withdrawn at any one time. It is at best a temporary relief as the fluid will rapidly accumulate again and the procedure may need to be repeated. Acute polyhydramnios managed by amnioreduction has a poor prognosis for the baby.
- Labour may need to be induced in late pregnancy if the woman's symptoms become worse.
- The lie must be corrected if it is not longitudinal and the membranes will be ruptured cautiously, allowing the amniotic fluid to drain out slowly in order to avoid altering the lie and to prevent cord prolapse.
- Placental abruption is also a hazard if the uterus suddenly diminishes in size.
- Labour is usually normal but the midwife should be prepared for the possibility of postpartum haemorrhage. The baby should be carefully examined for abnormalities and the patency of the oesophagus ascertained by passing a nasogastric tube.

OLIGOHYDRAMNIOS

Oligohydramnios is an abnormally small amount of amniotic fluid. At term it may be 300–500 ml but amounts vary and it can be even less. When diagnosed in the first half of pregnancy the condition is often found to be associated with renal agenesis (absence of kidneys) or Potter syndrome, in which the baby also has pulmonary hypoplasia. When diagnosed at any time in pregnancy before 37 weeks, it may be due to fetal abnormality or to preterm premature rupture of the membranes where the amniotic fluid fails to reaccumulate. The lack of amniotic fluid reduces the intrauterine space and over time will cause compression deformities. The baby has a squashed-looking face, flattening of the nose, micrognathia and talipes. The skin is dry and leathery in appearance. Oligohydramnios sometimes occurs in the post-term pregnancy.

Diagnosis
- On inspection, the uterus may appear smaller than expected for the period of gestation.
- The mother who has had a previous normal pregnancy may have noticed a reduction in fetal movements.
- When the abdomen is palpated, the uterus is small and compact and fetal parts are easily felt.
- Ultrasonic scanning will enable differentiation of oligohydramnios from intrauterine growth restriction. Renal abnormality may be visible on the scan.

Management
If the ultrasound scan demonstrates renal agenesis, the baby will not survive. Liquor volume will also be estimated from the ultrasound scan, and if renal agenesis is not present, then further investigations will include careful questioning of the woman to check the possibility of preterm rupture of the membranes. Placental function tests will also be performed.

- Where fetal anomaly is not considered to be lethal, or the cause of the oligohydramnios is not known, prophylactic amnioinfusion with normal saline, Ringer's lactate or 5% glucose may be performed in order to prevent compression deformities and hypoplastic lung disease, and prolong the pregnancy.
- Labour may occur spontaneously or be induced because of the possibility of placental insufficiency.
- Epidural analgesia may be indicated because uterine contractions are often unusually painful.
- Continuous fetal heart rate monitoring is desirable.

PRETERM PRELABOUR RUPTURE OF THE MEMBRANES (PPROM)

This condition occurs before 37 completed weeks of gestation where rupture of the fetal membranes takes place without the onset of spontaneous uterine activity resulting in cervical dilatation.

Risks of PPROM
See Box 12.7.

Management
If PPROM is suspected, the woman will be admitted to the labour suite. A careful history is taken and rupture of the membranes confirmed by a sterile

Box 12.7 Some risks involved in preterm prelabour rupture of the membranes (PPROM)

- Labour, which may result in a preterm birth
- Chorioamnionitis, which may be followed by fetal and maternal systemic infection if not treated promptly
- Oligohydramnios if prolonged PPROM occurs
- Psychosocial problems resulting from uncertain fetal and neonatal outcome and long-term hospitalisation
- Cord prolapse
- Malpresentation associated with prematurity
- Primary antepartum haemorrhage

speculum examination of any pooling of liquor in the posterior fornix of the vagina. A fetal fibronectin immunoenzyme test may be used to confirm rupture of the membranes.

Digital vaginal examination should be avoided to reduce the risk of introducing infection. Observations must also be made of the fetal condition from the fetal heart rate (an infected fetus may have a tachycardia) and maternal infection screen, temperature and pulse, uterine tenderness and any purulent or offensively smelling vaginal discharge. A decision on future management will then be made.

If the woman has a gestation of less than 32 weeks, the fetus appears to be uncompromised, and APH and labour have been excluded, she will be managed expectantly:

- Admit to hospital.
- Offer frequent ultrasound scans to check the growth of the fetus and the extent and complications of any oligohydramnios.
- Administer corticosteroids.
- If labour intervenes, consider tocolytic drugs to prolong the pregnancy.
- Treat known vaginal infection with antibiotics. Prophylactic antibiotics may be offered to women without symptoms of infection.

If the woman is more than 32 weeks pregnant, the fetus appears to be compromised and APH or intervening labour is suspected or confirmed, active management will ensue.

MALIGNANT DISEASE IN PREGNANCY

If cancer is discovered before pregnancy is embarked upon, it should be treated and followed up before pregnancy is attempted. Once successfully treated, and as long as the reproductive organs are not damaged, pregnancy is rarely contraindicated for medical reasons. However, cancer discovered during pregnancy leads to a host of management dilemmas. The options involve balancing the effects of the treatment, the disease and delivery on both the mother and her fetus.

OBESITY OR FAILURE TO GAIN WEIGHT IN PREGNANCY

Although evidence exists to refute strongly the value of routine weighing of pregnant women in predicting various perinatal outcomes, surprisingly little is known about optimal weight gain and the effects of large and low weight gain in pregnancy.

A woman who starts pregnancy while obese, or puts on an excessive amount of weight during pregnancy, appears to be:

- at greater risk of hypertensive disturbances, including pregnancy-induced hypertension, gestational diabetes, urinary tract infection, uncertain fetal position, postpartum haemorrhage and thrombophlebitis
- more likely to be delivered by caesarean section
- more likely to give birth to a baby who is either small or large for gestational age
- more prone to wound infection following operative delivery.

Obesity may also be associated with malnourishment from essential nutrient deficiency.

Ideally, all women should be given the opportunity to discuss diet, as well as other general lifestyle factors, from as early on in their pregnancy as possible, and at regular intervals thereafter. Referral to a dietitian may be helpful.

Blood pressure measurements should always be taken accurately with a correctly sized cuff, and screening carried out for gestational diabetes and urinary tract infection. Routine weighing is rarely of any practical benefit, and may only reduce a woman's self-esteem and make her dread her antenatal appointments. The midwife should also bear in mind that obesity can be a symptom of another disease.

Conversely, the midwife may observe that a woman appears to be thin during her pregnancy and not laying down healthy fat stores. Detailed discussion should attempt to elicit the quality and quantity of the woman's diet and her weight pattern over previous years.

Where a woman is suffering from nutritional deprivation she is at greater risk of:

- anaemia
- preterm birth
- intrauterine growth restriction and its sequelae, including birth asphyxia and perinatal death.

CHAPTER 13

Common Medical Disorders Associated with Pregnancy

CARDIAC DISEASE

In most pregnancies, heart disease is diagnosed before pregnancy. There is, however, a small but significant group of women who will present at an antenatal clinic with an undiagnosed heart condition. Cardiac disease takes a variety of forms. Those more likely to be seen in pregnancy are:

- rheumatic heart disease
- congenital heart disease.

The most common congenital heart defects found in pregnancy are shown in Box 13.1. Some acquired heart conditions are listed in Box 13.2.

CHANGES IN CARDIOVASCULAR DYNAMICS DURING PREGNANCY

In normal pregnancy the haemodynamic profile alters in order to meet the increasing demands of the growing fetoplacental unit. Although this increases the workload of the heart quite significantly, normal, healthy pregnant women are able to adjust to these physiological changes easily. In women with coexisting heart disease, however, the added workload can precipitate complications.

- The haemodynamic changes commence early in pregnancy and gradually reach their maximum effect between 28 and 32 weeks.
- During labour there is a significant increase in cardiac output as a result of uterine contractions.
- In the 12–24 hours following birth there is further alteration with the shift of blood (approximately 1 litre) from the uterine to the systemic circulation.

Diagnosis

The recognition of heart disease in pregnancy may be difficult, as many of the symptoms of normal pregnancy resemble those of heart disease. The signs and symptoms of cardiac compromise are listed in Box 13.3.

Box 13.1 Common congenital heart defects in pregnancy

- Atrial septal defect (ASD)
- Ventricular septal defect (VSD)
- Patent ductus arteriosus (PDA)
- Pulmonary stenosis
- Aortic stenosis
- Tetralogy of Fallot
- Eisenmenger syndrome
- Marfan syndrome

Box 13.2 Some acquired heart conditions

- Aortic dissection (acute)
- Rheumatic heart disease
- Ischaemic heart disease (IHD)
- Endocarditis
- Peripartum cardiomyopathy

Box 13.3 Common signs and symptoms of cardiac compromise in pregnancy

- Fatigue
- Shortness of breath (dyspnoea)
- Difficulty in breathing unless upright (orthopnoea)
- Palpitations
- Bounding/collapsing pulse
- Chest pain
- Development of peripheral oedema
- Distended jugular veins
- Progressive limitation of physical activity

Laboratory tests can assist with the diagnosis of cardiac disease and determine the type of lesion, together with giving an assessment of current functional capacity. Tests include:

- full blood count (FBC)
- electrocardiography (ECG)
- chest radiograph to assess cardiac size and outline, pulmonary vasculature and lung fields
- clotting studies
- echocardiography.

Risks to mother and fetus

The majority of pregnancies complicated by maternal heart disease can be expected to have a favourable outcome for both mother and fetus. The risk for morbidity and mortality depends on:

- the nature of the cardiac lesion
- its effect on the functional capacity of the heart
- the development of pregnancy-related complications such as hypertensive disorders of pregnancy, infection, thrombosis and haemorrhage.

PRECONCEPTION CARE

Women with known heart disease should seek advice from a cardiologist and an obstetrician before becoming pregnant, so that the risks of the condition can be discussed.

ANTENATAL CARE

The symptoms of normal pregnancy, together with the haemodynamic changes, can mimic the signs and symptoms of heart disease. Maternal investigations should be carried out prior to and at the onset of pregnancy in order to gain baseline referral points.

Management

All pregnant women with heart disease should be managed in obstetric units via a multidisciplinary approach involving midwives, obstetricians, cardiologists and anaesthetists. The aim is to maintain a steady haemodynamic state and prevent complications, as well as promote physical and psychological wellbeing. Visits to a joint clinic run by a cardiologist and obstetrician are usually made every 2 weeks until 30 weeks' gestation and weekly thereafter until birth. At each visit functional grading is made according to the New York Heart Association classification and the severity of the heart lesion is assessed by clinical examination. Evaluation of fetal wellbeing will include:

- ultrasound examination to confirm gestational age and congenital abnormality
- assessment of fetal growth and amniotic fluid volume, both clinically and by ultrasound
- monitoring the fetal heart rate by cardiotocography (CTG)
- measurement of fetal and maternal placental blood flow indices by Doppler ultrasonography.

INTRAPARTUM CARE

The first stage of labour

Vaginal birth is preferred unless there is an obstetric indication for caesarean section. Optimal management involves monitoring the maternal condition closely. This will include the measurement of:

- temperature
- pulse

- respiration
- blood pressure
- urine output.

Pulse oximetry, insertion of a central venous pressure (CVP) catheter and electrocardiogram (ECG) monitoring may be utilised.

Fluid balance

Women with significant heart disease require care to be taken concerning fluid balance in labour. Indiscriminate use of intravenous crystalloid fluids will lead to an increase in circulating blood volume, which women with heart disease will find difficult to cope with and they may easily develop pulmonary oedema.

Pain relief

It is important to consult a doctor before administering any form of pain-relieving drug to a woman with a heart condition. In the majority, an epidural would be the analgesia of choice.

Positioning

Cardiac output is influenced by the position of the labouring woman. It is preferable for an upright or left lateral position to be adopted.

Preterm labour

If a woman with heart disease should go into labour prematurely, then beta-sympathomimetic drugs are contraindicated.

Induction

The least stressful labour for a woman with cardiac disease will be spontaneous in onset; induction is considered safe only if the benefits outweigh the disadvantages.

The second stage of labour

This should be short without undue exertion on the part of the mother.

- The midwife should encourage the woman to breathe normally and follow her natural desire to push, giving several short pushes during each contraction.
- Forceps or ventouse may be used to shorten the second stage if the maternal condition deteriorates.
- Care should be taken when the woman is in the lithotomy position, as this produces a sudden increase in venous return to the heart, which may result in heart failure.

The third stage of labour

This is usually actively managed owing to the increased risk of postpartum haemorrhage (PPH).

- Oxytocin is the drug of choice but its use in the prevention of PPH must be balanced against the risk of oxytocin-induced hypotension and tachycardia in women with cardiovascular compromise.
- Ergot-containing preparations such as ergometrine are contraindicated.

POSTNATAL CARE

- During the first 48 hours following birth the heart must cope with the extra blood from the uterine circulation. Close observation should identify early signs of infection, thrombosis or pulmonary oedema.
- Breastfeeding is not contraindicated.
- Discharge planning is particularly important for women with heart disease. The woman and her partner will need to discuss the implications of a future pregnancy with the cardiologist and obstetrician.

RESPIRATORY DISORDERS

ASTHMA

Pregnancy does not consistently affect the maternal asthmatic status; some women experience no change in symptoms whereas others have a distinct worsening of the disease.

Antenatal care

The main anxiety for women and those providing care is generated by the use of medication and the fear that this may harm the fetus.

- To date all medications commonly used in the treatment of asthma, including systemic steroids, are considered safe and it is crucial that therapy is maintained during pregnancy in order to prevent deterioration of the condition and precipitation of adverse pregnancy events.
- The lynchpin of management is the use of peak expiratory flow rates (PEFR) to monitor the level of resistance in the airways caused by inflammation or bronchospasm, or both.

Intrapartum care

- If an asthma attack does occur, it should be treated with the same rapidity and medication as an attack outside of pregnancy.
- Intravenous, intra-amniotic and transcervical prostaglandins should be avoided in pregnancy and labour because of their bronchospasmic action.
- Any woman who has received corticosteroids in pregnancy should have increased doses for the stress of labour.

Postnatal care

- Breastfeeding should be encouraged, particularly as it may protect infants from developing certain allergic conditions.

CYSTIC FIBROSIS

Cystic fibrosis (CF) is an autosomal recessive disorder affecting the exocrine glands that causes production of excess secretions with abnormal electrolyte concentrations, resulting in the obstruction of the ducts and glands.

Prepregnancy care
- When planning a pregnancy, a woman with CF and her partner should have genetic counselling.
- Although pregnancy appears to be well tolerated in women with pre-existing mild pulmonary dysfunction, morbidity and mortality are increased in women with pancreatic insufficiency or moderate to severe lung disease, or both.

Antenatal care
- Once pregnancy is confirmed, a multidisciplinary approach combining midwifery, obstetric, dietetic, medical, nursing and physiotherapy expertise is essential.

Intrapartum care
- During labour close monitoring of cardiorespiratory function will be required and an anaesthetist should be involved at an early stage.
- Fluid and electrolyte management requires careful attention, as women with CF may easily become hypovolaemic from the loss of large quantities of sodium in sweat.
- Epidural analgesia is the recommended form of pain relief in labour and general anaesthesia should be avoided.

Postnatal care
- Women should be cared for in a high-dependency unit and should be closely monitored, as studies have highlighted that cardiorespiratory function often deteriorates following birth.
- Breastfeeding is not contraindicated; however, in order for this to be successful, women need to be well nourished and maintain an adequate calorie intake.

PULMONARY TUBERCULOSIS

Tuberculosis (TB) is caused by the tubercle bacillus, *Myobacterium tuberculosis*. The lungs are the organ most commonly affected, although the disease may involve any organ.

Management
Standard antituberculous therapy should be used to treat TB in pregnancy. TB is treated in two phases:
- In the first phase, rifampicin, isoniazid and pyrazinamide are given daily for the first 2 months.
- In the second (continuation) phase, rifampicin and isoniazid are taken for a further 4 months.

These drugs are considered to be safe and are not associated with human fetal malformations. Attention should also be given to rest, good nutrition and education with regard to preventing the spread of the disease. TB is usually rendered non-infectious after 2 weeks of treatment.

Postnatal care

- Babies born to mothers with infectious TB should be protected from the disease by the prophylactic use of isoniazid syrup 5 mg/kg/day for 6 weeks and should then be tuberculin tested.
- If the tuberculin test is negative, bacille Calmette–Guérin (BCG) vaccination should be given and drug therapy discontinued.
- If the test is positive, the baby should be assessed for congenital or perinatal infection, and drug therapy should be continued if these are excluded.
- Breastfeeding is contraindicated only if the mother has active TB.

It is advisable for a woman with TB to avoid further pregnancies until the disease has been quiescent for at least 2 years. The woman needs to be aware that rifampicin reduces the effectiveness of oral contraception.

RENAL DISEASE

ASYMPTOMATIC BACTERIURIA

A diagnosis of asymptomatic bacteriuria (ASB) is made when there are more than 100 000 bacteria per millilitre of urine. All women should be screened for bacteriuria using a clean voided specimen of urine at their first antenatal visit.

If ASB is not identified and treated with antibiotics, 20–30% of affected women will develop a symptomatic urinary tract infection such as cystitis or pyelonephritis. These infections represent a significant risk for both mother and fetus and there is evidence to suggest that they may play a role in the onset of preterm labour.

PYELONEPHRITIS

Clinical presentation
See Box 13.4.

Management
- Refer to a doctor; admit to hospital.
- Obtain a midstream specimen of urine (MSU) to test for culture and sensitivity.

Box 13.4 Clinical presentation of pyelonephritis

- Pyrexia, rigors and tachycardia
- Nausea and vomiting; dehydration
- Pain and tenderness over the loin area; muscle guarding
- Urine cloudy; infecting organism often found to be *Escherichia coli*

- Give intravenous antibiotics followed by oral antibiotics once the pyrexia has settled.
- Record fluid balance; intravenous fluids may be required.
- Maintain 4-hourly observation of temperature and pulse.
- Monitor uterine activity.
- Prevent complications of immobility, e.g. deep vein thrombosis.
- Repeat cultures 2 weeks after completion of antibiotics and monthly until birth.

CHRONIC RENAL DISEASE

In order to determine the impact of pregnancy on a woman with chronic renal disease, the following factors need to be considered:
- Type of pre-existing renal disease.
- General health status of the woman.
- Presence or absence of hypertension.
- Current renal function.
- Prepregnancy drug therapy.

If renal disease is under control, the maternal and fetal outcome is usually good. In some instances renal function may deteriorate and the chance of pregnancy complications subsequently rises.

Care and management

The aim of pregnancy care is to prevent deterioration in renal function. This will necessitate more frequent attendance for antenatal care and close liaison between the midwife, obstetrician and nephrologist.
- Renal function is assessed on a regular basis by measuring serum urate levels, serum electrolyte and urea, 24-hour creatinine clearance and serum creatinine.
- Screen for glycosuria, proteinuria, haematuria, urinary tract infection and anaemia.
- Monitor for the emergence and severity of hypertension and pre-eclampsia.
- Fetal surveillance includes fortnightly ultrasound scans from 24 weeks, Doppler flow studies and daily fetal activity charts.

THE ANAEMIAS

Anaemia may be caused by a decrease in red blood cell (RBC) production, or a reduction in haemoglobin (Hb) content of the blood, or a combination of these. Signs and symptoms are listed in Box 13.5. A low Hb concentration only indicates that anaemia is present; it does not reveal the cause.

PHYSIOLOGICAL ANAEMIA OF PREGNANCY

During pregnancy the maternal plasma volume gradually expands by 50%, an increase of approximately 1200 ml by term. The total increase in RBCs is 25%, or approximately 300 ml. This relative haemodilution produces a fall in Hb concentration, which reaches a nadir during the second trimester of pregnancy and then rises again in the third trimester.

Box 13.5 Common signs and symptoms of anaemia

- Pallor of the mucous membranes
- Fatigue
- Dizziness and fainting
- Headache
- Exertional shortness of breath
- Tachycardia
- Palpitations

IRON DEFICIENCY ANAEMIA

Iron deficiency anaemia in women is usually due to:

- reduced intake or absorption of iron; this includes dietary deficiency and gastrointestinal disturbances such as diarrhoea or hyperemesis
- excess demand, such as frequent, numerous or multiple pregnancies
- chronic infection, particularly of the urinary tract
- acute or chronic blood loss: e.g. menorrhagia, bleeding haemorrhoids, or antepartum or postpartum haemorrhage.

Investigation

- Mean cell volume (MCV): normal value 80–95 femtolitres.
- Mean cell haemoglobin concentration (MCHC): normal value 32–36 g/dl.
- Serum iron levels: normal value 10–30 µmol/l.
- Total iron-binding capacity (TIBC): normal range 40–70 µmol/l.
- Serum ferritin: normal range 10–300 µg/l.

Management

- Identify the woman at risk through clinical observation and by taking an accurate medical, obstetric and social history.
- Advice regarding the dietary intake of iron, taking account of how the intake of iron may be affected by social, religious and cultural preferences.
- Iron supplements may be prescribed where the Hb level is outside the UK range (11 g/dl at first contact, 10.5 g/dl at 28 weeks) and iron deficiency anaemia has been diagnosed. Oral iron supplementation should continue postnatally, particularly if the woman is breastfeeding. In women who are unable to take, tolerate or absorb oral preparations, iron can also be given intramuscularly or intravenously.

FOLIC ACID DEFICIENCY ANAEMIA

Folic acid is needed for the increased cell growth of both mother and fetus but there is a physiological decrease in serum folate levels in pregnancy. The Medical Research Council Vitamin Study Research Group (1991) found a positive correlation between folate deficiency and the development of neural tube defects in the fetus.

Causes
- A reduced dietary intake or reduced absorption, or a combination of these.
- An excessive demand and loss of folic acid, e.g. haemolytic anaemia, multiple pregnancy.
- Interference of some drugs with the utilisation of folic acid, e.g. anticonvulsants, sulphonamides and alcohol.

Investigation
Examination of the red cell indices will reveal that the red cells are reduced in number but enlarged in size.

Management
- Advise on the correct selection and preparation of foods that are high in folic acid.
- Recommend folic acid supplements for all pregnant women, 400 µg/day (National Institute for Clinical Excellence 2003). Additional supplements may be prescribed for women considered at risk.

HAEMOGLOBINOPATHIES

This term describes inherited conditions where the haemoglobin is abnormal. Defective genes lead to the formation of abnormal Hb; this may be as a result of impaired globin synthesis (thalassaemia syndromes) or from structural abnormality of globin (Hb variants such as sickle cell anaemia). These conditions are found mainly in people whose families come from Africa, the West Indies, the Middle East, the eastern Mediterranean and Asia.

As these conditions are inherited and in the homozygous form can be fatal, screening of the population at risk should be carried out. If both parents are carriers (i.e. heterozygous), there is a 1 in 4 chance that the fetus will be homozygous for the condition.

THALASSAEMIA

Thalassaemia is most common in people of Mediterranean, African, Middle and Far Eastern origin. The basic defect is a reduced rate of globin chain synthesis in adult Hb. This leads to ineffective erythropoiesis and increased haemolysis with a resultant inadequate Hb content. The red cell indices show a low Hb and MCHC level, but raised serum iron level. Definitive diagnosis is obtained by electrophoresis. The severity of the condition depends on whether the abnormal genes are inherited from one parent or from both. There are also different types of thalassaemia, depending on whether the alpha or beta globin chain synthesis is affected:
- alpha thalassaemia major
- beta thalassaemia major
- alpha and beta thalassaemia minor.

SICKLE-CELL DISORDERS

Sickle-cell disorders are found most commonly in people of African or West Indian origin. In these conditions defective genes produce abnormal Hb beta chains; the resulting Hb is called HbS.

- In sickle-cell anaemia (HbSS, or SCA) abnormal genes have been inherited from both parents.
- In sickle-cell trait (HbAS) only one abnormal gene has been inherited. Maternal and fetal/neonatal risks are listed in Box 13.6.

All women in the at-risk population are screened in early pregnancy, and where possible their partners are screened too. Those who are diagnosed as having SCA should be referred to a specialist sickle-cell centre with trained haemoglobinopathy and genetic counsellors.

Sickle-cell trait

This is usually asymptomatic. The blood appears normal, although the sickle screening test is positive. There is no anaemia, even under the additional stress of pregnancy.

DIABETES MELLITUS

The term 'diabetes mellitus' (DM) describes a metabolic disorder of multiple aetiology that affects the normal metabolism of carbohydrates, fats and protein.

Classification

See Box 13.7.

Diagnosis

Routine screening in pregnancy is not recommended. Increased thirst, increased urine volume, excessive tiredness, unexplained weight loss and a family history

---

Box 13.6 Common risks and complications of sickle-cell disorders

Maternal risks
- Antenatal and postnatal pain crisis
- Infections
- Pulmonary complications
- Anaemia
- Pre-eclampsia
- Caesarean section

Fetal and neonatal complications
- Preterm birth
- Smallness for gestational age
- Neonatal jaundice

> **Box 13.7 Classification of diabetes mellitus (DM)**
>
> *Type 1 DM*
> - Occurs when beta cells in the islets of Langerhans in the pancreas are destroyed, stopping insulin production
> - Insulin therapy is required in order to prevent the development of ketoacidosis, coma and death
>
> *Type 2 DM*
> - Results from a defect or defects in insulin action and insulin secretion
> - Insulin therapy is not needed to survive
> - The risk of developing this type of DM increases with age, obesity and lack of physical activity
>
> *Gestational diabetes mellitus (GDM)*
> - Carbohydrate intolerance resulting in hyperglycaemia of variable severity
> - Onset or first recognition is during pregnancy
>
> *Impaired glucose regulation*
> - Includes *impaired glucose tolerance* (IGT) and *impaired fasting glycaemia* (IFG), metabolic states intermediate between normal glucose homeostasis and diabetes

require further investigations. The World Health Organization (WHO) criteria for diagnosis after a 75 g glucose load are:

- Two-hour venous glucose <7.8 mmol/l = normal.
- Two-hour venous glucose 7.8–11 mmol/l = impaired glucose tolerance.
- Two-hour venous glucose >11 mmol/l = gestational diabetes.

However, these levels are based on a non-pregnant population and hence could lead to overdiagnosis.

Monitoring diabetes

The main objectives of diabetic therapy are:

- to maintain blood glucose levels as near to normal as possible
- to reduce the risk of long-term complications.

Long-term blood glucose control can be determined by undertaking a laboratory test to measure glycosylated haemoglobin (HbA1c). Between 5% and 8% of Hb in the red blood cells carries a glucose molecule and is said to be glycosylated. The degree of Hb glycosylation is dependent on the amount of glucose the red blood cells have been exposed to during their 120-day life. A random blood test measuring the percentage of Hb that is glycosylated will reflect the average blood glucose during the preceding 1–2 months. The higher the HbA1c, the poorer is the blood sugar control. Good diabetic control is defined as an HbA1c of <6.5%.

Carbohydrate metabolism in pregnancy

Pregnancy is characterised by several factors that produce a diabetogenetic state so that insulin and carbohydrate metabolism is altered in order to make glucose more readily available to the fetus. Women with DM do not have the capacity to increase insulin secretion in response to the altered carbohydrate metabolism in pregnancy and therefore glucose accumulates in the maternal and fetal system, leading to significant morbidity and mortality.

Prepregnancy care

- Assessment is made of current diabetic control, aiming for pre-meal glucose levels of <6 mmol/L and HbA1c of ≤7%.
- Insulin dosage is reviewed.
- Women on oral hypoglycaemics will need to discuss transfer to insulin to prevent the possibility of teratogenesis.
- Higher-dose folic acid supplementation is given.
- Smoking cessation support is arranged.
- Assessment and management are provided for diabetes complications.

Antenatal care

- Women and their partners should ideally be seen in a combined clinic by a team that includes a physician, an obstetrician with a special interest in diabetes in pregnancy, a specialist diabetes nurse, a specialist midwife and a dietitian. They will be seen as often as required in order to maintain good diabetic control and undertake relevant screening, e.g. retinal examination.
- Blood glucose levels should be monitored frequently (four times a day using a reflectance meter) and insulin levels adjusted to achieve pre-meal blood sugar levels of 5.0–6.0 mmol/l and post-meal levels of <7.5 mmol/l. Additional estimations of blood glucose control, such as monthly HbA1c measurements, are also recommended.
- A diet that is high in fibre is beneficial, as carbohydrates are released slowly and therefore a more constant blood glucose level can be achieved.
- Advise women on early recognition of the signs and symptoms of urinary and vaginal infections.
- Anomaly ultrasound screening should be offered at 20 weeks' gestation and fetal echocardiography at 20–22 weeks to detect cardiac abnormalities. Serum screening for Down syndrome is altered with maternal diabetes and care should be taken when interpreting the results.
- There is an increased risk of growth restriction due to maternal vascular disease, pre-eclampsia or a combination of both. A baseline measurement of the fetal abdominal circumference is taken at 20 weeks. This is followed by serial measurements every 2–4 weeks, commencing at 24 weeks. Serial ultrasound should also detect fetal macrosomia and whether polyhydramnios is present.

Intrapartum care

- Ideally, labour should be allowed to commence spontaneously at term for women with uncomplicated DM during pregnancy. Poor diabetic control or a deterioration in the maternal or fetal condition may necessitate earlier, planned birth. Induction of labour may also be considered where the fetus is judged to be macrosomic. Steroids such as dexamethasone may be used to aid lung maturation and surfactant production, but these will increase insulin requirements.

- The aim of intrapartum care is to maintain normoglycaemia in labour (i.e. <7.0 mmol/l).
- Continuous electronic fetal monitoring is recommended and fetal blood sampling should be utilised if acidosis is suspected.
- Adequate pain relief, such as epidural analgesia, assists in regulating the blood sugar levels and preventing the development of metabolic acidosis. It is also useful if difficulties should arise with the birth of the shoulders or an operative birth is required.

Postpartum care

- Immediately after the third stage of labour the insulin requirements will fall rapidly to prepregnancy levels. The insulin infusion rate should be reduced by at least 50%.
- Women with type 2 DM who were previously on oral hypoglycaemics or dietary control need to be reviewed prior to recommencing therapy.
- Breastfeeding should be encouraged in all women with diabetes. An additional carbohydrate intake of 40–50 g is recommended and insulin therapy may need to be adjusted accordingly.
- All women should be offered contraceptive advice so that optimum metabolic control is achieved prior to planning the next pregnancy.

Neonatal care

The development of complications in the neonate is related to maternal hyperglycaemia during pregnancy leading to fetal hyperinsulinaemia. This will result in the following conditions: macrosomia, hypoglycaemia, polycythaemia and respiratory distress syndrome.

Macrosomia

This is defined as a fetal birth weight >4500 g. The increased fetal size may cause prolonged labour and predisposes the infant to shoulder dystocia and birth injuries. As a consequence, asphyxia is common and these infants are more likely than babies of normal weight to die from an intrapartum-related event.

Hypoglycaemia

Beta-cell hyperplasia causes the baby to continue to produce more insulin than required for up to 24 hours following birth. To prevent hypoglycaemia the neonatal blood glucose needs to be assessed 1–2 hours after birth and then every 4–6 hours for the first 24–48 hours.

Regular feeding is encouraged to maintain a blood glucose of at least 2.6 mmol/l.

Polycythaemia

Fetal hyperinsulinaemia during pregnancy also leads to an increase in red cell production resulting in polycythaemia (venous haematocrit >65%). The rapid breakdown of the excess red blood cells, combined with the relative immaturity of the liver in the newborn, predisposes the baby to jaundice. This will be exacerbated if there is bruising as a result of birth trauma.

Respiratory distress syndrome

Hyperinsulinaemia is thought to impair the production of surfactant and delay lung maturation. Hence, babies born at term may display symptomatology of respiratory distress.

Observations of temperature, apex beat and respirations and monitoring of blood sugar levels are important in the first 24–48 hours. Clinical signs, together with symptomatology such as respiratory distress, apnoea or tachypnoea, cyanosis, jitteriness, irritability, seizures, feeding intolerance and temperature instability may all be indicative of respiratory distress syndrome, polycythaemia and hypoglycaemia; these will require further investigation and treatment in a neonatal unit.

GESTATIONAL DIABETES

Screening for GDM (including dipstick testing for glycosuria) is not a recommended intervention for *routine* antenatal care.

Diagnosis is based on the WHO recommendations. However, caution should be exercised if the following occur in the third trimester when glucose tolerance is known to be impaired:

- If the fasting venous plasma glucose is >7.0 mmol/l, *or*
- There is a fasting venous plasma glucose <7.0 mmol/l and a plasma glucose of >7.8 mmol/l 2 hours after a 75-g glucose load.

Treatment will depend on the blood glucose levels. Grossly abnormal results are likely to require insulin therapy, which will be discontinued immediately after the birth of the baby. It is recommended that a postnatal oral glucose tolerance test is performed at 6 weeks; if the results are abnormal, then appropriate referral should be made. Those with normal glucose levels require advice regarding the implications for future pregnancies and the development of type 1 or type 2 DM.

EPILEPSY

The prevalence of epilepsy in the general population is 1 in 200 and it affects 0.3–0.5% of pregnant women.

An epileptic seizure results from abnormal electrical activity in the brain, which is manifest by brief sensory, motor and autonomic dysfunction. These disturbances recur spontaneously and are classified according to the parts of the brain affected. Seizures may be described as shown in Box 13.8.

Identification of the type of epilepsy is important in the treatment of epilepsy. The aim of treatment is to identify the cause of the seizure and provide appropriate therapy to prevent recurrence. The control of seizures can be achieved for the majority of people through the use of antiepileptic drugs (AEDs).

Box 13.8 Classification of epilepsy

Partial
- Usually arising from the temporal or frontal lobe of the brain

Generalised
- Resulting from disturbances involving both halves of the brain:
  - Absence seizures (petit mal)
  - Myoclonic seizures
  - Tonic–clonic seizures (grand mal)
  - Atonic seizures
  - Status epilepticus

Prepregnancy care

Women on AEDs become folic acid deficient and may develop macrocytic anaemia. Folic acid deficiency has also been associated with neural tube defects and other congenital malformations.

There is a 1–2% risk of neural tube defects if a woman is taking sodium valproate (Epilim) or carbamazepine (Tegretol) in pregnancy. Of the other older AEDs, phenytoin gives rise to a combination of malformations termed 'fetal hydantoin syndrome', which comprises craniofacial dysmorphic features, digital defects, microcephaly and growth retardation. Preconception advice is therefore essential for women with epilepsy.

- AED therapy may be withdrawn gradually prior to pregnancy in order to reduce the risk of teratogenicity when women suffer from seizures that are unlikely to harm the fetus, such as absence, partial or myoclonic seizures, or have been seizure free for over 2 years.
- Folic acid supplementation (5 mg/day) should be commenced before pregnancy and continued throughout pregnancy.

Antenatal care

- Antenatal care should include a detailed anomaly scan at 18–22 weeks.
- Abnormalities are more common if AEDs are prescribed in high concentration and particularly if more than one is used.
- Some women may experience an increase in seizures; this is often due to non-compliance with the drug regimen, sleep deprivation during pregnancy and the decline in plasma concentrations of the AED as the pregnancy progresses.
- Particular emphasis should also be placed on the first-aid measures that should be adopted following an epileptic seizure in order to prevent aspiration, and the dangers of hot baths inducing fainting and consequent drowning.

Intrapartum care

- Care during labour and childbirth is not likely to be different from that of other mothers.

- Seizures are more likely to occur in conditions such as sleep deprivation, hypoglycaemia, anaemia, stress or hyperventilation – all of which may arise during labour. AEDs should therefore be maintained throughout labour.

Postnatal care

- Safety precautions in the home are important. The mother is given advice about how to minimise risks when feeding, bathing, changing and transporting the baby.
- AED therapy should be reviewed 6 weeks postnatally and the dosage adjusted to prepregnancy levels.

EFFECT OF EPILEPSY ON THE FETUS AND NEONATE

The majority of women with epilepsy will have uncomplicated pregnancies with normal births and healthy children.

When status epilepticus occurs, one-third of mothers and half of the fetuses do not survive. Convulsive status epilepticus is a medical emergency.

AEDs cross the placenta freely and decrease production of vitamin K, leading to the risk of haemorrhagic disease of the newborn. This can be prevented by routine administration of vitamin K to the mother from 36 weeks' gestation and to the baby shortly after birth. The rate of clearance of AEDs varies according to the drug. Newborn infants may therefore suffer harmful effects from the AED level and, as a group, tend to be less efficient at feeding and gain weight more slowly. A minority will suffer withdrawal symptoms such as tremor, excitability and convulsions. AEDs pass into the breast milk in relatively small quantities and therefore breastfeeding is recommended. Some AEDs, such as phenobarbital, primidone or benzodiazepines, may have a sedative effect, in which case bottle feeding or mixed feeding may be advised.

AUTOIMMUNE DISEASE

Autoimmune disease arises from a disruption in the function of the immune system of the body, resulting in the production of antibodies against the body's own cells. Antigens normally present on the body's cells stimulate the development of autoantibodies, which, unable to distinguish the self antigens from non-self or foreign antigens, act against the body's cells to cause localised and systemic reactions. The cause of this condition is unknown but it is thought to be multifactorial with genetic, environmental, hormonal and viral influences. Many autoimmune diseases are more prevalent in women, particularly between puberty and the menopause, which suggests that female hormonal factors may play a role. They broadly fall into two groups:

- multisystem disease, such as systemic lupus erythematosus (SLE)
- tissue- or organ-specific disorders, such as autoimmune thyroid disease.

These disorders are characterised by periods of remission interrupted by periods of crisis, which may require hospitalisation. Treatment is aimed at lessening the severity of the symptoms rather than effecting a cure.

- Mild cases usually respond to anti-inflammatory drugs.
- More severe illnesses may require steroids or immunosuppressant therapy.

SYSTEMIC LUPUS ERYTHEMATOSUS

SLE, or lupus, is an inflammatory disorder of the connective tissue, which forms the fibrous, elastic, fatty or cartilaginous matrix that connects and supports other tissues.

- The initial manifestation of SLE is often arthritis accompanied by fever, fatigue, malaise, weight loss, photosensitivity and anaemia.
- A wide range of skin lesions are seen and an erythematous facial 'butterfly' rash is characteristic of the disorder.
- Depending on the organs involved, inflammatory conditions such as pleuritis, pericarditis, glomerulonephritis, neuritis and gastritis may arise.
- Renal disease and neurological abnormalities are the most serious manifestations of the disease.

Most people with SLE have a normal life expectancy and serious complications are rare. Infection is the major cause of mortality.

Diagnosis

The diagnosis of SLE is based on a collection of the signs and symptoms, particularly when joint pain, skin conditions and fatigue occur in combination or evolve over time. Blood tests are used to confirm the diagnosis and comprise:

- full blood count
- erythrocyte sedimentation rate (ESR)
- testing for antinuclear antibody (ANA).

There is often normochromic normocytic anaemia, the ESR is elevated even when the disease is in remission and more than 95% of people with SLE will have ANA. Antiphospholipid syndrome (APS) is found in conjunction with SLE in 30% of cases. A blood test will detect antiphospholipid antibodies (aPL), lupus anticoagulant and anticardiolipin antibodies (anti-Ro and anti-La) if APS is present.

This will identify a group of people with SLE at particular risk of thromboembolic disorders and a high rate of fetal loss.

Effect of SLE on pregnancy

The effects of SLE on pregnancy is variable, although worsening of SLE symptoms is common and may occur at any trimester of pregnancy and in the postpartum period. The frequency of the 'flares' is, however, lower in women with mild and well controlled disease. Women with SLE should be counselled about planning a pregnancy and the importance of being in remission for at least 6 months before conception. Overall, pregnancies in SLE women have an increased incidence of adverse pregnancy outcome. Approximately one-third of pregnancies will result in fetal wastage owing to spontaneous abortion, therapeutic abortion, intrauterine death or stillbirth. The rate of preterm birth and intrauterine growth restriction is closely related to the incidence of pre-eclampsia.

Neonatal lupus syndrome is rare but may occur as a result of the transplacental passage of maternal anti-Ro/La antibodies.

Antenatal care

Women should be referred as soon as possible to a centre that specialises in the care of people with lupus disorders.

- Baseline haematological and immunological blood tests are performed at the first antenatal visit.
- A baseline 24-hour urine collection for creatinine clearance and total protein to assess renal function is also recommended.
- An early first trimester scan is undertaken to confirm fetal viability and an anomaly scan is performed at 18–20 weeks. Women with SLE and APS are offered a fetal cardiac anomaly scan at 24 weeks' gestation and echocardiography to detect congenital heart block.
- Serial ultrasound examinations for fetal growth, placental size and quality, and amniotic fluid volume should begin at 28–32 weeks.
- Doppler flow studies are performed at 20 and 24 weeks and thereafter according to fetal growth and wellbeing.

The aim is to control disease activity and achieve clinical remission while keeping drug therapy to a minimum.

- Women who have a mild form of the disease or are in remission require minimal to no medication.
- Avoidance of emotional stress and the promotion of a healthy lifestyle may play a part in reducing the likelihood of flares or exacerbations of SLE arising during pregnancy.
- If treatment is required, simple analgesics such as paracetamol and co-dydramol are used for symptomatic relief.
- Mild flares with joint pain, skin lesions and fatigue respond well to low-dose steroid therapy such as prednisone or prednisolone.
- Antimalarial drugs are effective as maintenance therapy in women with frequent flares and hydroxychloroquine is considered safe to use in pregnancy.
- Advanced renal disease requires immunosuppressants.
- Women with SLE and APS have associated recurrent miscarriage, thrombosis and thrombocytopenia and it is recommended that treatment with low-dose aspirin (75 mg daily) and heparin (5000 IU every 12 hours given subcutaneously) is commenced as soon as these women have a positive pregnancy test.

Intrapartum care

- The timing of birth depends on current activity of the disease and whether there are any complications.
- Women with SLE are particularly prone to infection, hypertension, thrombocytopenia and thromboembolic disorders. Close monitoring of the

maternal condition is required to evaluate cardiac, pulmonary and renal function. Blood tests should be undertaken to screen for haematological conditions, which may lead to clotting disorders. Comfort measures and thromboembolitic D (TED) stockings can reduce pressure sores and the development of deep vein thrombosis. Women who have been on long-term steroid therapy will require parenteral steroid cover during labour.

- As SLE may compromise the uteroplacental circulation, continuous fetal monitoring in conjunction with fetal blood gas estimation is recommended.

Postpartum care

- During the immediate postpartum period the midwife should observe closely for signs of SLE flares and signs and symptoms of infection, pre-eclampsia, renal disease, thrombosis and neurological changes.
- Careful consideration needs to be given to breastfeeding, as most of the drugs used to treat SLE are excreted in breast milk. Large doses of aspirin should be avoided and non-steroidal anti-inflammatory drugs (NSAIDs) are contraindicated when breastfeeding jaundiced neonates; paracetamol is the drug of choice for postpartum analgesia. Low-dose steroids such as prednisone and prednisolone and the antimalarial hydroxychloroquine are considered safe to use when breastfeeding. Immunosuppressive therapy is contraindicated and should be avoided.
- The choice of contraceptives for a woman with SLE may be limited.

THYROID DISEASE

In pregnancy, thyroid function is affected by three factors that increase the basal metabolic rate by 20%:

- Oestrogen stimulates the production of thyroid-binding globulin (TBG), which binds more of the thyroid hormones resulting in a doubling of the total serum levels of *thyroxine* (T4) and *tri-iodothyronine* (T_3).
- Human chorionic gonadotrophin (HCG) secreted by the placenta appears to stimulate the thyroid gland directly as *thyroid-stimulating hormone* (TSH) levels fall in early pregnancy and then increase in the second and third trimesters, with a corresponding rise and then fall in the level of HCG.
- A rise in the glomerular filtration rate in pregnancy leads to increased renal clearance of iodine, resulting in an increase in dietary iodine requirement.

Clinical assessment of thyroid dysfunction is difficult, as pregnancy-related symptoms are similar to hyperthyroidism and hypothyroidism. Thyroid function can be assessed by biochemical tests that measure total T_4, free thyroxine (FT_4), total T_3 and TSH. It is important to remember that thyroid function tests may appear abnormal in pregnancy despite normal activity of the thyroid gland.

HYPERTHYROIDISM

The most common cause of hyperthyroidism in pregnancy is *Graves' disease*, which is an autoimmune disorder that results in antibody activation of the thyroid gland. The gland becomes enlarged and secretes an increased amount of thyroid hormone. The metabolic processes of the body are accelerated, resulting in fatigue, heat intolerance, palpitations, diarrhoea and mood lability. Clinical diagnosis may be difficult, as the physiological signs and symptoms that pregnant women normally exhibit may mask this condition.

- The disease should be suspected in any woman who loses weight despite a good appetite.
- Other symptoms include an enlarged thyroid gland (goitre), exophthalmos, eyelid lag and persistent tachycardia.

A serious complication of untreated or poorly controlled hyperthyroidism is *thyroid storm*. This may occur spontaneously or be precipitated by infection or stress. It is characterised by signs and symptoms associated with a high metabolic rate:

- hyperthermia (temperature >41°C), leading to:
  - dehydration
  - tachycardia
  - acute respiratory distress
  - cardiovascular collapse.

This is a medical emergency requiring oxygen, cooling, hydration, antibiotics and drug therapy to stop the production and reduce the effect of thyroid hormone.

Hyperthyroidism in pregnancy is associated with an increase in the incidence of pre-eclampsia, preterm birth, low birth weight and fetal death.

Management

Treatment of hyperthyroidism is achieved through the use of antithyroid drugs.

- Propylthiouracil and carbimazole may be used in pregnancy. Propylthiouracil is the drug of choice, as less of it crosses the placenta and only small amounts are found in breast milk.
- The aim of management is to use the lowest dose possible, as these drugs may cause goitre and hypothyroidism in the fetus.
- During the antenatal period the pregnant woman should be seen monthly by the endocrinologist for clinical evaluation and monitoring of her thyroid levels.
- Factors that may precipitate thyroid storm include infection, the stress of labour and caesarean section.

HYPOTHYROIDISM

The most common cause of hypothyroidism in pregnancy is *autoimmune thyroiditis* (Hashimoto's disease). Slowing of the body's metabolic processes may occur, giving rise to mental and physical lethargy, excessive weight gain, constipation, cold intolerance and dryness of the skin. However, the symptoms may be non-specific and the condition can be difficult to diagnose. Hypothyroidism in pregnancy will result in reduced availability of the hormone for fetal requirements, leading to subsequent poor neurological development. Women should be encouraged to increase their dietary iodine intake during pregnancy and hypothyroidism should be treated with daily thyroxine. Following birth, the neonate's thyroid status should be checked to identify whether neonatal hypothyroidism is present. There is no contraindication to breastfeeding but the dose of thyroxine may need adjustment postpartum because of maternal weight loss following childbirth.

POSTPARTUM THYROIDITIS

This is an autoimmune disorder and is a form of Hashimoto's thyroiditis, which occurs in 5% of women during the first year following childbirth. It is a transient thyroid disorder, characterised by a period of mild hyperthyroidism occurring a few months after birth and followed by a phase of hypothyroidism. In both phases the disorder presents with fatigue and a painless goitre; the condition may also mimic postpartum depression. Treatment is not required, as recovery is usually spontaneous.

CHAPTER 14

Hypertensive Disorders of Pregnancy

Hypertension is the commonest medical condition encountered in pregnancy, complicating approximately 5% of all pregnancies; it is a significant cause of maternal and fetal/neonatal morbidity and mortality. Pregnancy may induce hypertension in women who have been normotensive prior to pregnancy, or may aggravate existing hypertensive conditions.

DEFINITION AND CLASSIFICATION

The definition and classification of the hypertensive disorders are complex (Box 14.1). It is important to recognise the distinction between:
- a woman whose hypertension antedates pregnancy (pre-existing or chronic hypertension)
- a woman who develops an increased blood pressure during pregnancy (new, gestational or pregnancy-induced hypertension).

An incremental rise in blood pressure is not included in this classification system. However, it is considered that women who have a rise of 30 mmHg systolic or 15 mmHg diastolic blood pressure require close observation especially if proteinuria and hyperuricaemia (raised uric acid level) are also present.

PATHOLOGICAL CHANGES

Blood

Hypertension, together with endothelial cell damage, affects capillary permeability. Plasma proteins leak from the damaged blood vessels, causing a decrease in the plasma colloid pressure and an increase in oedema within the extracellular space. The reduced intravascular plasma volume causes hypovolaemia and haemoconcentration, which is reflected in an elevated haematocrit. In severe cases the lungs become congested with fluid and pulmonary oedema develops, oxygenation is impaired and cyanosis occurs. With vasoconstriction and disruption of the vascular endothelium the coagulation cascade is activated.

Box 14.1 Classification and definition of hypertensive disorders in pregnancy

Chronic hypertension

- Hypertension before pregnancy or a diastolic blood pressure of 90 mmHg or more before 20 weeks' gestation, and persisting 6 weeks after delivery

New, gestational or pregnancy-induced hypertension

- Development of hypertension without other signs of pre-eclampsia
- Diagnosed when, after resting, the woman's blood pressure rises above 140/90 mmHg, on at least two occasions, no more than 1 week apart after the 20th week of pregnancy in a woman known to be normotensive
- Hypertension diagnosed for the first time in pregnancy, which does not resolve postpartum, is also classified as gestational hypertension

Pre-eclampsia

- Diagnosed on the basis of hypertension with proteinuria, when proteinuria is measured as >1+ on dipstick or >0.3 g/L of protein in a random clean catch specimen or an excretion of 0.3 g protein/24 hours
- In the absence of proteinuria, pre-eclampsia is suspected when hypertension is accompanied by symptoms including:
  - headache
  - blurred vision
  - abdominal/epigastric pain, *or*
  - altered biochemistry: specifically, low platelet counts, abnormal liver enzyme levels
- These signs and symptoms, together with blood pressure above 160 mmHg systolic or above 110 mmHg diastolic and proteinuria of 2+ or 3+ on a dipstick, demonstrate the more severe form of the disease

Eclampsia

- The new onset of convulsions during pregnancy or postpartum, unrelated to other cerebral pathological conditions, in a woman with pre-eclampsia

Pre-eclampsia superimposed on chronic hypertension

- This may occur in women with pre-existing hypertension (under 20 weeks' gestation) who develop:
  - new proteinuria (>0.3 g/24 hours)
  - sudden increases in pre-existing hypertension and proteinuria
  - thrombocytopenia (platelet count <100 × 10^9/L)
  - abnormal liver enzymes

Coagulation system

Increased platelet consumption produces thrombocytopenia. Disseminated intravascular coagulation (DIC) is characterized by low platelets and fibrinogen and prolonged prothrombin time. As the process progresses, fibrin and platelets are deposited, which will occlude blood flow to many organs, particularly the kidneys, liver, brain and placenta.

Kidneys

In the kidney, hypertension leads to vasospasm of the afferent arterioles, resulting in a decreased renal blood flow, which produces hypoxia and oedema of the endothelial cells of the glomerular capillaries. Glomeruloendotheliosis (glomerular endothelial damage) allows plasma proteins to filter into the urine, producing proteinuria. Renal damage is reflected by reduced creatinine clearance and increased serum creatinine and uric acid levels. Oliguria develops as the condition worsens, signifying severe and renal vasoconstriction.

Liver

Vasoconstriction of the hepatic vascular bed will result in hypoxia and oedema of the liver cells. In severe cases oedematous swelling of the liver causes epigastric pain and can lead to intracapsular haemorrhages and, in very rare cases, rupture of the liver. Altered liver function is reflected by falling albumin levels and a rise in liver enzyme levels.

Brain

Hypertension, combined with cerebrovascular endothelial dysfunction, increases the permeability of the blood–brain barrier, resulting in cerebral oedema and microhaemorrhaging characterised by the onset of headaches, visual disturbances and convulsions. Where the mean arterial pressure (MAP – i.e. the systolic blood pressure plus twice the diastolic pressure divided by 3) exceeds 125 mmHg, the autoregulation of cerebral flow is disrupted, resulting in cerebral vasospasm, cerebral oedema and blood clot formation. This is known as *hypertensive encephalopathy*; if left untreated, it can progress to cerebral haemorrhage and death.

Fetoplacental unit

In the uterus, vasoconstriction caused by hypertension reduces the uterine blood flow which can result in placental abruption and placental scarring. The amount of oxygen that diffuses through the cells of the syncytiotrophoblast and cytotrophoblast into the fetal circulation within the placenta is diminished, the placental tissue becomes ischaemic, the capillaries in the chorionic villi thrombose and infarctions occur, leading to fetal growth restriction.

THE MIDWIFE'S ROLE IN ASSESSMENT AND DIAGNOSIS

As the hypertensive disorders are unlikely to be prevented, early detection and appropriate management can minimise the severity of the condition. A comprehensive history will identify:

- adverse social circumstances or poverty, which could prevent the woman from attending for regular antenatal care
- the mother's age and parity
- primipaternity and partner-related factors
- a family history of hypertensive disorders

- a past history of pre-eclampsia
- the presence of underlying medical disorders: for example, renal disease, diabetes, systemic lupus erythematosus (SLE) and thromboembolic disorders.

The two essential features of pre-eclampsia, hypertension and proteinuria, are assessed for at regular intervals throughout pregnancy. Diagnosis is usually based on the rise in blood pressure and the presence of proteinuria after 20 weeks' gestation.

Blood pressure measurement

The mother's blood pressure is taken early in pregnancy to compare with all subsequent recordings, taking into account the normal pattern in pregnancy. It is important to consider several factors in assessing blood pressure.

- Blood pressure machines should be calibrated for use in pregnancy and regularly maintained.
- Blood pressure can be overestimated as a result of using a sphygmomanometer cuff of inadequate size relative to the arm circumference. The length of the bladder should be at least 80% of the arm circumference. Two cuffs should be available with inflation bladders of 35 cm for normal use and 42 cm for large arms.
- Rounding off of blood pressure measurements should be avoided and an attempt should be made to record the blood pressure as accurately as possible to the nearest 2 mmHg.
- The use of Korotkoff V (disappearance of sound) as a measure of the diastolic blood pressure has been found to be easier to obtain, more reproducible and closer to the intra-arterial pressure; therefore this reading should be used unless the sound is near zero, in which case Korotkoff IV (muffling sound) should be used instead.

Urinalysis

Proteinuria in the absence of urinary tract infection is indicative of glomerular endotheliosis. The amount of protein in the urine is frequently taken as an index of the severity of pre-eclampsia. A significant increase in proteinuria, coupled with diminished urinary output, indicates renal impairment. A 24-hour urine collection for total protein measurement will be required to be certain about the presence or absence of proteinuria and to provide an accurate quantitative assessment of protein loss.

- A finding of >300 mg/24 hours is considered to be indicative of mild to moderate pre-eclampsia.
- A finding of >3 g/24 hours is considered to be severe.

Oedema and excessive weight gain

These are variable findings and nowadays are usually considered only when a diagnosis of pre-eclampsia has been made based on other criteria. The sudden severe widespread appearance of oedema is suggestive of pre-eclampsia or some underlying pathology and further investigations are necessary. This oedema pits on pressure and may be found in non-dependent anatomical areas such as the face, hands, lower abdomen, and vulval and sacral areas.

Box 14.2 Laboratory findings in pre-eclampsia

- Increased haemoglobin (Hb) and haematocrit levels
- Thrombocytopenia
- Prolonged clotting times
- Raised serum creatinine and urea levels
- Raised serum uric acid level
- Abnormal liver function tests, particularly raised transaminases

Laboratory tests

The alterations in the haematological and biochemical parameters listed in Box 14.2 are suggestive of pre-eclampsia.

CARE AND MANAGEMENT

The aim of care is to monitor the condition of the woman and her fetus and, if possible, to prevent the hypertensive disorder worsening by using appropriate interventions and treatment. The ultimate aim is to prolong the pregnancy until the fetus is sufficiently mature to survive, while safeguarding the mother's life.

ANTENATAL CARE

Rest

It is preferable for the woman to rest at home and to be visited regularly by the midwife or GP. When proteinuria develops in addition to hypertension, the risks to the mother and fetus are considerably increased. Admission to hospital is required to monitor and evaluate the maternal and fetal condition.

Diet

There is little evidence to support dietary intervention for preventing or restricting the advance of pre-eclampsia.

Weight gain

Weight gain may be useful for monitoring the progression of pre-eclampsia in conjunction with other parameters.

Blood pressure and urinalysis

The blood pressure is monitored daily at home or every 4 hours when in hospital. Urine should be tested for protein daily. If protein is found in a midstream specimen of urine, a 24-hour urine collection is instigated in order to determine the amount of protein. The level of protein indicates the degree of vascular damage. Reduced kidney perfusion is indicated by:

- proteinuria
- reduced creatinine clearance
- increased serum creatinine and uric acid.

Abdominal examination

This is carried out daily. Any discomfort or tenderness may be a sign of placental abruption. Upper abdominal pain is highly significant and indicative of HELLP syndrome (see p. 148) associated with fulminating (rapid-onset) pre-eclampsia.

Fetal assessment

It is advisable to undertake a biophysical profile in order to determine fetal health and wellbeing. This is done by the use of:

- kick charts
- cardiotocography (CTG) monitoring
- serial ultrasound scans to check for fetal growth
- assessment of liquor volume and fetal breathing movements or Doppler flow studies, or both, to determine placental blood flow.

Laboratory studies

These include:

- a full blood count, platelet count and clotting profile
- urea and electrolytes
- creatinine and liver function tests, including albumin levels.

In severe pre-eclampsia blood samples should be taken every 12–24 hours.

Antihypertensive therapy

The use of antihypertensive therapy as prophylaxis is controversial, as this shows no benefit in significantly prolonging pregnancy or improving maternal or fetal outcome. Its use is, however, advocated as short-term therapy in order to prevent an increase in blood pressure and the development of severe hypertension, thereby reducing the risk to the mother of cerebral haemorrhage.

- Methyldopa is the most widely used drug in women with mild to moderate gestational hypertension and appears to be safe and effective for both mother and fetus.
- Alpha and beta blockers such as labetalol are considered safe in pregnancy. Atenolol used over the long term is not recommended as it may cause significant fetal growth restriction.

Antithrombotic agents

Early activation of the clotting system may contribute to the later pathology of pre-eclampsia; as a result the use of anticoagulants or antiplatelet agents has been considered for the prevention of pre-eclampsia and fetal growth restriction. Aspirin is thought to inhibit the production of the platelet-aggregating agent, thromboxane A_2; it is recommended for women at risk from 12 weeks.

INTRAPARTUM CARE

It is essential to monitor the maternal and fetal condition carefully.

Vital signs

- Blood pressure is measured half-hourly, or every 15–20 minutes in severe pre-eclampsia.
- Because of the potentially rapid haemodynamic changes in pre-eclampsia, a number of authors recommend the measurement of the MAP. MAP reflects the systemic perfusion pressure, and therefore the degree of hypovolaemia, whereas manual measurement of diastolic pressure alone is a better indicator of the degree of hypertension.
- Observation of the respiratory rate (>14/min) will be complemented with pulse oximetry in severe pre-eclampsia; this gives an indication of the degree of maternal hypoxia.
- Temperature should be recorded as necessary.
- In severe pre-eclampsia, examination of the optic fundi can give an indication of optic vasospasm. Cerebral irritability can be assessed by the degree of hyper-reflexia or the presence of clonus (significant if more than 3 beats).

Fluid balance

The reduced intravascular compartment in pre-eclampsia, together with poorly controlled fluid balance, can result in circulatory overload, pulmonary oedema, acute respiratory distress syndrome and ultimately death. In severe pre-eclampsia a central venous pressure (CVP) line may be considered; measurements are taken hourly.

- If the value is >10 mmHg, then 20 mg furosemide should be considered. Intravenous fluids are administered using infusion pumps; the total recommended fluid intake in severe pre-eclampsia is 85 ml/h.
- Oxytocin should be administered with caution, as it has an antidiuretic effect.
- Urinary output should be monitored and urinalysis undertaken every 4 hours to detect the presence of protein, ketones and glucose.
- In severe pre-eclampsia a urinary catheter should be in situ and urine output is measured hourly; a level >30 ml/h reflects adequate renal function.

Plasma volume expansion

Although women with pre-eclampsia have oedema, they are hypovolaemic. The blood volume of women with pre-eclampsia is reduced, as shown by a high haemoglobin (Hb) concentration and a high haematocrit level. This results in movement of fluid into the extravascular compartment, causing oedema. The oedema initially occurs in dependent tissues, but as the disease progresses oedema occurs in the liver and brain.

Pain relief

Epidural analgesia may procure the best pain relief, reduce the blood pressure and facilitate rapid caesarean section, should the need arise. It is important to ensure a normal clotting screen and a platelet count $>100 \times 10^9$/L prior to insertion of the epidural.

Fetal condition

The fetal heart rate should be monitored closely. Deviations from the normal must be reported and acted upon.

Birth plan

When the second stage commences, the obstetrician and paediatrician should be notified. A short second stage may be prescribed, depending on the maternal and fetal conditions.

- If the maternal or fetal condition shows significant deterioration during the first stage of labour, a caesarean section will be undertaken.
- Oxytocin is the preferred agent for the management of the third stage of labour.
- Ergometrine and syntometrine will cause peripheral vasoconstriction and increase hypertension; they should therefore not normally be used in the presence of any degree of pre-eclampsia, unless there is severe haemorrhage.

POSTPARTUM CARE

The maternal condition should continue to be monitored at least every 4 hours for the next 24 hours or more following childbirth, as there is still a potential danger of the mother developing eclampsia.

SIGNS OF IMPENDING ECLAMPSIA

See Box 14.3.

The aim of care at this time is to preclude death of the mother and fetus by controlling hypertension, inhibiting convulsions and preventing coma.

HELLP SYNDROME

The syndrome of haemolysis (H), elevated liver enzymes (EL) and low platelet count (LP) is generally thought to represent a variant of the pre-eclampsia/eclampsia syndrome. Pregnancies complicated by this syndrome have been associated with significant maternal and perinatal morbidity and mortality.

Box 14.3 Signs of impending eclampsia

- A sharp rise in blood pressure
- Diminished urinary output
- Increase in proteinuria
- Headache, which is usually severe, persistent and frontal in location
- Drowsiness or confusion
- Visual disturbances, such as blurring of vision or flashing lights
- Epigastric pain
- Nausea and vomiting

Clinical presentation

HELLP syndrome typically manifests itself between 32 and 34 weeks' gestation and 30% of cases will occur postpartum.

- The woman often complains of malaise, epigastric or right upper quadrant pain, and nausea and vomiting.
- Some will have non-specific viral syndrome-like symptoms.
- Hypertension and proteinuria may be absent or slightly abnormal.

Diagnosis

Pregnant women presenting with the above symptoms should have a full blood count, platelet count and liver function tests, irrespective of maternal blood pressure. The diagnosis of HELLP syndrome may be assisted by confirming:

- haemolysis
- elevated lactate dehydrogenase (LDH)
- raised bilirubin levels
- low ($<100 \times 10^9$/L) or falling platelets
- elevated liver transaminases (aspartate aminotransferase, alanine transaminase and gamma-glutamyl transferase – AST, ALT and GGT).

Complications

Subcapsular haematoma or rupture of the liver, or both together, is a rare but potentially fatal complication of the HELLP syndrome. The condition usually presents with severe epigastric pain, which may persist for several hours. In addition women may complain of neck and shoulder pain.

Management

Women with the HELLP syndrome should be admitted to a consultant unit with intensive or high-dependency care facilities available.

- In pregnancies of less than 32 weeks' gestation expectant management may be undertaken with appropriate safeguards and consent.
- In term pregnancies, or where there is a deteriorating maternal or fetal condition, immediate delivery is recommended.

ECLAMPSIA

Eclampsia is rarely seen in developed countries today; it has an incidence of 2.1 per 10 000 maternities in the UK.

Eclampsia is associated with increased risks of maternal and perinatal morbidity and mortality. Significant maternal life-threatening complications as a result of eclampsia include:

- pulmonary oedema
- renal and hepatic failure
- placental abruption and haemorrhage
- DIC
- HELLP syndrome
- brain haemorrhage.

There can be a problem in the prevention and treatment of eclampsia. A significant finding is that hypertension is not necessarily a precursor to the onset of eclampsia but will almost always be evident following a seizure. Detecting and managing imminent eclampsia is also made more difficult in that, unlike other types of seizure, warning symptoms are not always present before onset of the convulsion.

Care of a woman with eclampsia

The aims of immediate care are to:

- summon medical aid
- clear and maintain the mother's airway – this may be achieved by placing the mother in a semiprone position in order to facilitate the drainage of saliva and vomit
- administer oxygen and prevent severe hypoxia
- prevent the mother from being injured.

In the first instance all effort is devoted to the preservation of the mother's life; the wellbeing of the baby is secondary. The woman will require intensive/high-dependency care, as she may remain comatose for a time following the seizure or may be sleepy. Recordings should be carried out as for severe pre-eclampsia. Periodic restlessness associated with uterine contraction may indicate that labour has commenced. It is usual to expedite delivery of the baby when eclampsia occurs. In this instance caesarean section is the usual mode of delivery.

Anticonvulsant therapy

Magnesium sulphate is now the recommended drug of choice for routine anticonvulsant management of women with eclampsia; it is administered intravenously according to a protocol:

- A loading dose of 4 g is given over 5–10 minutes intravenously, followed by a maintenance dose of 5 g/500 ml normal saline given as an intravenous infusion at a rate of 1–2 g/h until 24 hours following delivery or the last seizure.
- Recurrent seizures should be treated with a further bolus of 2 g.
- Magnesium sulphate can be toxic and therefore the deep tendon reflexes should be monitored hourly. The respiratory rate and oxygen saturation levels are measured hourly and should remain >14/min and >95% respectively. In women with oliguria, serum magnesium levels should be monitored and maintained within the therapeutic range (2–3 mmol/l). Calcium gluconate is the antidote for magnesium toxicity and should be readily available.

Treatment of hypertension

Severe hypertension is defined as >160/110 mmHg or a MAP >125 mmHg.

- Intravenous hydralazine is the most useful agent to gain control of the blood pressure quickly; 5 mg should be administered slowly and the blood pressure measured at 5-minute intervals until the diastolic pressure reaches 90 mmHg. The diastolic blood pressure may be maintained at this level by titrating an intravenous infusion of hydralazine against the blood pressure.

- Labetalol may be used in preference to hydralazine, in which case 20 mg is given intravenously followed at 10-minute intervals by 40 mg, 80 mg and 80 mg up to a cumulative dose of 300 mg.

Fluid balance
Care must be taken not to overload the maternal system with intravenous fluids.

Anaesthesia
Both general and regional (epidural/spinal) anaesthesia carry a degree of risk in the eclamptic woman. In general, epidural is preferred in eclamptic women who are conscious, haemodynamically stable and cooperative.

Postnatal care
As almost half of eclamptic fits occur following childbirth, intensive surveillance of the woman is required in a high-dependency or intensive care unit. Parameters to monitor are:

- a return to normal blood pressure
- an increase in urine output and reduction in protein
- a reduction in oedema
- a return to normal laboratory indices.

Thromboelastic stockings should be worn to prevent deep vein thrombosis.

All the usual postpartum care is given, and as soon as the mother's condition permits, she should be taken to see her baby. Alternatively, if the baby's condition is good, he or she may be returned to the mother.

CHRONIC HYPERTENSION

Chronic hypertension has the following possible causes:

- It may be a pre-existing disorder: for example, essential hypertension.
- It may be secondary to existing medical problems, such as renal disease, SLE, coarctation of the aorta, Cushing syndrome or phaeochromocytoma.

Diagnosis
Consistent blood pressure recordings of 140/90 mmHg or more, on two occasions more than 24 hours apart during the first 20 weeks of pregnancy, suggest that the hypertension is a chronic problem and unrelated to the pregnancy. The diagnosis may be difficult to make because of the changes seen with blood pressure in pregnancy. This is a particular problem in women who present late in their pregnancy with no baseline blood pressure measurement.

Investigation
Women with chronic hypertension tend to be older, parous and have a family or personal history of hypertension.

Accurate measurement of blood pressure is important. Serial blood pressure recordings should be made in order to determine the true pattern, as even normotensive women show occasional peaks.

There may be long-term effects of hypertension, such as retinopathy, ischaemic heart disease and renal damage. Renal function tests may be performed; however, it is important to realise the extent to which the alterations in the physiological norms may affect clinical interpretation in pregnancy. Blood urate levels may help to differentiate between chronic hypertension and pre-eclampsia; they do not rise in the former as they do in the latter.

Complications

The perinatal outcome in mild chronic hypertension is good. However:

- The perinatal morbidity and mortality are increased in those women who develop severe chronic hypertension or superimposed pre-eclampsia.
- Other complications are independent of pregnancy and include renal failure and cerebral haemorrhage.
- Maternal mortality is high if phaeochromocytoma is not diagnosed and left untreated.

MANAGEMENT

Mild chronic hypertension

This is defined as a systolic blood pressure of <160 mmHg and a diastolic blood pressure of <110 mmHg. The woman is unlikely to need antenatal admission to hospital and may be cared for in the community. The woman's condition should be carefully monitored in order to identify any pre-eclampsia that develops.

Severe chronic hypertension

The systolic blood pressure is >160 mmHg and the diastolic blood pressure is >110 mmHg. Ideally, the woman will be cared for by the obstetric team in conjunction with the physician. Frequent antenatal visits are recommended in order to monitor the maternal condition.

Monitoring includes:

- blood pressure monitoring
- urinalysis to detect proteinuria
- blood tests to measure the haematocrit and renal function.

Antihypertensive drug therapy is used in order to prevent maternal complications but has no proven benefit for the fetus, nor in the prognosis of the pre-eclamptic process.

- The most commonly used agent is methyldopa 1–4 g/day in divided doses. It has a sedative effect lasting 2–3 days and is generally considered safe for mother and fetus.
- Other drugs in common usage include labetalol, nifedipine and oral hydralazine.
- Sedative drugs may be given to reduce anxiety and help the woman to rest, but are rarely recommended.

Monitoring of fetal wellbeing and of placental function should be carried out assiduously because of the risk of fetal compromise. This would include using serial growth scans and placental blood flow studies by Doppler ultrasound. If the maternal or fetal condition causes concern, the woman will be admitted to hospital. The timing of the birth is planned according to the needs of mother and fetus. If early delivery is deemed necessary, induction of labour is preferred to caesarean section.

Renal function should be reassessed postnatally and the woman should be seen by the physician with a view to long-term management of persistent hypertension. Antihypertensive therapy may be required.

CHAPTER 15

Sexually Transmissible and Reproductive Tract Infections in Pregnancy

TRENDS IN SEXUAL HEALTH

Trends of particular concern are the high rates of and increase in sexually transmitted infection (STI) diagnoses particularly in women aged 16–24. Most at risk are those who have high numbers of sexual partners, partner change and unprotected sexual intercourse.

Multidisciplinary team work

Joint management between an obstetrician and a genitourinary medicine (GUM) physician during pregnancy is essential for women with infections that are serious, life-threatening, or both, such as human immunodeficiency virus (HIV); in addition, a paediatrician is required in the care and management of the neonate infected through vertical transmission. The midwife plays a vital role in the provision of individualised care throughout pregnancy, labour and the puerperium.

INFECTIONS OF THE VAGINA AND VULVA

There are three main types of vaginal and vulval infection:
- trichomoniasis
- bacterial vaginosis
- candidiasis.

TRICHOMONIASIS

Trichomoniasis is almost exclusively sexually transmissible. It is caused by infection with the parasite *Trichomonas vaginalis*, a round or oval flagellated protozoan. Common symptoms include:
- vaginal discharge
- vulval pruritus
- inflammation.

However, 10–50% of women are asymptomatic. Vaginal discharge is present in up to 70% of cases and may vary in consistency from thin and scanty to profuse and thick. A classic frothy yellow–green discharge occurs in 10–30% of women. Dyspareunia, mild dysuria and lower abdominal pain may also be experienced.

Trichomoniasis in pregnancy
Trichomoniasis has been linked with a small risk of preterm birth and low birth weight, and an increase in the risk of HIV via sexual intercourse. Trichomoniasis may be acquired perinatally.

Diagnosis
In women:
- 95% of cases can be diagnosed by cultures
- 40–80% of cases by microscopic examination of a wet-film or acridine orange-stained slide from the posterior fornix.

Treatment
- The recommended treatment is metronidazole daily for 5–7 days or in a single dose. Although it is contraindicated, meta-analyses have concluded that there is no evidence of teratogenicity from its use in women during the first trimester of pregnancy.
- Clotrimazole pessaries daily for 7 days can be used in early pregnancy. High single-dose regimens should be avoided during pregnancy and breastfeeding.
- It is usual to treat the partner(s) and advise against sexual intercourse until the treatment is completed.
- In addition, patients should be advised not to take alcohol during the treatment and for at least 48 hours afterwards, as this may cause nausea and vomiting.

BACTERIAL VAGINOSIS

Bacterial vaginosis (BV) is the most common cause of vaginal discharge in women of childbearing age. It can arise and remit spontaneously in sexually active and non-sexually active women. It often coexists with other STIs. It is more common in:
- black women
- those with an intrauterine contraceptive device (IUCD)
- those who smoke
- pelvic inflammatory disease (PID).

In this condition the normal lactobacilli-predominant vaginal flora are replaced with a number of anaerobic bacteria. The vaginal epithelium is not inflamed; hence the term 'vaginosis' rather than 'vaginitis'. The main symptom is a malodorous and greyish watery vaginal discharge, although approximately 50% of women are asymptomatic. The odour is usually more pronounced following sexual intercourse owing to the release of amines by the alkaline semen. Vulval irritation may occur in about one-third of women.

BV in pregnancy

BV is present in up to 20% of women during pregnancy, although the majority are asymptomatic. BV during pregnancy is associated with preterm birth, low birth weight, preterm premature rupture of membranes, intra-amniotic infection and postpartum endometritis.

Diagnosis

A diagnosis of BV is confirmed if three of the following criteria are present:

- a thin, white to grey, homogeneous discharge
- 'clue cells' on microscopy (squamous epithelial cells covered with adherent bacteria)
- a vaginal pH of >4.7
- the release of a fishy odour when potassium hydroxide is added to a sample of the discharge.

A Gram-stained vaginal smear is another diagnostic technique.

Treatment

Antibiotic therapy is highly effective at eradicating infection and improving the outcome of pregnancy for women with a past history of preterm birth.

- The treatment regimen is the same as for trichomoniasis.
- Alternative treatments include oral clindamycin, intravaginal clindamycin cream or metronidazole gel.
- All these treatments have been shown in controlled trials to achieve cure rates of 70–80% after 4 weeks, but recurrences of infection are common.
- Women should be advised to avoid vaginal douching, use of shower gel and use of antiseptic agents or shampoo in the bath.

CANDIDIASIS

Candidiasis is a common cause of vulvitis, vaginitis and vaginal discharge. The causative organism is usually *Candida albicans*, a fungal parasite. It is a commensal and is found in the flora of the mouth, gastrointestinal tract and vagina. Colonisation of the vagina and vulva may be introduced from the lower intestinal tract or through sexual intercourse. During the reproductive years 10–20% of women may harbour *Candida* species but remain asymptomatic and do not require treatment. Predisposing factors that encourage *C. albicans* to convert from a commensal to a parasitic role are listed in Box 15.1.

The signs and symptoms of candidiasis include:

- intense vulval pruritus and soreness
- often, a thick, white curdy discharge (not always present)
- erythema and oedema of the vulva, vagina and cervix may be erythematous and oedematous
- white plaques of the vulva, vagina and cervix
- dyspareunia.

Box 15.1 Factors that provoke the conversion of *Candida albicans* from a commensal to a parasite

- Local changes to the vaginal immunity (e.g. vaginal douches)
- Immunosuppressant disease or treatment (e.g. acquired immunodeficiency syndrome (AIDS), chemotherapy)
- Drug therapy (e.g. antibiotics)
- Endocrine disease (e.g. diabetes mellitus)
- Physiological changes (e.g. pregnancy)
- Miscellaneous disorders (e.g. iron deficiency)

Candidiasis in pregnancy

Vaginal candidiasis is found 2–10 times more frequently in pregnant than in non-pregnant women and it is more difficult to eradicate.

Diagnosis

Vaginal culture is the most sensitive method currently available for detecting *Candida* cells.

Treatment

Candidiasis is treated primarily with antifungal pessaries or cream inserted high into the vagina at night. Preparations that may be given include:

- clotrimazole pessaries
- nystatin pessaries or gel
- oral fluconazole (Diflucan).

Diflucan is available from chemists without a prescription but this form of treatment has not been tested in pregnancy and it cannot be assumed to be safe. It should also be used with caution whilst breastfeeding owing to toxic effects in high doses.

Recurrence is common. This may be due to resistant cases or failure to complete the treatment. It is usual to treat the partner and advise against sexual intercourse until the treatment is completed. Vaginal douches and perfumed products should be avoided and tight-fitting synthetic clothing should be discouraged.

BACTERIAL INFECTIONS

CHLAMYDIA

Chlamydia trachomatis is an intracellular bacterium. It is the most common cause of sexually transmitted bacterial infection and a leading cause of PID.

- Serotypes D–K are sexually transmitted and are important causes of morbidity in both sexes.
- Serotypes A, B and C cause trachoma and blindness

- Serotypes L1–L3 cause the genital disease lymphogranuloma venereum.

Chlamydial infection is asymptomatic in approximately 80% of cases. Some women may have a purulent vaginal discharge, postcoital or intermenstrual bleeding, lower abdominal pain, mucopurulent cervicitis and/or contact bleeding. Chlamydial infection of the cervix is found in 15–30% of women attending GUM clinics, and concurrently in 35–40% of women with gonorrhoea. Specific high-risk groups include:

- women aged less than 25
- those with a new sexual partner or more than one sexual partner in recent years
- those not using barrier contraception
- those using oral contraception
- those presenting for termination of pregnancy.

Chlamydial infection has been estimated to account for 40% of ectopic pregnancies.

Chlamydia in pregnancy

It can cause amnionitis and postpartum endometritis.

Fetal and neonatal infections

The major risk to the infant is from passing through an infected cervix during birth. Up to 70% of babies born to mothers with chlamydial infection will become infected, with 30–40% developing conjunctivitis and 10–20% a characteristic pneumonia. The incubation period of chlamydial ophthalmia is 6–21 days. Chlamydial pneumonia usually occurs between the 4th and 11th weeks of life. It affects about half the babies who develop conjunctivitis but is not always preceded by it. The pharynx, middle ear, rectum and vagina are also targets for infection, with a delay of up to 7 months before cultures become positive.

Diagnosis

Nucleic acid amplification (NAA) tests should be used to screen women for genital chlamydial infection.

Treatment

Genital chlamydial infections are sensitive to three classes of antibiotic:

- the tetracyclines
- macrolides (e.g. erythromycin)
- the fluorinated quinolones, especially ofloxacin.

The tetracyclines and the fluoroquinolones are currently contraindicated in pregnancy. Erythromycin has long been the preferred treatment for cervical chlamydial infection despite its gastrointestinal effects. Erythromycin is also used for chlamydial infections in infants, young children and pregnant and lactating women. Single-dose azithromycin is expensive but gaining favour because of its effectiveness, low incidence of adverse gastrointestinal effects and enhanced compliance.

GONORRHOEA

Gonorrhoea is caused by *Neisseria gonorrhoeae*, a Gram-negative diplococcus. Transmission is by sexual contact. This organism adheres to mucous membranes. The primary sites of infection are therefore the mucous membranes of the urethra, endocervix, rectum, pharynx and conjunctiva. Gonorrhoea may coexist with other genital mucosal pathogens, notably *T. vaginalis, C. albicans* and *C. trachomatis.* Gonorrhoea is a major cause of PID. The sequelae of PID include:

- infertility
- ectopic pregnancy
- chronic pelvic pain.

Although uncommon, gonorrhoea may also cause disseminated systemic disease and arthritis.

- The most common symptom is an increased or altered vaginal discharge, although up to 50% of women are asymptomatic.
- Lower abdominal pain, dysuria, intermenstrual uterine bleeding and menorrhagia may also be experienced, ranging in intensity from minimal to severe.

Gonorrhoea in pregnancy

The incidence of gonorrhoea in pregnancy is low but its presence has been associated with:

- spontaneous abortion
- very low birth weight
- prelabour rupture of the membranes
- chorioamnionitis
- preterm birth
- postpartum endometritis
- pelvic sepsis.

Fetal and neonatal infections

N. gonorrhoeae can be transmitted during birth, or occasionally in utero when there is prolonged rupture of the membranes. The risk of transmission is between 30% and 47%. Infection usually manifests as gonococcal ophthalmia neonatorum, a notifiable condition. A profuse, purulent discharge is usually evident within a few days of birth. It can be diagnosed by microscopy and culture of an eye swab. The eyes may be cleaned with saline but systemic antibiotics are required. If left untreated, the condition will eventually lead to blindness, and occasionally the neonate may develop further infection such as gonococcal arthritis.

Diagnosis

Culture on antibiotic-containing medium is used for detecting *N. gonorrhoeae*. The sensitivity is almost 100% in specialised clinics, but isolation rates are lower in non-specialised settings.

Treatment

- The antibiotic regimen of penicillin and probenicid remains effective. Oral, single-dose preparations are now most commonly given.
- In the case of penicillin allergy or penicillin-resistant organisms, spectinomycin or ceftriaxone are also effective.

SYPHILIS

Syphilis is caused by the bacterium *Treponema pallidum*, a spiral organism (spirochaete), and is usually acquired by sexual contact. It can also be congenitally transmitted. It is a complex systemic disease that can involve virtually any organ in the body.

Acquired syphilis is divided into the stages shown in Box 15.2.

Syphilis in pregnancy

Although sequelae are dependent on the stage of infection in the mother, untreated syphilis in pregnancy may result in:

- spontaneous abortion
- preterm birth
- stillbirth
- neonatal death
- significant infant or later morbidity.

Vertical transmission may occur at any time during pregnancy, but is more likely if the mother has primary, secondary or early latent syphilis. The infection does not usually occur before the 4th month of pregnancy because treponemes from the maternal circulation are unable to pass through the Langhans cell layer of the early placenta.

Congenital syphilis

Approximately two-thirds of live-born infected infants do not have any signs or symptoms at birth, but they present over the following weeks, months or years. Lesions develop only after the 4th month when immunological competence

---

Box 15.2 Stages of acquired syphilis

Early infectious

- *Primary*: 9–90 days after exposure (mean 21 days)
- *Secondary*: 6 weeks to 6 months after exposure (4–8 weeks after primary lesion)
- *Latent (early)*: 2 years after exposure

Late non-infectious

- *Latent (late)*: ≥2 years after exposure with no symptoms or signs
- *Neurosyphilis, cardiovascular syphilis, gummatous syphilis*: 3–20 years after exposure

becomes established. Serology at birth is unreliable owing to passive transfer from the mother and the treponemal-specific IgM test is prone to false positive and negative results.

Diagnosis

Women in the UK are screened for syphilis at antenatal booking and treated if need be. However, this does not detect women who acquire the infection during pregnancy, or women who are incubating syphilis at the time of serological testing. A range of serological tests is used for screening (Box 15.3).

Treatment

- The preferred treatment is intramuscular penicillin.
- In the case of penicillin allergy, the alternative is erythromycin, as tetracycline is contraindicated in pregnancy.
- The poor placental transfer of erythromycin does not reliably cure the fetus and as a precaution the baby may be given a course of penicillin at birth.

GROUP B STREPTOCOCCUS (GBS)

GBS (*Streptococcus agalactiae*) is a Gram-positive bacterium that naturally colonises the body. It is harboured primarily in the gastrointestinal tract, with approximately 30% of adults asymptomatically carrying the organism at any one time. It also colonises the vagina in up to 25% of women.

GBS in pregnancy

In pregnant women colonised with GBS, high-risk factors associated with vertical transmission include:

- preterm birth
- prolonged rupture of membranes
- maternal pyrexia during labour
- GBS cultured in a urine sample
- known carriage of GBS
- a history of a GBS infection in a previous pregnancy.

GBS is able to infiltrate the amniotic cavity, whether or not the membranes are intact, and infects the fetus through the lung epithelium. Postpartum endometritis and postcaesarean wound infection may also occur in the mother.

Box 15.3 Serological tests for syphilis

- Venereal Diseases Research Laboratory (VDRL)
- Rapid plasma reagin (RPR) test
- *Treponema pallidum* haemagglutination assay (TPHA)
- *Treponema pallidum* particle agglutination (TPPA) assay
- Fluorescent treponemal antibody absorption (FTA-abs) test
- Treponemal enzyme immunoassay (EIA)

Fetal and neonatal infections

GBS is the commonest cause of overwhelming sepsis in newborns during the first days of life, occurring at a rate of approximately 1–2 per 1000 live births. The respiratory infection rapidly progresses to sepsis and shock and causes significant morbidity and mortality. GBS infection in the neonate may be:

- early onset, in which case the infection starts in utero
- late onset, which usually presents between 7 days and 3 months of age.

Diagnosis

- Vaginal and rectal swabs can detect colonisation with GBS, although higher rates are detected with a special enrichment culture medium. The degree of colonisation is extremely variable and the tendency for recolonisation after treatment makes control difficult.
- Swabs taken late in pregnancy at around 35 weeks are effective in predicting whether or not GBS will be carried during labour.

Treatment

Intrapartum antibiotic treatment of women colonised with GBS appears to reduce neonatal infection.

- The usual regimen is intravenous ampicillin during labour.
- Alternatives include benzyl penicillin or erythromycin.

VIRAL INFECTIONS

GENITAL WARTS

Genital warts are caused by human papillomavirus (HPV) types 6 and 11. Transmission is most often by sexual contact, although infants and young children may develop laryngeal papillomas after being infected from maternal genital warts at birth.

In pregnancy genital warts may dramatically increase in size and appear as cauliflower-like masses, although they usually diminish in size following the birth. Occasionally they can obstruct a vaginal birth; therefore a caesarean section would be indicated.

- Genital warts are difficult and time-consuming to treat.
- They are usually treated initially with locally applied caustic agents such as podophyllum. However, this is contraindicated in pregnancy because of possible teratogenic effects.
- It is recommended that no treatment be offered during pregnancy, although there are alternatives such as trichloroacetic acid, cryotherapy or electrocautery.

Women presenting with genital warts should be fully investigated to exclude other STIs. In addition, colposcopy should be performed to exclude flat warts on the cervix. Most genital warts are benign, but cervical intraepithelial neoplasia (CIN) is strongly associated with HPV types 16, 18, 31, 33 and 35; therefore an annual cervical smear is recommended.

HEPATITIS B VIRUS (HBV)

HBV infection is an important cause of morbidity and mortality from acute infection and chronic sequelae that include chronic active hepatitis, cirrhosis and primary liver cancer. HBV can be transmitted sexually or parenterally mainly through infected blood or blood products. It can be transmitted by means of unsterilised equipment, such as may be used when injecting drug users share needles and syringes, or in tattooing or acupuncture, or as a consequence of needle-stick injury in healthcare workers. Vertical transmission is a major mode of transmission, most frequently occurring perinatally. Acute HBV infection during pregnancy is associated with an increased rate of spontaneous abortion and preterm labour. There are usually two phases of symptoms:

- The prodromal phase, characterised by flu-like symptoms.
- The icteric phase, characterised by jaundice, anorexia, nausea and fatigue.

The infection may be asymptomatic in 10–50% of adults in the acute phase and in virtually all infants and children. If chronic infection occurs, there are often no physical signs but there may be signs of chronic liver disease.

In the acute early phase the hepatitis B surface antigen (HBsAg, formally called Australia antigen) is produced by the infected hepatocytes and appears in the sera of most patients. The presence of the hepatitis Be antigen (HBeAg) in the serum indicates viral activity, which can persist over days or weeks. IgM- and IgG-type antibodies to the core antigen develop. IgG antibodies may be detectable for many years after recovery. As the infection resolves, HBeAg becomes undetectable; once infection is cleared, the antibody to the surface antigen component, anti-HBs, appears, indicating immunity. If HBsAg remains detectable for more than 6 months, the patient is usually referred to as a hepatitis B virus carrier.

All pregnant women should be offered antenatal screening for HBV and babies born to infected mothers should be vaccinated.

- The injections should be administered at birth and at 1 and 6 months.
- In addition, the babies of mothers who have become infected with HBV during pregnancy and those who do not have anti-HBe antibodies should also receive hepatitis B-specific immunoglobulin (HBIg) at birth. This should be injected at a different site to the vaccine (the anterolateral thigh is the preferred site in infants). This confers immediate immunity and reduces vertical transmission by 90%.
- Infected mothers should continue to breastfeed, as there is no additional risk of transmission.

HEPATITIS C VIRUS (HCV)

HCV infection is another type of viral hepatitis that occurs throughout the world.

- The principal route of transmission is by percutaneous inoculation, blood and blood products.
- The incidence of transmission by sexual contact is low.
- Vertical transmission is also low, occurring at 5% or less, but higher rates are seen if the mother is HIV- and HCV-positive.

At present there is no known way of reducing the risk of vertical transmission. There is no firm evidence that breastfeeding constitutes an additional risk of transmission unless the mother is symptomatic with a high viral load.

HERPES SIMPLEX VIRUS (HSV)

There are two types of HSV: HSV-1 and HSV-2.

- HSV-1 causes the majority of orolabial infections, and is often acquired during childhood through direct physical contact with oral secretions.
- HSV-2 is the most common cause of genital herpes and is sexually transmitted via genital secretions.

Infections may be primary or non-primary. Once infected, the virus remains in the individual for life, causing recurrent infection. Prior infection with HSV-1 modifies the clinical manifestations of first infection by HSV-2. The incidence of HSV infection depends on factors such as:

- age
- duration of sexual activity
- number of sexual partners
- socioeconomic status
- previous genital infections
- race.

In adults, HSV infection may be asymptomatic, but painful, vesicular or ulcerative lesions of the skin and mucous membranes occur frequently. Dysuria and vaginal or urethral discharge may also occur. There may be systemic symptoms of fever and myalgia. Symptoms are more common in primary infection.

Genital herpes infection

This is defined as:

- *First episode primary infection* – first infection with either HSV-1 or HSV-2 in an individual with no pre-existing antibodies to either type. The local symptoms tend to be severe and lesions may last for 2–3 weeks.
- *First episode non-primary infection* – first infection with either HSV-1 or HSV-2 in an individual with pre-existing circulating antibodies to the other type.
- *Recurrent infection* – recurrence of clinical symptoms due to reactivation of pre-existent HSV-1 or HSV-2 infection after a period of latency.

HSV in pregnancy

The most important complication of HSV infection in pregnancy is neonatal herpes, a rare but potentially very serious condition. Congenital infection, a consequence of primary infection early in pregnancy, can cause severe abnormalities that in the absence of vesicles are difficult to distinguish from similar syndromes caused by rubella, toxoplasmosis or cytomegalovirus. The risk of neonatal infection is about 40% with active primary infection, but less than 8% with recurrent infections at the time of delivery and rare with asymptomatic shedding.

Diagnosis

- Viral cultures from open lesions are one of the best methods of diagnosing infection but they have a significant false negative rate. Culture levels are normally available within 48–96 hours.
- Serological tests that demonstrate rising titres of HSV antibodies can be used for the diagnosis of primary infections only by confirming seroconversion. The presence of antibody titre in an initial specimen or the presence of a typical lesion is suggestive of non-primary first episode or recurrent disease.
- These tests cannot reliably distinguish between HSV-1 and HSV-2 except by using HSV-type specific glycoprotein G as the antigen.

Treatment

The treatment and management in pregnancy include:

- antiviral therapy
- saline bathing
- analgesia
- topical anaesthetic gels.

Primary infection acquired during the first or second trimester should be treated with oral or intravenous antiviral therapy, depending on the clinical condition. Aciclovir reduces viral shedding, reduces pain and promotes the healing of lesions. It is not licensed for use in pregnancy. The recommended dose is the same as for non-pregnant adults, but higher doses may be required for immunocompromised women. Continuous aciclovir in the last 4 weeks of pregnancy reduces the risk of clinical recurrence at term and delivery by caesarean section.

In the third trimester, women with active genital lesions after 34 weeks should be delivered by caesarean section, as the risk of viral shedding and vertical transmission is high. Recurrent HSV infection during pregnancy is also treated with aciclovir. Caesarean section is not indicated unless genital lesions or prodromal symptoms of an impending outbreak, such as vulval pain or burning, are present.

CYTOMEGALOVIRUS (CMV)

Cytomegalovirus is a member of the herpes virus family. Seroepidemiological studies show that CMV infection is common. Most CMV infections are subclinical. However, the clinical manifestations of CMV infection vary with age, route of transmission and the immune competence of the subject. Primary infection may cause generally mild mononucleosis-type symptoms such as malaise, myalgia and fever in immunocompetent adults, whereas it is particularly pathogenic among immunosuppressed individuals, recipients of organ transplants, premature infants and patients with AIDS.

CMV infection in pregnancy

Several studies have shown that primary infection occurs in all trimesters, with about 37% of neonates being born with congenital infection. As the majority of these do not develop the disease, it is not a sufficient criterion to recommend TOP (Termination of Pregnancy).

Fetal and neonatal infections

CMV is the most common intrauterine infection, affecting from 0.4% to 2.3% of all live births. Unlike rubella, which has a teratogenic effect, CMV allows fetal organs to develop normally but causes disease by the secondary destruction of the cells. Up to 18% of infants born to mothers with primary infection may be symptomatic at birth. The prognosis is thus poor. More than 90% of all symptomatic patients develop sensorineural hearing loss, mental retardation, chorioretinitis and other more subtle complications in later years. In infants with subclinical infection the outlook is much better, but 5–15% will develop some sequelae that are generally less severe than in infants with symptomatic infection at birth.

Perinatal infections result from exposure to CMV in the maternal genital tract at birth or from breast milk. The majority of infants are asymptomatic; occasionally, however, perinatally acquired infection is associated with pneumonitis in preterm and sick full-term infants, neurological sequelae and psychomotor retardation.

Diagnosis

CMV infections can be diagnosed by direct methods such as:
- viral cultures (from urine, saliva, breast milk, cervical secretions, biopsy and autopsy specimens)
- polymerase chain reaction (PCR)
- antigen detection.

Treatment

Ganciclovir and foscarnet have been used with encouraging results in life-threatening CMV infections in immunocompromised hosts. Both drugs are, however, extensively toxic.

HUMAN IMMUNODEFICIENCY VIRUS (HIV)

There are two types of HIV: HIV-1 and HIV-2.
- HIV-1 is the cause of the worldwide spread of AIDS.
- HIV-2 is largely confined to West Africa.

The three principal means of HIV transmission are by:
- blood or blood products
- sexual contact
- passage from mother to child.

Two to 6 weeks after exposure to HIV, 50–70% of those infected develop a transient non-specific illness with fever, myalgia, malaise, lymphadenopathy and pharyngitis. Over 50% develop a rash. Oral and genital ulcers have also been reported. The illness begins abruptly and usually lasts for 1–2 weeks, but could be more protracted. Seroconversion is usually followed by an asymptomatic period lasting on average 10 years without antiretroviral therapy. However, although the infection is latent clinically, there is intense viral and lymphocyte turnover with worsening immunodeficiency. Approximately one-third of patients will experience persistent generalised lymphadenopathy. The average time for progression from HIV to AIDS is between 5 and 20 years.

HIV in pregnancy

HIV-1 infection is associated with poor pregnancy outcomes. The most serious effect of HIV-1 infection during pregnancy is vertical transmission. This can occur during pregnancy, in the intrapartum period or postnatally. In non-breastfed infants, up to 75% of transmission is thought to occur in late pregnancy and the period covering labour and birth.

HIV-1 DNA is present in breast milk and so postnatal transmission can occur during breastfeeding. Avoidance of breastfeeding by HIV-1-infected women is therefore recommended if safe and affordable alternatives are available. Other factors associated with an increased risk of transmission are listed in Box 15.4.

Diagnosis

- Acute infection is accompanied by the development of serum antibodies in the case of core and surface proteins of the virus in 2–6 weeks. Over 90% of seroconversions occur within 3 months of infection. In a minority of cases seroconversion may be delayed to more than 6 months; therefore negative diagnostic tests need to be repeated 3 months after possible exposure and after 6–9 months where there has been a high risk of transmission. Following seroconversion, antibody persists indefinitely in the serum and forms a highly specific test for HIV infection. One or more enzyme immunoassays (EIAs) directed towards HIV-1 and HIV-2 are used as the initial screening tests.
- Positive screening tests are confirmed by serum titre tests, a Western blot or immunofluorescence assay.
- Babies born to infected mothers may have maternal HIV antibody. A specific test such as PCR can confirm HIV infection in 95% of infected infants by 1 month of age.

Box 15.4 Factors associated with an increased risk of transmission in HIV

- Breastfeeding
- Advanced clinical HIV disease
- Impaired maternal immunocompetence
- Maternal nutritional status
- Resistant viral strains
- Vaginal birth
- Prolonged rupture of membranes
- Invasive obstetric procedures
- Maternal ulcerative genital infection
- Recreational drug use during pregnancy
- Prematurity
- Low birth weight

Treatment

- The incidence of mother-to-child transmission can be significantly reduced as a result of measures that include counselling, testing, antiretroviral treatment and infant formula feeding.
- Antiviral drugs include zidovudine, lamivudine and nevirapine. Regimens involve different combinations over different time periods.
- Antiretroviral medication may be given antenatally, intrapartum, postnatally and prophylactically to babies. Highly active antiretroviral therapy (HAART) has significantly reduced vertical transmission rates.
- In the event of labour, measures can be taken to avoid situations known to predispose to vertical transmission of HIV. Amniotomy is contraindicated and labour should be augmented if contractions are either weak or absent to avoid a prolonged interval between membrane rupture and birth. Invasive techniques, such as direct cardiotocography monitoring through scalp clips and fetal blood sampling, should be avoided and the restrictive use of episiotomy is recommended. Instrumental delivery should be avoided to minimise abrasions to both mother and baby.
- Elective caesarean section should be recommended and breastfeeding avoided in developed countries.

HIV antibody testing and counselling in pregnancy

An HIV test is offered to all pregnant women. Post-test counselling will involve the giving of positive, negative or indeterminate results. Issues for discussion include the natural history of the infection, treatment options and safe sex to avoid transmission to an HIV-negative partner(s) and acquisition of other STIs. The diagnosis should be confirmed by a second test and an immediate referral should be made for specialist medical assessment.

CHAPTER 16

Multiple Pregnancy

The term 'multiple pregnancy' is used to describe the development of more than one fetus in utero at the same time.

TWIN PREGNANCY

TYPES OF TWIN PREGNANCY

Twins will be either monozygotic (MZ) or dizygotic (DZ) (Box 16.1). Of all twins born in the UK, two-thirds will be DZ and one-third MZ.

Superfecundation is the term used when twins are conceived from sperm from different men if a woman has had more than one partner during a menstrual cycle. It is not known how often this happens, but if suspected then paternity can be checked by DNA testing.

Superfetation is the term used for twins conceived as the result of two coital acts in different menstrual cycles. This is thought to be very rare.

Determination of zygosity and chorionicity

Determination of zygosity means determining whether or not the twins are identical.

- In about one-third of all twins born this will be obvious, as the children will be of a different sex.
- At birth, identical twins tend to have a greater weight variation than non-identical ones.
- In approximately two-thirds of identical twins a monochorionic placenta will confirm monozygosity. If the babies have a single outer membrane, the chorion, they must be MZ.
- In one-third of identical twins the placenta will have two chorions and two amnions, and either fused placentae or two separate placentae (dichorionic); this situation is indistinguishable from that in non-identical twins. It occurs when the fertilised oocyte splits within the first 3 or 4 days after fertilisation and while it is still in the uterine tube.
- When these entities are seen on an early scan they appear as two separate placentae and are dichorionic and diamniotic, exactly the same as non-identical twins.

Box 16.1 Monozygosity and dizygosity

Monozygotic or uniovular twins
- Also referred to as 'identical twins'
- Develop from the fusion of one oocyte and one spermatozoon, which after fertilisation splits into two
- Are of the same sex and have the same genes, blood groups and physical features such as eye and hair colour, ear shapes and palm creases; may be of different sizes and sometimes have different personalities

Dizygotic or binovular twins
- Also referred to as 'non-identical twins'
- Develop from two separate oocytes that are fertilised by two different spermatozoa
- Are no more alike than any brother or sister and can be of the same or different sex

---

- In about two-thirds of cases the division occurs up to approximately 10–12 days after fertilisation; these will be monochorionic and diamniotic.
- Monoamniotic twins occur in about 1% of cases, when the embryo divides after 12 days.

Monochorionic twin pregnancies have a 3–5 times higher risk of perinatal mortality and morbidity than dichorionic twin pregnancies.

Zygosity determination after birth

The most accurate method of determining zygosity is to compare DNA. DNA can be extracted from cells taken from a cheek swab from inside the mouth. Specific genetic markers extracted from different chromosomes are compared and the results are up to 99.99% accurate.

Zygosity determination should be routinely offered to all same-sex twins for the reasons listed in Box 16.2.

Box 16.2 Reasons for determining zygosity

- Most parents will want to know whether or not their twins are identical
- If parents are considering further pregnancies, they will want to know the likelihood of having twins again:
  - DZ twins tend to run in families and the increased likelihood is approximately five-fold
  - MZ twins do not run in families and the likelihood does not change
- It will help the twins in establishing their sense of identity; it will influence their life and family relationships
- The information is important for genetic reasons: not just the monogenic disorders but with any serious illness later in life
- Twins are frequently asked to be involved in research where knowledge of zygosity is essential

DIAGNOSIS OF TWIN PREGNANCY

This is usually through ultrasound examination. Diagnosis can be made as early as 6 weeks into the pregnancy, or later at the routine detailed structural scan between the 18th and 20th weeks. A family history of twins should alert the midwife to the possibility of a multiple pregnancy. Occasionally (1 in 12 000 live births), one fetus may die in the second trimester and become a fetus papyraceous, which becomes embedded in the surface of the placenta and expelled with the placenta at delivery.

Abdominal examination
See Box 16.3.

THE PREGNANCY

A multiple pregnancy tends to be shorter than a single pregnancy. The average gestation for twins is 37 weeks, for triplets 34 weeks, and for quadruplets 33 weeks.

Box 16.3 Abdominal examination in the diagnosis of multiple pregnancy

Inspection

- The size of the uterus may be larger than expected for the period of gestation, particularly after the 20th week. The uterus may look broad or round
- Fetal movements may be seen over a wide area, although the findings are not diagnostic of twins
- Fresh striae gravidarum may be apparent
- Up to twice the amount of amniotic fluid is normal in a twin pregnancy but polyhydramnios is not an uncommon complication of a twin pregnancy, particularly with monochorionic twins

Palpation

- The fundal height may be greater than expected for the period of gestation
- The presence of two fetal poles (head or breech) in the fundus of the uterus may be noted; multiple fetal limbs may also be palpable
- The head may be small in relation to the size of the uterus
- Lateral palpation may reveal two fetal backs or limbs on both sides
- Pelvic palpation may give findings similar to those on fundal palpation, although one fetus may lie behind the other and make detection difficult
- Location of three poles in total is diagnostic of at least two fetuses

Auscultation

- Hearing two fetal hearts is not diagnostic; however, if simultaneous comparison of the heart rates reveals a difference of at least 10 beats per minute, it may be assumed that two hearts are being heard

Effects of pregnancy

Exacerbation of common disorders

More than one fetus and the higher levels of circulating hormones often exacerbate the common disorders of pregnancy. Sickness, nausea and heartburn may be more persistent and more troublesome than in a singleton pregnancy.

Anaemia

Iron deficiency and folic acid deficiency anaemias are common. Early growth and development of the uterus and its contents make greater demands on the maternal iron stores; in later pregnancy (after the 28th week) fetal demands may lead to anaemia. Routine prescription of iron and folic acid supplements is not necessary.

Polyhydramnios

This is particularly associated with monochorionic twins and with fetal abnormalities. Polyhydramnios will add to any discomfort that the woman is already experiencing. Acute polyhydramnios can lead to miscarriage or premature labour.

Pressure symptoms

Impaired venous return from the lower limbs increases the tendency to varicose veins and oedema of the legs. Backache is common and the increased uterine size may also lead to marked dyspnoea and to indigestion.

Other effects

There can be an increase in complications of pregnancy.

Antenatal screening

- Nuchal translucency for Down syndrome is accurate only if performed between 11 and 13 weeks.
- Serum screening is not usually performed in multiple pregnancy, as results are too complex to interpret.
- Chorionic villus sampling (CVS) is not usually recommended in multiple pregnancy, as loss rates are high.
- Amniocentesis can be performed in twin pregnancies, usually between 15 and 20 weeks. It should be performed in a specialist fetal medicine unit. Most obstetricians prefer to do a dual needle insertion so there is no chance of contamination between the two sacs.
- Chorionicity should be determined in the first trimester.
- All MZ twins should have echocardiography performed at approximately 20 weeks' gestation, as there is a much higher risk of cardiac anomalies in these babies.

Ultrasound examination

- Monochorionic twin pregnancies should be scanned every 2 weeks from diagnosis to check for discordant fetal growth and signs of twin-to-twin transfusion syndrome (TTTS).

- Dichorionic twin pregnancies should be scanned at 20 weeks for anomalies, and then usually every 4 weeks.

ANTENATAL PREPARATION

Early diagnosis of a twin pregnancy and of chorionicity is extremely important in order to support and advise the parents.

Preparation for breastfeeding

Mothers should be advised not only that it is possible to breastfeed two, and in some cases three, babies, but also that, nutritionally, this is the best way for her to feed her babies.

LABOUR AND BIRTH

ONSET OF LABOUR

The higher the number of fetuses the mother is carrying, the earlier the labour is likely to start. Term for twins is usually considered to be 37 weeks rather than 40, and approximately 30% of twins are born preterm. In addition to being preterm the babies may be small for gestational age and therefore prone to the associated complications of both conditions. If spontaneous labour begins very early the mother may be given drugs to inhibit uterine activity. Known causes of preterm labour, for example urinary tract infection, should be treated with antibiotics.

It is very unusual for a twin pregnancy to last more than 40 weeks; many obstetricians advise induction of labour at 38 weeks. If the first twin is in a cephalic presentation, labour is usually allowed to continue normally to a vaginal birth, but if the first twin is presenting in any other way (Fig. 16.1), an elective caesarean section is usually recommended.

MANAGEMENT OF LABOUR

- Induction of labour usually occurs around 38 weeks' gestation. The presence of complications such as pregnancy-induced hypertension, intrauterine growth restriction or twin-to-twin transfusion syndrome may be reasons for earlier induction.
- The majority will go into labour spontaneously. There is an increased incidence of dysfunctional labour in twin pregnancies, possibly because of overdistension of the uterus.
- Continuous fetal heart monitoring of both babies is advocated. This can be achieved:
  - with two external transducers, *or*
  - once the membranes are ruptured, with a scalp electrode on the presenting twin and an external transducer on the second.

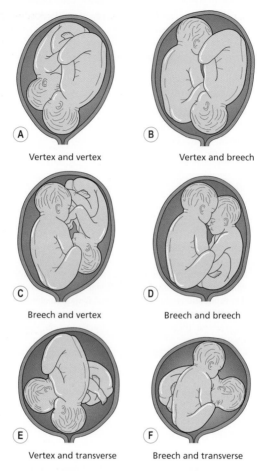

Fig. 16.1: Presentation of twins before birth. (After Bryan 1984, with permission of Edward Arnold.)

- If a 'twin monitor' is available, both heartbeats can be monitored simultaneously to give a more reliable reading. Uterine activity will also need to be monitored.
- If cardiotocography (CTG) is not available, use of the Doptone or Sonicaid may give more accurate recordings of the fetal heart rates than a fetal stethoscope. If the latter has to be used, two people must auscultate simultaneously so that fetal heart rates are counted over the same minute.

- Mobilisation is encouraged or the adoption of whichever position the mother finds most comfortable. A foam rubber wedge under the side of the mattress will help to prevent supine hypotensive syndrome by giving a lateral tilt. A birthing chair or a reclining chair may be more comfortable than a delivery bed.
- Regional epidural block provides excellent analgesia and, if necessary, allows easier instrumental deliveries and also manipulation of the second twin. The use of inhalation analgesia may be helpful, either before the epidural is in situ or during the second stage if the effect of the epidural is wearing off.
- If fetal compromise occurs during labour, delivery will need to be expedited, usually by caesarean section. Action may also need to be taken if the mother's condition gives cause for concern.
- If uterine activity is poor, the use of intravenous oxytocin may be required once the membranes have been ruptured.
- If the babies are expected to be premature and of low birth weight or known to have any other problems, the neonatal unit must be informed.

MANAGEMENT OF THE BIRTHS

- The second stage of labour may be confirmed by a vaginal examination. The obstetrician, paediatric team and anaesthetist should be present for the births because of the risk of complications.
- If epidural analgesia has been used, it may be 'topped up'.
- The possibility of emergency caesarean section is ever-present and the operating theatre should be ready to receive the mother at short notice.
- Monitoring of both fetal hearts should continue.
- Provided that the first twin is presenting by the vertex, the birth can be expected to proceed normally.
- When the first twin is born, the time of birth and the sex are noted. This baby and cord must be labelled as 'twin one' immediately.
- The baby may be put to the breast because suckling stimulates uterine contractions.
- If the first baby requires active resuscitation, the paediatric team will take over.
- After the birth of the first twin, abdominal palpation is carried out to ascertain the lie, presentation and position of the second twin and to auscultate the fetal heart:
  - If the lie is not longitudinal, an attempt may be made to correct it by external cephalic version.
  - If it is longitudinal, a vaginal examination is made to confirm the presentation.
  - If the presenting part is not engaged, it should be guided into the pelvis by fundal pressure before the second sac of membranes is ruptured.

- The fetal heart should be auscultated again once the membranes are ruptured.
- If uterine activity does not recommence, intravenous oxytocin may be used to stimulate it.
- When the presenting part becomes visible, the mother should be encouraged to push with contractions to birth the second twin.
- Owing to the reduced size of the placental site following the birth of the first twin, the second fetus may be somewhat deprived of oxygen.
- The birth of the second twin should be completed within 45 minutes of the first twin as long as there are no signs of fetal distress in the second twin; if there are, the birth must be expedited and the second twin may need to be delivered by caesarean section.
- A uterotonic drug (usually Syntocinon or Syntometrine) is usually given intramuscularly or intravenously, depending on local policy, after the birth of the anterior shoulder.
- This baby and cord are labelled as 'twin two'. A note of the time of birth and the sex of the child is made.
- The risk of asphyxia is greater for the second twin. The baby may need to be transferred to the neonatal unit but shown to the mother prior to transfer.
- Once the uterotonic drug has taken effect, controlled cord traction is applied to both cords simultaneously and the placentae should be delivered without delay. Emptying the uterus enables bleeding to be controlled and postpartum haemorrhage (PPH) is prevented. An infusion of 40 IU of Syntocinon in 500 ml of normal saline should be prepared for prophylactic use in the management of PPH.
- The placenta(e) should be examined and the number of amniotic sacs, chorions and placentae noted. Pathological examination of placentae and membranes may be needed to confirm chorionicity.

COMPLICATIONS ASSOCIATED WITH MULTIPLE PREGNANCY

The high perinatal mortality associated with twinning is largely due to complications of pregnancy, such as the premature onset of labour, intrauterine growth restriction and complications of delivery.

Polyhydramnios

Acute polyhydramnios may occur as early as 18–20 weeks. It may be associated with fetal abnormality but it is more likely to be due to TTTS.

Twin-to-twin transfusion syndrome

Also known as fetofetal transfusion syndrome (FFTS), this can be acute or chronic. The acute form usually occurs during labour and is the result of a blood transfusion from one fetus (donor) to the other (recipient) through vascular anastomosis in a monochorionic placenta. Both fetuses may die of cardiac failure if not treated immediately.

Chronic TTTS can occur in up to 35% of monochorionic twin pregnancies and accounts for 15–17% of perinatal mortality in twins. The placenta in TTTS transfuses blood from one twin fetus to the other. These cases are characterised by one or more deep unidirectional arteriovenous anastomoses. This results in anaemia and growth restriction in the donor twin and polycythaemia with circulatory overload in the recipient twin (hydrops). The fetal and neonatal mortality is high but some infants may be saved by early diagnosis and prenatal treatment with either amnioreduction, which may have to be repeated regularly as fluid can reaccumulate rapidly, or laser coagulation of communicating placental vessels. Selective fetocide is sometimes considered.

Fetal abnormality
This is particularly associated with MZ twins.

Conjoined twins
This extremely rare malformation of MZ twinning results from the incomplete division of the fertilised oocyte. Delivery has to be by caesarean section. Separation of the babies is sometimes possible and will depend on how they are joined and which internal organs are involved.

Acardiac twins (twin reversed arterial perfusion – TRAP)
One twin presents without a well-defined cardiac structure and is kept alive through placental anastomoses to the circulatory system of the viable fetus.

Fetus-in-fetu (endoparasite)
Parts of one fetus may be lodged within another fetus; this can happen only in MZ twins.

Malpresentations
The fetuses can restrict each other's movements, which may result in malpresentations, particularly of the second twin. After the birth of the first twin, the presentation of the second twin may change.

Premature rupture of the membranes
Malpresentations due to polyhydramnios may predispose to preterm rupture of the membranes.

Prolapse of the cord
This is associated with malpresentations and polyhydramnios and is more likely if there is a poorly fitting presenting part. The second twin is particularly at risk.

Prolonged labour
Malpresentations are a poor stimulus to good uterine action and a distended uterus is likely to lead to poor uterine activity and consequently prolonged labour.

Monoamniotic twins
Monoamniotic twins risk cord entanglement with occlusion of the blood supply to one or both fetuses. Delivery is usually at around 32–34 weeks and by caesarean section.

Locked twins

This is a rare but serious complication. There are two types: one occurs when the first twin presents by the breech and the second by the vertex, the other when both are vertex presentations (Fig. 16.2). In both instances the head of the second twin prevents the continued descent of the first.

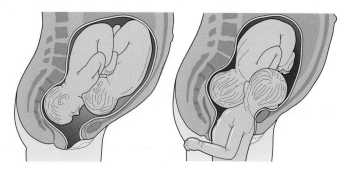

Fig. 16.2: Locked twins.

Delay in the birth of the second twin

After delivery of the first twin, uterine activity should recommence within 5 minutes. Birth of the second twin is usually completed within 45 minutes of the first birth. In the past the birth interval was limited to 30 minutes in an attempt to minimise complications. With the introduction of fetal heart rate monitoring the interval time between babies is not so crucial as long as the fetal condition is monitored. Poor uterine action as a result of malpresentation may be the cause of delay. The risks of delay are:

● intrauterine hypoxia
● birth asphyxia following premature separation of the placenta
● sepsis as a result of ascending infection from the first umbilical cord, which lies outside the vulva.

After the birth of the first twin the lower uterine segment begins to reform and the cervical canal may have to dilate fully again.

The midwife may need to 'rub up' a contraction and to put the first twin to the mother's breast to stimulate uterine activity.

● If there appears to be an obstruction, a caesarean section may be necessary.
● If there is no obstruction, oxytocin infusion may be commenced or forceps delivery considered.

Premature expulsion of the placenta

The placenta may be expelled before delivery of the second twin.

● In dichorionic twins with separate placentae, one placenta may be delivered separately.

- In monochorionic twins, the shared placenta may be expelled. The risks of severe asphyxia and death of the second twin are then very high.
- Haemorrhage is also likely if one twin is retained in utero, as this prevents adequate retraction of the placental site.

Postpartum haemorrhage
Poor uterine tone as a result of overdistension or hypotonic activity is likely to lead to postpartum haemorrhage.

Undiagnosed twins
The possibility of an unexpected undiagnosed second baby should be considered if the uterus appears larger than expected after the birth of the first baby or if the baby is surprisingly smaller than expected. If a uterotonic drug has been given after the birth of the anterior shoulder of the first baby, the second baby is in great danger and delivery should be expedited. He or she will require active resuscitation because of severe asphyxia.

POSTNATAL PERIOD

CARE OF THE BABIES

Immediate care at delivery is the same as for a single baby. Identification of the infants should be clear and the parents should be given the opportunity to check the identity bracelets and cuddle their babies.

Nutrition
Both babies may be breastfed, either simultaneously or separately. The mother may choose to feed artificially.

- If the babies are small for gestational age or preterm, the paediatrician may recommend that the babies be 'topped up' after a breastfeed. Expressed breast milk is the best form of nutrition for these babies.
- If the babies are not able to suck adequately at the breast, then the mother should be encouraged to express her milk regularly for her babies.
- If she does not have sufficient milk for them, milk from a human milk bank can be used, which is much better for preterm babies than formula milk.

The more stimulation the breasts are given, the more plentiful is the milk supply.

CARE OF THE MOTHER

- Involution of the uterus will be slower because of its increased bulk. 'Afterpains' may be troublesome and analgesia should be offered.
- A good diet is essential, and if the mother is breastfeeding, she requires a high-protein, high-calorie diet. It is quite common for breastfeeding mothers to feel hungry between meals.

- Once the mother is at home she must be encouraged to rest and eat a well-balanced diet. Routine is the essence of coping with new babies.

Isolation can be a real problem for new mothers. The incidence of postnatal depression has been shown to be significantly higher in twin mothers.

TRIPLETS AND HIGHER-ORDER BIRTHS

The rapidly increasing number of surviving triplets and higher-order births will produce many more families needing special advice and support from healthcare workers.

A woman expecting three or more babies is at risk of all the same complications as one expecting twins, but more so. She is more likely to have a period in hospital resting before the babies are born and they will almost certainly be delivered prematurely. Perinatal mortality rates are higher for triplets than twins and the incidence of cerebral palsy is also increased.

The mode of delivery for triplets or more babies is usually by caesarean section. It is essential that the paediatric team be present. The special dangers associated with these births are:

- asphyxia
- intracranial injury
- perinatal death.

If the family need extra outside help, the organisation of this must start before the babies are born.

DISABILITY AND BEREAVEMENT

Perinatal mortality and long-term morbidity are both more common among multiple births than singletons. The perinatal mortality rate for twins is about four times that of singletons, and that of triplets 12 times higher.

The grief of parents following the death of one of a multiple set is often underestimated. Addresses of organisations that offer support should be made available to the parents.

Where one or more of a multiple set has a disability, it is often the healthy child who needs special attention. He or she may feel guilt about doing something that caused the twin's disability and may be resentful of the attention that the other one needs, or of the loss of twinship.

EMBRYO REDUCTION

This is the reduction of an apparently healthy higher-order multiple pregnancy down to two or even one embryo so the chances of survival are much higher. The procedure may be offered to parents who have conceived triplets or more.

The procedure is usually carried out between the 10th and 12th weeks of the pregnancy. Various techniques may be used, involving the insertion of a needle under ultrasound guidance either via the vagina or, more commonly, through the abdominal wall into the fetal thorax. Potassium chloride is usually used, although some doctors prefer saline. All embryos remain in the uterus until birth.

SELECTIVE FETOCIDE

This may be offered to parents with a multiple pregnancy when one of the babies has a serious abnormality. The affected fetus is injected as described in embryo reduction, so allowing the healthy fetus to grow and develop normally.

The full impact of either of these procedures on the parents and their feelings of bereavement will often not be felt until the birth of their remaining baby (or babies) many weeks later.

SOURCES OF HELP

In the UK the support provided by social services varies greatly, so it is always advisable for families with triplets to apply. Home Start, or the local colleges with nursery training courses, may be able to offer assistance.

- *Tamba (Twins and Multiple Births Association).* The umbrella organisation for the 250 or so local twins clubs throughout the country. The clubs are run by parents of twins.
- *Multiple Births Foundation (MBF).* Offers advice and support to families as soon as their multiple pregnancy is diagnosed, as well as to couples considering treatment for infertility. It offers information and support for couples and professionals.

Section 3

Labour

CHAPTER 17

The First Stage of Labour

Normal labour is spontaneous in onset between 37 and 42 weeks' gestation with the fetus presenting by the vertex, culminating in a healthy mother and baby.

Phases of the first stage
These are described in Box 17.1.

THE ONSET OF SPONTANEOUS NORMAL LABOUR

The onset of labour appears to be initiated by a combination of hormonal and mechanical factors.

- Levels of maternal oestrogen rise sharply during the last weeks of pregnancy, resulting in changes that overcome the inhibiting effects of progesterone.
- High levels of oestrogens cause uterine muscle fibres to display oxytocic receptors and form gap junctions with each other.
- Oestrogen also stimulates the placenta to release prostaglandins that induce a production of enzymes that will digest collagen in the cervix, helping it to soften.

It is thought that both fetal and placental factors are involved in the process. Uterine activity may also result from mechanical stimulation of the uterus and cervix, brought about by overstretching or pressure from a presenting part that is well applied to the cervix.

When the woman is in labour, contractions will often be accompanied or preceded by a blood-stained mucoid 'show'; this results from the operculum, which formed the cervical plug during pregnancy, being lost when the cervix dilates.

Occasionally the membranes will rupture; this should always be reported to the midwife, who will check that there are no changes in the fetal heart rate and that meconium is not present in the liquor.

Spurious labour
Many women experience contractions before the onset of labour; these may be painful and may even be regular for a time, causing a woman to think that labour has started. The two features of true labour that are absent here are:

- effacement of the cervix
- dilatation of the cervix (see below).

Box 17.1 Phases of the first stage of labour

The latent phase

- Precedes the active first stage of labour
- May last 6–8 hours in first-time mothers
- The cervix dilates from 0 cm to 3–4 cm
- The cervical canal shortens from 3 cm long to less than 0.5 cm

The active first stage

- Begins when the cervix is 3–4 cm dilated
- In the presence of rhythmic contractions, is complete when the cervix is fully dilated (10 cm)
- Usually completed within 6–12 hours

The transitional phase

- The cervix expands from around 8 cm dilated until it is fully dilated (or until the expulsive contractions during the second stage are felt by the woman)
- There is often a brief lull in the intensity of uterine activity at this time

PHYSIOLOGICAL PROCESSES

UTERINE ACTION

Fundal dominance (Fig. 17.1)

Each uterine contraction starts in the fundus near one of the cornua and spreads across and downwards. The contraction lasts longest in the fundus where it is also most intense, but the peak is reached simultaneously over the whole uterus and the contraction fades from all parts together and is weakest in the lower segment.

Polarity

Polarity is the neuromuscular harmony that prevails between the two poles or segments of the uterus throughout labour. During each uterine contraction:

- the upper pole contracts strongly and retracts to expel the fetus
- the lower pole contracts slightly and dilates to allow expulsion to take place.

If polarity is disorganised, then the progress of labour is inhibited.

Contraction and retraction

Retraction is when muscle fibres retain some of the shortening of the contraction instead of becoming completely relaxed (Fig. 17.2). It assists in the progressive expulsion of the fetus; the upper segment of the uterus becomes gradually shorter and thicker and its cavity diminishes.

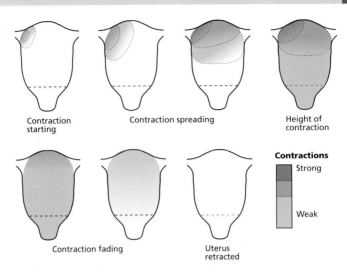

Fig. 17.1: Fundal dominance during uterine contractions.

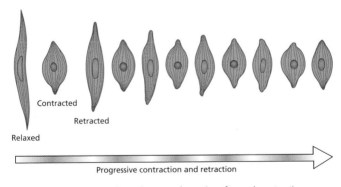

Fig. 17.2: How uterine muscle retains some shortening after each contraction.

Before labour becomes established, uterine contractions may occur every 15–20 minutes and may last for about 30 seconds; they may be imperceptible to the mother. By the end of the first stage they occur at 2–3-minute intervals, last for 50–60 seconds and are very powerful.

Formation of upper and lower uterine segments

By the end of pregnancy, the body of the uterus is described as having divided into two anatomically distinct segments:

● The upper uterine segment is formed from the body of the uterus.
● The lower uterine segment is formed from the isthmus and the cervix, and is about 8–10 cm in length.

The muscle content reduces from the fundus to the cervix, where it is thinner. When labour begins, the retracted longitudinal fibres in the upper segment pull on the lower segment, causing it to stretch; this is aided by the force applied by the descending presenting part. A ridge forms between the upper and lower uterine segments; this is known as the *physiological retraction ring*.

Cervical effacement

'Effacement' refers to the inclusion of the cervical canal into the lower uterine segment (Fig. 17.3).

Effacement may occur late in pregnancy, or it may not take place until labour begins.

● In the nulliparous woman, the cervix will not usually dilate until effacement is complete.
● In the parous woman, effacement and dilatation may occur simultaneously and a small canal may be felt in early labour. This is often referred to as a 'multips os'.

Cervical dilatation

Dilatation of the cervix is the process of enlargement of the os uteri from a tightly closed aperture to an opening large enough to permit passage of the fetal head.

● Dilatation is measured in centimetres and full dilatation at term equates to about 10 cm.
● Dilatation occurs as a result of uterine action and the counterpressure applied by either the intact bag of membranes or the presenting part, or both.
● A well-flexed fetal head closely applied to the cervix favours efficient dilatation.
● Pressure applied evenly to the cervix causes the uterine fundus to respond by contraction and retraction.

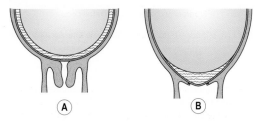

Fig. 17.3: (A) The cervix before effacement. (B) The cervix after effacement. The cervical canal is now part of the lower uterine segment.

MECHANICAL FACTORS

Formation of the forewaters

As the lower uterine segment forms and stretches, the chorion becomes detached from it; the increased intrauterine pressure causes this loosened part of the sac of fluid to bulge downwards into the internal os. The well-flexed head fits snugly into the cervix and cuts off the fluid in front of the head, the 'forewaters', from that which surrounds the body, the 'hindwaters'.

General fluid pressure

While the membranes remain intact, the pressure of the uterine contractions is exerted on the fluid and, as fluid is not compressible, the pressure is equalised throughout the uterus and over the fetal body; it is known as 'general fluid pressure'. Preserving the integrity of the membranes optimises the oxygen supply to the fetus and helps to prevent intrauterine and fetal infection.

Rupture of the membranes

- The optimum physiological time for the membranes to rupture spontaneously is at the end of the first stage of labour after the cervix becomes fully dilated and no longer supports the bag of forewaters.
- The uterine contractions are also applying increasing force at this time.
- Membranes may sometimes rupture days before labour begins or during the first stage.
- If there are no other signs of labour but the history of ruptured membranes is convincing or obvious liquor is draining, then digital examination should be avoided owing to an increased risk of ascending infection.
- If the diagnosis is not obvious, then one sterile speculum examination should be performed to try to visualise pooling of liquor in the posterior fornix; endocervical swabs may also be taken at this time.
- The majority of women will labour spontaneously within 48 hours. After 48 hours an obstetrician may consider augmentation of labour.
- Women with prelabour ruptured membranes should have their temperature recorded and be monitored for signs of fetal compromise associated with infection.
- Occasionally, the membranes do not rupture, even in the second stage, and appear at the vulva as a bulging sac covering the fetal head as it is born; this is known as the 'caul'.

Fetal axis pressure

During each contraction the uterus rises forward and the force of the fundal contraction is transmitted to the upper pole of the fetus and down the long axis of the fetus, and applied by the presenting part to the cervix. This is known as 'fetal axis pressure' and becomes much more significant after rupture of the membranes and during the second stage of labour.

OBSERVATIONS AND CARE IN LABOUR

MATERNAL WELLBEING

Women must be enabled to be in control throughout labour, with the midwife providing evidence-based information, listening to the woman and ensuring consent is given before any intervention.

Past history and reaction to labour

Factors of particular relevance at the onset of labour are listed in Box 17.2.

Pulse rate

This is recorded every 1–2 hours during early labour and every 30 minutes when labour is more advanced. If the rate increases to more than 100 beats per minute it may be indicative of:

- anxiety
- pain
- infection
- ketosis
- haemorrhage.

Temperature

This is recorded at least every 4 hours in normal labour. Pyrexia is indicative of infection or ketosis, or may be associated with epidural analgesia.

Blood pressure

This is measured every 2–4 hours, unless it is abnormal. The blood pressure must be monitored very closely following epidural or spinal anaesthetic. Hypotension may be caused by:

- the supine position
- shock
- epidural anaesthesia.

Box 17.2 Important factors in the history at the onset of labour

- The birth plan – whatever choices the woman makes, she must be the focus of the care, and should be able to feel she is in control of what is happening to her and able to make decisions about her care
- Parity and age
- Character and outcomes of previous labours
- Weights and condition of previous babies
- Attendance at any specialist clinics
- Any known problems – social or physical
- Blood results, including Rhesus isoimmunisation and haemoglobin (Hb)

Urinalysis and bladder care

The woman should be encouraged to empty her bladder every 1–2 hours during labour. The urine passed should be tested for glucose, ketones and protein.

- A low level of ketones is very common during labour and is not thought to be significant.
- A trace of protein may be a contaminant following rupture of the membranes or a sign of a urinary infection, but more significant proteinuria may indicate pre-eclampsia.

A full bladder may prevent the fetal head from entering the pelvic brim and can increase the risk of postpartum haemorrhage. If the bladder is incompletely emptied or the woman is unable to void for some hours, it may become necessary to pass a catheter.

Fluid balance

A record should be kept of all urine passed and fluids administered.

Abdominal examination

This is undertaken at the initial assessment and then repeated at intervals throughout labour to assess the length, strength and frequency of contractions and the descent of the presenting part. Contractions that are unduly long or very strong and coming in quick succession should give cause for concern. Hyperstimulation should be considered if oxytocin is being infused. Descent of the presenting part is usually described in terms of fifths of the head which can still be palpated above the brim.

Vaginal examination and progress in labour

Although it is not essential to examine the woman vaginally at frequent intervals, it may be useful to do so when progress is in doubt or another indication arises. The features that are indicative of progress are:

- effacement and dilatation of the cervix
- descent, flexion and rotation of the fetal head.

Progressive dilatation is monitored as labour continues and charted on either the partograph or the cervicograph.

The level or station of the presenting part is estimated in relation to the ischial spines; during normal labour the head descends progressively (Fig. 17.4). Moulding or a large caput will give a false impression of the level of the fetal head.

In vertex presentations, progress depends partly on increased flexion. Flexion is assessed by the position of the sutures and fontanelles:

- If the head is fully flexed, the posterior fontanelle becomes almost central (Fig. 17.5).
- If the head is deflexed, both anterior and posterior fontanelles may be palpable.

Rotation is assessed by noting changes in the position of the fetus between one examination and the next. The sutures and fontanelles are palpated in order to determine position.

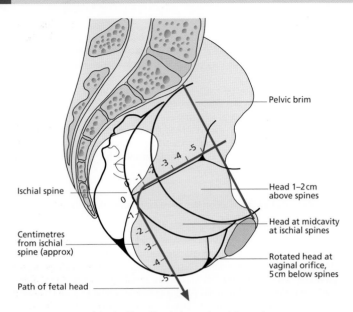

Fig. 17.4: Stations of the fetal head in relation to the pelvic canal.

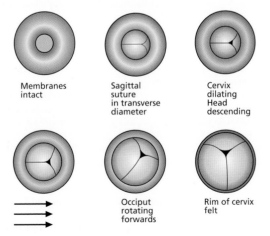

Fig. 17.5: Dilatation of the cervix and rotation of the fetal head, as felt on vaginal examination.

Under no circumstances should a midwife make a vaginal examination if there is any frank bleeding, unless the placenta is positively known to be in the upper uterine segment.

Nutrition

In normal labour women may take a low-fat, low-residue diet according to appetite. The vigorous muscle contractions of the uterus during labour demand a continuous supply of glucose. If this is not obtained from the diet, the body will start to metabolise protein and fat stores in an effort to provide glucose (gluconeogenesis). This relatively inefficient method of producing glucose results in the occurrence of ketoacidosis.

In an effort to reduce gastric volume and decrease the gastric acidity of the labouring woman, prophylactic antacids may be administered.

Prevention of infection

Invasive procedures should be kept to a minimum. Personal hygiene is important for both the woman and her attendants.

The fetal membranes should be preserved intact unless there is a positive indication for their rupture that would outweigh the advantage of their protective functions. Women whose labours are prolonged are at particular risk of infection and are often subjected to a number of invasive procedures.

Some women will need specialised care, especially women with any transmissible infection such as gastroenteritis, hepatitis or HIV infection.

Bowel preparation

If there has been no bowel action for 24 hours or the rectum feels loaded on vaginal examination, the woman should be asked if she would like an enema or suppositories. This is never done as a routine procedure.

Position and mobility

Mobility in labour should be encouraged, as it lessens the need for pharmacological analgesia.

Pain management

The biological, psychological, social, spiritual, cultural and educational dimensions of each woman have an impact on how she expresses herself and how she perceives pain during labour.

Midwives should work with women to encourage them to maintain control and be as mobile as possible throughout labour.

Non-pharmacological methods of pain control

These are listed in Box 17.3.

Pharmacological methods of pain control

Opiate drugs

Three systemic opioids are commonly used for pain relief in labour:

- *Pethidine*: usually administered intramuscularly in doses of 50–150 mg; takes about 20 minutes to have an effect.

Box 17.3 Non-pharmacological methods of pain control

- Breathing and relaxation techniques
- Massage
- Hydrotherapy
- Aromatherapy
- Transcutaneous electrical nerve stimulation (TENS)
- Reflexology
- Homeopathy
- Music therapy
- Acupuncture
- Herbal medicine.

- *Diamorphine*: usual dosage 10 mg given via intramuscular injection.
- *Meptazinol*: usually given in doses of 100–150 mg intramuscularly.

Inhalation analgesia

The most commonly used inhalation analgesia in labour is a premixed gas made up of 50% nitrous oxide and 50% oxygen administered through a piped system or via the Entonox apparatus. It takes effect within 20 seconds, maximum efficacy occurring after about 45–50 seconds.

Regional (epidural) analgesia

- A local anaesthetic is administered via a catheter into the epidural space of the lumbar region, usually between vertebrae L1 and L2, or between L2 and L3, or between L3 and L4.
- Bolus injections of bupivacaine (Marcain) or continuous infusion of dilute bupivacaine and opioids (usually fentanyl) may be used.
- An intravenous infusion of crystalloid fluids is commenced prior to siting the epidural.
- After the administration of the first dose of bupivacaine and any subsequent top-up doses of local anaesthetic, the blood pressure and pulse should be measured and recorded every 5 minutes for 20–30 minutes, and then every 30 minutes. The fetal heart is usually monitored electronically.
- The mother may sit up in bed once it has been established that her blood pressure is stable, but should be tilted to one side to prevent aortocaval compression.
- The spread of the block is checked regularly by the midwife.

Table 17.1 shows contraindications to regional analgesia and Table 17.2 lists the advantages and disadvantages of epidural analgesia.

FETAL WELLBEING

Fetal condition during labour can be assessed by obtaining information about:

- the fetal heart rate and patterns
- the pH of the fetal blood
- the amniotic fluid.

Table 17.1 Contraindications to regional analgesia, with...

Contraindication	Risk
Uncorrected anticoagulation or coagulopathy	Vertebral canal haer...
Local or systemic sepsis (pyrexia above 38°C not treated with antibiotics)	Vertebral canal absc...
Hypovolaemia or active haemorrhage	Cardiovascular collapse secondary to sympathetic blockade
Patient refusal	Legal action
Lack of sufficient trained midwives for continuous care and monitoring of mother and fetus for the duration of the epidural blockade	Maternal collapse, convulsion, respiratory arrest; fetal compromise

Table 17.2 Advantages and disadvantages of epidural analgesia

Disadvantages	Advantages
Ineffective blocks	Effective pain relief
More frequent monitoring of vital signs	Tendency to lower blood pressure can be advantageous in cases of pregnancy-induced hypertension
Lengthens first stage of labour	
Mother less able to adopt different birth positions	If labour is prolonged, gives effective pain relief, allowing mother to rest
Less sensation of expulsive efforts and lengthens second stage of labour	Does not depress respiratory centre of fetus
Increase in instrumental vaginal delivery	

The fetal heart

Women with an uncomplicated pregnancy should have intermittent auscultation with a Pinard stethoscope or hand-held Doppler device. There is no evidence to support an admission cardiotocography (CTG); it should therefore not be done as routine.

For women with problems in their pregnancy or other risk factors, including the use of oxytocin or epidural analgesia, electronic fetal monitoring (EFM) is appropriate.

The use of a CTG may limit the choice of position.

Intermittent monitoring

The heart rate should be counted over a complete minute.

● The baseline rate should be between 110 and 160 beats per minute (bpm).
● Variability of more than 5 bpm should be maintained throughout labour.

If decelerations are heard in the first stage of labour with a Pinard or Doppler instrument, then electronic monitoring may be indicated to assess their extent.

tinuous EFM

ntinuous recording usually combines a fetal cardiograph and a maternal ocograph in a CTG apparatus. This presents a graphic record of the response of the fetal heart to uterine activity, as well as information about its rate and variability.

Findings

The CTG provides information on:

- baseline fetal heart rate
- baseline variability
- accelerations from baseline rate
- decelerations from baseline rate
- uterine activity.

Response of the fetal heart to uterine contractions

The fetal heart rate will normally remain steady or accelerate during uterine contractions during the first stage of labour. Compression of the umbilical cord or fetal head will result in some decelerations, particularly if the membranes are not intact. These would be early or variable decelerations lasting less than 3 minutes, with good recovery to predeceleration rate.

A late or variable deceleration lasting longer than 3 minutes begins during or after a contraction, reaches its nadir (lowest point) after the peak of the contraction and has not recovered by the time that the contraction has ended. The *time lag* between the peak of the contraction and the nadir of the deceleration is more significant in terms of severity than the drop in the fetal heart rate.

Interpretation of CTG

'Darth Vader' is a useful mnemonic for thorough evaluation of a CTG (Box 17.4).

Box 17.4 The 'Darth Vader' mnemonic

- **D** details (name, time, etc.)
- **A** assess quality
- **R** recorded fetal movements
- **T** tocograph
- **H** heart rate
- **V** variability
- **A** accelerations
- **D** decelerations
- **E** evaluation
- **R** response

Only four variables are considered when interpreting a CTG:

- baseline rate
- baseline variability
- whether accelerations are present
- presence or absence of decelerations.

This makes a CTG interpretable using the three categories recommended by the National Institute for Health and Clinical Excellence (NICE) in 2001 (Fig. 17.6):

- normal
- suspicious
- pathological.

All areas that use EFM should have ready 24-hour access to fetal blood sampling (FBS) facilities. All CTG traces should be secured in the notes.

Fetal blood sampling

When the fetal heart rate pattern is suspicious or pathological and fetal acidosis is suspected, then FBS should be carried out unless the birth is imminent.

- An FBS result of 7.25 or below should be repeated usually within 30 minutes to an hour.
- An FBS below 7.20 indicates that the fetus should be delivered.

Amniotic fluid

- If the fetus becomes hypoxic, meconium may be passed, causing the amniotic fluid to be stained green.
- Amniotic fluid that is a muddy yellow colour or is only slightly green may signify a previous event from which the fetus has recovered; it is also common and of no significance in postdates babies.
- If the breech is presenting, the fetus may pass meconium because of the compression of the abdomen or as a result of hypoxia.
- Bleeding of sudden onset at the time of rupture of the membranes may be the result of ruptured vasa praevia and is an acute emergency.

Fetal compromise

Signs of fetal compromise resulting from oxygen deprivation are:

- fetal tachycardia
- a pathological CTG and corresponding poor FBS result
- fetal bradycardia or a severe change in fetal heart rate or decelerations related to uterine contractions, or both
- passage of meconium-stained amniotic fluid.

Midwife's management of fetal compromise

- Summon medical assistance.
- Stop oxytocin if it is being administered.
- Place the woman in a more favourable position, usually on her left side.
- In cases of maternal oxygen lack, give oxygen.
- Assist with arrangements to expedite the birth.

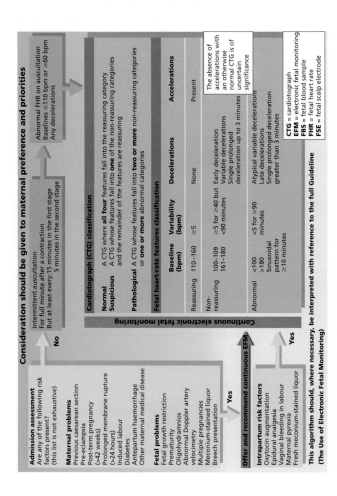

Consideration should be given to maternal preference and priorities

Admission assessment
Are any of the following risk factors present?
(this list is not exhaustive)

Maternal problems
Previous caesarean section
Pre-eclampsia
Post-term pregnancy (>42 weeks)
Prolonged membrane rupture (>24 hours)
Induced labour
Diabetes
Antepartum haemorrhage
Other maternal medical disease

Fetal problems
Fetal growth restriction
Prematurity
Oligohydramnios
Abnormal Doppler artery velocimetry
Multiple pregnancies
Meconium-stained liquor
Breech presentation

No → Intermittent auscultation
For full minute after a contraction
But at least every:15 minutes in the first stage
5 minutes in the second stage

Abnormal FHR on auscultation
Baselines ≤110 bpm or ≥60 bpm
Any decelerations

Yes → **Offer and recommend continuous EFM**

Intrapartum risk factors
Oxytocin augmentation
Epidural analgesia
Vaginal bleeding in labour
Maternal pyrexia
Fresh meconium-stained liquor

Yes → **Continuous electronic fetal monitoring**

Cardiotograph (CTG) classification

Normal A CTG where all four features fall into the reassuring category
Suspicious A CTG whose features fall into one of the non-reassuring categories and the remainder of the features are reassuring
Pathological A CTG whose features fall into two or more non-reassuring categories or one or more abnormal categories

Fetal heart-rate features classification

	Baseline (bpm)	Variability (bpm)	Decelerations	Accelerations
Reassuring	110–160	≥5	None	Present
Non-reassuring	100–109 161–180	≥5 for ≥40 but <90 minutes	Early deceleration Variable decelerations Single prolonged deceleration up to 3 minutes	The absence of accelerations with an otherwise normal CTG is of uncertain significance
Abnormal	<100 >180 Sinusoidal pattern for ≥10 minutes	<5 for ≥90 minutes	Atypical variable decelerations Late decelerations Single prolonged deceleration greater than 3 minutes	

CTG = cardiotograph
EFM = electronic fetal monitoring
FBS = fetal blood sample
FHR = fetal heart rate
FSE = fetal scalp electrode

This algorithm should, where necessary, be interpreted with reference to the full Guideline
(The Use of Electronic Fetal Monitoring)

Fig. 17.6: Guidelines for fetal monitoring in labour.

PRETERM LABOUR

Preterm labour is defined as labour commencing after 24 weeks' gestation and before the 37th completed week of pregnancy.

A woman who is at risk of giving birth preterm should be transferred to a unit with intensive neonatal facilities, preferably with the fetus in utero. Tocolytic drugs may be used in very early labour to try to delay the birth. Antenatal administration of steroids has been shown to reduce the incidence of hyaline membrane disease, intraventricular haemorrhage and necrotising enterocolitis in fetuses of 26–34 weeks' gestation. Two doses given over 24 hours last for at least 7 days.

RECORDS

The record of labour is a legal document and must be kept meticulously. It provides current, comprehensive and concise information regarding:

- the woman's observations
- her physical, psychological and sociological state
- any problems that arose
- the midwife's response to that problem, including any interventions.

An accurate record during labour provides the basis on which clinical improvements, progress or deterioration of the mother or fetus can be judged. For this reason the notes should be kept in chronological order. Key points for practice are summarised in Box 17.5.

Box 17.5 Key points for practice

- Women should be well informed and offered choice founded on evidence-based information where possible
- A competent woman can give or withhold consent for any procedure
- Another adult cannot consent or withhold consent on behalf of a competent woman
- Good communication between women and midwives and between professionals is a fundamental component of maternity services
- The latent phase of labour should be more widely acknowledged in hospital settings
- The use of strict time limits for first and second stages of labour should be reviewed in problem-free pregnancies
- Good record keeping and care plans are an essential aspect of care

CHAPTER 18

The Second Stage of Labour

THE NATURE OF TRANSITION AND SECOND-STAGE PHASES OF LABOUR

The second stage of labour is the phase between full dilatation of the cervical os and the birth of the baby. However, most midwives and labouring women are aware of a transitional period between the dilatation, or first stage of labour, and the time when active maternal pushing efforts begin. This period is typically characterised by maternal restlessness, discomfort, desire for pain relief, a sense that the process is never-ending and demands to attendants to get the birth over with as quickly as possible. Some women may experience the urge to push before the cervix is fully dilated, and others may have a lull in activity before the full expulsive nature of the second-stage contractions becomes evident. This latter phenomenon is termed the *resting phase* of the second stage of labour.

The onset of the second stage of labour is traditionally confirmed with a vaginal examination, however it may not be necessary unless there are signs that the labour is not progressing as anticipated.

Uterine action

Contractions become stronger and longer but may be less frequent. The membranes often rupture spontaneously towards the end of the first stage or during transition to the second stage. Fetal axis pressure increases flexion of the head, which results in smaller presenting diameters, more rapid progress and less trauma to both mother and fetus. If the mother is upright during this time, these processes are optimised.

The contractions become expulsive as the fetus descends further into the vagina. Pressure from the presenting part stimulates nerve receptors in the pelvic floor (this is termed the 'Ferguson reflex') and the woman experiences the need to push. This reflex may initially be controlled to a limited extent but becomes increasingly compulsive, overwhelming and involuntary during each contraction. The mother's response is to employ her secondary powers of expulsion by contracting her abdominal muscles and diaphragm.

Soft tissue displacement

With descent of the head, the soft tissues of the pelvis become displaced.

- Anteriorly, the bladder is pushed upwards; this results in the stretching and thinning of the urethra so that its lumen is reduced.

- Posteriorly, the rectum becomes flattened into the sacral curve and the pressure of the advancing head expels any residual faecal matter.
- The levator ani muscles dilate, thin out and are displaced laterally, and the perineal body is flattened, stretched and thinned.

The fetal head becomes visible at the vulva, advancing with each contraction and receding between contractions until crowning takes place. The head is then born. The shoulders and body follow with the next contraction, accompanied by a gush of amniotic fluid and sometimes of blood. The second stage culminates in the birth of the baby.

Duration of the second stage

The time taken to complete the second stage will vary considerably. Although many maternity units do currently impose routine limits on the duration of the second stage, beyond which medical help should be called, these are not based on good evidence.

MATERNAL RESPONSE TO TRANSITION AND THE SECOND STAGE

PUSHING

The urge to push may come before the vertex is visible. Traditionally, in order to conserve maternal effort and allow the vaginal tissues to stretch passively, the mother is encouraged to avoid active pushing at this stage. It is now accepted that managed active pushing accompanied by breath holding (the *Valsalva manœuvre*) has adverse consequences. Whenever active pushing commences, the woman should be encouraged to follow her own inclinations in relation to expulsive effort. Few women need instruction on how to push unless they are using epidural analgesia. Some mothers vocalise loudly as they push.

Position

If the mother lies flat on her back, then vena caval compression is increased, resulting in hypotension. This can lead to reduced placental perfusion and diminished fetal oxygenation and the efficiency of uterine contractions may be reduced.

The mother's instinctive preference is the primary consideration:

- *Semirecumbent or supported sitting position, with the thighs abducted.* This is the posture most commonly used in Western cultures.
- *Squatting, kneeling, all fours or standing.* Radiological evidence demonstrates an average increase of 1 cm in the transverse diameter and 2 cm in the anteroposterior diameter of the pelvic outlet when the squatting position is adopted.
- *Left lateral position.* An assistant may be required to support the right thigh, which may not be ergonomic. It is an alternative position for women who find it difficult to abduct their hips.

THE MECHANISM OF NORMAL LABOUR

As the fetus descends, soft tissue and bony structures exert pressures that lead to descent through the birth canal by a series of movements, called *mechanism of labour*. During vaginal birth, the fetal presentation, position and size will govern the exact mechanism, as the fetus responds to external pressures. Principles common to all mechanisms are:

● Descent takes place.
● Whichever part leads and first meets the resistance of the pelvic floor will rotate forwards until it comes under the symphysis pubis.
● Whichever part emerges from the pelvis will pivot around the pubic bone.

During the mechanism of normal labour the fetus turns slightly to take advantage of the widest available space in each plane of the pelvis. The widest diameter of the pelvic brim is the transverse; at the pelvic outlet the greatest space lies in the anteroposterior diameter.

At the onset of labour, the most common presentation is the vertex and the most common position either left or right occipitoanterior. When these conditions are met, the way that the fetus is normally situated can be described as follows:

● The lie is longitudinal.
● The presentation is cephalic.
● The position is right or left occipitoanterior.
● The attitude is one of good flexion.
● The denominator is the occiput.
● The presenting part is the posterior part of the anterior parietal bone.

MAIN MOVEMENTS
Descent
Throughout the first stage of labour the contraction and retraction of the uterine muscles allow less room in the uterus, exerting pressure on the fetus to descend. Following rupture of the forewaters and the exertion of maternal effort, progress speeds up.

Flexion
Pressure exerted down the fetal axis will increase flexion, resulting in smaller presenting diameters that will negotiate the pelvis more easily.

● At the onset of labour the suboccipitofrontal diameter (10 cm) is presenting.
● With flexion the suboccipitobregmatic diameter (9.5 cm) presents.
● The occiput becomes the leading part.

Internal rotation of the head
During a contraction the leading part is pushed downwards onto the pelvic floor. The resistance of this muscular diaphragm brings about rotation.

● In a well-flexed vertex presentation the occiput leads and meets the pelvic floor first and rotates anteriorly through one-eighth of a circle.

- This causes a slight twist in the neck of the fetus, as the head is no longer in direct alignment with the shoulders.
- The anteroposterior diameter of the head now lies in the widest (anteroposterior) diameter of the pelvic outlet.
- The occiput slips beneath the subpubic arch and crowning occurs when the head no longer recedes between contractions and the widest transverse diameter (biparietal) is born.
- While flexion is maintained, the suboccipitobregmatic diameter (9.5 cm) distends the vaginal orifice.

Extension of the head

Once crowning has occurred, the fetal head can extend, pivoting on the suboccipital region around the pubic bone. The sinciput, face and chin sweep the perineum and are born.

Restitution

The twist in the neck of the fetus that resulted from internal rotation is corrected by a slight untwisting movement. The occiput moves one-eighth of a circle towards the side from which it started (Fig. 18.1A and B).

Internal rotation of the shoulders

The anterior shoulder is the first to reach the levator ani muscle and it therefore rotates anteriorly to lie under the symphysis pubis. This movement can be clearly seen as the head turns at the same time (external rotation of the head) (Fig. 18.1C).

Lateral flexion

The anterior shoulder is usually born first, although it has been noted by midwives who commonly use upright or kneeling positions that the posterior shoulder is commonly seen first. In the former case the anterior shoulder slips beneath the subpubic arch and the posterior shoulder passes over the perineum. The remainder of the body is born by lateral flexion as the spine bends sideways through the curved birth canal.

OBSERVATIONS AND CARE DURING THE SECOND STAGE OF LABOUR

PRINCIPLES OF CARE

See Box 18.1.

- Surgical gloves should be worn during the birth for the protection of both mother and midwife from infection. In some units, goggles or plain glasses are also advised to minimise the risk of transmission of infection through blood splashes to the eyes.
- A uterotonic agent (commonly Syntometrine 1 ml or oxytocin 5 or 10 units) may be prepared, either in readiness for the active management of the third stage if this is acceptable to the woman, or for use during an emergency.

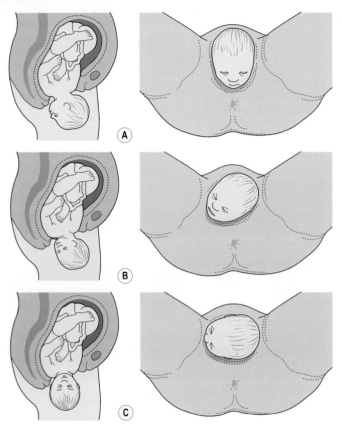

Fig. 18.1: (A) Birth of the head. (B) Restitution. (C) External rotation.

- Neonatal resuscitation equipment should be thoroughly checked and readily accessible and blood bottles prepared if, for example, the mother is Rhesus negative.
- A warm cot and clothes should be prepared for the baby.

Box 18.1 Principles of care during the second stage of labour

- Observation of progress
- Prevention of infection
- Emotional and physical comfort of the mother
- Anticipation of normal events
- Recognition of abnormal developments

OBSERVATIONS

At least five factors determine whether the second stage is continuing optimally, and these must be carefully observed:

- uterine contractions
- descent, rotation and flexion
- fetal condition
- suspicious/pathological changes in the fetal heart
- maternal condition.

Uterine contractions

The strength, length and frequency of contractions should be assessed continuously by observation of maternal responses, and regularly by uterine palpation.

Descent, rotation and flexion

If there is a delay in progress despite regular strong contractions and active maternal pushing, a vaginal examination may be performed:

- to confirm whether or not internal rotation of the head has taken place
- to assess the station of the presenting part
- to determine whether a caput succedaneum has formed.

In the absence of good rotation and flexion, or a weakening of uterine contractions, or both, then a change of position, nutrition and hydration or use of optimal fetal positioning techniques may be considered. If there is evidence that either the fetal or maternal condition is compromised, an experienced obstetrician must be consulted. A full bladder impedes progress.

Fetal condition

If the membranes are ruptured, the liquor amnii is observed to ensure that it is clear.

- Thick, fresh meconium is always ominous.
- Thin, old meconium staining is not always regarded as a sign of fetal compromise.

As the fetus descends, fetal oxygenation may be less efficient owing either to cord or head compression or to reduced perfusion at the placental site. A well-grown healthy fetus will not be compromised by this transitory hypoxia. This will tend to be manifest in early decelerations of the fetal heart, with a swift return to the normal baseline after a contraction. During the second stage the fetal heart is usually auscultated immediately after a contraction, with some readings being taken through a contraction if the woman can tolerate this.

Suspicious/pathological changes in the fetal heart

Signs for concern include:

- late decelerations
- lack of return to the normal baseline
- a rising baseline
- diminishing beat-to-beat variation.

If these are heard for the first time in second stage, they may be due to cord or head compression, which may be helped by a change in position. If they persist following such a change, then medical advice must be sought. If the labour is taking place in a unit that is distant from an obstetric unit, an episiotomy may be considered if the birth is imminent. Midwives who are trained and experienced in ventouse birth may consider expediting the birth at this point. Otherwise, transfer to an obstetric unit should be arranged.

Maternal condition

Monitoring includes an appraisal of the mother's ability to cope emotionally, as well as an assessment of her physical wellbeing. Maternal pulse rate is usually recorded every half hour and blood pressure every hour, provided that these remain within normal limits. The woman should be encouraged to pass urine at the beginning of the second stage, unless she has recently done so.

BIRTH OF THE HEAD

- Once the birth is imminent, the perineum may be swabbed and a clean pad placed under the woman on the bed or floor as appropriate.
- With each contraction the head descends. As it does so, the superficial muscles of the pelvic floor can be seen to stretch. The head recedes between contractions, which allows these muscles to thin gradually. The skill of the midwife in ensuring that the active phase is unhurried helps to safeguard the perineum from trauma. She must either watch the advance of the fetal head or control it with light support from her hand, or both.
- Once the head has crowned, the mother can achieve control by gently blowing or 'sighing' out each breath in order to minimise active pushing.
- The head is born by extension as the face appears.
- During the resting phase before the next contraction, the midwife may check that the cord is not around the baby's neck.
- If it is, then the usual practice is to slacken it to form a loop through which the shoulders may pass.
- If the cord is very tightly wound around the neck, it is common practice to apply two artery forceps approximately 3 cm apart and to sever the cord between the two clamps.
- Once severed, the cord may be unwound from around the neck.
- The mother may now be able to see and touch her baby's head and assist in the birth of the trunk.

BIRTH OF THE SHOULDERS

- Restitution and external rotation of the head usually occurs, maximising the smooth birth of the shoulders and minimising the risk of perineal laceration.
- If the woman is in an upright position, the shoulders may be left to birth spontaneously with the help of gravity.

- During a water birth, it is important not to touch the emerging baby to avoid stimulating it to gasp underwater.
- Once restitution has occurred fully; a hand is placed on each side of the baby's head, over the ears, and gentle downward traction is applied. The anterior shoulder escapes under the symphysis pubis. When the axillary crease is seen, the head and trunk are guided in an upward curve to allow the posterior shoulder to pass over the perineum. (These manoeuvres are reversed if the mother is, for example, on 'all fours'). The midwife or mother may now grasp the baby around the chest to aid the birth of the trunk and lift the baby towards the mother's abdomen.
- The time of birth is noted.
- The cord is severed between two clamps and a cord clamp is applied close to the umbilicus.
- The baby is dried and placed in the skin-to-skin position with the mother, unless she requests otherwise.
- A warm cover is placed over the exposed areas of the baby to prevent cooling.

EPISIOTOMY

As the perineum distends, a decision to undertake an episiotomy may very occasionally be necessary. This is an incision through the perineal tissues to enlarge the vulval outlet during the birth. The rationale for its use depends largely on the need to minimise the risk of severe, spontaneous, maternal trauma and to expedite the birth when there is evidence of fetal compromise. The mother needs to give consent prior to the procedure.

- The perineum should be adequately anaesthetised prior to the incision. Lidocaine is commonly used, either 0.5% 10 ml or 1% 5 ml.
- The incision is made during a contraction when the tissues are stretched so that there is a clear view of the area and bleeding is less likely to be severe.
- Birth of the head should follow immediately and its advance must be controlled in order to avoid extension of the episiotomy.

Types of incision
- *Mediolateral*. Begins at the midpoint of the fourchette and is directed at a 45° angle to the midline towards a point midway between the ischial tuberosity and the anus (Fig. 18.2).
- *Median*. A midline incision that follows the natural line of insertion of the perineal muscles. It is associated with reduced blood loss but a higher incidence of damage to the anal sphincter.

PERINEAL TRAUMA

Spontaneous trauma may be of the labia anteriorly, the perineum posteriorly or both. A gentle, thorough examination must be carried out to assess the extent of the trauma accurately and to determine who should carry out the repair.
- *Anterior labial tears*. A suture may be necessary to secure haemostasis.

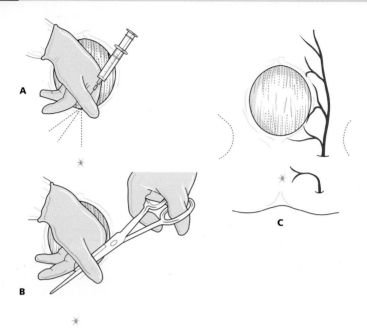

Fig. 18.2: (A) Infiltrating the perineum. (B) Performing an episiotomy. (C) Innervation of the vulval area and perineum.

- *Posterior perineal trauma.* Spontaneous tears are usually classified in degrees (Box 18.2). Third- and fourth-degree tears should be repaired by an experienced obstetrician. A general anaesthetic or effective epidural or spinal anaesthetic is necessary.

Box 18.2 Classification of spontaneous posterior perineal tears

First-degree tear
- Involves the fourchette only

Second-degree tear
- Involves the fourchette and the perineal muscles

Third-degree tear
- Involves the fourchette, the perineal muscles and the anal sphincter

Fourth-degree tear
- Sometimes used to describe trauma that extends into the rectal mucosa

RECORDS

Records should include:

- details of any drugs administered
- duration and progress of labour
- reason for performing an episiotomy
- perineal repair.

The birth notification must be completed within 36 hours of the birth.

See Box 18.3 for key points relating to the second stage of labour.

Box 18.3 Key points for practice

- The transitional and second-stage phases of labour are emotionally intense and physically hard
- The vast majority of labours will progress physiologically
- Maternal behaviour is usually a good indication of progress during this time
- The core midwifery skill is to support the mother in the context of a sound knowledge of the physiology and the mechanisms of this phase of labour
- Support should be unobtrusive
- The woman is the central player
- Clear, comprehensive record keeping is essential
- There are many gaps in the research evidence in this area

CHAPTER 19

The Third Stage of Labour

PHYSIOLOGICAL PROCESSES

During the third stage of labour, separation and expulsion of the placenta and membranes occur as the result of an interplay of mechanical and haemostatic factors. The time at which the placenta actually separates from the uterine wall can vary. It may shear off during the final expulsive contractions accompanying the birth of the baby or remain adherent for some considerable time. The third stage usually lasts between 5 and 15 minutes, but any period up to 1 hour may be considered to be within normal limits.

SEPARATION AND DESCENT OF THE PLACENTA
Mechanical factors (Fig. 19.1)
Separation usually begins centrally so that a retroplacental clot is formed (Fig. 19.2). Two methods of separation are described:
- Schultze (Fig. 19.3A).
- Matthews Duncan (Fig. 19.3B).

Once separation has occurred, the uterus contracts strongly, forcing the placenta and membranes to fall into the lower uterine segment and finally into the vagina.

Haemostasis
The three factors that are critical to control of bleeding are the following:
- *Retraction* of the oblique uterine muscle fibres in the upper uterine segment through which the tortuous blood vessels intertwine.
- The presence of vigorous uterine *contraction* following separation – this brings the walls into apposition so that further pressure is exerted on the placental site.
- The achievement of *haemostasis* – following separation, the placental site is rapidly covered by a fibrin mesh utilising 5–10% of the circulating fibrinogen.

MANAGEMENT OF THE THIRD STAGE

UTEROTONICS OR UTEROTONIC AGENTS

These are drugs (e.g. Syntometrine, Syntocinon, ergometrine and prostaglandins) that stimulate the smooth muscle of the uterus to contract. They may be administered with crowning of the baby's head, at the time of

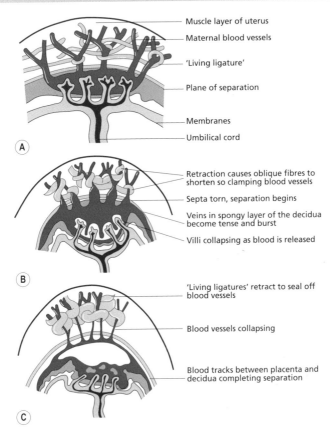

Fig. 19.1: The placental site during separation. (A) Uterus and placenta before separation. (B) Separation begins. (C) Separation is almost complete.

birth of the anterior shoulder of the baby, at the end of the second stage of labour or following the delivery of the placenta.

Information related to the best available research information on the use of uterotonic drugs during the third stage of labour should be provided in an objective manner.

Expectant or physiological management

In the event of expectant management:

- routine administration of the uterotonic drug is withheld

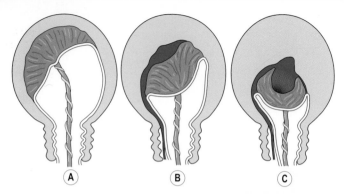

Fig. 19.2: The mechanism of placental separation. (A) Uterine wall is partially retracted, but not sufficiently to cause placental separation. (B) Further contraction and retraction thicken the uterine wall, reduce the placental site and aid placental separation. (C) Complete separation and formation of the retroplacental clot. *Note:* the thin lower segment has collapsed like a concertina following the birth of the baby.

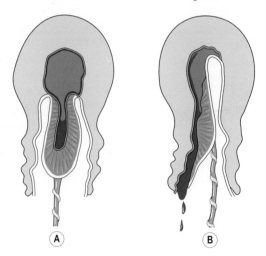

Fig. 19.3: Expulsion of the placenta. (A) Schultze method. (B) Matthews Duncan method.

- the umbilical cord is left unclamped until cord pulsation has ceased or the mother requests it to be clamped, or both
- the placenta is expelled by use of gravity and maternal effort.

With this approach, *therapeutic* uterotonic administration would be administered either to stop bleeding once it has occurred or to maintain the uterus in a contracted state when there are indications that excessive bleeding is likely to occur.

Active management

This is a policy whereby *prophylactic* administration of a uterotonic is applied, regardless of the assessed obstetric risk status of the woman. This is undertaken in conjunction with clamping of the umbilical cord shortly after birth of the baby and delivery of the placenta by the use of controlled cord traction. One of the following uterotonic drugs is usually used:

- ergometrine
- oxytocin
- combined ergometrine and oxytocin.

Intravenous ergometrine 0.25 mg

- This drug acts within 45 seconds; therefore it is particularly useful in securing a rapid contraction where hypotonic uterine action results in haemorrhage.
- If a doctor is not present in such an emergency, a midwife may give the injection.

Combined ergometrine and oxytocin

(A commonly used brand is Syntometrine.)

- A 1-ml ampoule contains 5 IU of oxytocin and 0.5 mg ergometrine and is administered by intramuscular injection.
- The oxytocin acts within 2.5 minutes, and the ergometrine within 6–7 minutes.
- Their combined action results in a rapid uterine contraction enhanced by a stronger, more sustained contraction lasting several hours.
- Administered, normally, at birth of the anterior shoulder.
- *Caution.* No more than two doses of ergometrine 0.5 mg should be given, as it can cause headache, nausea and an increase in blood pressure; it is normally contraindicated where there is a history of hypertensive or cardiac disease.

Oxytocin

(A commonly used brand is Syntocinon.)

- Oxytocin can be administered as both an intravenous and an intramuscular injection. However, an intravenous bolus of oxytocin can cause profound, fatal hypotension, especially in the presence of cardiovascular compromise.
- No more than 5 IU should be given by slow intravenous injection.

CLAMPING OF THE UMBILICAL CORD

This may have been carried out during birth of the baby if the cord was tightly around the neck. Early clamping is carried out in the first 1–3 minutes immediately after birth, regardless of whether cord pulsation has ceased.

Proponents of late clamping suggest that no action be taken until cord pulsation ceases or the placenta has been completely delivered, thus allowing the physiological processes to take place without intervention.

DELIVERY OF THE PLACENTA AND MEMBRANES
Controlled cord traction (CCT)

This manœuvre is believed to reduce blood loss and shorten the third stage of labour, therefore minimising the time during which the mother is at risk from haemorrhage. It is designed to enhance the normal physiological process. Before starting CCT check that the conditions listed in Box 19.1 have been met. At the beginning of the third stage, a strong uterine contraction results in the fundus being palpable below the umbilicus. It feels broad, as the placenta is still in the upper segment. As the placenta separates and falls into the lower uterine segment there is a small fresh blood loss, the cord lengthens and the fundus becomes rounder, smaller and more mobile as it rises in the abdomen. (*Note*: there is a school of thought that does not believe it is necessary to wait for signs of separation and descent *but* the uterus must be well contracted and care exerted with cord traction.)

It is important not to manipulate the uterus in any way, as this may precipitate incoordinate action. No further step should be taken until a strong contraction is palpable. If tension is applied to the umbilical cord without this contraction, uterine inversion may occur (see Ch. 23).

When CCT is the preferred method of management, the following sequence of actions is usually undertaken:

- Once the uterus is found on palpation to be contracted, one hand is placed above the level of the symphysis pubis with the palm facing towards the umbilicus and exerting pressure in an upwards direction. This is countertraction.
- Grasping the cord, traction is applied in a downward and backward direction following the line of the birth canal.
- Some resistance may be felt but it is important to apply steady tension by pulling the cord firmly and maintaining the pressure. Jerky movements and force should be avoided.
- The aim is to complete the action as one continuous, smooth, controlled movement. However, it is only possible to exert this tension for 1 or 2 minutes, as it may be an uncomfortable procedure for the mother and the midwife's hand will tire.
- Downward traction on the cord must be released *before* uterine countertraction is relaxed, as sudden withdrawal of countertraction while tension is still being applied to the cord may also cause uterine inversion.

Box 19.1 Conditions for starting controlled cord traction

- A uterotonic drug has been administered
- It has been given time to act
- The uterus is well contracted
- Countertraction is applied
- Signs of placental separation and descent are present

- If the manœuvre is not immediately successful, there should be a pause before uterine contraction is again checked and a further attempt is made.
- Should the uterus relax, tension is temporarily released until a good contraction is again palpable.
- Once the placenta is visible, it may be cupped in the hands to ease pressure on the friable membranes.
- A gentle upward and downward movement or twisting action will help to coax out the membranes and increase the chances of delivering them intact. Great care should be taken to avoid tearing the membranes.

Expectant management

This management policy allows the physiological changes within the uterus that occur at the time of birth to take their natural course with minimal intervention; it excludes the administration of uterotonic drugs. The processes of placental separation and expulsion are quite distinct from one another and the signs of separation and descent must be evident before maternal effort can be used to expedite expulsion.

- If sitting or squatting, gravity will aid expulsion.
- If good uterine contractions are sustained, maternal effort will usually bring about expulsion. The mother simply pushes, as during the second stage of labour.
- Encouragement is important, as by now she may be exhausted and the contractions will feel weaker and less expulsive than those during the second stage of labour.
- Providing that fresh blood loss is not excessive, the mother's condition remains stable and her pulse rate normal, there need be no anxiety. This spontaneous process can take from 20 minutes to an hour to complete.
- It is important that the midwife monitors uterine action by placing a hand lightly on the fundus. She can thus palpate the contraction while checking that relaxation does not result in the uterus filling with blood.
- Vigilance is crucial, as it should be remembered that the longer the placenta remains undelivered, the greater is the risk of bleeding because the uterus cannot contract down fully while the bulk of the placenta is in situ.
- Early attachment of the baby to the breast may enhance these physiological changes by stimulating the release of oxytocin from the posterior lobe of the pituitary gland.

ASEPSIS

The need for asepsis is even greater now than in the preceding stages of labour. Laceration and bruising of the cervix, vagina, perineum and vulva provide a route for the entry of micro-organisms. The placental site, a raw wound, provides an ideal medium for infection. Strict attention to the prevention of sepsis is therefore vital.

CORD BLOOD SAMPLING

This may be required:
- when the mother's blood group is Rhesus negative or her Rhesus type is unknown
- when atypical maternal antibodies have been found during an antenatal screening test
- where a haemoglobinopathy is suspected (e.g. sickle cell disease).

The sample should be taken from the fetal surface of the placenta where the blood vessels are congested and easily visible.

COMPLETION OF THE THIRD STAGE

- Once the placenta is delivered, the uterus should be well contracted and fresh blood loss minimal.
- Perineum and lower vagina checked for trauma.
- Blood loss is estimated; including blood that has soaked into linen and swabs as well as measurable fluid loss and clot formation.
- A thorough inspection of the placenta or membranes must be carried out to make sure that no part has been retained.
- If there is any suspicion that the placenta or membranes are incomplete, they must be kept for inspection and a doctor informed immediately.

IMMEDIATE CARE

It is advisable for mother and infant to remain in the midwife's care for at least an hour after birth, regardless of the birth setting.
- The woman should be encouraged to pass urine because a full bladder may impede uterine contraction.
- Uterine contraction and blood loss should be checked on several occasions during this first hour.
- Throughout this same period the midwife should pay regard to the baby's general wellbeing. She should check the security of the cord clamp and observe general skin colour, respirations and temperature.
- The warmest place for a baby to be placed is in a direct skin-to-skin contact position with the mother or wrapped and cuddled, whichever she prefers.
- Most women intending to breastfeed will wish to put their baby to the breast during these early moments of contact.

COMPLICATIONS OF THE THIRD STAGE OF LABOUR

POSTPARTUM HAEMORRHAGE

Postpartum haemorrhage (PPH) is defined as excessive bleeding from the genital tract at any time following the baby's birth up to 12 weeks after birth.

- If it occurs during the third stage of labour or within 24 hours of delivery, it is termed *primary postpartum haemorrhage*.
- If it occurs subsequent to the first 24 hours following birth up until the 12th week postpartum, it is termed *secondary postpartum haemorrhage*.

Primary postpartum haemorrhage

A measured loss that reaches 500 ml or any loss that adversely affects the mother's condition constitutes a PPH.

There are several reasons why a PPH may occur, including:
- atonic uterus
- retained placenta
- trauma
- blood coagulation disorder.

Atonic uterus

This is a failure of the myometrium at the placental site to contract and retract, and to compress torn blood vessels and control blood loss by a living ligature action. Causes of atonic uterine action resulting in PPH are listed in Box 19.2.

There are, in addition, a number of factors that do not directly *cause* a PPH, but do increase the likelihood of excessive bleeding (Box 19.3).

Signs of PPH

These may be obvious, such as:
- visible bleeding
- maternal collapse.

However, more subtle signs may present, such as:
- pallor
- rising pulse rate
- falling blood pressure
- altered level of consciousness; the mother may become restless or drowsy
- an enlarged uterus that feels 'boggy' on palpation (i.e. soft, distended and lacking tone); even if little visible blood loss.

Prophylaxis

- During the antenatal period, identify risk factors, e.g. previous obstetric history, anaemia.
- During labour, prevent prolonged labour and ketoacidosis.
- Ensure the mother does not have a full bladder at any stage.
- Give prophylactic administration of a uterotonic agent.
- If a woman is known to have a placenta praevia, keep 2 units of cross-matched blood available.

Box 19.2 Causes of atonic uterine action

- Incomplete separation of the placenta
- Retained cotyledon, placental fragment or membranes
- Precipitate labour
- Prolonged labour resulting in uterine inertia
- Polyhydramnios or multiple pregnancy causing overdistension of uterine muscle
- Placenta praevia
- Placental abruption
- General anaesthesia, especially halothane or cyclopropane
- Mismanagement of the third stage of labour
- A full bladder
- Aetiology unknown

Box 19.3 Predisposing factors which might increase the risks of postpartum haemorrhage

- Previous history of postpartum haemorrhage or retained placenta
- High parity, resulting in uterine scar tissue
- Presence of fibroids
- Maternal anaemia
- Ketoacidosls
- Multiple pregnancy

Management of PPH

Three basic principles of care:
- Call for medical aid.
- Stop the bleeding:
  - Rub up a contraction
  - Give a uterotonic
  - Empty the bladder
  - Empty the uterus
  - Apply pressure if there is trauma.
- Resuscitate the mother.

See Figure 19.4 for a summary of management; at the same time as taking these measures, check the blood is clotting.

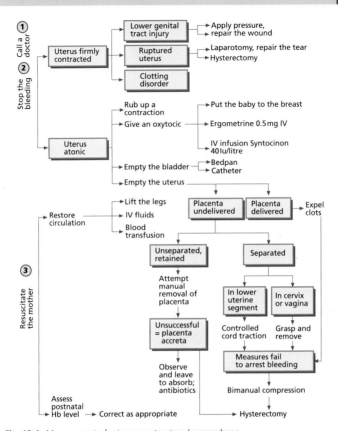

Fig. 19.4: Management of primary postpartum haemorrhage.

Secondary postpartum haemorrhage
See Chapter 25.

CHAPTER 20

Prolonged Pregnancy and Disorders of Uterine Action

POST-TERM OR PROLONGED PREGNANCY

Risks and clinical implications of post-term pregnancy
- Post-term pregnancy is one that is in excess of 287 days (although 42 weeks is often considered acceptable).
- Accurate dating of a pregnancy is essential, as incorrect diagnosis that a pregnancy has gone beyond term may lead to inappropriate or unnecessary intervention.
- Post-term pregnancy is associated with an increase in perinatal mortality and neonatal morbidity rates.
- Possible fetal consequences include macrosomia or fetal compromise due to placental demise.
- Prolonged pregnancy is the largest single indication for induction of labour.

Management of post-term pregnancy
Two forms of care are offered:
- Expectant management with fetal surveillance.
- Elective induction of labour after 41 weeks of gestation.

Antenatal surveillance
- *Biophysical profile*. A combined ultrasound assessment of fetal breathing, fetal movement, fetal tone, reactivity of the heart rate and amniotic fluid volume is used to predict fetal wellbeing in a high-risk pregnancy. A total score of 8–10 indicates the fetus is in good condition.
- *Doppler ultrasound of umbilical artery*.
- Twice weekly *cardiotocography* (CTG), also known as non-stress testing (NST).
- *Amniotic fluid measurement*.

INDUCTION OF LABOUR

Indications for induction

Induction is indicated when the benefits to the mother or the fetus outweigh those of continuing the pregnancy. It is associated with the maternal and fetal factors described in Box 20.1.

Contraindications to induction

These include:

- placenta praevia
- transverse or compound fetal presentation
- cord presentation or cord prolapse
- cephalopelvic disproportion
- severe fetal compromise
- active genital herpes.

If delivery is imperative, it should be effected by caesarean section.

CERVICAL RIPENING

Structural changes in ripening

Successful induction occurs when the cervix is favourable or so-called 'ripe'. The cervix is then more compliant, offering less soft tissue resistance to the actions of the myometrium and the presenting part.

Prostaglandins

Pre-induction prostaglandin can be used to prime or mature the cervix for induction. A low-dose prostaglandin is administered to bring about effacement and dilatation without stimulating contractions.

Box 20.1 Indications for induction of labour

Maternal

- Prolonged or post-term pregnancy
- Hypertension, including pre-eclampsia
- Diabetes
- Medical problems, e.g. renal, respiratory or cardiac disease
- Placental abruption
- Obstetric history, such as previous stillbirth or previous caesarean section
- Prelabour rupture of membranes
- Maternal request

Fetal

- Suspected fetal compromise
- Multiple pregnancy
- Intrauterine death
- Some breech presentations

METHODS OF INDUCING LABOUR

Prostaglandins and induction

Prior to prescribing prostaglandin, the cervix is assessed using the Bishop's score (Table 20.1). PGE_2 preparations are available in gels, tablets or controlled-release pessary form; they are inserted close to the cervix within the posterior fornix of the vagina. Fetal heart rate and uterine contractions should be monitored continuously for 30–60 minutes thereafter. The mother remains recumbent or resting for 1 hour. Changes in the cervix can be assessed by an increase in the Bishop's score.

Recommended prescribed doses of PGE_2 are shown in Table 20.2.

Sweeping or stripping of membranes

Sweeping the membranes can be an effective method of inducing labour where there is an uncomplicated pregnancy. During a vaginal examination the clinician inserts a finger through the cervical os, and using a sweeping or circular movement releases the fetal membranes from the lower uterine segment. The woman should be made aware that it may cause some discomfort and bleeding.

Amniotomy

Amniotomy is the artificial rupture of the fetal membranes (ARM), resulting in drainage of liquor. It is performed to induce labour when the cervix is favourable or during labour to augment contractions. ARM may also be

Table 20.1 Modified Bishop's pre-induction pelvic scoring system

Inducibility features	0	1	2	3
Dilatation of cervix in cm	<1	1–2	2–4	>4
Consistency of cervix	Firm	Firm	Medium	Soft
Cervical canal length in cm	>4	2–4	1–2	<1
Position of cervix	Posterior	Mid	Anterior	–
Position of presenting part in cm above or below ischial spine	–3	–2	–1	+1, +2

Table 20.2 Recommended prescribed doses of prostaglandin E_2

Form	Dose
Slow-release pessary	One dose (10 mg of dinoprostone), string left accessible, removed after 24 hours
Tablets	3 mg 6–8 hourly, maximum dose 6 mg
Gels	Nulliparous women with an unfavourable cervix: 2 mg (maximum 4 mg)
	All other women: 1 mg (maximum 3 mg)
	Repeat doses of 1–2 mg 6 hourly may be given

Box 20.2 Amniotomy procedures

Prior to intervention

- Informed maternal consent is obtained
- The reason for the amniotomy is clearly stated in the records
- Presentation and degree of engagement of the presenting part are confirmed by abdominal palpation
- The fetal heart rate is auscultated
- The presence of a low-lying placenta or cord is excluded

Following intervention

- Note the colour and quantity of liquor
- Check the presentation, position and station of the fetus
- Ensure no cord has prolapsed
- Auscultate the fetal heart rate

carried out to visualise the colour of the liquor or to attach a fetal scalp electrode for the purposes of continuous electronic monitoring of the fetal heart rate. A well-fitting presenting part is essential to prevent cord prolapse.

ARM is carried out using an amnihook or an amnicot. Procedures are shown in Box 20.2.

Hazards of ARM

These include:

- intrauterine infection
- early decelerations of the fetal heart
- cord prolapse
- bleeding from fetal vessels in the membranes (vasa praevia); friable vessels in the cervix; or placenta praevia.

Oxytocin

Oxytocin is used in conjunction with amniotomy and may be commenced at the same time as ARM or after a delay of several hours.

Administration of oxytocin to induce labour

- Oxytocin is used intravenously, diluted in an isotonic solution such as normal saline.
- The infusion should be controlled through a pump to enable accurate assessment of volume and rate.
- Dosage should be recorded in milliunits per minute, with the suggested dilution being 30 IU in 500 ml of normal saline. (*Note*: 1 ml per hour delivers 1 milliunit per minute.) The midwife should aim to administer the lowest dose required to maintain effective, well-spaced uterine contractions, with a maximum of 3–4 contractions every 10 minutes (Table 20.3).
- Oxytocin should not be started within 6 hours of the administration of prostaglandins.

Table 20.3 Suggested regimen for intravenous oxytocin in the presence of ruptured membranes

Time in minutes after starting	Dose delivery (milliunits per minute)	Notes
0	1	Most women should have adequate contractions at 12 milliunits per minute
30	2	
60	4	
90	8	Maximum licensed dose is 20 milliunits per minute
120	12	
150	16	If regular contractions are not established after 5 IU (5 hours on suggested regimen), then induction should be stopped
180	20	
210	24	
240	28	
270	32	

Side-effects of oxytocin

● Hyperstimulation of the uterus, which could cause fetal hypoxia and uterine rupture.
● Water retention.
● Prolonged use may contribute to uterine atony postpartum.

RESPONSIBILITIES OF THE MIDWIFE AND CARE OF A MOTHER IN INDUCTION OF LABOUR

The role of the midwife is to monitor the wellbeing of the mother and fetus throughout the process of induction, assess progress in labour and observe for signs of side effects of oxytocin. The parameters listed in Box 20.3 should be monitored.

The midwife should be aware of the risk of uterine rupture associated with excessive use of oxytocin, particularly if there is a previous history of caesarean section.

PROLONGED LABOUR

Prolonged labour is associated with the medical model of management of childbirth and for many women – and midwives – the attempts to place time limits on the physiological process of labour is problematic. However, prolonged labour is associated with increasing risks to mother and fetus.

Prolonged labour is most common in primigravidae and may be caused by:
● ineffective uterine contractions
● cephalopelvic disproportion
● an occipitoposterior position.

Box 20.3 The midwife's responsibilities in induction of labour

Baseline observations
- Maternal pulse rate, blood pressure and temperature are recorded

Uterine contractions
- Frequency, duration and strength are monitored every 15–30 minutes
- Continuous tocography is recommended when oxytocin is in use and for an hour following insertion of prostaglandins

Fetal wellbeing
- Fetal heart rate is recorded every 15 minutes
- There should be continuous monitoring in conjunction with oxytocin, using an abdominal ultrasound transducer or a fetal scalp electrode

Assessment of pain
- The rapid build-up of contractions can be difficult to cope with

Assessment of progress
- Position and station of the presenting part are noted
- Length, consistency, position and dilatation of the cervix are monitored
- Vaginal examinations are usually carried out every 4 hours

Dystocia literally means 'difficult labour' and is associated with slowness or lack of progress in labour. Possible problems include:
- contractions being ineffective in dilating and effacing the cervix
- uncoordinated contractions, where the two segments of the uterus fail to work in harmony
- contractions giving inadequate involuntary expulsion.

Other causes of dystocia are abnormalities of fetal presentation and position, the pelvis, the birth canal and congenital abnormalities.

Prolonged latent phase
The latent phase of labour is still poorly understood and its duration difficult to define; therefore, a diagnosis of a prolonged latent phase may be arbitrary and result in inappropriate intervention.

Prolonged active phase
Slow progress may be defined either as total duration of hours in labour or as failure of the cervix to dilate at a fixed rate per hour. A rate of 1 cm per hour is most commonly taken as normal, but use of a standardised progress rate is now being questioned. A prolonged active phase is caused by a combination of factors, including the cervix, the uterus, the fetus and the mother's pelvis.

Inefficient uterine action
In the absence of effective contractions, descent of the presenting part and dilatation of the cervix may be delayed.

Factors that may affect uterine action
- Restricting food and fluids to mothers in labour may have a detrimental effect.
- Ambulation may promote more effective uterine activity.
- An upright position improves the application of the presenting part on to the cervix, and may trigger the neuroendocrine Ferguson reflex.
- Stress and psychosocial factors can adversely affect contractions.

AUGMENTATION OF LABOUR

Augmentation of labour refers to intervention to correct slow progress in labour. Correction of ineffective uterine contractions includes amniotomy, administration of oxytocin and amniotomy or administration of oxytocin in the presence of the previously ruptured membranes. Cephalopelvic disproportion should be excluded before attempts are made to speed up the contractions.

Incoordinate uterine activity
This may be hypertonic and also inefficient. Possible signs include the following:
- Fundal dominance is lacking.
- Polarity is reversed.
- Resting tone of the uterus is raised.
- Pain is intense and out of proportion to the effect of the contraction on the dilatation of the cervix.

Where coordination of the contractions is completely lacking, different areas of the uterus contract independently, causing a 'colicky' uterus. The mother suffers severe generalised pain. Fetal compromise may occur due to diminished placental perfusion.

Constriction ring dystocia
This is a localised spasm of a ring of muscle fibres that occurs at the junction of the upper and lower segments of the uterus. It is associated with the use of oxytocin.

MANAGEMENT OF PROLONGED LABOUR

Determining the cause is necessary before deciding on management. Hypotonic uterine activity may be corrected with amniotomy or oxytocin infusion, or both. If, however, there have been strong contractions and slow progress, a caesarean section is likely. Obvious disproportion or malpresentation is an indication for caesarean section.

Principles of care are summarised in Box 20.4.

PROLONGED SECOND STAGE OF LABOUR

Provided that there is evidence of descent of the fetus and in the absence of fetal or maternal distress, there is no basis for placing a time limit on the duration of the second stage of labour.

Box 20.4 Principles of care in prolonged labour

Comfort and analgesia
- Adequate analgesia should be offered
- An epidural block may be beneficial

Observations
- Temperature is recorded every 4 hours
- Vaginal swabs may be taken and broad-spectrum antibiotics commenced if infection is suspected
- Pulse and blood pressure recorded hourly, or more frequently if the woman's condition dictates this

Fluid balance
- Input and output should be recorded
- The mother should be encouraged to empty her bladder every 2 hours; a full bladder may affect the uterine action in labour
- Reduced urinary output and ketones may indicate dehydration

Assessment of progress
- Vaginal examination is usually carried out 4 hourly

Fetal wellbeing
- Fetal heart is monitored continuously
- The presence of meconium-stained liquor and an abnormal fetal heart tracing are suggestive of fetal hypoxia; fetal blood sampling may be carried out
- A paediatrician may be required, and if the mother is in labour at home it may be necessary for her to be transferred into hospital

Causes of delay in the second stage
These are listed in Box 20.5.

Management of a prolonged second stage of labour
- Confirm the position, attitude and station of the presenting part by vaginal examination.
- Auscultate the fetal heart after every contraction or use electronic monitoring.

Box 20.5 Causes of delay in the second stage of labour

- Ineffective contractions
- Poor maternal effort
- Loss or absence of a desire to push caused by epidural analgesia
- A large fetus, malpresentation or malposition
- A full bladder or a full rectum
- A reduced pelvic outlet, in association with an occipitoposterior position may result in deep transverse arrest

- In the presence of inefficient uterine contractions, an infusion of oxytocin should be commenced.
- Where the mother is in labour at home, arrange for transfer to hospital or seek support from the supervisor of midwives.
- Birth may be expedited where the conditions alter and maternal or fetal wellbeing become compromised. Ventouse or forceps will be utilised where the pelvic outlet is adequate and vaginal birth can be safely carried out. Caesarean section may be necessary where there is evidence of cephalopelvic disproportion.

CERVICAL DYSTOCIA

This occurs rarely and is often acquired as a consequence of scarring of the cervix or a congenital structural abnormality. Despite effective contractions the cervix fails to dilate, although it may efface. Caesarean section is necessary to deliver the baby.

OVEREFFICIENT UTERINE ACTIVITY (PRECIPITATE LABOUR)

The contractions are strong and frequent from the onset of labour. Resistance from the soft tissue is low, resulting in rapid completion of the first and second stages. The mother may be distressed by the intensity of the contractions and the unexpected speed of the birth. Soft tissue damage to the cervix or perineum may complicate the birth. The uterus may fail to retract during the third stage, leading to retained placenta or postpartum haemorrhage.

Fetal hypoxia and rapid moulding can occur. The speed of the birth may result in the baby being born in an inappropriate place and sustaining injury.

Precipitate labour tends to recur.

TRIAL OF LABOUR

A trial of labour is offered to mothers when there is a minor degree of cephalopelvic disproportion. Review of place of birth may be necessary. If, despite good uterine contractions, cervical dilatation is slow and the head fails to descend, the outlook for vaginal birth is poor and the decision must be made whether to allow labour to continue.

If at any stage during this labour the mother or fetus is under stress, then a caesarean section will be performed. A trial of labour for vaginal birth may also be considered following previous caesarean section (VBAC).

OBSTRUCTED LABOUR

Labour is obstructed when there is no advance of the presenting part despite strong uterine contractions. The obstruction usually occurs at the pelvic brim but may occur at the outlet.

Causes of obstructed labour

- Cephalopelvic disproportion.
- Deep transverse arrest.
- Malpresentation, e.g. shoulder or brow presentation, or in persistent mentoposterior position.
- Pelvic mass, e.g. fibroids, ovarian or pelvic tumours.
- Fetal abnormalities, e.g. hydrocephalus, conjoined twins.

Signs of obstructed labour

These are listed in Box 20.6.

On examination the vagina feels hot and dry; the presenting part is high and feels wedged and immovable. It may be difficult to assess the station of the presenting part accurately due to excessive moulding of the fetal skull and a large caput succedaneum.

Management of obstructed labour

- An intravenous infusion to correct dehydration.
- Blood is taken for cross-matching in case a transfusion is needed.
- Antibiotics should be given to overcome any infection.
- If obstructed labour is recognised in the first stage of labour, delivery should be by caesarean section.

Box 20.6 Signs of obstructed labour

Early signs

- The presenting part does not enter the pelvic brim despite good contractions (exclude full bladder, loaded rectum or excessive liquor)
- Cervical dilatation is slow; the cervix hangs loosely like 'an empty sleeve'
- Pressure may result in early rupture or formation of a large elongated sac of forewaters

Late signs

- The mother is dehydrated, ketotic and in constant pain
- The mother is pyrexial
- Urinary output is poor and haematuria may be present
- There is evidence of fetal compromise
- The uterus becomes moulded round the fetus and fails to relax properly between contractions
- Contractions continue to build in strength and frequency until the uterus is in a continuous state of tonic contraction
- A visible retraction ring (Bandl's ring), similar in appearance to a full bladder, appears at an oblique angle across the abdomen
- In a primigravida, uterine contractions may cease for a while before recommencing with renewed vigour

- In the second stage of labour, failure to progress and descend may be due to deep transverse arrest. If rotation and assisted birth fail, caesarean section should be performed.
- If the mother is in labour at home, arrangements should be made to transfer her to the nearest maternity unit with facilities for an immediate caesarean section. Blood is taken for cross-matching and an intravenous infusion is sited prior to transfer.
- The paediatrician should be present at the birth.

Complications of obstructed labour

Complications are listed in Box 20.7.

Box 20.7 Complications of obstructed labour

Maternal

- There is trauma to the bladder, e.g. vesicovaginal fistula
- There is intrauterine infection due to prolonged rupture of membranes
- Neglected obstruction will result in rupture of the uterus, leading to haemorrhage and possible death of the mother and the fetus

Fetal

- Intrauterine asphyxia may result in a fresh stillbirth or, if the baby is born alive, permanent brain damage
- Ascending infection can cause neonatal pneumonia; this may also develop as a consequence of meconium aspiration

CHAPTER 21

Malpositions of the Occiput and Malpresentations

OCCIPITOPOSTERIOR POSITIONS

Occipitoposterior positions are the most common type of malposition of the occiput and occur in approximately 10% of labours. A persistent occipitoposterior position results from a failure of internal rotation prior to delivery. The vertex is presenting, but the occiput lies in the posterior rather than the anterior part of the pelvis. As a consequence, the fetal head is deflexed and larger diameters of the fetal skull present.

CAUSES

The direct cause is often unknown, but it may be associated with an android- or anthropoid-shaped pelvis.

ANTENATAL DIAGNOSIS

Abdominal examination

Inspection
- There is a saucer-shaped depression at or just below the umbilicus.

Palpation
- The back is difficult to palpate; it is well out to the side.
- Limbs can be felt on both sides of the midline.
- The head is usually high.
- The occiput and sinciput are on the same level.

Auscultation
- The fetal heart can be heard in the midline or in the flank.

DIAGNOSIS DURING LABOUR

- The woman may complain of continuous and severe backache worsening with contractions.
- Spontaneous rupture of the membranes may occur at an early stage of labour.
- Contractions may be incoordinate.
- There is slow descent of the head, even with good contractions.
- The woman may have a strong desire to push early in labour.

Vaginal examination

The findings will depend upon the degree of flexion of the head; locating the anterior fontanelle in the anterior part of the pelvis is diagnostic. The direction of the sagittal suture and location of the posterior fontanelle will help to confirm the diagnosis.

MANAGEMENT OF LABOUR

Labour with a fetus in an occipitoposterior position can be long and painful. The deflexed head does not fit well onto the cervix and therefore does not produce optimal stimulation.

Management is described in Box 21.1.

MECHANISM OF THE RIGHT OCCIPITOPOSTERIOR POSITION (LONG ROTATION)

See Figures 21.1–21.4 and Table 21.1.
- *Flexion*. Descent takes place with increasing flexion. The occiput becomes the leading part.
- *Internal rotation of the head*. The occiput reaches the pelvic floor first and rotates forwards three-eighths of a circle along the right side of the pelvis to lie under the symphysis pubis. The shoulders follow, turning two-eighths of a circle from the left to the right oblique diameter.

Box 21.1 Management of labour: occipitoposterior positions

First stage of labour

- Assist with pain management techniques, such as massage, changes of posture and position. Offer pharmacological pain control methods as appropriate
- Prevent dehydration and ketosis
- Correct any incoordinate uterine action or ineffective contractions with an oxytocin infusion
- The urge to push long before the cervix has become fully dilated may be eased by a change in position and the use of breathing techniques or nitrous oxide and oxygen to enhance relaxation

Second stage of labour

- Full dilatation of the cervix may need to be confirmed by a vaginal examination
- Encourage the woman to remain upright
- If contractions are weak and ineffective, an oxytocin infusion may be commenced
- The length of the second stage of labour is increased when the occiput is posterior, and there is an increased likelihood of operative delivery

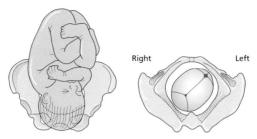

Fig. 21.1: Head descending with increased flexion. Sagittal suture in right oblique diameter of the pelvis.

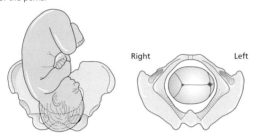

Fig. 21.2: Occiput and shoulders have rotated one-eighth of a circle forwards. Sagittal suture in transverse diameter of the pelvis.

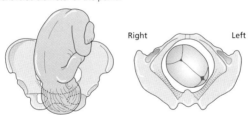

Fig. 21.3: Occiput and shoulders have rotated two-eighths of a circle forwards. Sagittal suture in the left oblique diameter of the pelvis. The position is right occipitoanterior.

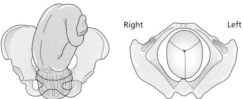

Fig. 21.4: Occiput has rotated three-eighths of a circle forwards. Note the twist in the neck. Sagittal suture in the anteroposterior diameter of the pelvis.

Table 21.1 Terminology for mechanisms of the right occipitoposterior, left mentoanterior and left sacroanterior positions

	Right occipitoposterior	Left mentoanterior	Left sacroanterior
Lie	Longitudinal	Longitudinal	Longitudinal
Attitude	Deflexion of head	Extension of head and back	Complete flexion
Presentation	Vertex	Face	Breech
Denominator	Occiput	Mentum	Sacrum
Presenting part	Middle or anterior area of left parietal bone	Left malar bone	Anterior (left) buttock
Diameter	Occipitofrontal diameter (11.5 cm) lies in right oblique diameter of pelvic brim Occiput points to right sacroiliac joint and sinciput to left iliopectineal eminence		Bitrochanteric diameter (10 cm) enters pelvis in the oblique diameter of brim Sacrum points to left iliopectineal eminence

- *Crowning*. The occiput escapes under the symphysis pubis and the head is crowned.
- *Extension*. The sinciput, face and chin sweep the perineum and the head is born by a movement of extension.
- *Restitution*. The occiput turns one-eighth of a circle to the right and the head realigns itself with the shoulders.
- *Internal rotation of the shoulders*. The shoulders enter the pelvis in the right oblique diameter; the anterior shoulder reaches the pelvic floor first and rotates forwards one-eighth of a circle to lie under the symphysis pubis.
- *External rotation of the head*. At the same time the occiput turns a further one-eighth of a circle to the right.
- *Lateral flexion*. The anterior shoulder escapes under the symphysis pubis, the posterior shoulder sweeps the perineum and the body is born by a movement of lateral flexion.

POSSIBLE COURSE AND OUTCOMES OF LABOUR

Long internal rotation

This is the most common outcome, with good uterine contractions producing flexion and descent of the head so that the occiput rotates forward three-eighths of a circle, as described above.

Short internal rotation (persistent occipitoposterior position)

This results from failure of flexion.

● The sinciput reaches the pelvic floor first and rotates forwards.
● The occiput goes into the hollow of the sacrum.
● The baby is born facing the pubic bone (face to pubis).

Diagnosis

In the first stage of labour:

● There is slow descent with a deflexed head and fetal heart audible in the flank or in the midline.

In the second stage of labour:

● Delay is common.
● On vaginal examination the anterior fontanelle is felt behind the symphysis pubis.
● Dilatation of the anus and gaping of the vagina may occur while the fetal head is barely visible; there may also be excessive bulging of the perineum.

The birth

The sinciput will first emerge from under the symphysis pubis; the midwife maintains flexion to prevent it from escaping further than the glabella. The occiput sweeps the perineum and is born. The head is then extended to bring the face down from under the symphysis pubis. An episiotomy may be required to prevent excessive perineal trauma.

Deep transverse arrest

● This occurs when the occiput begins to rotate forwards but flexion is not maintained; the occipitofrontal diameter becomes caught at the narrow bispinous diameter of the outlet.
● Arrest may be due to weak contractions, a straight sacrum or a narrowed outlet.

Diagnosis

On vaginal examination:

● The sagittal suture is in the transverse diameter of the pelvis and both fontanelles are palpable.
● The head is at the level of the ischial spines and there is no advance.

Management

Pushing may not resolve the problem, though a change of position and sighing out slowly (SOS) breathing may help to overcome the urge to bear down.

An operative delivery may be required to rotate the head to an occipitoanterior position before birth. Adequate analgesia or anaesthesia should be given.

Conversion to face or brow presentation

● This occurs when the head is deflexed at the onset of labour and extension occurs instead of flexion.
● Complete extension results in a face presentation; incomplete extension leads to a brow presentation.

COMPLICATIONS

- Prolonged labour with increased likelihood of instrumental delivery.
- Obstructed labour.
- Maternal perineal trauma.
- Neonatal trauma/cerebral haemorrhage.
- Cord prolapse.

FACE PRESENTATION

The attitude of the head is one of complete extension. It may be primary (presents before labour) or secondary (develops during labour). The denominator is the mentum and the presenting diameters are the submentobregmatic (9.5 cm) and the bitemporal (8.2 cm) (Figs 21.5–21.10).

CAUSES

- Anterior obliquity of the uterus.
- Contracted pelvis.
- Polyhydramnios.
- Congenital abnormality, e.g. anencephaly.

DIAGNOSIS DURING LABOUR

Abdominal palpation

Face presentation may be difficult to diagnose.

- The occiput feels prominent, with a groove between head and back.
- The limbs may be palpated on the side opposite to the occiput.
- The fetal heart is best heard through the fetal chest on the same side as the limbs. It is difficult in a mentoposterior position.

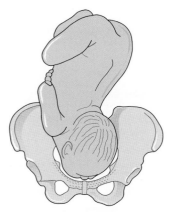

Fig. 21.5: Right mentoposterior.

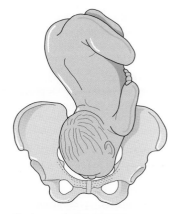

Fig. 21.6: Left mentoposterior.

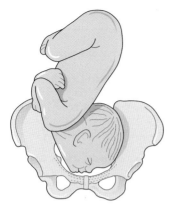

Fig. 21.7: Right mentolateral.

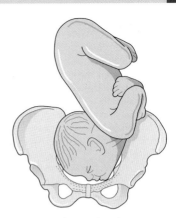

Fig. 21.8: Left mentolateral.

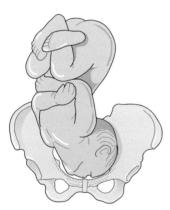

Fig. 21.9: Right mentoanterior.

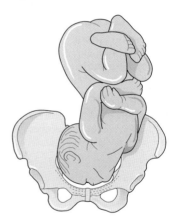

Fig. 21.10: Left mentoanterior.

Vaginal examination
- The presenting part is high, soft and irregular.
- The orbital ridges, eyes, nose and mouth may be felt.
- As labour progresses the face becomes oedematous, making it more difficult to distinguish from a breech presentation.
- Care must be taken not to injure or infect the eyes.

MECHANISM OF THE LEFT MENTOANTERIOR POSITION

See Table 21.1 (p. 232).
- *Extension*. Descent takes place with increasing extension. The mentum becomes the leading part.

- *Internal rotation of the head*. This occurs when the chin reaches the pelvic floor and rotates forwards one-eighth of a circle. The chin escapes under the symphysis pubis.
- *Flexion*. Flexion takes place when the sinciput, vertex and occiput sweep the perineum; the head is born.
- *Restitution*. This occurs when the chin turns one-eighth of a circle to the woman's left.
- *Internal rotation of the shoulders*. The shoulders enter the pelvis in the left oblique diameter, and the anterior shoulder reaches the pelvic floor first and rotates forwards one-eighth of a circle along the right side of the pelvis.
- *External rotation of the head*. This occurs simultaneously. The chin moves a further one-eighth of a circle to the left.
- *Lateral flexion*. The anterior shoulder escapes under the symphysis pubis, the posterior shoulder sweeps the perineum and the body is born by a movement of lateral flexion.

POSSIBLE COURSE AND OUTCOMES OF LABOUR

Prolonged labour

This is due to an ill-fitting presenting part and facial bones that do not mould. The fetal axis pressure is directed to the chin and the head is extended almost at right angles to the spine, increasing the diameters to be accommodated in the pelvis.

Mentoanterior positions

With good uterine contractions, descent and rotation of the head occur and labour progresses to a spontaneous birth.

Mentoposterior positions

If the head is completely extended and the contractions are effective, the mentum will rotate forwards and the position becomes anterior.

Persistent mentoposterior position

If the head is incompletely extended and the sinciput reaches the pelvic floor first and rotates forwards one-eighth of a circle, bringing the chin into the hollow of the sacrum, no further mechanism is possible and labour becomes obstructed.

MANAGEMENT OF LABOUR

See Box 21.2.

COMPLICATIONS

- Obstructed labour.
- Cord prolapse.

Box 21.2 Management of labour: face presentations

First stage of labour

- Inform the obstetrician
- Do not apply a fetal scalp electrode and take care not to infect or injure the eyes during vaginal examinations
- Following rupture of the membranes, exclude cord prolapse
- Observe descent of the head by abdominal palpation
- Assess cervical dilatation and descent of the head by vaginal examination every 2–4 hours. In mentoposterior positions, note whether the mentum is lower than the sinciput. If the head remains high in spite of good contractions, caesarean section is likely

Birth of the head

- When the face appears at the vulva, maintain extension by holding back the sinciput and permitting the mentum to escape under the symphysis pubis before the occiput is allowed to sweep the perineum. In this way the submentovertical diameter (11.5 cm), instead of the mentovertical diameter (13.5 cm), distends the vaginal orifice
- Because the perineum is also distended by the biparietal diameter (9.5 cm), an elective episiotomy may be performed
- If the head does not descend in the second stage and is in a mentoanterior position, it may be possible for the obstetrician to deliver the baby with forceps; when rotation is incomplete, or the position remains mentoposterior, a rotational forceps delivery may be feasible
- If the head has become impacted, or there is any suspicion of disproportion, a caesarean section will be necessary

- Facial bruising/oedema.
- Cerebral haemorrhage.
- Maternal perineal and vaginal trauma.

BROW PRESENTATION

The fetal head is partially extended with the frontal bone (bounded by the anterior fontanelle and the orbital ridges) lying at the pelvic brim. The presenting diameter is the mentovertical (13.5 cm).

CAUSES

These are the same as for a secondary face presentation; during extension from a vertex presentation to a face presentation, the brow will present temporarily and in a few cases this will persist.

DIAGNOSIS

Brow presentation is not usually detected before the onset of labour.

Abdominal palpation

- The head is high, appears unduly large and does not descend into the pelvis despite good uterine contractions.

Vaginal examination

- The presenting part is high.
- The anterior fontanelle may be felt on one side of the pelvis and the orbital ridges, and possibly the root of the nose, at the other.
- A large caput succedaneum may mask these landmarks if the woman has been in labour for some hours.

MANAGEMENT

Management of brow presentations is summarised in Box 21.3.

COMPLICATIONS

These are the same as in a face presentation, except that obstructed labour requiring caesarean section is the probable outcome.

BREECH PRESENTATION

Here the fetus lies longitudinally with the buttocks in the lower pole of the uterus. There are six positions (Figs 21.11–21.16).

TYPES OF BREECH PRESENTATION POSITION

- Breech with extended legs (frank breech) (Fig. 21.17).
- Complete breech (Fig. 21.18).
- Footling breech (Fig. 21.19).
- Knee presentation (Fig. 21.20).

CAUSES

Often no cause is identified, but the following circumstances favour breech presentation:

- extended legs
- preterm labour

Box 21.3 Management of labour: brow presentations

- Inform the obstetrician immediately this presentation is suspected; vaginal birth is extremely rare unless the woman has a large pelvis and a small baby
- If there is no evidence of fetal compromise, the woman may be allowed to labour for a short while in case further extension of the head converts the brow presentation to a face presentation
- Occasionally, spontaneous flexion may occur, resulting in a vertex presentation

- multiple pregnancy
- polyhydramnios
- hydrocephaly
- uterine abnormalities
- placenta praevia.

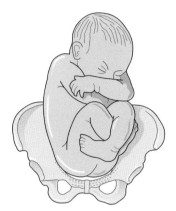

Fig. 21.11: Right sacroposterior.

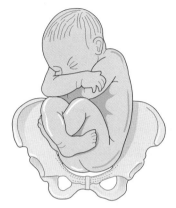

Fig. 21.12: Left sacroposterior.

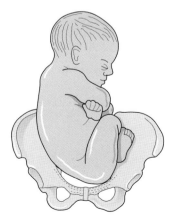

Fig. 21.13: Right sacrolateral.

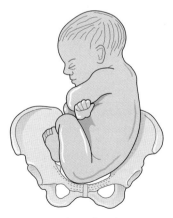

Fig. 21.14: Left sacrolateral.

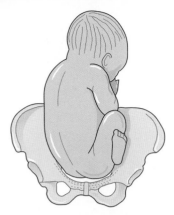

Fig. 21.15: Right sacroanterior.

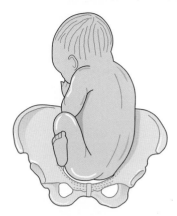

Fig. 21.16: Left sacroanterior.

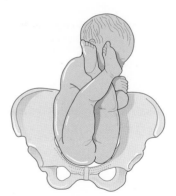

Fig. 21.17: Frank breech.

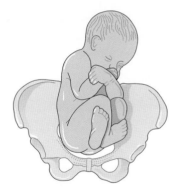

Fig. 21.18: Complete breech.

ANTENATAL DIAGNOSIS

Abdominal examination

Palpation

- The lie is longitudinal with a soft presentation, which is more easily felt using Pawlik's grip.
- The head can usually be felt in the fundus as a round hard mass, which may be made to move independently of the back by ballottement with one or both hands.
- If the legs are extended, the feet may prevent such nodding.

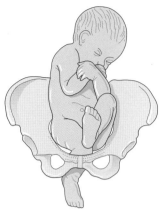
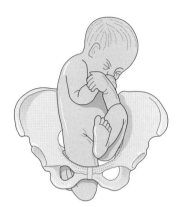

Fig. 21.19: Footling presentation. **Fig. 21.20:** Knee presentation.

- When the breech is anterior and the fetus well flexed, it may be difficult to locate the head, but use of the combined grip, in which the upper and lower poles are grasped simultaneously, may aid diagnosis.
- The woman may complain of discomfort under her ribs, especially at night, owing to pressure of the head on the diaphragm.

Auscultation
- When the breech has not passed through the pelvic brim, the fetal heart is heard most clearly above the umbilicus.
- When the legs are extended, the breech descends into the pelvis easily. The fetal heart is then heard at a lower level.

Ultrasound examination
- This may be used to demonstrate a breech presentation.

X-ray examination
- Although largely superseded by ultrasound, X-ray has the added advantage of allowing pelvimetry to be performed at the same time.

DIAGNOSIS DURING LABOUR
Abdominal examination
- Breech presentation may be diagnosed on admission in labour.

Vaginal examination
- The breech feels soft and irregular with no sutures palpable.
- The anus may be felt and fresh meconium on the examining finger is usually diagnostic.

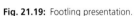

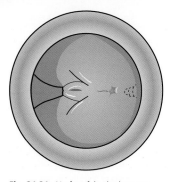

Fig. 21.21: No feet felt; the legs are extended.

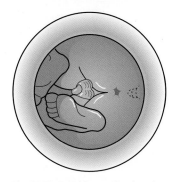

Fig. 21.22: Feet felt; complete breech presentation.

- If the legs are extended (Fig. 21.21), the external genitalia are very evident but it must be remembered that these become oedematous.
- A foot must be differentiated from a hand (Fig. 21.22).

Presentation may be confirmed by ultrasound scan or X-ray.

ANTENATAL MANAGEMENT

If the midwife suspects or detects a breech presentation at 36 weeks' gestation or later, she should refer the woman to an obstetrician. There are differing opinions among obstetricians as to the management of breech presentation during pregnancy and a decision on management is usually deferred until near term.

External cephalic version

External cephalic version (ECV) involves external manipulation on the mother's abdomen to convert a breech to a cephalic presentation. ECV may be offered at term and should only be undertaken in a unit where there are facilities for emergency delivery. Contraindications include:

- pre-eclampsia or hypertension
- multiple pregnancy
- oligohydramnios
- ruptured membranes
- a hydrocephalic fetus
- any condition that would require delivery by caesarean section.

PERSISTENT BREECH PRESENTATION

At 37 weeks' gestation a discussion of the available options should take place between the mother and an experienced practitioner, and a decision made as to whether to perform an elective caesarean section or to attempt a vaginal birth.

Assessment for vaginal birth

Any doubt as to the capacity of the pelvis to accommodate the fetal head must be resolved before the buttocks are delivered and the head attempts to enter the pelvic brim.

Fetal size

This, especially in relation to maternal size, can be assessed on abdominal palpation but is more accurately judged in association with an ultrasound examination.

Pelvic capacity

This can be judged on vaginal assessment. This will show the shape of the sacrum and give accurate measurements of the anteroposterior diameters of the pelvic brim, cavity and outlet. In a multigravida, information about the type of birth and the size of previous babies when compared with the size of the present fetus can be helpful.

MECHANISM OF THE LEFT SACROANTERIOR POSITION

This is described in Table 21.1 (p. 232).

- *Compaction.* Descent takes place with increasing compaction, owing to increased flexion of the limbs.
- *Internal rotation of the buttocks.* The anterior buttock reaches the pelvic floor first and rotates forwards one-eighth of a circle along the right side of the pelvis to lie underneath the symphysis pubis. The bitrochanteric diameter is now in the anteroposterior diameter of the outlet.
- *Lateral flexion of the body.* The anterior buttock escapes under the symphysis pubis, the posterior buttock sweeps the perineum and the buttocks are born by a movement of lateral flexion.
- *Restitution of the buttocks.* The anterior buttock turns slightly to the mother's right side.
- *Internal rotation of the shoulders.* The shoulders enter the pelvis in the same oblique diameter as the buttocks, the left oblique. The anterior shoulder rotates forwards one-eighth of a circle along the right side of the pelvis and escapes under the symphysis pubis, the posterior shoulder sweeps the perineum and the shoulders are born.
- *Internal rotation of the head.* The head enters the pelvis with the sagittal suture in the transverse diameter of the brim. The occiput rotates forwards along the left side and the suboccipital region (the nape of the neck) impinges on the undersurface of the symphysis pubis.
- *External rotation of the body.* At the same time the body turns so that the back is uppermost.
- *Birth of the head.* The chin, face and sinciput sweep the perineum and the head is born in a flexed attitude.

MANAGEMENT OF LABOUR

Careful assessment should be made at the start of labour and anticipated labour management should be reviewed (Box 21.4). A consultant obstetrician should be informed of a breech presentation in labour.

Types of vaginal birth

- *Spontaneous breech birth*. The birth occurs with little assistance from the attendant.
- *Assisted breech birth*. The buttocks are born spontaneously, but some assistance is necessary for delivery of extended legs or arms and the head.
- *Breech extraction*. This is a manipulative delivery carried out by an obstetrician and is performed to hasten delivery in an emergency situation such as fetal compromise.

Management of breech birth

- *When the buttocks are distending the perineum*, the woman is upright or in the lithotomy position. The bladder must be empty and it is usually catheterised at this stage. If epidural analgesia is not being used, the perineum is infiltrated with up to 10 ml of 0.5% plain lidocaine if an episiotomy is to be performed. (Pudendal block is sometimes used by an obstetrician.)
- The buttocks are born spontaneously.
- If the legs are flexed, the feet disengage at the vulva and the baby is born as far as the umbilicus.

Box 21.4 Management of labour: breech presentations

First stage of labour

- Basic care during this stage is the same as in normal labour
- Meconium-stained liquor is sometimes found owing to compression of the fetal abdomen and is not always a sign of fetal compromise
- A vaginal examination should be performed to exclude cord prolapse as soon as the membranes rupture. If they do not rupture spontaneously at an early stage, it is considered safer to leave them intact until labour is well established and the breech is at the level of the ischial spines.

Second stage of labour

- Full dilatation of the cervix should always be confirmed by vaginal examination before the woman commences active pushing.
- In hospital, inform the obstetrician of the onset of the second stage
- A paediatrician should be present for the birth
- Inform the anaesthetist too in case a general anaesthetic is required
- Active pushing is commenced when the buttocks are distending the vulva. Failure of the breech to descend onto the perineum in the second stage despite good contractions may indicate a need for caesarean section

- A loop of cord may be gently pulled down to avoid traction on the umbilicus.
- The midwife should feel for the elbows, which are usually on the chest. If so, the arms will escape with the next contraction. If the arms are not felt, they are extended.

Birth of the shoulders

- The shoulders should rotate into the anteroposterior diameter of the outlet. (It is helpful to wrap a small towel around the baby's hips, which preserves warmth and improves the grip.)
- Grasp the baby by the iliac crests with thumbs held parallel over the sacrum and tilt the baby towards the maternal sacrum in order to free the anterior shoulder.
- When the anterior shoulder has escaped, the buttocks are lifted towards the mother's abdomen to enable the posterior shoulder and arm to pass over the perineum.
- The head enters the pelvic brim and descends through the pelvis with the sagittal suture in the transverse diameter.
- The back must remain lateral until this has happened but afterwards will be turned uppermost. If the back is turned upwards too soon, the anteroposterior diameter of the head will enter the anteroposterior diameter of the brim and may become extended. The shoulders may then become impacted at the outlet and the extended head may cause difficulty.

Birth of the head

- When the back has been turned, the infant is allowed to hang from the vulva without support.
- The baby's weight brings the head onto the pelvic floor on which the occiput rotates forwards. The sagittal suture is now in the anteroposterior diameter of the outlet.
- If rotation of the head fails to take place, two fingers should be placed on the malar bones and the head rotated.
- The baby can be allowed to hang for 1 or 2 minutes.
- Gradually the neck elongates, the hairline appears and the suboccipital region can be felt.

Controlled birth of the head is vital to avoid any sudden change in intracranial pressure and subsequent cerebral haemorrhage. There are three methods:

- Forceps delivery.
- Burns Marshall method (if the head is flexed).
- Mauriceau–Smellie–Veit manoeuvre (jaw flexion and shoulder traction).

Forceps delivery

Most breech births are performed by an obstetrician, who will apply forceps to the after-coming head to achieve a controlled delivery.

Burns Marshall method

- Stand facing away from the mother and, with the left hand, grasp the baby's ankles from behind with forefinger between the two (Fig. 21.23A).
- The baby is kept on the stretch with sufficient traction to prevent the neck from bending backwards and being fractured.
- The suboccipital region, and not the neck, should pivot under the apex of the pubic arch or the spinal cord may be crushed.
- The feet are taken up through an arc of 180° until the mouth and nose are free at the vulva.
- The right hand may guard the perineum in order to prevent sudden escape of the head. The mother should be asked to take deliberate, regular breaths that allow the vault of the skull to escape gradually (Fig. 21.23B).

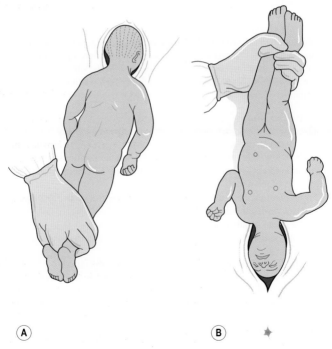

(A)   (B)

Fig. 21.23: Burns Marshall method of delivering the after-coming head of a breech presentation. (A) The baby is grasped by the feet and held on the stretch. (B) The mouth and nose are free. The vault of the head is delivered slowly.

Mauriceau–Smellie–Veit manoeuvre

- This is mainly used when there is delay in descent of the head because of extension.
- The baby is laid astride the right arm with the palm supporting the chest. Two fingers are placed on the malar bones.
- Two fingers of the left hand are hooked over the shoulders, with the middle finger pushing on the occiput to aid flexion.
- Traction is applied to draw the head out of the vagina and, when the suboccipital region appears, the body is lifted to assist the head to pivot around the symphysis pubis.
- The speed of delivery of the head must be controlled so that it does not emerge suddenly.

Alternative positions

When the woman has chosen to birth in an alternative position, it is the upright or supported squat that is the most suitable. The techniques described above will be adapted accordingly and the midwife will observe and encourage the spontaneous mechanism of birth.

Use of uterotonics for third stage

These are withheld until the head is born.

Delivery of extended legs

- Delay may occur at the outlet because the legs splint the body and impede lateral flexion of the spine.
- When the popliteal fossae appear at the vulva, two fingers are placed along the length of one thigh with the fingertips in the fossa.
- The leg is swept to the side of the abdomen (abducting the hip) and the knee is flexed by the pressure on its undersurface. As this movement is continued, the lower part of the leg will emerge from the vagina (Fig. 21.24).
- Repeat to deliver the second leg. The knee is a hinge joint, which bends in one direction only. If the knee is pulled forwards from the abdomen, severe injury to the joint can result.

Delivery of extended arms

Extended arms are diagnosed when the elbows are not felt on the chest after the umbilicus is born. This may be dealt with by using the Løvset manoeuvre (Figs 21.25 and 21.26). This is a combination of rotation and downward traction to deliver the arms, whatever position they are in. The direction of rotation must always bring the back uppermost and the arms are delivered from under the pubic arch.

- When the umbilicus is born and the shoulders are in the anteroposterior diameter, the baby is grasped by the iliac crests with the thumbs over the sacrum.
- Downward traction is applied until the axilla is visible.

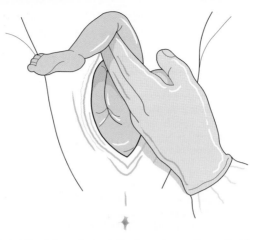

Fig. 21.24: Assisting delivery of extended leg by pressure on the popliteal fossa.

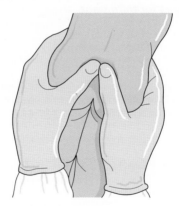

Fig. 21.25: Correct grasp for Løvset manoeuvre.

- Maintaining downward traction throughout, the body is rotated through a half-circle, 180°, starting by turning the back uppermost. The friction of the posterior arm against the pubic bone as the shoulder becomes anterior sweeps the arm in front of the face. The movement allows the shoulders to enter the pelvis in the transverse diameter.
- The first two fingers of the hand that is on the same side as the baby's back are used to splint the humerus and draw it down over the chest as the elbow is flexed.
- The body is now rotated back in the opposite direction and the second arm delivered in a similar fashion.

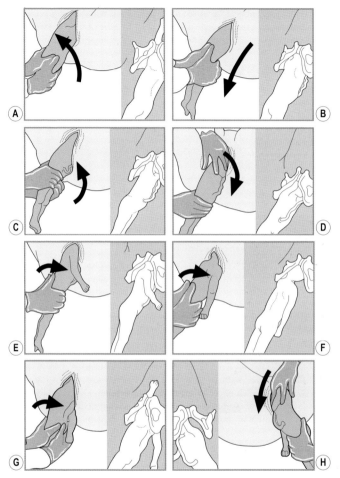

Fig. 21.26: Løvset manoeuvre for delivery of extended arms (see text).

Delay in birth of the head

- *Extended head*. If, when the body has been allowed to hang, the neck and hairline are not visible, it is probable that the head is extended. This may be dealt with by the use of forceps or the Mauriceau–Smellie–Veit manœuvre.
- *Posterior rotation of the occiput*. This malrotation of the head is rare and is usually the result of mismanagement. To deliver the head with the occiput posterior, the chin and face are permitted to escape under

the symphysis pubis as far as the root of the nose, and the baby is then lifted up towards the mother's abdomen to allow the occiput to sweep the perineum.

COMPLICATIONS

Apart from those difficulties already mentioned, other complications can arise, most of which affect the fetus. Many of these can be avoided by allowing only an experienced operator, or a closely supervised learner, to deliver the baby:

- Impacted breech.
- Cord prolapse.
- Birth injury:
  - superficial tissue damage
  - fractures of humerus, clavicle or femur or dislocation of shoulder or hip
  - Erb's palsy
  - trauma to internal organs
  - damage to the adrenals
  - spinal cord damage or fracture of the spine
  - intracranial haemorrhage
  - fetal hypoxia
  - premature separation of the placenta
  - maternal trauma.

The maternal complications of a breech delivery are the same as those found in other operative vaginal deliveries.

SHOULDER PRESENTATION

When the fetus lies with its long axis across the long axis of the uterus (*transverse lie*), the shoulder is most likely to present. Occasionally the lie is oblique but this does not persist, as the uterine contractions during labour make it longitudinal or transverse.

CAUSES

Maternal

- Lax abdominal and uterine muscles.
- Uterine abnormality.
- Contracted pelvis.

Fetal

- Preterm pregnancy.
- Multiple pregnancy.
- Polyhydramnios.
- Macerated fetus.
- Placenta praevia.

ANTENATAL DIAGNOSIS
Abdominal palpation
- The uterus appears broad and the fundal height is less than expected for the period of gestation.
- On pelvic and fundal palpation, neither head nor breech is felt. The mobile head is found on one side of the abdomen and the breech at a slightly higher level on the other.

Ultrasound
An ultrasound scan may be used to confirm the lie and presentation.

DIAGNOSIS DURING LABOUR
Abdominal palpation
- The findings are as above but when the membranes have ruptured the irregular outline of the uterus is more marked.
- If the uterus is contracting strongly and becomes moulded around the fetus, palpation is very difficult.
- The pelvis is no longer empty, the shoulder being wedged into it.

Vaginal examination
- This should not be performed without first excluding placenta praevia.
- In early labour, the presenting part may not be felt.
- The membranes usually rupture early.
- If the labour has been in progress for some time, the shoulder may be felt as a soft irregular mass.
- It is sometimes possible to palpate the ribs, their characteristic grid-iron pattern being diagnostic.
- When the shoulder enters the pelvic brim, an arm may prolapse; this should be differentiated from a leg.

POSSIBLE OUTCOMES OF LABOUR
If shoulder presentation persists in labour, delivery must be by caesarean section to avoid obstructed labour and subsequent uterine rupture.

MANAGEMENT
Antenatal
A cause must be sought before deciding on a course of management. Once placenta praevia or uterine abnormalities have been excluded, ECV may be attempted. If this fails, or if the lie is again transverse at the next antenatal visit, the woman is admitted to hospital while further investigations into the cause are made. She frequently remains there until birth because of the risk of cord prolapse.

Intrapartum

If a transverse lie is detected in early labour while the membranes are still intact, the obstetrician or competent health professional may attempt an ECV, followed, if this is successful, by a controlled rupture of the membranes. If the membranes have already ruptured spontaneously, a vaginal examination must be performed immediately to exclude cord prolapse.

Immediate caesarean section must be performed:
- if the cord prolapses
- when the membranes are already ruptured
- when ECV is unsuccessful
- when labour has already been in progress for some hours.

COMPLICATIONS

- Prolapsed cord.
- Prolapsed arm.
- Impacted shoulder presentation leading to obstructed labour, ruptured uterus and stillbirth.

UNSTABLE LIE

The lie is defined as unstable when, after 36 weeks' gestation, instead of remaining longitudinal, it varies from one examination to another between longitudinal and oblique or transverse.

CAUSES

Conditions that increase the mobility of the fetus or prevent the head from entering the pelvic brim can cause an unstable lie.

Maternal causes include:
- lax uterine muscles in multigravidae
- contracted pelvis.

Fetal causes include:
- polyhydramnios
- placenta praevia.

MANAGEMENT

Antenatal

- Advise the woman to go to the labour ward as soon as labour commences or membranes rupture.
- Exclude placenta praevia.
- Attempts to correct the abnormal presentation by ECV may be made. If unsuccessful, caesarean section is considered.

Intrapartum

Labour may be induced after 38 weeks' gestation, having first ensured that the lie is longitudinal; the induction may be performed by commencing an intravenous infusion of oxytocin to stimulate contractions. An empty bladder and rectum are important. A controlled rupture of the membranes is performed so that the head enters the pelvis.

The abdomen is palpated at frequent intervals to ensure that the lie remains longitudinal and to assess the descent of the head.

COMPLICATIONS

If labour commences with the lie other than longitudinal, the complications are the same as for a transverse lie.

COMPOUND PRESENTATION

A compound presentation is when a hand, or occasionally a foot, lies alongside the head. If diagnosed during the first stage of labour, medical aid must be sought. If, during the second stage, the midwife sees a hand presenting alongside the vertex, she could try to hold the hand back.

CHAPTER 22

Assisted Births

BIRTH BY FORCEPS

Forceps are most commonly employed to expedite delivery of the fetal head or to protect the fetus or the mother, or both, from trauma and exhaustion. They are also used to assist the delivery of the after-coming head of the breech or to draw the head of the baby up and out of the pelvis at caesarean section birth.

The three main indications for the use of forceps are:

- delay in the second stage of labour
- fetal compromise
- maternal distress.

TYPES OF OBSTETRIC FORCEPS

- *Wrigley's forceps*. These are designed for use when the head is on the perineum. They are also used for the after-coming head of a breech delivery, or at caesarean section.
- *Neville-Barnes or Simpson's forceps*. These are generally used for a low or mid-cavity forceps delivery when the sagittal suture is in the anteroposterior diameter of the cavity/outlet of the pelvis.
- *Kielland's forceps*. These are generally used for the rotation and extraction of the head that is arrested in the deep transverse or the occipitoposterior position.

PREREQUISITES FOR FORCEPS DELIVERY

'Forceps' is a useful mnemonic (Box 22.1).

The paediatrician may not be required at birth, but should be kept informed of circumstances. Neonatal resuscitation equipment must be checked and prepared in case it is needed.

COMPLICATIONS

These are listed in Box 22.2.

BIRTH BY THE VENTOUSE METHOD

The ventouse vacuum extractor is an instrument that applies traction. It can be used as an alternative to forceps. The cup cleaves to the fetal scalp by suction and is used to assist maternal effort. It may be employed when there is a delay in labour, when the cervix is not quite fully dilated. It may also be useful in the case of a second twin, when the head remains relatively high.

Box 22.1 The 'forceps' mnemonic

- **F**ull dilatation of the cervix
- **O**-fifths of the head palpable abdominally
- **R**oom in pelvis and ruptured membranes
- **C**ephalic presentation
- **E**mpty bladder
- **P**osition recognised
- **S**uitable pain relief – epidural or pudendal block plus perineal infiltration of local anaesthetic

Box 22.2 Some complications of forceps delivery

Maternal

- Trauma or soft tissue damage, which may occur to the perineum, vagina or cervix
- Haemorrhage from the above
- Dysuria or urinary retention, which may result from bruising or oedema to the urethra
- Painful perineum

Neonatal

- Marks on the baby's face caused by the pressure of the forceps; these resolve quite rapidly
- Excessive bruising
- Facial palsy

PROCEDURE

- The woman is usually in the lithotomy position and the same precautions are observed as for a forceps birth.
- The cup of the ventouse is placed as near as possible to, or on, the flexing point of the fetal head.
- The vacuum in the cup is increased gradually so as to achieve a close application to the fetal head. Usually a vacuum of $0.8\,\mathrm{kg/cm^2}$ is reached, by an increase of $0.2\,\mathrm{kg/cm^2}$ in stages, or an increase from 0.2 to $0.8\,\mathrm{kg/cm^2}$ is achieved directly.
- When the vacuum is achieved, traction is applied with a contraction and with maternal effort. This traction is applied in a downwards and backwards direction, then forwards and upwards, thus following the natural curve of the pelvis.
- The vacuum is released and the cup is removed at the crowning of the fetal head.
- The mother can then push the baby for the final part of the birth.

COMPLICATIONS

Prolonged traction will increase the likelihood of:

- scalp abrasions
- cephalhaematoma
- subaponeurotic bleeding.

CAESAREAN SECTION

Caesarean section is an operative procedure that is carried out under anaesthesia, whereby the fetus, placenta and membranes are delivered through an incision in the abdominal wall and the uterus. This is usually carried out after viability has been reached (i.e. 24 weeks of gestation onwards).

PREPARATION

Women expect to be actively involved in their care and the midwife must ensure that recent, valid and relevant information is provided.

The usual preoperative preparation is observed, including:

- an anaesthetic chart/preoperative assessment
- measurement of weight
- baseline observations of blood pressure, pulse and temperature
- gowning and removal of make-up and jewellery.

Results are obtained of any blood tests that have been requested and a full blood count is carried out. Blood is grouped and saved. In the case of pre-eclampsia, urea and electrolyte levels will be examined and clotting factors assessed. The woman will have fasted and taken the prescribed antacid therapy. Attitudes and practices vary regarding pubic shaving.

The woman may choose to be catheterised in theatre under epidural or general anaesthetic, or in her room where it may be more private.

Positioning of the woman

As the woman will need to lie flat, it is essential that a wedge or cushion is used, or the table is tilted, to direct the weight of the gravid uterus away from the inferior vena cava and so avoid supine hypotensive syndrome.

Elective caesarean section

This implies that the decision to carry out the procedure has been taken during the pregnancy; therefore before labour has commenced.

Indications for elective caesarean section are shown in Box 22.3.

Emergency caesarean section

This is carried out when adverse conditions develop during pregnancy or labour. Some examples of urgent/emergency reasons for caesarean birth are given in Box 22.4.

Box 22.3 Some indications for elective caesarean section

Definite

- Cephalopelvic disproportion
- Major degree of placenta praevia
- High-order multiple pregnancy

Possible

- Breech presentation
- Moderate to severe pre-eclampsia
- A medical condition that warrants the exclusion of maternal effort
- Diabetes mellitus
- Intrauterine growth restriction
- Antepartum haemorrhage
- Certain fetal abnormalities (e.g. hydrocephalus)

Box 22.4 Some indications for emergency caesarean section

- Antepartum haemorrhage
- Cord prolapse
- Uterine rupture (dramatic/scar dehiscence)
- Cephalopelvic disproportion diagnosed in labour
- Fulminating pre-eclampsia, eclampsia
- Failure to progress in the first or second stage of labour.
- Fetal compromise if birth is not imminent

Vaginal birth after caesarean section (VBAC)

If the indication for caesarean section has been a non-recurring one – for example, placenta praevia – VBAC may be attempted. Repeat caesarean section may be indicated in, for example, cephalopelvic disproportion, or on a uterus that has been scarred twice.

Trial of labour

A trial of labour is carried out whenever there is doubt about the outcome of the labour because of a previous caesarean section. Criteria include the following:

- It is established that the presenting part is capable of flexing adequately to pass through the brim of the pelvis.
- All the facilities for assisted birth are readily available.
- Progress of the labour is sufficient, observed both in the descent of the presenting part and by the dilatation of the cervix.
- Time limits as to the duration of the trial are set.

ANAESTHESIA

Regional anaesthesia normally remains the safer option for caesarean birth; however, general anaesthesia is sometimes required.

- Regional anaesthesia is incompatible with any maternal coagulation disorder.
- General anaesthesia can be more rapidly administered.
- Some women choose general rather than regional anaesthesia.

Mendelson's syndrome

This is caused if acid gastric contents are inhaled and result in a chemical pneumonitis. This regurgitation may occur during the induction of a general anaesthetic. The acidic gastric contents damage the alveoli, impairing gaseous exchange, and death may result.

Prevention of Mendelson's syndrome

- *Antacid therapy*. A usual regimen is for women having an elective operation to be given two doses of oral ranitidine 150 mg approximately 8 hours apart, plus 30 ml sodium citrate immediately before transfer to theatre. Women in labour who are thought to have a high risk of caesarean section should have ranitidine 150 mg every 8 hours.
- *Cricoid pressure*. This is applied during intubation.

COMPLICATIONS ASSOCIATED WITH CAESAREAN SECTION

- Infection, e.g. wound, intrauterine, urinary tract and pelvic infections, thrombophlebitis.
- Thromboembolic disorders.

POSTOPERATIVE CARE

Immediate care

If the mother intends to breastfeed, the baby should be put to the breast as soon as possible. Ideally, the baby should remain with the mother and they should be transferred to the postnatal ward together.

Observations

- Blood pressure and pulse should be recorded every quarter of an hour in the immediate recovery period.
- Temperature should be recorded every 2 hours.
- Lochia and the wound should be inspected every half hour.
- Following general anaesthesia, level of consciousness and respirations should be monitored.

Analgesia and antiemetics

Analgesia is prescribed and given as required, for example:

- an epidural opioid
- rectal analgesia (e.g. diclofenac)

- intramuscular analgesia
- oral medications (e.g. dihydrocodeine, paracetamol).

Antiemetics (e.g. cyclizine, prochlorperazine) are usually prescribed.

Care following regional block

- Following epidural or spinal anaesthesia the woman may sit up as soon as she wishes, provided her blood pressure is not low.
- Fluids are introduced gradually, followed by a light diet.
- The intravenous infusion remains in progress for about 12 hours.
- Care must be taken to avoid any damage to the legs, which will gradually regain sensation and movement.
- As it is possible that an opiate administered via the epidural route may cause some respiratory depression, the woman's respiratory rate must be recorded. This means of pain relief offers the advantage of excellent analgesia without motor block and also seems to give a feeling of wellbeing. Women are usually able to become mobile very quickly, which reduces the risk of deep venous thrombosis.

Care in the postnatal ward

- Blood pressure, temperature and pulse are usually checked every 4 hours.
- The urinary catheter may remain in situ until the woman is able to get up to the toilet. Urinary output should be monitored after removal of the catheter. Haematuria is reported to the doctor.
- The wound and lochia must initially be observed at least hourly.
- Leg and breathing exercises are encouraged.
- Prophylactic low-dose heparin and TED antiembolism stockings are often prescribed.
- Appropriate analgesia must be given as frequently as necessary.
- Help may be needed with care for the baby.
- The woman may value talking about her feelings.

SYMPHYSIOTOMY

This is an incision of the fibrocartilage partly through the symphysis pubis and is performed in labour to enlarge the transverse diameter of the pelvis. It is rarely seen in the UK, but is carried out in countries where the risk of caesarean section is particularly high for the management of cephalopelvic disproportion.

CHAPTER 23

Obstetric Emergencies

VASA PRAEVIA

The term *vasa praevia* is used when a fetal blood vessel lies over the os, in front of the presenting part. This occurs when fetal vessels from a velamentous insertion of the cord cross the area of the internal os to the placenta. Vasa praevia may sometimes be palpated on vaginal examination when the membranes are still intact. It may also be visualised on ultrasound. If it is suspected, a speculum examination should be made.

RUPTURED VASA PRAEVIA

When the membranes rupture in a case of vasa praevia, a fetal vessel may also rupture. This leads to exsanguination of the fetus unless birth occurs within minutes.

Diagnosis
- Slight fresh vaginal bleeding, particularly if it commences at the same time as rupture of the membranes.
- Fetal distress disproportionate to blood loss.

Management
See Box 23.1.

PRESENTATION AND PROLAPSE OF THE UMBILICAL CORD

See Box 23.2 for definitions.

Predisposing factors
Any situation where the presenting part is neither well applied to the lower uterine segment nor well down in the pelvis may make it possible for a loop of cord to slip down in front of the presenting part. Such situations include:
- high or ill-fitting presenting part
- high parity
- prematurity
- malpresentation
- multiple pregnancy
- polyhydramnios.

Box 23.1 Management of vasa praevia

- Request urgent medical aid
- Monitor the fetal heart rate
- If the mother is in the first stage of labour and the fetus is still alive, an emergency caesarean section is carried out
- If in the second stage of labour, delivery should be expedited and a vaginal birth may be achieved
- A paediatrician should be present at delivery. If the baby is alive, haemoglobin (Hb) estimation will be necessary after resuscitation

Box 23.2 Definitions

Cord presentation

- The umbilical cord lies in front of the presenting part, with the fetal membranes still intact

Cord prolapse

- The cord lies in front of the presenting part and the fetal membranes are ruptured

Occult cord prolapse

- The cord lies alongside, but not in front of, the presenting part

CORD PRESENTATION

This is diagnosed on vaginal examination when the cord is felt behind intact membranes. It is, however, rarely detected but may be associated with aberrations in fetal heart monitoring such as decelerations, which occur if the cord becomes compressed.

Management
See Box 23.3.

Box 23.3 Management of cord presentation

- Under no circumstances should the membranes be ruptured
- Summon medical aid
- Assess fetal wellbeing, using continuous electronic fetal monitoring if available
- Help the mother into a position that will reduce the likelihood of cord compression
- Caesarean section is the most likely outcome

CORD PROLAPSE

Diagnosis

- Diagnosis is made when the cord is felt below or beside the presenting part on vaginal examination.
- A loop of cord may be visible at the vulva.
- Whenever there are factors present that predispose to cord prolapse, a vaginal examination should be performed immediately on spontaneous rupture of membranes. Variable decelerations and prolonged decelerations of the fetal heart are associated with cord compression, which may be caused by cord prolapse.

Immediate action and management

See Box 23.4.

Box 23.4 Management of cord prolapse

Immediate action

- Call for urgent assistance
- If an oxytocin infusion is in progress, this should be stopped
- A vaginal examination is performed to assess the degree of cervical dilatation and identify the presenting part and station. If the cord can be felt pulsating, it should be handled as little as possible
- If the cord lies outside the vagina, replace it gently to try to maintain temperature
- Auscultate the fetal heart rate
- Relieve pressure on the cord
- Keep your fingers in the woman's vagina and, especially during a contraction, hold the presenting part off the umbilical cord
- Help the mother to change position so that her pelvis and buttocks are raised. The knee–chest position causes the fetus to gravitate towards the diaphragm, relieving the compression on the cord
- Alternatively, help the mother to lie on her left side, with a wedge or pillow elevating her hips (exaggerated Sims' position)
- The foot of the bed may be raised
- These measures need to be maintained until the delivery of the baby, either vaginally or by caesarean section
- Consider inserting 500 ml of warm saline into the bladder to relieve the pressure if transfer to an obstetric unit is required

Treatment

- Delivery must be expedited with the greatest possible speed
- Caesarean section is the treatment of choice if the fetus is still alive and delivery is not imminent, or vaginal birth cannot be indicated
- In the second stage of labour the mother may be able to push and you may perform an episiotomy to expedite the birth
- Where the presentation is cephalic, assisted birth may be achieved through ventouse or forceps

SHOULDER DYSTOCIA

Definition

The term 'shoulder dystocia' is used to describe failure of the shoulders to traverse the pelvis spontaneously after delivery of the head. The anterior shoulder becomes trapped behind or on the symphysis pubis, while the posterior shoulder may be in the hollow of the sacrum or high above the sacral promontory. This is, therefore, a bony dystocia, and traction at this point will further impact the anterior shoulder, impeding attempts at delivery.

Risk factors

These can only give a high index of suspicion:

- post-term pregnancy
- high parity
- maternal obesity (weight over 90 kg)
- fetal macrosomia (birth weight over 4000 g)
- maternal diabetes and gestational diabetes
- prolonged labour (first and second stages)
- operative delivery.

Warning signs and diagnosis

The birth may have been uncomplicated initially, but the head may have advanced slowly and the chin may have had difficulty in sweeping over the perineum. Once the head is born, it may look as if it is trying to return into the vagina.

Shoulder dystocia is diagnosed when manoeuvres normally used by the midwife fail to accomplish birth.

Management

See Box 23.5 and Figs 23.1–23.3.

The mnemonic HELPERR is widely used in obstetric drills (Box 23.6). An algorithm (Fig. 23.4) can also be helpful.

Complications associated with shoulder dystocia

- Postpartum haemorrhage.
- Uterine rupture.
- Neonatal asphyxia.
- Erb's palsy.
- Intrauterine death.

Box 23.6 The 'HELPERR' mnemonic

- **H**elp
- **E**pisiotomy need assessed
- **L**egs in McRoberts position
- **P**ressure suprapubically
- **E**nter vagina (internal rotation)
- **R**emove posterior arm
- **R**oll over and try again

Box 23.5 Management of shoulder dystocia

- Summon help – an obstetrician, an anaesthetist and a person proficient in neonatal resuscitation
- Attempt to disimpact the shoulders and accomplish delivery. An accurate and detailed record of the type of manoeuvre(s) used, the time taken, the amount of force used and the outcome of each attempted manoeuvre should be made
- Try the procedures for 30–60 seconds; if the baby is not born, move on to the next procedure

Non-invasive procedures

- *Change in maternal position*
- *McRoberts manoeuvre.* Involves helping the woman to lie flat and to bring her knees up to her chest as far as possible to rotate the angle of the symphysis pubis superiorly and use the weight of her legs to create gentle pressure on her abdomen, releasing the impaction of the anterior shoulder
- *Suprapubic pressure* (Fig. 23.1). Pressure is exerted on the side of the fetal back and towards the fetal chest to adduct the shoulders and push the anterior shoulder away from the symphysis pubis. Can be used with the McRoberts manoeuvre.

Manipulative procedures

Where non-invasive procedures have not been successful, direct manipulation of the fetus must now be attempted:

- *Positioning of the mother.* McRoberts or the all-fours position may be used
- *Episiotomy.* May be necessary to gain access to the fetus and reduce maternal trauma
- *Rubin's manoeuvre.* The posterior shoulder is pushed in the direction of the fetal chest, thus rotating the anterior shoulder away from the symphysis pubis into the oblique diameter
- *Wood's manoeuvre* (Fig. 23.2). A hand is inserted into the vagina, pressure is exerted on the posterior fetal shoulder, and rotation is achieved
- *Reverse Wood's manoeuvre.* Fingers on the back of the posterior shoulder apply pressure to rotate in opposite direction
- *Delivery of the posterior arm* (Fig. 23.3). A hand is inserted into the vagina, and two fingers splint the humerus of the posterior arm, flex the elbow and sweep the forearm over the chest to deliver the hand. If the rest of the delivery is not then accomplished, the second arm can be delivered following rotation of the shoulder using either Wood's or Rubin's manoeuvre or by reversing the Løvset manoeuvre. Has a high complication rate

Box 23.5 Management of shoulder dystocia—cont'd

- *Zavanelli manoeuvre*. If the manoeuvres described above have been unsuccessful, the obstetrician may consider the Zavanelli manoeuvre. Requires the reversal of the mechanisms of delivery so far and success rates vary

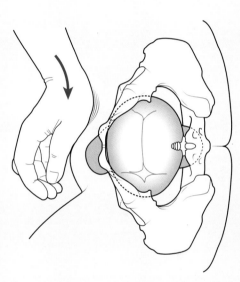

Fig. 23.1: Correct application of suprapubic pressure for shoulder dystocia. (After Pauerstein C 1987, with permission.)

Continued

Box 23.5 Management of shoulder dystocia—cont'd

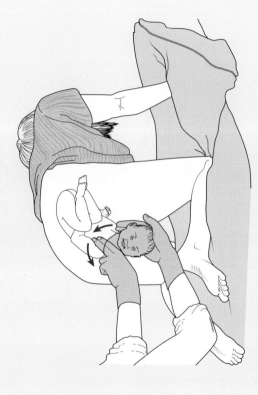

Fig. 23.2: The Woods manoeuvre. (After Sweet & Tiran 1996, p. 664, with permission.)

Box 23.5 Management of shoulder dystocia—cont'd

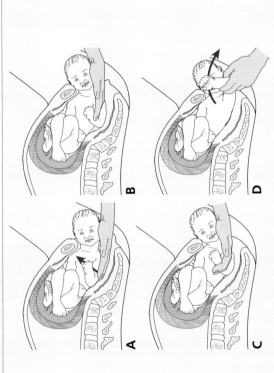

Fig. 23.3: Delivery of the posterior arm. (A) Location of the posterior arm. (B) Directing the arm into the hollow of the sacrum. (C) Grasping and splinting the wrist and forearm. (D) Sweeping the arm over the chest and delivering the hand.

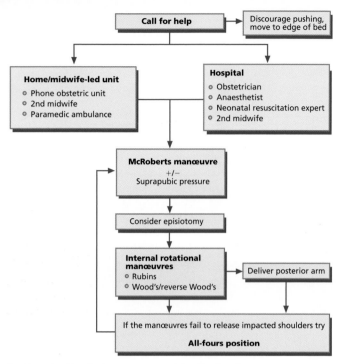

Fig. 23.4: Algorithm for the management of shoulder dystocia.

RUPTURE OF THE UTERUS

Rupture of the uterus is defined as:

- *complete rupture* – involves a tear in the wall of the uterus with or without expulsion of the fetus.
- *incomplete rupture* – involves tearing of the uterine wall but not the perimetrium.

The life of both mother and fetus may be endangered in either situation.

Dehiscence of an existing uterine scar may also occur.

Causes

- High parity.
- Injudicious use of oxytocin, particularly where the mother is of high parity.
- Obstructed labour.
- Neglected labour, where there is previous history of caesarean section.

- Extension of severe cervical laceration upwards into the lower uterine segment.
- Trauma, as a result of a blast injury or an accident.
- Antenatal rupture of the uterus, where there has been a history of previous classical caesarean section.

Signs of rupture of the uterus
- Maternal tachycardia.
- Scar pain and tenderness (where there has been previous caesarean section).
- Abnormalities of the fetal heart rate and pattern.
- Poor progress in labour.
- Vaginal bleeding.

Management
- Immediate caesarean section.
- Repair of the rupture or a hysterectomy, depending on the extent of the trauma and the mother's condition.

AMNIOTIC FLUID EMBOLISM/ANAPHYLACTOID SYNDROME OF PREGNANCY

This rare but potentially catastrophic condition occurs when amniotic fluid enters the maternal circulation via the uterus or placental site. The presence of amniotic fluid in the maternal circulation triggers an anaphylactoid response and the term 'embolus' is a misnomer.

The body responds in two phases:
- The initial phase is one of pulmonary vasospasm causing hypoxia, hypotension, pulmonary oedema and cardiovascular collapse.
- The second phase sees the development of left ventricular failure, with haemorrhage and coagulation disorder and further uncontrollable haemorrhage.

Amniotic fluid embolism can occur at any time, but during labour and its immediate aftermath is most common. It should be suspected in cases of sudden collapse or uncontrollable bleeding. Maternal and fetal/neonatal mortality and morbidity are high.

ACUTE INVERSION OF THE UTERUS

This is a rare but potentially life-threatening complication of the third stage of labour.

Classification of inversion
Inversion can be classified according to severity as follows:
- *First-degree*. The fundus reaches the internal os.
- *Second-degree*. The body or corpus of the uterus is inverted to the internal os.
- *Third-degree*. The uterus, cervix and vagina are inverted and are visible.

Causes

Causes of acute inversion are associated with uterine atony and cervical dilatation, and include:

- mismanagement in the third stage of labour, involving excessive cord traction to manage the delivery of the placenta actively
- combining fundal pressure and cord traction to deliver the placenta
- use of fundal pressure while the uterus is atonic, to deliver the placenta
- pathologically adherent placenta
- spontaneous occurrence of unknown cause
- short umbilical cord
- sudden emptying of a distended uterus.

Warning signs and diagnosis

- There is haemorrhage, the amount of which will depend on the degree of placental adherence to the uterine wall.
- There is shock and sudden onset of pain.
- The fundus will not be palpable on abdominal examination.
- A mass may be felt on vaginal examination.
- The fundus may be visible at the introitus.

Management

See Box 23.7.

Box 23.7 Management of acute inversion of the uterus

Immediate action

- Summon appropriate medical support
- Attempt to replace the uterus by pushing the fundus with the palm of the hand, along the direction of the vagina, towards the posterior fornix. The uterus is then lifted towards the umbilicus and returned to position with a steady pressure (Johnson's manoeuvre)
- Give hydrostatic pressure with warm saline
- Insert an intravenous cannula and commence fluids. Take blood for cross-matching prior to starting the infusion
- If the placenta is still attached, it should be left in situ as attempts to remove it at this stage may result in uncontrollable haemorrhage
- Once the uterus is repositioned, the operator should keep the hand in situ until a firm contraction is palpated. Oxytocics should be given to maintain the contraction

Medical management

- If manual replacement fails, then medical or surgical intervention is required

BASIC LIFE-SUPPORT MEASURES

Before starting any resuscitation, assessment of any risk to the carer and the patient is needed. The basic principles of life support are:

- *A* – airway
- *B* – breathing
- *C* – circulation.

The level of consciousness is established by shaking the woman's shoulders and enquiring whether she can hear.

- Summon assistance.
- Lie the woman flat; if she is pregnant, position with a left lateral tilt to prevent aortocaval compression.
- Airway check – remove obstructions, tilt head back and lift chin upwards.
- Breathing – look, listen and feel for up to 10 seconds.
- Circulation – check carotid pulse; if no pulse felt, commence cardiopulmonary resuscitation (CPR).

CPR

- Thirty chest compressions (rate of 100/min at a depth of 4–5 cm).
- Two mouth-to-mouth ventilations (insert airway if one available, rate of 10 breaths/min).
- Maintain ratio 30:2 (*note*: ratios may change in light of evidence; check resuscitation council guidelines).

SHOCK

Shock can be classified as follows:

- *Hypovolaemic* – the result of a reduction in intravascular volume.
- *Cardiogenic* – impaired ability of the heart to pump blood.
- *Distributive* – an abnormality in the vascular system that produces a maldistribution of the circulatory system; this includes septic and anaphylactic shock.

HYPOVOLAEMIC SHOCK

This is caused by any loss of circulating fluid volume that is not compensated for, as in haemorrhage, but may also occur when there is severe vomiting. The body reacts to the loss of circulating fluid in stages, as described below.

Initial stage

The reduction in fluid or blood decreases the venous return to the heart. The ventricles of the heart are inadequately filled, causing a reduction in stroke volume and cardiac output. As cardiac output and venous return fall, the blood pressure is reduced. The drop in blood pressure decreases the supply of oxygen to the tissues and cell function is affected.

Compensatory stage

The drop in cardiac output produces a response from the sympathetic nervous system through the activation of receptors in the aorta and carotid arteries. Blood is redistributed to the vital organs. Vessels in the gastrointestinal tract, kidneys, skin and lungs constrict. This response is seen as the skin becomes pale and cool. Peristalsis slows, urinary output is reduced and exchange of gas in the lungs is impaired as blood flow diminishes. The heart rate increases in an attempt to improve cardiac output and blood pressure. The pupils of the eyes dilate. The sweat glands are stimulated and the skin becomes moist and clammy. Adrenaline (epinephrine) is released from the adrenal medulla and aldosterone from the adrenal cortex. Antidiuretic hormone (ADH) is secreted from the posterior lobe of the pituitary. Their combined effect is to cause vasoconstriction, an increased cardiac output and a decrease in urinary output. Venous return to the heart will increase but, unless the fluid loss is replaced, will not be sustained.

Progressive stage

This stage leads to multisystem failure. Compensatory mechanisms begin to fail, with vital organs lacking adequate perfusion. Volume depletion causes a further fall in blood pressure and cardiac output. The coronary arteries suffer lack of supply. Peripheral circulation is poor, with weak or absent pulses.

Final, irreversible stage of shock

Multisystem failure and cell destruction are irreparable. Death ensues.

Management

The priorities are listed in Box 23.8.

SEPTIC SHOCK

The most common form of sepsis in childbearing in the UK is reported to be that caused by beta-haemolytic *Streptococcus pyogenes* (Lancefield group A). This is a Gram-positive organism, responding to intravenous antibiotics, specifically those that are penicillin based. In the general population, infections from Gram-negative organisms such as *Escherichia coli*, *Proteus* or *Pseudomonas pyocyaneus* are predominant; these are common pathogens in the female genital tract.

The placental site is the main point of entry for an infection associated with pregnancy and childbirth. This may occur following prolonged rupture of fetal membranes, obstetric trauma or septic abortion, or in the presence of retained placental tissue. Endotoxins present in the organisms release components that trigger the body's immune response, culminating in multiple organ failure.

Clinical presentation

The mother may present with a sudden onset of tachycardia, pyrexia, rigors and tachypnoea. She may also exhibit a change in her mental state. Signs of shock, including hypotension, develop as the condition takes hold. Haemorrhage may develop as a result of disseminated intravascular coagulation.

Box 23.8 Priorities in the management of hypovolaemic shock

- Call for help

  Shock is a progressive condition and delay in correcting hypovolaemia can ultimately lead to maternal death

- Maintain the airway

  If the mother is severely collapsed, she should be turned on to her side and 40% oxygen administered at a rate of 4–6 l per minute
  If she is unconscious, an airway should be inserted

- Replace fluids

  Two wide-bore intravenous cannulae should be inserted to enable fluids and drugs to be administered swiftly
  Blood should be taken for cross-matching prior to commencing intravenous fluids
  A crystalloid solution such as Hartmann's or Ringer's lactate is given until the woman's condition has improved
  To maintain intravascular volume, colloids (e.g. Gelofusine, Haemaccel) are recommended

- Ensure warmth

  It is important to keep the woman warm, but not overwarmed or warmed too quickly, as this will cause peripheral vasodilatation and result in hypotension

- Arrest haemorrhage

  The source of the bleeding needs to be identified and stopped

- Monitor vital signs

Management

This is based on preventing further deterioration by restoring circulatory volume and eradication of the infection (Box 23.9).

Box 23.9 Management of septic shock

- Replacement of fluid volume will restore perfusion of the vital organs
- Satisfactory oxygenation is also needed
- Rigorous treatment with intravenous antibiotics, after blood cultures have been taken, is necessary to halt the illness
- Retained products of conception can be detected on ultrasound, and these can then be removed

Section 4

Puerperium

CHAPTER 24

Physiology and Care in the Puerperium

DEFINING THE PUERPERIUM AND THE POSTNATAL PERIOD

Following the birth of the baby and expulsion of the placenta, the mother enters a period of physical and psychological recuperation. From a medical and physiological viewpoint this period, called the *puerperium*, starts immediately after delivery of the placenta and membranes and continues for 6 weeks.

MIDWIVES AND THE MANAGEMENT OF POSTPARTUM CARE

The *postnatal period* means the period after the end of labour during which the attendance of a midwife upon the woman and baby is required, being not less than 10 days and for a longer period if the midwife considers it necessary (Nursing and Midwifery Council (NMC) Rule).

PHYSIOLOGICAL OBSERVATIONS

THE UTERUS AND VAGINAL FLUID LOSS

After the birth, oxytocin is secreted from the posterior pituitary gland to act upon the uterine muscle and assist separation of the placenta. Following expulsion of the placenta, the uterine cavity collapses inwards; the now-opposed walls of the uterus compress the newly exposed placental site and effectively seal the exposed ends of the major blood vessels. The muscle layers of the myometrium are said to simulate the action of ligatures that compress the large sinuses of the blood vessels exposed by placental separation. These occlude the exposed ends of the large blood vessels and contribute further to reducing blood loss. In addition, vasoconstriction in the overall blood supply to the uterus results in the tissues being denied their previous blood supply; deoxygenation and a state of ischaemia arise. Through the process of autolysis, autodigestion of the ischaemic muscle fibres by proteolytic enzymes occurs, resulting in an overall reduction in their size. There is phagocytic action of polymorphs and macrophages in the blood and lymphatic systems upon the waste products of autolysis, which are then excreted via the renal system in the urine. Coagulation takes place through platelet aggregation and the release of thromboplastin and fibrin.

Renewal of the uterine lining and renewal of the placental site involve different physiological processes. What remains of the inner surface of the uterine lining, apart from the placental site, regenerates rapidly to produce a covering of epithelium. Partial coverage is said to have occurred within 7–10 days of the birth; total coverage is complete by the 21st day.

Once the placenta is expelled, the circulating levels of oestrogen, progesterone, human chorionic gonadotrophin and human placental lactogen are reduced. This leads to further physiological changes in muscle and connective tissues, as well as having a major influence on the secretion of prolactin from the anterior pituitary gland.

Once empty, the uterus can be likened to an empty sac, although it retains its muscular structure. It is therefore important to remember that the uterus, although at this point markedly reduced in size, still retains the potential to be a much larger cavity. This underpins the requirement to undertake immediate and then regular observations of fundal height and the degree of uterine contraction in the first few hours after the birth. Abdominal palpation of the uterus is usually performed soon after placental expulsion to ensure that the physiological processes described above are beginning to take place. On abdominal palpation, the fundus of the uterus should be located centrally, at the same level or slightly below the umbilicus, and should be in a state of contraction, feeling firm under the palpating hand. The woman may experience some uterine or abdominal discomfort, especially where uterotonic drugs have been administered to augment the physiological process.

The physiological process of the uterus returning to its non-pregnant state is known as *involution*. A well-contracted uterus will gradually reduce in size until it is no longer palpable above the symphysis pubis. The rate at which this occurs and the duration of time taken have been demonstrated to be highly individual. The uterus should not be tender during this process, although the woman may be experiencing afterpains.

The observations obtained by the midwife about the state of involution of the uterus should be placed into context alongside the colour, amount and duration of the woman's vaginal fluid loss and her general state of health at that time.

Postpartum vaginal fluid loss (lochia)

Blood products constitute the major part of the vaginal loss immediately after the birth of the baby and expulsion of the placenta. As involution progresses, the vaginal loss reflects this and changes from a predominantly fresh blood loss to one that contains stale blood products, lanugo, vernix and other debris from the unwanted products of the conception. This loss varies from woman to woman, being lighter or darker in colour, but for any woman the shade and density tend to be consistent.

Assessment of vaginal blood loss

The mother should be asked about the current vaginal loss:

- Whether this is more or less than previously.
- Whether it is lighter or darker than previously.
- Whether she herself has any concerns about it.

It is of particular importance to record any clots passed and when these occurred.

PERINEAL PAIN

Regardless of whether the birth resulted in actual perineal trauma, women are likely to feel bruised around the vaginal and perineal tissues for the first few days after the birth. Women who have undergone any degree of actual perineal injury will experience pain for several days until healing takes place.

All women should be asked about discomfort in the perineal area, regardless of whether there is a record of actual perineal trauma. Where women appear to have no discomfort or anxieties about their perineum, it is not essential for the midwife to examine this area. For the majority of women, the perineal wound gradually becomes less painful and healing should occur by 7–10 days after the birth.

Advice on what might help perineal pain

- Appropriate information and advice are important components in pain management and should take into account women's individual experiences of their pain and their preferences for its relief.
- Women may find soaking in a bath of great comfort to them regardless of any additive, and relief may be derived from the use of a bidet or cool water poured over the area that is tender.
- There is increasing interest in complementary therapeutic preparations and more and more research is being undertaken into their use. Essential oils such as lavender and tea tree have been found to be beneficial when used as bath additives or topical compresses. Homeopathic remedies such as arnica, calendula and *Bellis perennis* can be applied topically or taken orally.

VITAL SIGNS AND GENERAL HEALTH

Observations of pulse, temperature, respiration and blood pressure

While monitoring the pulse rate the midwife can also observe a number of related signs of wellbeing, as well as just listening to what the woman is saying:

- respiratory rate
- overall body temperature
- any untoward body odour
- skin condition
- overall colour and complexion.

Observation of temperature is unnecessary in women who are well and without symptoms that could be associated with an infection. Where the woman complains of feeling unwell with flu-like symptoms, or there are signs of possible infection, then the temperature must be taken.

Blood pressure

Following the birth of the baby, a baseline recording of the woman's blood pressure will be made. In the absence of any previous history of morbidity associated with hypertension, it is usual for the blood pressure to return to a normal range within 24 hours of the birth. Routine observations of blood pressure is not required.

Circulation

The body has to reabsorb a quantity of excess fluid following the birth. For the majority of women this results in passing large quantities of urine, particularly in the first day, as diuresis is increased. Women may also experience oedema of their ankles and feet and this swelling may be greater than that experienced in pregnancy. These are variations of normal physiological processes and should resolve within the puerperal time scale as the woman's activity levels also increase. Advice should be related to:

- taking reasonable exercise
- avoiding long periods of standing
- elevating the feet and legs when sitting, where possible.

Swollen ankles should be bilateral and not accompanied by pain; the midwife should note particularly if this is present in one calf only, as it could indicate pathology associated with a deep vein thrombosis.

Skin and nutrition

Women who have suffered from urticaria of pregnancy or cholestasis of the liver should experience relief once the pregnancy is over. The pace of life once the baby is born might lead to women having a reduced fluid intake than formerly or to taking a different diet. This in turn might affect their skin and overall physiological state. Women should be encouraged to maintain a balanced fluid intake and to eat a diet that has a greater proportion of fresh food in it.

Urine and bowel function

Minor disorders of urinary and bowel function are common. These may be associated with retention or incontinence of urine or constipation, or both. The midwife should explore the possible cause of this and decide whether it will resolve spontaneously or requires further investigation.

Exercise and healthy activity versus rest, relaxation and sleep

Exploring each woman's level of activity will encourage advice in relation to appropriate exercise and, by association, nutritional intake and rest or relaxation and sleep. Undertaking regular pelvic floor exercises is of benefit to women's long-term health.

AFTERPAINS

Management of afterpains is by an appropriate analgesic; where possible, this should be taken prior to breastfeeding, as it is the production of oxytocin in relation to the let-down response that initiates the contraction in the uterus and causes pain. Pain in the uterus that is constant or present on abdominal palpation is unlikely to be associated with afterpains and further enquiry should be made into this. Women might also confuse afterpains with flatus pain, especially after an operative birth or where they are constipated. Relief of the cause is likely to relieve the symptoms.

FUTURE HEALTH, FUTURE FERTILITY

Midwives need to be aware of a range of different needs with regard to women's sexuality and should be able to offer sensitive and appropriate advice on contraception where this is needed.

CHAPTER 25

Physical Problems and Complications in the Puerperium

THE NEED FOR WOMEN-CENTRED AND WOMEN-LED POSTPARTUM CARE

The woman's social and ethnic environment should take into account their individual perceptions and experiences surrounding the pregnancy and the birth event. Where the birth involved complications, postpartum care is likely to differ from that of women whose pregnancy and labour are considered straightforward; the role of the midwife in these cases is:

● to identify whether a potentially pathological condition exists
● if so, to refer the woman for appropriate investigations and care.

IMMEDIATE UNTOWARD EVENTS FOR THE MOTHER FOLLOWING THE BIRTH OF THE BABY

POSTPARTUM HAEMORRHAGE

● *Immediate (primary) postpartum haemorrhage (PPH).* This is the most immediate and potentially life-threatening event occurring at the point, or within 24 hours, of delivery of the placenta and membranes. It presents as a sudden and excessive vaginal blood loss of 500 ml or more. (See Ch. 19 for management.)
● *Secondary or delayed PPH.* This is where there is excessive or prolonged vaginal loss from 24 hours after delivery of the placenta and for up to 12 weeks postpartum. Unlike primary PPH, which includes a specified volume of blood loss as part of its definition, there is no such volume defined for secondary PPH.

Regardless of the timing of any haemorrhage, it is most frequently the placental site that is the source. Alternatively, a cervical or deep vaginal wall tear or trauma to the perineum might be the cause in women who have recently given birth. Retained placental fragments or other products of conception are likely to inhibit the process of involution, or reopen the placental wound. The diagnosis is likely to be determined by the woman's condition and pattern of events and is also often complicated by the presence of infection (see Box 25.1).

Box 25.1 Secondary PPH

Signs of secondary PPH

- Lochial loss is heavier than normal
- Lochia returns to a bright red loss and may be offensive
- Subinvolution of the uterus
- Pyrexia and tachycardia
- Haematoma formation

Treatment

- Call a doctor
- Reassure the woman and her support person(s)
- Rub up a contraction by massaging the uterus if it is still palpable
- Express any clots
- Encourage the mother to empty her bladder
- Give an uterotonic drug, such as ergometrine maleate, by the intravenous or intramuscular route
- Keep all pads and linen to assess the volume of blood lost
- Antibiotics may be prescribed
- If retained products of conception are seen on an ultrasound scan, it may be appropriate to transfer the woman to hospital and prepare her for theatre

MATERNAL COLLAPSE WITHIN 24 HOURS OF THE BIRTH WITHOUT OVERT BLEEDING

Consider:

- inversion of the uterus
- amniotic fluid embolism
- cerebrovascular accident.

POSTPARTUM COMPLICATIONS AND IDENTIFYING DEVIATIONS FROM THE NORMAL

The midwife needs to establish whether there are any signs of possible morbidity and determine whether these might indicate the need for referral. Figure 25.1 suggests a model for linking together key observations that suggest potential risk of, or actual, morbidity.

The central point, as with any personal contact, is the midwife's initial review of the woman's appearance, psychological state and vital signs.

- A rise in temperature above 37.8°C is usually considered to be of clinical significance. A mildly raised temperature may be related to normal physiological hormonal responses: e.g. the increasing production of breast milk.

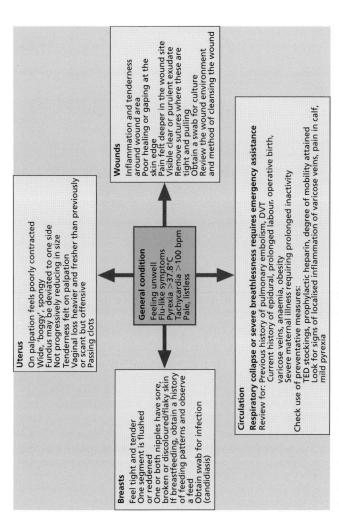

Uterus
On palpation feels poorly contracted
Wide, 'boggy', spongy
Fundus may be deviated to one side
Not progressively reducing in size
Tenderness felt on palpation
Vaginal loss heavier and fresher than previously
or scant but offensive
Passing clots

Wounds
Inflammation and tenderness
around wound area
Poor healing or gaping at the
skin edge
Pain felt deeper in the wound site
Visible clear or purulent exudate
Remove sutures where these are
tight and pulling
Obtain a swab for culture
Review the wound environment
and method of cleansing the wound

General condition
Feeling unwell
Flu-like symptoms
Pyrexia >37.8°C
Tachycardia >100 bpm
Pale, listless

Breasts
Feel tight and tender
One segment is flushed
or reddened
One or both nipples have sore,
broken or discoloured/flaky skin
If breastfeeding, obtain a history
of feeding patterns and observe
a feed
Obtain swab for infection
(candidiasis)

Circulation
Respiratory collapse or severe breathlessness requires emergency assistance
Review for: Previous history of pulmonary embolism, DVT
        Current history of epidural, prolonged labour, operative birth,
        varicose veins, anaemia, obesity
        Severe maternal illness requiring prolonged inactivity
Check use of preventative measures:
        TED stockings, prophylactic heparin, degree of mobility attained
        Look for signs of localised inflammation of varicose veins, pain in calf,
        mild pyrexia

Fig. 25.1: Diagrammatic demonstration of the relationship between deviation from normal physiology and potential morbidity.

- A weak and rapid pulse rate in a woman who is in a state of collapse with signs of shock and a low blood pressure, but no evidence of vaginal haemorrhage, may indicate the formation of a haematoma. A rapid pulse rate in an otherwise well woman might suggest that she is anaemic but could also indicate increased thyroid or other dysfunctional hormonal activity.
- The midwife needs to be alert to any possible relationship between the observations overall and their potential cause, keeping common illnesses in mind – e.g. the woman may have a common cold.

THE UTERUS AND VAGINAL LOSS FOLLOWING VAGINAL BIRTH

Assessment of uterine involution is needed where the woman:
- is feeling generally unwell
- has abdominal pain
- has a vaginal loss that is markedly brighter red or heavier than previously
- is passing clots
- reports her vaginal loss to be offensive.

Where palpation of the uterus identifies deviation to one side, this might be the result of a full bladder. Where the woman had emptied her bladder prior to palpation, the presence of urinary retention must be considered. Catheterisation of the bladder in these circumstances is indicated for two reasons: to remove any obstacle that is preventing the process of involution taking place and to provide relief to the bladder itself. If deviation is not the result of a full bladder, further investigations need to be undertaken to determine the cause.

Morbidity might be suspected where the uterus:
- fails to follow the expected progressive reduction in size
- feels wide or 'boggy' on palpation
- is less well contracted than expected.

This might be described as subinvolution of the uterus, which can indicate postpartum infection, or the presence of retained products of the placenta or membranes, or both.

Treatment involves:
- antibiotics
- oxytocic drugs
- hormonal preparations
  or
- evacuation of the uterus (ERPC).

Vulnerability to infection: potential causes and prevention

Causes include:
- poor immunity
- pre-existing resistance to the invading organism
- virulence of the organism
- presence of hospital 'superbugs'.

The bacteria responsible for the majority of puerperal infections belong to the streptococcal or staphylococcal species.

- The *Streptococcus* bacterium may be haemolytic or non-haemolytic, aerobic or anaerobic; e.g. beta-haemolytic *S. pyogenes* (Lancefield group A).
- The *Staphylococcus* bacterium has a grape-like structure; the most important species are *Staph. aureus* or *pyogenes*. Staphylococci are the most frequent cause of wound infections; where these bacteria are coagulase-positive they form clots on the plasma, which can lead to more widespread systemic morbidity. There is additional concern about their resistance to antibiotics and about subsequent management to control spread of the infection.

THE UTERUS AND VAGINAL LOSS FOLLOWING OPERATIVE DELIVERY

It may be some hours after the operation before the woman sits up or moves about. Blood and debris will have been slowly released from the uterus during this time and, when the woman begins to move, this will be expelled though the vagina and may appear as a substantial fresh-looking red loss. Following this initial event, it is usual for the amount of vaginal loss to lessen and for further fresh loss to be minimal. All this can be observed without actually palpating the uterus, which is likely to be very painful in the first few days after the operation.

Where clinically indicated – for example, where vaginal bleeding is heavier than expected – the uterine fundus can be gently palpated. If the uterus is not well contracted, then medical intervention is needed. The following may be required:

- Uterotonics (e.g. intravenous infusion of oxytocin, intravenous ergometrine, intramuscular Syntometrine).
- Blood tests for clotting factors.
- Exploration of the uterine cavity.

WOUND PROBLEMS

Perineal problems

Severe perineal pain might be the result of:

- the analgesia no longer being effective
- increased oedema in the surrounding tissues
- haematoma formation.

The blood contained within a haematoma can exceed 1000 ml and may significantly affect the overall state of the woman, who can present with signs of acute shock. Treatment is by evacuation of the haematoma and resuturing of the perineal wound, usually under a general anaesthetic.

Oedema can cause the stitches to feel excessively tight. Local application of cold packs, oral analgesia, as well as complementary medicines such as arnica and witch hazel, may bring relief.

Pain in the perineal area that occurs at a later stage or pain that reoccurs might be associated with an infection. The skin edges are likely to have a moist, puffy and dull appearance; there may also be an offensive odour and evidence of pus in the wound.

- A swab should be obtained for micro-organism culture and referral should be made to a GP.
- Antibiotics might be commenced immediately when there is specific information about any infective agent.
- Advice should be given about cleaning the area, using cotton underwear, avoiding tights and trousers and changing sanitary pads frequently.
- Women should also be advised to avoid using perfumed bath additives or talcum powder.

If the perineal area fails to heal or continues to cause pain by the time the initial healing process should have begun, resuturing or refashioning might be advised. Women should be pain free and able to resume sexual intercourse without pain by 6 weeks after the birth; some discomfort might still be present, however, depending on the degree of trauma experienced.

Caesarean section wounds

It is now common practice for women undergoing an operative birth to be given prophylactic antibiotics at the time of the surgery. This has been demonstrated to reduce the incidence of subsequent wound infection and endometritis significantly. It is usual for the wound dressing to be removed after the first 24 hours, as this also aids healing and reduces infection.

A wound that is hot, tender and inflamed and is accompanied by a pyrexia is highly suggestive of an infection. Where this is observed:

- a swab should be obtained for micro-organism culture
- medical advice should be sought.

Haematoma and abscesses can also form underneath the wound, and women may identify increased pain around the wound where these are present. Rarely, a wound may need to be probed to reduce the pressure and to allow infected material to drain, reducing the likelihood of the formation of an abscess.

CIRCULATION PROBLEMS

Pulmonary embolism remains a major cause of maternal deaths in the UK. Women at higher risk include those with the factors listed in Box 25.2.

Women who undergo surgery and have these pre-existing factors should be:

- provided with TED stockings during, or as soon as possible after, the birth
- prescribed prophylactic heparin until they attain normal mobility.

Clinical signs that women might report include the following conditions (the most common given first, progressing to the most serious):

- Signs of circulatory problems related to varicose veins usually include localised inflammation or tenderness around the varicose vein, sometimes accompanied by a mild pyrexia. This is superficial thrombophlebitis, which is usually resolved by applying support to the affected area and

Box 25.2 Risk factors for postpartum pulmonary embolism

- Previous history of pulmonary embolism
- Deep vein thrombosis
- Varicose veins
- Epidural anaesthetic
- Anaemia
- Prolonged labour
- Operative birth

administering anti-inflammatory drugs, where these do not conflict with other medication being taken or with breastfeeding.

- Unilateral oedema of an ankle or calf, accompanied by stiffness or pain and a positive Homan's sign, might indicate a deep vein thrombosis that has the potential to cause a pulmonary embolism. Urgent medical referral must be made to confirm the diagnosis and commence anticoagulant or other appropriate therapy.
- The most serious outcome is the development of a pulmonary embolism. The first sign might be the sudden onset of breathlessness, which may not be associated with any obvious clinical sign of a blood clot. Women with this condition are likely to become seriously ill and could suffer respiratory collapse with very little prior warning.

Some degree of oedema of the lower legs, ankles and feet can be viewed as being within normal limits where it is not accompanied by calf pain (especially unilaterally), pyrexia or raised blood pressure.

Hypertension

Women who have had previous episodes of hypertension in pregnancy may continue to demonstrate this postpartum. Mothers with clinical signs of pregnancy-induced hypertension still run the risk of developing eclampsia in the hours and days following the birth, although this is a relatively rare outcome in the normal population. Some degree of blood pressure monitoring should be continued for women who suffered hypertension antenatally, and postpartum management should proceed on an individual basis. For these women the medical advice should cover:

- optimal systolic and diastolic levels
- instructions for treatment with antihypertensive drugs if the blood pressure exceeds these levels.

Occasionally, women can develop postnatal pre-eclampsia without associated antenatal problems. Therefore, if a postpartum woman presents with signs associated with pre-eclampsia, the midwife should:

- undertake observations of the blood pressure and urine
- obtain medical advice.

For women with essential hypertension, management of their overall medical condition will be reviewed postpartum by their usual caregivers.

HEADACHE

Concern about postpartum morbidity should centre around the history of:
- the severity, duration and frequency of the headaches
- the medication being taken to alleviate them
- how effective this is.

If an epidural anaesthetic was administered for the birth (or at any time postpartum), medical advice should be sought and the anaesthetist who sited the epidural might need to be contacted. Headaches from a dural tap typically arise once the woman has become mobile after the birth; these headaches are at their most severe when the woman is standing, lessening when she lies down. They are often accompanied by:
- neck stiffness
- vomiting
- visual disturbances.

These headaches are very debilitating and are best managed by stopping the leakage of cerebrospinal fluid (CSF) by the insertion of 10–20 ml of blood into the epidural space; this should resolve the clinical symptoms. If women have returned home after the birth, they would need to return to the hospital to have this procedure carried out.

Headaches might also be precursors of psychological distress.

BACKACHE

Many women experience pain or discomfort from backache in pregnancy as a result of separation or diastasis of the abdominal muscles (rectus abdominis diastasis, RAD). It might be sufficient to:
- give advice on skeletal support to attain a good posture when feeding and lifting
- suggest a feasible personal exercise plan and how to achieve this
- discuss a range of relaxation techniques.

Where backache is causing pain that affects the woman's activities of daily living, referral can be made to local physiotherapy services. If the symphysis pubis has been affected in pregnancy, this should resolve in the weeks after the baby is born.

URINARY PROBLEMS

A short period of poor bladder control may be present for a few days after the birth, but this should resolve within a week. Epidural or spinal anaesthetic can have an effect on the neurological sensors that control urine release and flow; this might cause acute retention. Women with perineal trauma may have difficulty in deciding whether they have normal urinary control; retention of urine might be detected by the midwife as a result of abdominal palpation of the uterus. Abdominal tenderness in association with other urinary symptoms – for example, poor output, dysuria or offensive urine, and a pyrexia or general flu-like symptoms – might indicate a urinary tract infection. Very rarely, urinary incontinence might be a result of a urethral fistula following complications from the labour or birth.

The main complication of any form of urine retention is that the uterus might be prevented from effective contraction, which leads to increased vaginal blood loss. There is also increased potential for the development of a urine infection.

It is not uncommon for some women to have a small degree of leakage or retention of urine within the first 2 or 3 days after the birth while the tissues are recovering, but this should resolve with the practice of postnatal exercise and healing of any localised trauma. Referral to a physiotherapist might be appropriate. Specific enquiry about these issues should be made when women attend for their 6-week postnatal examination.

BOWELS AND CONSTIPATION

Normal bowel pattern should return within days of the birth. Women who have haemorrhoids or difficulty with constipation should be given:
- advice on following a diet high in fibre and fluids, preferably water
- instructions on the use of appropriate laxatives to soften the stools
- topical applications to reduce the oedema and pain.

It is also a matter of concern if women experience a loss of bowel control or faecal incontinence. It is important to determine the nature of the incontinence and distinguish it from an episode of diarrhoea. Women who identify any change to their prepregnant bowel pattern by the end of the puerperal period should have this reviewed.

ANAEMIA

The impact of the events of the labour and birth may leave many women looking pale and tired for a day or so afterwards.
- Where it is evident that a larger than normal blood loss has occurred, red blood cell volume and haemoglobin (Hb) can be assessed and appropriate treatment provided to reduce the effects of anaemia.
- Where the Hb level is less than 9.0 g/dl, a blood transfusion might be appropriate; oral iron and appropriate dietary advice are advocated when women decline a blood transfusion or when the Hb level is less than 11.0 g/dl.
- If Hb values have not been assessed, clinical symptoms such as lethargy, tachycardia, breathlessness or pale mucous membranes may suggest anaemia; a blood profile should then be considered.

BREAST PROBLEMS

Regardless of whether women are breastfeeding, they may experience tightening and enlargement of their breasts towards the 3rd or 4th day, as hormonal influences encourage the breasts to produce milk.

- For women who are breastfeeding, the general advice is to feed the baby and avoid excessive handling of the breasts. Simple analgesics may be required to reduce discomfort.
- For women who are not breastfeeding, the advice is to ensure that the breasts are well supported but that the support is not too constrictive; again, taking regular analgesia for 24–48 hours should reduce any discomfort. Heat and cold applied to the breasts via a shower or soaking in the bath may temporarily relieve acute discomfort.

It is important to gauge whether the duration of the engorgement is excessive and whether there are any other signs of a possible infection, such as overt tenderness or inflammation, pyrexia or flu-like symptoms. If infective mastitis is suspected, then antibiotics should be prescribed. If a woman is breastfeeding, it is important that this continues or that the breast milk is expressed.

CHAPTER 26

Perinatal Mental Health

STRESS/ANXIETY AND DOMESTIC ABUSE

Women are affected emotionally and socially on many levels. Women in abusive relationships are particularly vulnerable. Approximately 30% of domestic violence and abuse begins or escalates during pregnancy or following childbirth.

THE TRANSITION TO MOTHERHOOD

Postnatally, parents may find coping with the demands of a new baby, infant feeding, financial constraints and adjusting to changes in roles and relationships particularly testing emotionally. Disturbed sleep is inevitable. Soreness and pain from perineal trauma will affect libido; so too will the feelings of exhaustion, despair and unhappiness that may be associated with the round-the-clock demands of caring for a new baby.

NORMAL EMOTIONAL CHANGES DURING PREGNANCY, LABOUR AND THE PUERPERIUM

It is perfectly normal for women to have periods of self-doubt and crises of confidence. They may experience fluctuations between positive and negative emotions, as described below.

First trimester
- Pleasure, excitement, elation.
- Dismay, disappointment.
- Ambivalence.
- Emotional lability.
- Increased femininity.

Second trimester
- A feeling of wellbeing.
- A sense of increased attachment to the fetus.
- Stress and anxiety about antenatal screening and diagnostic tests.
- Increased demand for knowledge and information.
- Feelings relating to the need for increasing detachment from work commitments.

Third trimester

- Loss of or increased libido.
- Altered body image.
- Psychological effects from physiological discomforts such as backache and heartburn.
- Anxiety about labour (e.g. pain).
- Anxiety about fetal abnormality.
- Increased vulnerability to major life events.

LABOUR

For many women, labour will be greeted with varied emotional responses such as:

- great excitement and anticipation to utter dread
- fear of the unknown
- fear of technology, intervention
- fear of hospitals, illness and death
- tension, fear and anxiety about pain and lack of control
- concerns about the baby and ability of their partner to support/cope
- a fear of lack of privacy or embarrassment.

Women's perceptions of control during labour are influenced by:

- continuity of care by the midwife
- one-to-one care in labour
- not being left for long periods
- being involved in decision making.

THE PUERPERIUM

Normal emotional changes are complex and may encompass the following:

- Relief labour is over – others may convey a cool detachment from events.
- Contradictory and conflicting feelings from joy and elation to exhaustion and helplessness.
- Closeness to partner and/or baby or disinterest.
- Desire for prolonged skin-to-skin contact and early breastfeeding.
- Fear of the unknown and realisation of overwhelming responsibility.
- Exhaustion and increased emotionality.
- Pain (e.g. perineal, nipples).
- Increased vulnerability and indecisiveness.
- Loss of libido, disturbed sleep, anxiety.

Postnatal 'blues'

This normal and transient phase is experienced by 50–80%, of women depending on parity. The onset typically occurs between 3 and 4 days postpartum, but may last up to a week or more, though rarely persisting for longer than a few days. The features of this state are mild and transitory and may include a state in which women usually experience labile emotions. The actual aetiology is unclear but hormonal influences seem to be implicated, as the period of increased emotionality appears to coincide with the production of milk. Although the condition is self-limiting, the midwife must be vigilant as persistent features could be indicative of depressive illness.

EMOTIONAL DISTRESS ASSOCIATED WITH TRAUMATIC BIRTH EVENTS

Over recent years the label 'post-traumatic stress disorder' (PTSD) has emerged in midwifery practice. Many women will eventually overcome the stress, pain and trauma that might have been their birth experience. However, others may find their birth experience blights their life and affects relationships with their partner and baby.

PERINATAL PSYCHIATRIC DISORDERS

Perinatal psychiatric disorders encompass those that develop during the perinatal period as well as pre-existing disorders. Midwives are recommended to routinely ask at early pregnancy assessment about previous mental health problems, their severity and care. For example:

- During the past months, have you often been bothered by feeling down, depressed or hopeless?
- During the past months, have you often been bothered by having little interest or pleasure in doing things?

A third question should be considerd if the woman answers 'yes' to initial question.

- Is this something you feel you need or want help with?

TYPES OF PSYCHIATRIC DISORDER

Psychiatric disorders are conventionally grouped into the following categories:
- Serious mental illness, e.g. schizophrenia, bipolar illness, depressive illness.
- Mild to moderate psychiatric disorders, e.g. mild to moderate depressive illness, anxiety disorders, panic disorders, obsessive compulsive disorder, post-traumatic stress disorder.
- Adjustment reactions, e.g. distressing reactions to death, adversity.
- Substance misuse, e.g. dependence on alcohol or drugs.
- Personality disorders – should only be used for those with persistent severe problems, e.g. maintaining satisfactory relationships, controlling their behaviour.
- Learning disability when people have lifetime evidence of intellectual and cognitive impairment.

PSYCHIATRIC DISORDER IN PREGNANCY

New onset of psychiatric disorder in pregnancy is mostly accounted for by mild depressive illness, mixed anxiety and depression or anxiety states. Most conditions are likely to improve as pregnancy progresses. Caution needs to be exercised before pharmacological intervention.

New onset psychosis in pregnancy is relatively rare but if the condition appears it requires urgent and expert treatment.

Pre-existing psychiatric disorders require individualised care plans.

- Well, stable, not on medication – risk of becoming psychotic postnatally.
- Relatively well and stable but taking medication – need expert advice on risks and benefits of treatment.
- Chronically mentally ill and on medication – need careful monitoring by maternity, psychiatric and social services.

PSYCHIATRIC DISORDERS AFTER BIRTH

Conventionally, three postpartum disorders are described:

- The 'blues'.
- Puerperal psychosis.
- Postnatal depression.

The blues is a common dysphoric, self-limiting state, occurring in the first week postpartum.

Puerperal psychosis

This is the most severe form of postpartum affective disorder. The onset is very sudden, the majority presenting in the first 14 days postpartum, most commonly between day 3 and day 7.

Features may include:

- restlessness and agitation
- confusion and perplexity
- suspicion and fear, even terror
- insomnia
- episodes of mania making the woman hyperactive (e.g. talking rapidly and incessantly, and being very overactive and elated)
- neglect of basic needs (e.g. nutrition and hydration)
- hallucinations and morbid delusional thoughts involving self and baby
- major behavioural disturbance
- profound depressive mood.

Care and management should be based on:

- preventive measures preconception/antenatally
- interprofessional collaboration
- care in a specialist mother and baby unit.

Postnatal depressive illness

Postnatal depression should only be used for a nonpsychotic depressive illness of mild to moderate severity which arises within 3 months of childbirth.

Where a screening tool such as the Edinburgh Postnatal Depression Scale is used, a score of 14 is said to correlate with a clinical diagnosis of major depression (Box 26.1).

Box 26.1 Value and limitations of the Edinburgh Postnatal Depression Scale

Value

- Useful screening tool
- Acceptable to women
- Takes minutes to complete and score
- Results can be discussed immediately, leading to early identification of problems
- A score of 12+ indicates the likelihood of depression
- Provides women with tangible 'permission' to talk, be listened to and have feelings validated

Limitations

- May lead to misdiagnosis, i.e. false positives and medicalisation of low moods and situational distress
- Depression about depression
- Only predictive, not diagnostic
- Is not a magic wand
- Does not and should not replace clinical judgement
- Does not give women the opportunity to describe symptoms fully

Severe postnatal depression is an early-onset condition that develops over 2–4 weeks, unlike the abrupt onset of puerperal psychosis. The more severe illnesses tend to present by 4–6 weeks postpartum but the majority tend to present later, between 8 and 12 weeks postpartum.

The main characteristics are the following:

- 'Biological syndrome' of sleep disturbance – waking early in the morning; the woman will feel most depressed and her symptoms will be worst at the start of the day.
- Impaired concentration, disturbed thought processes, indecisiveness and an inability to cope with everyday life.
- Emotional detachment and profound lowering of mood.
- Loss of ability to feel pleasure (anhedonia).
- Feelings of guilt, incompetence and of being a 'bad' mother.
- In approximately one-third of women, distressing intrusive obsessional thoughts and ruminations.
- Commonly, extreme anxiety and even panic attacks.
- Impaired appetite and weight loss.
- In a small number, a depressive psychosis and morbid, delusional thoughts and hallucinations.

TREATMENT OF PERINATAL PSYCHIATRIC DISORDERS

There are three components to management:
- Psychological treatment and social intervention.
- Pharmacological treatment.
- Services and resources.
  Some or all will be required

PHARMACOLOGICAL TREATMENT

Given that there is a paucity of systematic research into the efficacy and risks of pharmacological intervention in the management of postnatal depression, balancing risk to the fetus against the risk of not treating the mother is a challenge. Women should be actively supported to breastfeed their baby, if this is their wish.

General principles
- Whenever possible, conception and birth should be medication free.
- Most new episodes of mental illness in pregnancy are early and improve as pregnancy progresses with appropriate psychosocial interventions.
- Liaison between the midwife, GP, obstetrician, psychiatrist, community psychiatric nurse, health visitor and, where necessary, social worker is of great importance.
- No medication is of proven safety.
- Medications that carry a significant risk of teratogenesis have been shown to affect 1–2% of exposed pregnancies, so may be considered of low risk. Nevertheless they may contribute to fetal demise, intrauterine growth restriction, organ dysgenesis and adverse effects on the neonate, such as withdrawal.
- Serious mental illness requires robust treatment; the more serious the illness is, the more likely it is that the risks of not treating outweigh the risks of treating.
- Babies more than 12 weeks old are at low risk of exposure to antidepressants in breast milk.
- Breast milk levels will reflect the serum levels of the medication. Therefore women should be advised to avoid feeding at times of peak plasma level, and preferably should time their medication after a feed and before the baby's longest sleep.
- The baby should be monitored for any deleterious effects, particularly weight gain and drowsiness.

A summary of key recommendations for best practice is given in Box 26.2.

Antidepressants
- *Tricyclic antidepressants* (e.g. imipramine, lofepramine, amitryptyline, dosulepin) have shown no harmful effects in pregnancy but babies are at risk of withdrawal effects.

- *Selective serotonin reuptake inhibitors* (SSRIs) (e.g. fluoxetine, paroxetine, citalopram) have given concerns as to their use in early pregnancy. This risk has to be balanced with potential reoccurrence of the woman's condition.
- Tricyclic antidepressants should be the medication of choice during breastfeeding.

Antipsychotics
As antipsychotic medication passes through the placenta and into breast milk, the dose should be reduced as far as possible.

Mood stabilizers
Lithium carbonate is not recommended in pregnancy or while breastfeeding. Close monitoring is essential if it has to be taken. Abrupt cessation is associated with substantial risk of recurrence of the condition.

Anticonvulsants
All anticonvulsants are associated with a risk of fetal abnormality. Folic acid reduces the risk of neural tube defects.

Box 26.2 Summary of key recommendations for best practice

Prevention of perinatal psychiatric disorders

- Prepare couples realistically to aim for achievable birth expectations and to deal ably with the demands and challenges of parenthood
- Recognise the value of interagency networking to afford more responsive helplines and points of contact for parents in crisis
- Develop an evidence base of effective mental health promotion strategies
- Be aware that the risk of recurrence of a severe mental illness is at its greatest in the first 30 days postpartum
- Antenatally, screen for risk factors that may culminate in antenatal or postnatal depression: personal or family history of mental illness, history of substance (drug or alcohol) abuse, domestic violence, and self-harm and suicidal traits
- Be vigilant with record keeping to ensure good communication and continuity of care. Promote good liaison between members of the interprofessional team
- Avoid misdiagnosis and prevent errors and missed opportunities in care by employing the correct terminology. Use of the umbrella term, 'PND', to describe all types of postpartum mental health problems must cease; use it only when referring to nonpsychotic depressive illness of mild to moderate severity that has an onset following childbirth

Standards and targets

- Set national targets for perinatal mental health services
- Develop clear care pathways for women with a history of mental health problems, substance abuse and abusive relationships

Box 26.2 Summary of key recommendations for best practice—cont'd

- Set targets to establish the incidence of antenatal depression and reduce the prevalence of postnatal depression; one way of achieving this is to standardise the criteria used for screening

Services

- Improve access to perinatal mental health services
- Increase consultants specialising in perinatal mental health problems
- Increase specialist activities to avoid risk of mother and baby being admitted to a general psychiatric ward
- Form a strategy group reflective of all key members of the multiprofessional team to review services for the childbearing woman with perinatal mental health problems
- Ensure interprofessional and interagency collaboration, especially within the primary and secondary care sectors

Research, education and training

- Evaluate perinatal mental health services
- Develop interprofessional or interagency education programmes to aid learning and to improve and understand lines of communication or delineate professional boundaries
- Distinguish between psychology and pathology in order to avoid or reduce inappropriate referrals

Section 5

The Newborn Baby

CHAPTER 27

The Baby at Birth

A newborn baby's survival is dependent on adaptations in cardiopulmonary circulation and other physiological adjustments to replace placental function and maintain homeostasis. Birth is also the commencement of the early parent/baby relationship.

ADAPTATION TO EXTRAUTERINE LIFE

Subjected to intermittent diminution of the oxygen supply during uterine contractions, compression followed by decompression of the head and chest, and extension of the limbs, hips and spine during birth, the baby emerges from the mother to encounter light, noises, cool air, gravity and tactile stimuli for the first time. Simultaneously, the baby has to make major adjustments in the respiratory and circulatory systems, as well as controlling body temperature.

Respiratory and cardiovascular changes are interdependent and concurrent.

PULMONARY ADAPTATION

Prior to birth, the fetus makes breathing movements and the lungs will be mature enough, both biochemically and anatomically, to produce surfactant and will have adequate numbers of alveoli for gas exchange. The fetal lung is full of fluid, which is excreted by the lung itself.

- During birth, this fluid leaves the alveoli, either by being squeezed up the airway and out of the mouth and nose, or by moving across the alveolar walls into the pulmonary lymphatic vessels and into the thoracic duct, or to the lung capillaries.
- Stimuli to respiration include the mild hypercapnia, hypoxia and acidosis that result from normal labour, due partially to the intermittent cessation of maternal–placental perfusion with contractions. The rhythm of respiration changes from episodic shallow fetal respiration to regular deeper breathing, as a result of a combination of chemical and neural stimuli: notably, a fall in pH and PaO_2 and a rise in $PaCO_2$. Other stimuli include cold, light, noise, touch and pain.
- Considerable negative intrathoracic pressure of up to 9.8 kPa (100 cm water) is exerted as the first breath is taken. Pressure exerted to effect inhalation diminishes with each breath taken until only 5 cm water pressure is required to inflate the lungs. This is an effect of surfactant, which lines the alveoli, lowering surface tension thus permitting residual air to remain in the alveoli between breaths. Surfactant is a complex of

lipoproteins and proteins produced by the alveolar type 2 cells in the lungs; it is primarily concerned with the reduction in surface tension at the alveolar surface, thus reducing the work of breathing.

CARDIOVASCULAR ADAPTATION

The baby's circulatory system must make major adjustments in order to divert deoxygenated blood to the lungs for reoxygenation.

- With the expansion of the lungs and lowered pulmonary vascular resistance, virtually all of the cardiac output is sent to the lungs.
- Oxygenated blood returning to the heart from the lungs increases the pressure within the left atrium.
- Pressure in the right atrium is lowered because blood ceases to flow through the cord.
- A functional closure of the foramen ovale takes place. During the first days of life this closure is reversible and reopening may occur if pulmonary vascular resistance is high – e.g. when crying – resulting in transient cyanotic episodes in the baby.
- The septa usually fuse within the first year of life to form the interatrial septum, though in some individuals perfect anatomical closure may never be achieved.
- Contraction of the muscular walls of the ductus arteriosus takes place; this is thought to occur because of sensitivity of the muscle of the ductus arteriosus to increased oxygen tension and reduction in circulating prostaglandin. As a result of altered pressure gradients between the aorta and pulmonary artery, a temporary reverse left-to-right shunt through the ductus may persist for a few hours, though there is usually functional closure of the ductus within 8–10 hours of birth.
- The remaining temporary structures of the fetal circulation – the umbilical vein, ductus venosus and hypogastric arteries – close functionally within a few minutes after birth and constriction of the cord. Anatomical closure by fibrous tissue occurs within 2–3 months, resulting in the formation of the ligamentum teres, ligamentum venosum and the obliterated hypogastric arteries. The proximal portions of the hypogastric arteries persist as the superior vesical arteries.

THERMAL ADAPTATION

The baby enters a much cooler atmosphere, the birthing room temperature of 21°C contrasting sharply with an intrauterine temperature of 37.7°C. Heat loss can be rapid, and takes place through the mechanisms listed in Box 27.1.

The heat-regulating centre in the baby's brain has the capacity to promote heat production in response to stimuli received from thermoreceptors. However, this is dependent on increased metabolic activity, compromising the baby's ability

Box 27.1 Mechanisms of heat loss in the newborn baby

Evaporation

- Amniotic fluid evaporates from the skin. Each millilitre that evaporates removes 560 calories of heat. The baby's large surface area:body mass ratio potentiates heat loss, especially from the head, which comprises 25% of body mass

Poor insulation

- The subcutaneous fat layer is thin, allowing rapid transfer of core heat to the skin and the environment

Conduction

- Conduction takes place when the baby is in contact with cold surfaces

Radiation

- Heat radiates to cold objects in the environment that are not in contact with the baby

Convection

- This is caused by currents of cool air passing over the surface of the body

to control body temperature, especially in adverse environmental conditions. The baby has a limited ability to shiver and is unable to increase muscle activity voluntarily in order to generate heat. Therefore the baby must depend on his or her ability to produce heat by metabolism.

The neonate has brown adipose tissue, which assists in the rapid mobilisation of heat resources (namely, free fatty acids and glycerol) in times of cold stress. This mechanism is called non-shivering thermogenesis. Babies derive most of their heat production from the metabolism of brown fat. The term baby has sufficient brown fat to meet minimum heat needs for 2–4 days after birth, but cold stress results in increased oxygen consumption as the baby strives to maintain sufficient heat for survival. Brown fat uses up to three times as much oxygen as other tissue, with the undesired effect of diverting oxygen and glucose from vital centres such as the brain and cardiac muscle. In addition, cold stress causes vasoconstriction, thus reducing pulmonary perfusion, and respiratory acidosis develops as the pH and PaO_2 of the blood decrease and the $PaCO_2$ increases, leading to respiratory distress, exhibited by tachypnoea, and grunting respirations. This, together with the reduction in pulmonary perfusion, may result in the reopening or maintenance of the right-to-left shunt across the ductus arteriosus. Anaerobic glycolysis (i.e. the metabolism of glucose in the absence of oxygen) results in the production of acid, compounding the situation by adding a metabolic acidosis. Protraction of cold stress, therefore, should be avoided. The peripheral vasoconstrictor mechanisms of the baby are unable to prevent the fall in core body temperature that occurs within the first few hours after birth. It is important, therefore, to minimise heat loss at birth.

IMMEDIATE CARE OF THE BABY AT BIRTH

Prevention of heat loss

It is important to provide an ambient temperature in the range 21–25°C. The baby's temperature can drop by as much as 3–4.5°C within the first minute. Measures to conserve heat include:

- drying the baby at birth
- removing wet towels
- encouraging skin-to-skin contact with the mother
- wrapping the baby in dry, prewarmed towels.

Clearing the airway

As the baby's head is born, excess mucus may be wiped gently from the mouth. Care must be taken to avoid touching the nares, as such action may stimulate reflex inhalation of debris in the trachea. Although fetal pulmonary fluid is present in the mouth, most babies will achieve a clear airway unaided. Only rarely will it be necessary to clear the airway with the aid of a soft suction catheter attached to low-pressure (10 cm water) mechanical suction. It is important to aspirate the oropharynx prior to the nasopharynx so that, if the baby gasps as the nasal passages are aspirated, mucus or other material is not drawn down into the respiratory tract. Suction at the back of the pharynx can result in vagal stimulation, with laryngospasm and bradycardia.

Cutting the cord

The optimal time for umbilical cord clamping after birth remains unknown. Delaying cord clamping for at least 2 minutes in a term neonate can be beneficial. What is agreed is that a term baby at birth can be drawn up onto the mother's abdomen but raised no higher, and a preterm baby should be kept at the level of the placenta. This is because:

- if a preterm baby is held above the placenta, blood can drain from the baby to the placenta, resulting in anaemia
- if the baby is held below the placenta, it can cause him or her to receive a blood transfusion.

Early clamping and cutting of the cord is advocated in preterm babies.

Identification

The time of birth and sex of the baby are noted and recorded.

Babies born in hospital must be readily identifiable from one another. In the UK each baby is issued with a National Unique Reference Number for receipt of Health and Social Care services.

Assessment of the baby's condition

At 1 minute and 5 minutes after the birth, an assessment is made of the baby's general condition using the Apgar score (Table 27.1).

- The assessment at 1 minute is important for the further management of resuscitation.

Table 27.1 The Apgar score

Sign	Score		
	0	1	2
Heart rate	Absent	<100 bpm	>100 bpm
Respiratory effort	Absent	Slow, irregular	Good or crying
Muscle tone	Limp	Some flexion of limbs	Active
Reflex response to stimulus	None	Minimal grimace	Cough or sneeze
Colour	Blue, pale	Body pink, extremities blue	Completely pink

The score is assessed at 1 minute and 5 minutes after birth. Medical aid should be sought if the score is less than 7.
'Apgar minus colour' score omits the fifth sign. Medical aid should be sought if the score is less than 6.

- An assessment at 5 minutes provides a record of response to resuscitation and immediate care needs.
- The higher the score, the better the outcome for the baby. A mnemonic – APGAR – for the Apgar score is given in Box 27.2.

Continued early care

Prior to leaving the mother's home or transferring the baby to the ward, the midwife undertakes a detailed examination of the baby, checking for obvious abnormalities such as:

- spina bifida
- imperforate anus
- cleft lip or palate
- abrasions
- fractures
- haemorrhage due to trauma.

The initial cord clamp is replaced by the application of a disposable plastic clamp (or rubber band or three cord ligatures) approximately 2–3 cm from the

Box 27.2 A mnemonic for the Apgar score

- **A**ppearance, i.e. colour
- **P**ulse, i.e. heart rate
- **G**rimace, i.e. response to stimuli
- **A**ctive, i.e. tone
- **R**espirations

umbilicus and the cutting off of the redundant cord. The baby's temperature is now recorded. The first bath and other non-urgent procedures may be deferred in order to minimise thermal stress.

Vitamin K

Depending on local policy and the mother's informed choice, vitamin K may be given intramuscularly or orally, as prophylaxis against bleeding disorders. Vitamin K is fat soluble and can only be absorbed from the intestine in the presence of bile salts. The body's capacity to store vitamin K is very low and the half-life of the vitamin K-dependent coagulation factors is short. A single dose (1.0 mg) of intramuscular vitamin K after birth has been found to be effective in the prevention of classic haemorrhagic disease of the newborn. Either intramuscular or oral (1.0 mg) vitamin K prophylaxis improves biochemical indices of coagulation status at 1–7 days. When three doses of oral vitamin K are compared to a single dose of intramuscular vitamin K, the plasma vitamin K levels are higher in the oral group at 2 weeks and 2 months, but again there is no evidence of a difference in coagulation studies.

FAILURE TO ESTABLISH RESPIRATION AT BIRTH

Although the majority of babies gasp and establish respirations within 60 seconds of birth, some do not, mainly as a consequence of intrauterine hypoxia.

INTRAUTERINE HYPOXIA

Possible causes include:
- maternal cardiac or respiratory disease
- eclamptic fit
- delayed intubation for induction of general anaesthesia
- hypertension
- hypotension due to haemorrhage or shock
- hypertonic uterine action
- prolapsed or compressed umbilical cord
- abnormal fetal cardiac function
- reduced fetal haemoglobin, e.g. Rhesus incompatibility, ruptured vasa praevia.

The fetus responds to hypoxia by accelerating the heart rate in an effort to maintain supplies of oxygen to the brain. If hypoxia persists, glucose depletion will stimulate anaerobic glycolysis, resulting in a metabolic acidosis. Cerebral vessels will dilate and some brain swelling may occur. Peripheral circulation will be reduced. As the fetus becomes acidotic and cardiac glycogen reserves are depleted, bradycardia develops, the anal sphincter relaxes and the fetus may pass meconium into the liquor. Gasping breathing movements triggered by hypoxia may result in the aspiration of meconium-stained liquor into the lungs, which presents an additional problem after birth.

The length of time during which the fetus or neonate is subjected to hypoxia determines the outcome.

- The initial response of gasping respirations is followed by a period of apnoea lasting 1.5 minutes – *primary apnoea*.
- If this is not resolved by means of intervention techniques, it is followed by a further episode of gasping respirations. These accelerate while diminishing in depth until, approximately 8 minutes after birth, respirations cease completely – *secondary apnoea*.

The essential difference between primary and secondary apnoea is the baby's circulatory status.

- During primary apnoea, the circulation and heart rate are maintained and such babies respond quickly to simple resuscitation measures.
- In secondary apnoea, the circulation is impaired, the heart rate is slow and the baby looks shocked (Table 27.2).

RESPIRATORY DEPRESSION

Obstruction of the baby's airway by mucus, blood, liquor or meconium is one of the most common reasons for a baby failing to establish respirations. Depression of the respiratory centre may be due to:

- the effects of drugs administered to the mother, e.g. narcotics or diazepam
- cerebral hypoxia during labour or traumatic delivery
- immaturity of the baby, which causes mechanical dysfunction because of underdeveloped lungs, lack of surfactant and a soft pliable thoracic cage
- intranatal pneumonia, which can inhibit successful establishment of respirations and should be considered, especially if the membranes have been ruptured for some time

Table 27.2 Degrees of respiratory depression	
Mildly depressed	**Severely depressed**
Heart rate not severely depressed (60–80 bpm)	Slow feeble heart rate (<40 bpm)
Short delay in onset of respiration	No attempt to breathe
Good muscle tone	Poor muscle tone
Responsive to stimuli	Limp, unresponsive to stimuli
Deeply cyanosed	Pale, grey
Apgar score 5–7	Apgar score <5
No significant deprivation of oxygen during labour (primary apnoea)	Oxygen lack has been prolonged before or after delivery, circulatory failure is present, baby is shocked (secondary apnoea)

- severe anaemia, caused by fetomaternal haemorrhage or Rhesus incompatibility, which diminishes the oxygen-carrying capacity of the blood
- respiratory function, which may be compromised by major congenital abnormalities, particularly by abnormalities of the central nervous system or within the respiratory tract
- a congenital abnormality such as choanal or tracheal atresia which may be present. (Choanal atresia should be suspected when a baby is pink when crying but becomes cyanosed at rest.)

RESUSCITATION OF THE NEWBORN

The aims of resuscitation are to:
- establish and maintain a clear airway, by ventilation and oxygenation
- ensure effective circulation
- correct acidosis
- prevent hypothermia, hypoglycaemia and haemorrhage.

As soon as the baby is born, the clock timer should be started. The Apgar score is assessed in the normal manner at 1 minute. In the absence of any respiratory effort, resuscitation measures are commenced. The baby's upper airways may be cleared by gentle suction of the oropharynx and nasopharynx and the presence of a heart beat verified. The baby is dried quickly, transferred to a well-lit resuscitaire and placed on a flat, firm surface at a comfortable working height and under a radiant heat source to prevent hypothermia. The baby's shoulders may be elevated on a small towel, which causes slight extension of the head and straightens the trachea. Hyperextension may cause airway obstruction owing to the short neck of the neonate and large, ill-supported tongue.

STIMULATION

Rough handling of the baby merely serves to increase shock and is unnecessary. Gentle stimulation by drying the baby may initiate breathing.

WARMTH

Hypothermia exacerbates hypoxia, as essential oxygen and glucose are diverted from the vital centres in order to create heat for survival. Wet towels are removed and the baby's body and head should be covered with a prewarmed blanket, leaving only the chest exposed. *Note that it is hazardous to use a silver swaddler under a radiant heater because it could cause burning.*

CLEARING THE AIRWAY

Most babies require no airway clearance at birth; however, if there is obvious respiratory difficulty a suction catheter may be used (size 10FG, or 8FG in preterm).
- The catheter tip should not be inserted further than 5 cm and each suction attempt should not last longer than 5 seconds. Even with a soft catheter, it is still possible to traumatise the delicate mucosa, especially in the preterm baby.

- If meconium is present in the airway, suction under direct vision should be performed by the passage of a laryngoscope blade and visualising the larynx. Care should be taken to avoid touching the vocal cords, as this may induce laryngospasm, apnoea and bradycardia. Thick meconium may need to be aspirated out of the trachea through an endotracheal tube.

VENTILATION AND OXYGENATION

If the baby fails to respond to these simple measures, assisted ventilation is necessary.

Facemask ventilation

- An appropriately sized mask (usually 00 or 0/1) is positioned on the face so that it covers the nose and mouth and ensures a good seal.
- A 500 ml bag is used, as a smaller 250 ml bag does not permit sustained inflation.
- Care should be taken not to apply pressure on the soft tissue under the jaw, as this may obstruct the airway.
- To aerate the lungs five sustained inflations are delivered, using oxygen or air or a combination of both, with a pressure of 30 cm H_2O applied for 2–3 seconds and repeated five times; then continue to ventilate at a rate of 40 respirations per minute.
- Insertion of a neonatal airway helps to prevent obstruction by the baby's tongue.
- Note that overextension of the baby's head causes airway obstruction. A longer inspiration phase improves oxygenation. Higher inflation pressures may be required to produce chest movement.

Endotracheal intubation

If the baby fails to respond to intermittent positive pressure ventilation (IPPV) by bag and mask, or if bradycardia is present, an endotracheal tube should be passed without delay. Intubating a baby requires special skill that, once acquired, must be practised if it is to be retained.

Technique for intubation

The equipment listed in Box 27.3 must be available and in working order.

- Position the baby on a flat surface, preferably a resuscitaire, and extend the neck into the 'neutral position'. A rolled-up towel placed under the shoulders will help maintain proper alignment.
- The blade of the laryngoscope is introduced over the baby's tongue into the pharynx until the epiglottis is seen.
- Elevation of the epiglottis with the tip of the laryngoscope reveals the vocal cords.
- Any mucus, blood or meconium which is obstructing the trachea should be cleared by careful suction prior to passing the endotracheal tube a distance of 1.5–2 cm into the trachea. (Pressure on the cricoid cartilage may facilitate visualisation of the larynx.)

Box 27.3 Resuscitation equipment

- Resuscitaire with overhead radiant heater (switched on) and light, piped oxygen, manometer, suction and clock timer
- Two straight-bladed infant laryngoscopes, spare batteries and bulbs (size 0 and 1)
- Neonatal endotracheal tubes (2.0, 2.5, 3.0 and 3.5 mm) and connectors
- Neonatal airways (sizes 0, 00 and 000)
- Suction catheters (sizes 6, 8 and 10FG)
- Neonatal bag and mask and facemasks of assorted sizes (clear, soft masks)
- Magill's forceps
- Endotracheal tube introducer
- Syringes (1 ml, 2 ml, 5 ml and 20 ml) and assorted needles
- Drugs:
  - Naloxone hydrochloride 1 ml ampoules 400 μg/ml (adult Narcan)
  - Adrenaline (epinephrine) 1:10 000 and 1:1000
  - THAM (tris-hydroxymethyl-amino-methane) 7%
  - Sodium bicarbonate 4.2%
  - Dextrose 10%
  - Vitamin K_1 1 mg ampoules
  - Normal saline 0.9%
- Stethoscope
- Cord clamps
- Warmed dry towels
- Adhesive tape for tube fixation

- Intubation may be easier if a tracheal introducer made of plastic-covered soft metal wire is used. This will increase the stiffness and curvature of the tube.
- After the laryngoscope is removed, oxygen is administered by IPPV to the endotracheal tube via the Ambu bag. A maximum of 30 cm water pressure should be applied, as there is risk of rupture of alveoli or tension pneumothorax with higher pressures.

The rise and fall of the chest wall should indicate whether the tube is in the trachea. This can be confirmed by auscultation of the chest. Distension of the stomach indicates oesophageal intubation, necessitating resiting of the tube.

Mouth-to-face/nose resuscitation

In the absence of specialised equipment, assisted ventilation can be achieved by mouth-to-face resuscitation.

- With the baby's head in the 'sniffing' position, the operator places her mouth over the baby's mouth and nose.
- Using only the air in her buccal cavity, she breathes gently into the baby's airway at a rate of 20–30 breaths per minute, allowing the infant to exhale between breaths.

It may be easier with larger babies to use mouth-to-face resuscitation.

EXTERNAL CARDIAC MASSAGE

Chest compressions should be performed if the heart rate is less than 60 bpm, or between 60 and 100 bpm and falling despite adequate ventilation. The most effective way of performing chest compressions is to:

- encircle the baby's chest with your fingers on the baby's spine and your thumbs on the lower mid-sternum (Fig. 27.1)
- depress the chest at a rate of 100–120 times per minute, at a ratio of three compressions to one ventilation, and at a depth of one-third (2–3 cm) of the baby's chest.

(Excessive pressure over the lower end of the sternum may cause rib, lung or liver damage.)

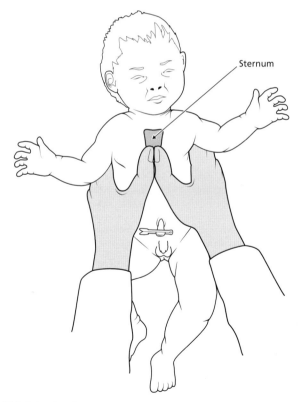

Sternum

Fig. 27.1: External cardiac massage.

USE OF DRUGS

If the baby's response is slow or he/she remains hypotonic after ventilation is achieved, consideration will be given to the use of drugs. In specialist obstetric units, pulse oximetry may be employed to monitor hypoxia and blood obtained through the umbilical artery or vein to ascertain biochemical status. Results will enable appropriate administration of resuscitation drugs, as discussed below.

Naloxone hydrochloride

- This should be used with caution and only in specific circumstances.
- It is a powerful anti-opioid drug for the reversal of the effects of maternal narcotic drugs given in the preceding 3 hours.
- Ventilation should be established prior to its use.
- *It must not be given to apnoeic babies.*
- A dose of up to 100 μg/kg body weight may be administered intramuscularly for prolonged action.
- As opioid action may persist for some hours, the midwife must be alert for signs of relapse when a repeat dose may be required.
- *It should not be administered to babies of narcotic-addicted mothers, as this may precipitate acute withdrawal.*

Sodium bicarbonate

- This is not recommended for brief periods of cardiopulmonary resuscitation.
- Once tissues are oxygenated by lung inflation with 100% oxygen and cardiac compression, the acidosis will self-correct unless asphyxia is very severe.
- If the heart rate is less than 60 bpm despite effective ventilation, chest compression and two intravenous doses of adrenaline (epinephrine) then sodium bicarbonate 4.2% solution (0.5 mmol/ml) can be administered using 2–4 ml/kg (1–2 mmol/kg) by slow intravenous injection
- It should be given at a rate of 1 ml/minute in order to avoid rapid elevation of serum osmolality with the attendant risk of intracranial haemorrhage.
- *It should not be given prior to ventilation being established.*
- THAM 7% (tris-hydroxymethyl-amino-methane) 0.5 mmol/kg may be used in preference to sodium bicarbonate.

Adrenaline (epinephrine)

- This is indicated if the heart rate is less than 60 bpm despite 1 minute of effective ventilation and chest compression.
- An initial dose of 0.1–0.3 ml/kg of 1:10 000 solution (10–30 μg/kg) can be given intravenously; this may be repeated after 3 minutes for a further two doses.
- The Royal College of Paediatrics and Child Health (1997) recommends a higher dose of 100 μg/kg intravenously, if there is no response to the boluses. It is reasonable to try giving one dose of adrenaline (epinephrine) 0.1 ml/kg of 1:1000 via the endotracheal tube, as this sometimes has an immediate effect.

Hypoglycaemia is not usually a problem unless resuscitation has been prolonged. A solution of dextrose 10% 3 ml/kg may be given intravenously to correct a blood sugar of less than 2.5 mmol/l.

OBSERVATIONS AND AFTER-CARE

Throughout the resuscitation procedure the baby's response is monitored and recorded. An accurate written record detailing the resuscitation events is essential. The endotracheal tube may be left in place for a few minutes after the baby starts to breathe spontaneously. Suction may be applied through the endotracheal tube as it is removed.

Explanation must be given to the parents about the resuscitation and the need for transfer to hospital (if the baby was born at home) or to the neonatal unit. The principles of resuscitation of the newborn are applicable wherever and whenever apnoea occurs. The midwife must be able to implement emergency care while awaiting medical assistance (Box 27.4 and Table 27.3).

Box 27.4 Key points for practice

- Anticipation of problems
- Checking of resuscitation equipment
- Starting clock
- Suctioning
- Keeping baby warm
- Apgar score
- Bag and mask ventilation
- Endotracheal ventilation
- Cardiac massage
- Drugs
- Other problems

Table 27.3 Resuscitation action plan

A	Anticipation	Assessment (Apgar)	Airway – clear debris
B	Breathing	Bag + mask	
C	Circulation	Cardiac massage	Caring – warmth, comfort
D	Doctor	Drugs	Documentation
E	Explanation	Environment	Endotracheal tube
F	Follow-up care	Family	

CHAPTER 28

The Normal Baby

GENERAL CHARACTERISTICS

APPEARANCE

Salient points relating to the newborn baby's general appearance are listed in Box 28.1.

PHYSIOLOGY

Respiratory system

- The normal baby has a respiratory rate of 40–60 breaths per minute.
- Breathing is diaphragmatic, the chest and abdomen rising and falling synchronously.
- The breathing pattern is erratic. Respirations are shallow and irregular, being interspersed with brief 10–15-second periods of apnoea. This is known as periodic breathing.
- Babies are obligatory nose breathers and do not convert automatically to mouth breathing when nasal obstruction occurs.
- Babies have a lusty cry, which is normally loud and of medium pitch.

Cardiovascular system and blood

- The heart rate is rapid: 110–160 beats per minute.
- Blood pressure fluctuates from 50–55/25–30 mmHg to 80/50 mmHg in the first 10 days of life.
- The total circulating blood volume at birth is 80 ml/kg body weight.
- The haemoglobin (Hb) level is high (13–20 g/dl), of which 50–85% is fetal Hb.
- Breakdown of excess red blood cells in the liver and spleen predisposes to jaundice in the first week.
- Vitamin K-dependent clotting factors II (prothrombin), VII, IX and X are low.
- Platelet levels equal those of the adult but there is a reduced capacity for adhesion and aggregation.

Temperature regulation

The baby's normal core temperature is 36.5–37.3°C. A healthy, clothed, term baby will maintain this body temperature satisfactorily, provided the environmental temperature is sustained between 18 and 21°C, nutrition is adequate and movements are not restricted by tight swaddling.

Box 28.1 The appearance of the newborn baby

- Weight is highly variable but is normally around 3.5 kg
- Length is in the region of 50 cm from the crown of the head to the heels
- Occipitofrontal head circumference is 34–35 cm
- In an attitude of flexion, with arms extended, babies' fingers reach upper thigh level
- Vernix caseosa, a white sticky substance, is present on the baby's skin at birth
- Lanugo, downy hair, covers areas of the skin
- Colour is according to ethnic origin
- Cartilage of the ears is well formed
- Milia, distended glands in the skin, are often found over nose and cheeks

Renal system

The glomerular filtration rate is low and tubular reabsorption capabilities are limited. The baby is not able to concentrate or dilute urine very well in response to variations in fluid intake nor compensate for high or low levels of solutes in the blood. The first urine is passed at birth or within the first 24 hours, and thereafter with increasing frequency as fluid intake rises.

- The urine is dilute, straw coloured and odourless.
- Cloudiness caused by mucus and urates may be present initially until fluid intake increases.
- Urates may cause pink staining, which is insignificant.

Gastrointestinal system

The mucous membrane of the mouth is pink and moist. The teeth are buried in the gums and ptyalin secretion is low. Small epithelial pearls are sometimes present at the junction of the hard and soft palates. Sucking pads in the cheeks give them a full appearance. Sucking and swallowing reflexes are coordinated.

The stomach has a small capacity (15–30 ml), which increases rapidly in the first weeks of life. The cardiac sphincter is weak, predisposing to regurgitation or posseting. Gastric acidity, equal to that of the adult within a few hours after delivery, diminishes rapidly within the first few days and by the 10th day the baby is virtually achlorhydric, which increases the risk of infection. Gastric emptying time is normally 2–3 hours.

The gut is sterile at birth but is colonised within a few hours. Bowel sounds are present within 1 hour of birth. Meconium, present in the large intestine from 16 weeks' gestation, is passed within the first 24 hours of life and is totally excreted within 48–72 hours.

- This first stool is blackish–green in colour, is tenacious and contains bile, fatty acids, mucus and epithelial cells.
- From the 3rd to the 5th days the stools undergo a transitional stage and are brownish–yellow in colour.

- Once feeding is established, yellow faeces are passed.
- The consistency and frequency of stools reflect the type of feeding.
- Breast milk results in loose, bright yellow and inoffensive acid stools. The baby may pass 8–10 stools a day or alternatively pass stools as infrequently as every 2 or 3 days.
- The stools of the bottle-fed baby are paler in colour, semiformed and less acidic, and have a slightly sharp smell.

Physiological immaturity of the liver results in low production of glucuronyl transferase for the conjugation of bilirubin. This, together with a high level of red cell breakdown and stimulation of hepatic blood flow, may result in a transient jaundice which is manifest on the 3rd to 5th days. Glycogen stores are rapidly depleted, so early feeding is required to maintain normal blood glucose levels (2.6–4.4 mmol/l). Feeding stimulates liver function and colonisation of the gut, which assists in the formation of vitamin K.

Immunological adaptations

Neonates demonstrate a marked susceptibility to infections. The baby has some immunoglobulins at birth. There are three main immunoglobulins – IgG, IgA and IgM.

- Only IgG is small enough to cross the placental barrier. It affords immunity to specific viral infections. At birth the baby's levels of IgG are equal to or slightly higher than those of the mother. This provides passive immunity during the first few months of life.
- IgM and IgA do not cross the placental barrier but can be manufactured by the fetus. Levels of IgM at term are 20% those of the adult, taking 2 years to attain adult levels. (Elevation of IgM levels at birth is suggestive of intrauterine infection.) Breast milk, especially colostrum, provides the baby with IgA passive immunity.

The thymus gland, where lymphocytes are produced, is relatively large at birth and continues to grow until 8 years of age.

Reproductive system: genitalia and breasts

- In boys, the testes are descended into the scrotum by 37 weeks. The urethral meatus opens at the tip of the penis and the prepuce is adherent to the glans.
- In girls born at term, the labia majora normally cover the labia minora. The hymen and clitoris may appear disproportionately large.
- In both sexes, withdrawal of maternal oestrogens results in breast engorgement sometimes accompanied by secretion of 'milk' by the 4th or 5th day. Baby girls may develop pseudomenstruation for the same reason. Both boys and girls have a nodule of breast tissue around the nipple.

Skeletomuscular system

The muscles are complete, subsequent growth occurring by hypertrophy rather than by hyperplasia. The long bones are incompletely ossified to facilitate growth at the epiphyses. The bones of the vault of the skull also reveal lack of ossification. This is essential for growth of the brain and facilitating moulding during labour. Moulding is resolved within a few days of birth.

- The posterior fontanelle closes at 6–8 weeks.
- The anterior fontanelle remains open until 18 months of age, making assessment of hydration and intracranial pressure possible by palpation of fontanelle tension.

PSYCHOLOGY AND PERCEPTION

The newborn baby is alert and aware of his or her surroundings when awake.

SPECIAL SENSES

Vision

Babies are sensitive to bright lights, which cause them to frown or blink. They demonstrate a preference for bold black and white patterns and the shape of the human face, focusing at a distance of approximately 15–20 cm. No tears are present in the eyes of the newborn; therefore they become infected easily.

Hearing

Newborn babies' eyes turn towards sound. On hearing a high-pitched sound they first blink or startle and then become agitated, and are comforted by low-pitched sounds. They prefer the sound of the human voice to other sounds.

Smell and taste

Babies prefer the smell of milk to that of other substances and show a preference for human milk. They turn away from unpleasant smells and show preference for sweet taste, as demonstrated by vigorous and sustained sucking and a speedy grimacing response to bitter, salty or sour substances.

Touch

Babies are acutely sensitive to touch, enjoying:
- skin-to-skin contact
- immersion in water
- stroking, cuddling and rocking movements.

SLEEPING AND WAKING

Sleeping and waking rhythms show marked variations. Initially, waking periods are related to hunger, but within a few weeks the waking periods last longer and meet the need for social interaction.

CRYING

The crying repertoire of babies distinguishes different needs and is the way in which they communicate discomfort and summon assistance. With experience it is possible to differentiate the cry and identify the need, which may be hunger, thirst, pain, general discomfort (for example, wanting a change of position or feeling too cold or too hot), boredom, loneliness or a desire for physical and social contact.

EXAMINATION AT BIRTH

Overall symmetry should be verified and skin blemishes or abrasions noted.

Colour and respirations

Babies are obligatory nose breathers; bilateral nasal obstruction is of major significance if due to bilateral choanal atresia, which is a major medical emergency. Observe the colour of the baby's skin and mucous membranes. In the normal baby, the lips and mucous membranes are pink and well perfused.

Face, head and neck

Each eye should be visualised to confirm that it is present and that the lens is clear. The eyes open spontaneously if the baby is held in an upright position. Any slight oedema or bruising is noted but may be insignificant. The normal space between the eyes is up to 3 cm.

The skull should be palpated to determine the degree of moulding by the amount of over-riding of the bones at the sutures and fontanelles.

- The bones should feel hard in a term baby.
- A wide anterior fontanelle and splayed sutures may indicate hydrocephalus or immaturity.
- An oedematous swelling, caput succedaneum, may be noted overlying the part that was presenting.
- The short thick neck of the baby must be examined to exclude the presence of swellings and to ensure that rotation and flexion of the head are possible.

The mouth

The mouth can be opened easily by pressing against the angle of the jaw. This allows visual inspection of the tongue, gums and palate.

- The palate should be high arched and intact, and the uvula should be central.
- Epithelial pearls (Epstein's pearls) may be observed. They are of no significance, though occasionally mistaken for infection, and they disappear spontaneously.
- Feel the palate for any submucous cleft. A normal baby will respond by sucking the finger.
- A tight frenulum will give the appearance of tongue-tie; no treatment is necessary for this.

The ears

The ears are inspected, noting their position.

- The upper notch of the pinna should be level with the canthus of the eye.
- Patency of the external auditory meatus is verified.
- Accessory auricles, small tags of tissue, are sometimes noted lying in front of the ear.

Ear abnormalities can be associated with chromosomal anomalies and syndromes, and should be reported to a paediatrician.

Chest and abdomen

- Chest and abdominal movements are synchronous. The respirations may still be irregular at this stage.
- The space between the nipples should be noted, widely spaced nipples being associated with chromosomal abnormality.
- The shape of the abdomen should be rounded.
- Haemostasis of the umbilical cord is vital. A blood loss of 30 ml from a baby is equivalent to almost 0.5 litre of blood from an adult.
- Normally, three cord vessels are present. Absence of one of the arteries is occasionally associated with renal anomalies and must be reported to the paediatrician.

Genitalia and anus

If the sex is uncertain, the paediatrician will initiate investigations.

Limbs and digits

- The hands should be opened fully, as any accessory digits may be concealed in the clenched fist.
- The feet are examined for any deformity such as talipes equinovarus, as well as looking for extra digits.
- The axillae, elbows, groins and popliteal spaces should also be examined for abnormalities.
- Normal flexion and rotation of the wrist and ankle joints should be confirmed.

Spine

With the baby lying prone, the midwife should inspect and palpate the baby's back. Any swellings, dimples or hairy patches may signify an occult spinal defect.

Temperature

The baby's temperature may be taken, normally in the axilla (underarm), tympanum (ear) or groin. The normal baby's skin temperature should range from 36.5 to 37.3°C.

Documentation

The midwife records her findings in the case notes. Any abnormalities are brought to the attention of the paediatrician, or GP if birth in the community.

OBSERVATION AND GENERAL CARE

The name bands must remain on the baby until discharge from hospital. During the first few hours after birth, the midwife should observe the baby frequently for any colour changes, patency of airway and haemorrhage from the umbilical cord. Temperature should also be monitored to ensure that it is maintained within the normal range.

NEONATAL CARE

In caring for the normal baby it is important to ensure protection from:
- airway obstruction
- hypothermia
- infection
- injury and accident.

Prevention of airway obstruction

It is important for a baby to sleep in the supine position (on the back) with the feet at the foot of the cot.

Prevention of hypothermia

- Where possible, the room temperature should be maintained at 18–21°C.
- Bath water should be warm (36°C), and wet clothing should be changed as soon as possible.
- It is essential also to avoid overheating.
- Parents should be advised to take account of environmental temperature when dressing their baby. Swaddling should be loose enough to permit movement of arms and legs.

Prevention of infection

- Members of staff who are liable to be a source of infection should not handle babies and friends and relatives who have colds or sore throats (especially children) should not visit.
- Hand washing before and after handling babies is essential.

Skin care

Promotion of skin integrity is enhanced by avoiding friction against hard fabrics or soiled or wet clothing.

The timing of the first bath is not critical, although it has been suggested that removal of blood and liquor reduces the risk of transmission of HIV and other organisms to staff.

Daily bathing is not essential.

- The baby's eyes do not need to be cleansed unless a discharge is present.
- Attention should be paid to the washing and drying of skin flexures to prevent excoriation.
- The buttocks must be washed and dried carefully at every napkin change. Sore buttocks may occur if the stools are loose, if there is protracted delay in changing a soiled napkin or if the skin is traumatised by overenthusiastic rubbing. Regular use of a barrier cream is recommended by some but may interfere with the 'one-way' membrane in disposable nappies.
- Cleanliness of the umbilical cord is essential.
- Hand washing is required before and after handling the cord.

- No specific cord treatment is required, although a wide variety of preparations have been used to promote early separation. Cleansing with tap water and keeping the cord dry have been shown to promote separation.
- The cord clamp may be removed on the third day, provided the cord is dry and necrosed.

Vaccination and immunisation

- BCG vaccination may be given during the early neonatal period in some areas where early protection is desirable.
- Vaccination against hepatitis B and poliomyelitis may also be given in some parts of the world.

Prevention of injury and accident

Advice should also be given to parents about baby care and safety in the home. This should address such issues as:

- bed sharing
- the use of cat nets
- fireguards
- cooker guards
- stair gates
- pram brakes
- car seats.

'Smoking', 'back to sleep' and 'feet-to-foot' advice should be included.

Assessing the baby's wellbeing

At every contact the mother is asked about the baby's health and feeding. Examination of the baby is at the discretion of the midwife and when the mother has any concerns.

- Weight loss is normal in the first few days but more than 10% body weight loss is abnormal and requires investigation.
- Most babies regain their birth weight in 7–10 days, thereafter gaining weight at a rate of 150–200 g per week.

FULL EXAMINATION WITHIN 72 HOURS OF BIRTH

This is usually performed by a competent professional (usually paediatrician or midwife) (Box 28.2).

Blood tests

- Certain inborn errors of metabolism and endocrine disorders are detected by means of a blood test, obtained from a heel prick made with a stilette on the lateral aspect of the heel to avoid nerves and blood vessels. Blood is dripped onto circles on an absorbent card, onto which full details of the baby's identity are entered.

- For detection of phenylketonuria, hypothyroidism and cystic fibrosis the baby must have had at least 4–6 days of milk feeding, and if for any reason the baby or mother is receiving antibiotics, this information should be recorded on the card.
- Some centres also test routinely for galactosaemia.

Box 28.2 Examination of the baby within 72 hours of birth

Appearance
- Activity
- Behaviour
- Breathing
- Colour
- Cry
- Posture

Skin
- Colour
- Texture
- Rashes
- Birthmarks

Head
- Symmetry and facial features
- Face
- Fontanelles
- Mouth
- Eyes
- Ears
- Neck

Neck, limbs and joints
- Proportions
- Symmetry
- Digits
- Movements

Heart
- Position
- Rate
- Rhythm
- Sounds
- Murmurs
- Femoral pulses

Lungs
- Rate
- Effort
- Sounds

Abdomen
- Shape
- Palpation for organ enlargement
- Umbilical cord

Genitalia and anus
- Sex clear
- Complete and patent
- Testes descended or not
- Meconium within 24 hours
- Urinary output

Spine
- Length felt for integrity and skin cover

Central nervous system
- Behaviour
- Tone
- Movements
- Posture
- Reflexes as appropriate

Hips
- Barlow and Ortolani's manoeuvres
- Symmetry of limbs

Feeding
- Ask mother, carers

Measurements
- Weight
- Length
- Head circumference

PROMOTING FAMILY RELATIONSHIPS

Parent–infant attachment

Parents develop their relationship with their babies in individual ways and at their own pace. It is suggested that the parents' relationship with one another is enhanced when the father is encouraged to be involved in discussions, choices and decisions about baby care and to share the responsibility for care.

Promoting confidence and competence

Total care should be delegated to the parents as soon as possible. In hospital, especially, procedures can be rendered unnecessarily complicated for new mothers.

Promoting communication

The increasing interest in baby massage in recent years capitalises on the knowledge that the baby is sensitive and responsive to touch.

- Grapeseed or equivalent oil is used rather than baby oils, which stick to the skin.
- Aromatherapy oils should not be used, as the extent of their absorption is not known.

CHAPTER 29

Infant Feeding

ANATOMY AND PHYSIOLOGY OF THE BREAST

The breasts are compound secreting glands, composed mainly of glandular tissue, which is arranged in lobes.

- Each lobe is divided into lobules that consist of alveoli and ducts.
- The alveoli contain acini cells, which secrete the components of milk and are surrounded by myoepithelial cells, which contract and propel the milk out.
- Small lactiferous ducts, carrying milk from the alveoli, unite to form larger ducts.
- Myoepithelial cells are oriented longitudinally along the ducts; under the influence of oxytocin, these smooth muscle cells contract and the tubule becomes shorter and wider.
- The nipple is composed of erectile tissue and plain muscle fibres, which have a sphincter-like action in controlling the flow of milk.
- Surrounding the nipple is an area of pigmented skin called the areola, which contains Montgomery's glands. These produce a sebum-like substance, which acts as a lubricant during pregnancy and throughout breastfeeding.
- The breast is supplied with blood from the internal and external mammary arteries with corresponding venous drainage.
- Lymph drains freely between the two breasts and into lymph nodes in the axillae and the mediastinum.

During pregnancy, oestrogens and progesterone induce alveolar and ductal growth, as well as stimulating the secretion of colostrum. When the levels of placental hormones fall, this allows the already high levels of prolactin to initiate milk secretion. Continued production of prolactin is caused by the baby feeding at the breast, with concentrations highest following night feeds.

Prolactin is particularly important in the initiation of lactation. As lactation progresses, the milk removal becomes the driving force behind milk production, due to a protein feedback inhibitor of lactation. This protein accumulates in the breast as the milk accumulates and it exerts negative feedback control on the continued production of milk. Removal of this autocrine inhibitory factor, by removing the milk, allows milk production to be stepped up again.

Milk release is under neuroendocrine control. Tactile stimulation of the breast also stimulates the oxytocin, causing contraction of the myoepithelial cells. This process is known as the 'let-down' or 'milk ejection' reflex and makes the milk available to the baby. This occurs in discrete pulses throughout the feed and may well trigger the bursts of active feeding.

In the early days of lactation this reflex is unconditioned. Later, it becomes a conditioned reflex, which can be enhanced or suppressed by environmental factors.

PROPERTIES AND COMPONENTS OF BREAST MILK

Human milk varies in its composition. The most dramatic change in the composition of milk occurs during the course of a feed.

- At the beginning of the feed the baby receives a high volume of relatively low-fat milk.
- As the feed progresses, the volume of milk decreases but the proportion of fat in the milk increases, sometimes to as much as five times the initial value.

The baby's ability to obtain this fat-rich milk is *not* determined by the length of time spent at the breast, but by the quality of attachment to the breast. The baby needs to be well attached so that he or she can use the tongue to maximum effect, stripping the milk from the breast, rather than relying solely on the mother's milk ejection reflex.

FATS AND FATTY ACIDS

For the human infant, with a unique and rapidly growing brain, it is the fat and not the protein in human milk that has particular significance.

- Ninety-eight per cent of the lipid in human milk is in the form of triglycerides: three fatty acids linked to a single molecule of glycerol.
- Over 100 fatty acids have so far been identified, about 46% being saturated fat and 54% unsaturated fat.
- Fat provides the baby with more than 50% of calorific requirements.
- It is utilised very rapidly because *the milk itself* contains the enzyme (bile salt-stimulated lipase) needed for fat digestion, but in a form that only becomes active when it reaches the infant's intestine.
- Pancreatic lipase is not plentiful in the newborn, so a baby who is not fed human milk is less able to digest fat.

CARBOHYDRATE

- The carbohydrate component of human milk is provided chiefly by lactose, which supplies the baby with about 40% of calorific requirements.
- Lactose is converted into galactose and glucose by the action of the enzyme lactase and these sugars provide energy to the rapidly growing brain.
- Lactose enhances the absorption of calcium and also promotes the growth of lactobacilli which increase intestinal acidity, thus reducing the growth of pathogenic organisms.

PROTEIN

Human milk contains less protein than any other mammalian milk. Human milk is whey dominant (the whey being mainly alpha-lactalbumin) and forms soft, flocculent curds when acidified in the stomach.

VITAMINS

All the vitamins required for good nutrition and health are supplied in breast milk, although the actual amounts vary from mother to mother.

Fat-soluble vitamins
Vitamin A

This is present in human milk as retinol, retinyl esters and beta-carotene. Colostrum contains twice the amount present in mature human milk, and it is this which gives colostrum its yellow colour.

Vitamin D

This is the name given to two fat-soluble compounds:
- calciferol (vitamin D2)
- cholecalciferol (vitamin D3).

Vitamin D3 plays an essential role in the metabolism of calcium and phosphorus in the body and prevents rickets in children. Adults can obtain these substances from dietary sources and the conversion of 7-dehydrocholesterol in the skin to vitamin D3 from exposure to sunlight.

- For light-skinned babies, exposure to sunlight for 30 minutes per week wearing only a nappy, or 2 hours per week fully clothed but without a hat, will keep vitamin D requirements within the lower limits of the normal range.
- The babies of dark-skinned mothers living in temperate zones and preterm babies may be at risk of vitamin D deficiency.

Vitamin E

Although vitamin E is present in human milk, its role is uncertain. It appears to prevent the oxidisation of polyunsaturated fatty acids and may prevent certain types of anaemia to which preterm infants are susceptible.

Vitamin K

This vitamin (83% of which is present as alpha-tocopherol) is essential for the synthesis of blood-clotting factors. It is present in human milk and absorbed efficiently. Because it is fat soluble, it is present in greater concentrations in colostrum and in the high-fat hind-milk, although the increased volume of milk as lactation progresses means that the infant obtains twice as much vitamin K from mature milk as from colostrum.

Water-soluble vitamins

Unless the mother's diet is seriously deficient, breast milk will contain adequate levels of all the vitamins. An improved diet is always more beneficial than artificial supplements. With some vitamins, particularly vitamin C, a plateau may be reached where increased maternal intake has no further impact on breast milk composition.

MINERALS AND TRACE ELEMENTS

Iron

Normal term babies are usually born with a high haemoglobin (Hb) level (16–22 g/dl), which decreases rapidly after birth. The iron recovered from Hb breakdown is utilised again. Babies also have ample iron stores, sufficient for at least 4–6 months. Although the amounts of iron are lower than those found in formula, the bioavailability of iron in breast milk is very much higher:

- 70% of the iron in breast milk is absorbed.
- Only 10% is absorbed from formula.

Zinc

A deficiency of this essential trace mineral may result in failure to thrive and typical skin lesions.

- Although there is more zinc present in formula than in human milk, the bio-availability is greater in human milk.
- Breastfed babies maintain high plasma zinc values when compared with formula-fed infants, even when the concentration of zinc is three times that of human milk.

Calcium

- Calcium is more efficiently absorbed from human milk than from formula milks because of human milk's higher calcium:phosphorus ratio.
- Infant formulas, which are based on cow's milk, inevitably have a higher phosphorous content than human milk.

Other minerals

Human milk has significantly lower levels of calcium, phosphorus, sodium and potassium than formula. Copper, cobalt and selenium are present at higher levels. The higher bioavailability of these minerals and trace elements ensures that the infant's needs are met while also imposing a lower solute load on the neonatal kidney than do breast milk substitutes.

ANTI-INFECTIVE FACTORS

Leucocytes

During the first 10 days of life there are more white cells per ml in breast milk than there are in blood. Macrophages and neutrophils are among the most common leucocytes in human milk and they surround and destroy harmful bacteria by their phagocytic activity.

Immunoglobulins

Five types of immunoglobulin have been identified in human milk: IgA, IgG, IgE, IgM and IgD. Of these the most important is IgA, which appears to be both synthesised and stored in the breast. Although some IgA is absorbed by the infant, much of it is not. Instead it 'paints' the intestinal epithelium and protects the mucosal surfaces against entry of pathogenic bacteria and enteroviruses. It affords protection against:

- *Escherichia coli*
- salmonellae
- shigellae
- streptococci
- staphylococci
- pneumococci
- poliovirus
- the rotaviruses.

Lysozyme

This kills bacteria by disrupting their cell walls. The concentration of lysozyme increases with prolonged lactation.

Lactoferrin

This binds to enteric iron, thus preventing potentially pathogenic *E. coli* from obtaining the iron needed for survival. It also has antiviral activity (HIV, cytomegalovirus, herpes simplex virus), acting by interfering with virus absorption and/or penetration.

Bifidus factor

The bifidus factor in human milk promotes the growth of Gram-positive bacilli in the gut flora, particularly *Lactobacillus bifidus*, which discourages the multiplication of pathogens.

Hormones and growth factors

Epidermal growth factor (and insulin-like growth factor) found in breast milk and colostrum stimulate the baby's digestive tract to mature more quickly and strengthen the barrier properties of the gastrointestinal epithelium. Once the initially leaky membrane lining the gut matures, it is less likely to allow the passage of large molecules and becomes less vulnerable to micro-organisms. The timing of the first feed also has a significant effect on gut permeability, which drops markedly if the first feed takes place soon after birth.

MANAGEMENT OF BREASTFEEDING

THE FIRST FEED

Early feeding contributes to the success of breastfeeding. The first feed should be supervised by the midwife. It should proceed without pain and the baby allowed to terminate the feed spontaneously.

ATTACHMENT AND POSITIONING

There are two main positions for the mother to adopt while she is breastfeeding:
- lying on her side
- sitting up – back upright and at a right angle to her lap.

The baby's body should be *turned towards* the mother's body so that he/she is coming up to her breast at the same angle as her breast is coming down to him/her (Fig. 29.1). If the baby's nose is opposite the mother's nipple before the baby is brought to the breast and his/her neck is slightly extended, the baby's mouth will be in the correct relationship to the nipple. In attaching the baby to the breast:
- the baby should be supported across the shoulders to allow slight extension of the neck
- encourage the baby to open the mouth wide by gently but persistently moving it against the mother's nipple
- aim the bottom lip as far away from the base of the nipple as is possible to draw breast tissue as well as the nipple into the mouth with the tongue
- the baby's lower jaw moves up and down, following the action of the tongue
- swallowing is visible and audible
- the mother may be startled by the physical sensation but should not experience pain.

FEEDING BEHAVIOUR

When babies first go to the breast, they feed vigorously, with few pauses. As the feed progresses, pausing occurs more frequently and lasts longer. Pausing is an integral part of the baby's feeding rhythm and should not be interrupted. The change in the pattern probably relates to milk flow. The fore-milk, which is obtained first, is more generous in quantity but lower in fat than the hind-milk delivered at the end, which is thus higher in calories. An excessive quantity of fore-milk is the most common cause of colic in breastfed babies; the problem is resolved by improving attachment and allowing babies to release the first breast when they have had sufficient milk.

The baby *should be offered* the second breast after being given the opportunity to bring up wind. Sometimes in the early days the baby will not need to feed from the second breast.

Provided that the baby starts each feed on alternate sides, both breasts will be used equally. If the baby does not release the breast or will not settle after a feed, the most likely reason is that he or she was not correctly attached to the breast and was therefore unable to strip the milk efficiently. Other reasons for coming off the breast are:
- The baby may need to let go and pause if the milk flow is very fast.
- The baby may have swallowed air with the generous flow of milk that occurs at the beginning of a feed and needs an opportunity to burp.

There is no justification for imposing either one breast per feed or both breasts per feed as a feeding regime.

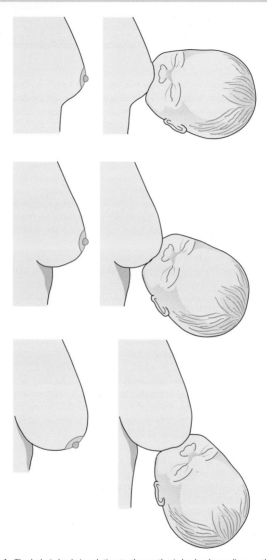

Fig. 29.1: The baby's body in relation to the mother's body, depending on the angle of the breast. (From an original drawing by Hilary English.)

Timing and frequency of feeds

- It is not unusual in the first day or two for the baby to feed infrequently, and to have 6–8-hour gaps between good feeds, each of which may be quite long. This is normal and provides the mother with the opportunity to sleep if she needs to.
- As the milk volume increases, the feeds tend to become more frequent and a little shorter. It is unusual for a baby to feed less often than six times in 24 hours from the 3rd day, and most babies ask for between six and eight feeds per 24 hours by the time they are a week old.
- Babies who feed infrequently may be consuming less milk than they need, and/or they may be unwell.
- Babies who feed very often (10–12 feeds in 24 hours after the first week) may be poorly attached.

The feeding technique and the weight should be monitored. However, mother–baby pairs develop their own unique pattern of feeding and, provided the baby is thriving and the mother is happy, there is no need to change it.

EXPRESSING BREAST MILK

Although all breastfeeding mothers should know how to hand-express milk, *routine* expression of the breasts should not be part of the normal management of lactation. The situations where expressing is appropriate are listed in Box 29.1.

CARE OF THE BREASTS

- Daily washing is all that is necessary for breast hygiene. The normal skin flora are beneficial to the baby.
- Brassieres may be worn in order to provide comfortable support and are useful if the breasts leak and breast pads (or breast shells) are used.

Box 29.1 Appropriate situations for expressing breast milk

- There is concern about the interval between feeds in the early newborn period (expressed colostrum should always be given in preference to formula to healthy term babies)
- There are problems in attaching the baby to the breast
- The baby is separated from the mother, owing to prematurity or illness
- There is concern about the baby's rate of growth or the mother's milk supply (expressing to top up with the mother's own milk may be necessary in the short term while the cause of the problem is resolved)
- Later in lactation, the mother may need to be separated from her baby for periods (occasionally or regularly)

BREAST PROBLEMS

Sore and damaged nipples

- The cause is almost always trauma from the hard palate of the baby's mouth and tongue, which results from incorrect attachment of the baby to the breast. Correcting this will provide immediate relief from pain and will also allow rapid healing to take place. Epithelial growth factor, contained in fresh human milk and saliva, may aid this process.
- 'Resting' the nipple is not advised as, although this enables healing to take place, it makes the continuation of lactation much more complicated.
- Nipple shields should be used with extreme caution, and never before the mother has begun to lactate.

Other causes of soreness

Infection with *Candida albicans* (thrush) can occur, although it is not common during the first week. The sudden development of pain, when the mother has had a period of trouble-free feeding, is suggestive of thrush. The nipple and areola are often inflamed and shiny, and pain typically persists throughout the feed. The baby may show signs of oral or anal thrush. Both mother and baby should receive concurrent fungicidal treatment.

One breast only

It is perfectly possible to feed a baby well using just one breast, as each breast works independently.

Anatomical variations

These are described in Box 29.2.

PROBLEMS WITH BREASTFEEDING

Engorgement

This condition occurs around the 3rd or 4th day postpartum. The breasts are hard (often oedematous), painful and sometimes flushed. The mother may be pyrexial. Engorgement is usually an indication that the baby is not in step with the stage of lactation. Engorgement may occur if feeds are delayed or restricted or if the baby is unable to feed efficiently because he or she is not correctly attached to the breast.

Management should be aimed at enabling the baby to feed well. In severe cases the only solution will be hand expression. This will reduce the tension in the breast and *will not* cause excessive milk production. The mother's fluid intake should not be restricted, as this has no direct effect on milk production.

Deep breast pain

In most cases this responds to improvement in breastfeeding technique and is thus likely to be due to raised intraductal pressure caused by inefficient milk removal.

Box 29.2 Anatomical nipple variations

Long nipples

- These can lead to poor feeding because the baby is able to latch on to the nipple without drawing breast tissue into his or her mouth
- The mother may need to be shown how to help the baby to draw in a sufficient portion of the breast

Short nipples

- As the baby has to form a teat from both the breast and nipple, short nipples should not cause problems
- The mother should be reassured

Abnormally large nipples

- If the baby is small, his/her mouth may not be able to get beyond the nipple and on to the breast
- Lactation could be initiated by expressing, either by hand or by pump, provided that the nipple fits into the breast cup
- As the baby grows and the breast and nipple become more protractile, breastfeeding may become possible

Inverted and flat nipples

- If the nipple is deeply inverted it may be necessary to initiate lactation by expressing
- Attempts to attach the baby to the breast are delayed until lactation is established and the breasts have become soft and the breast tissue more protractile

Although it may occur during the feed, it typically occurs afterwards and thus can be distinguished from the sensation of the let-down reflex, which some mothers experience as a fleeting pain. Very rarely, deep breast pain may be the result of ductal thrush infection.

Mastitis

Mastitis means inflammation of the breast. In the majority of cases it is the result of milk stasis, not infection, although infection may supervene. Typically, one or more adjacent segments are inflamed and appear as a wedge-shaped area of redness and swelling. In some cases flu-like symptoms, including shivering attacks or rigors, may occur.

Non-infective (acute intramammary) mastitis

This condition results from milk stasis. It may occur during the early days as the result of unresolved engorgement or at any time when poor feeding technique results in the milk from one or more segments of the breast not being efficiently removed by the baby. It occurs much more frequently in the breast that is opposite the mother's preferred side for holding her baby. It is extremely important that breastfeeding from the affected breast continues; otherwise milk stasis will increase further and provide ideal conditions for pathogenic bacteria to replicate.

Infective mastitis

The main cause of superficial breast infection is damage to the epithelium, which allows bacteria to enter the underlying tissues. The damage results from incorrect attachment of the baby to the breast, which has caused trauma to the nipple. The mother therefore urgently needs help to improve her technique, as well as the appropriate antibiotic. Multiplication of bacteria may be enhanced by the use of breast pads or shells. In spite of antibiotic therapy, abscess formation may occur. Infection may also enter the breast via the milk ducts if milk stasis remains unresolved.

Breast abscess

A fluctuant swelling develops in a previously inflamed area. Pus may be discharged from the nipple. Simple needle aspiration may be effective or incision and drainage may be necessary. It may not be possible to feed from the affected breast for a few days but milk removal should continue and breastfeeding should recommence as soon as practicable to reduce the chances of further abscess formation. A sinus that drains milk may form but it is likely to heal in time.

Blocked ducts

Lumpy areas in the breast are not uncommon – the mother is usually feeling distended glandular tissue. If they become very firm and tender (and sometimes flushed), they are often described as 'blocked ducts'. The solution is to improve milk removal (improved attachment, and possibly milk expression as well) and to treat the accompanying pain and inflammation. Massage, which is often advocated to clear the imagined 'blockage', may make matters worse by forcing more milk into the surrounding tissue.

White spots

Very occasionally, a ductal opening in the tip of the nipple may become obstructed by a white granule or by epithelial overgrowth.

- White granules appear to be caused by the aggregation and fusion of casein micelles, to which further materials become added. This hardened lump may obstruct a milk duct as it slowly makes its way down to the nipple, where it may be removed by the baby during a feed or expressed manually.
- Epithelial overgrowth seems to be the more common cause of a physical obstruction. A white blister is evident on the surface of the nipple, and it effectively closes off one of the exit points in the nipple, which leads from one or more milk-producing sections of the breast.

This problem may also be resolved if the baby feeds. Alternatively, after the baby has fed (and the skin is softened), the spot may be removed with a clean fingernail, a rough flannel or a sterile needle.

True blockages of this sort tend to recur, but once the woman understands how to deal with them, progression to mastitis can be avoided.

Feeding difficulties due to the baby
Cleft lip
Provided that the palate is intact, the presence of a cleft in the lip should not interfere with breastfeeding because the vacuum that is necessary to enable the baby to attach to the breast is created between the tongue and the hard palate, not the breast and the lips.

Cleft palate
Babies are only able to obtain milk as the result of the mother's milk ejection reflex. Because of the cleft, the baby is unable to create a vacuum and thus form a teat out of the breast and nipple. The use of an orthodontic plate has limited success. The mother should be encouraged to put the baby to the breast – for comfort, pleasure or food – provided that she is aware that expressed breast milk will also be required.

Tongue-tie
If the baby cannot extend the tongue over the lower gum he or she is unlikely to be able to draw the breast deeply into the mouth, which is necessary for effective feeding. Sometimes this is because the tongue is short, and sometimes this is because the frenulum, the whitish strip of tissue which attaches the tongue to the floor of the mouth, is preventing it. As the baby lifts the tongue, the tip becomes heart shaped as the frenulum pulls on it. Frenotomy is now recommended.

Blocked nose
Babies normally breathe through their noses. If there is an obstruction, they have great difficulty with feeding because they have to interrupt the process in order to breathe.

Down syndrome
Babies with this condition can be successfully breastfed, although extra help and encouragement may be necessary initially.

Prematurity
Preterm infants who are sufficiently mature to have developed sucking and swallowing reflexes may successfully breastfeed. Babies who are too immature to breastfeed may be able to cup feed, as an alternative to being tube fed.

CONTRAINDICATIONS TO BREASTFEEDING
Medication
Breastfeeding may have to be suspended temporarily following the administration of certain drugs or following diagnostic techniques. Breast milk expression must continue to maintain lactation.

Cancer
If the mother has cancer, the treatment she receives will make it impossible to breastfeed without harming the baby. If she has had a mastectomy, she may

feed successfully from the other breast. Following a lumpectomy for cancer, she may also be able to breastfeed. She should seek advice from her surgeon.

Breast surgery
Neither breast reduction nor augmentation are an inevitable contraindication to breastfeeding and much depends on the technique used.

HIV infection
HIV may be transmitted in breast milk.
- In developed countries, where artificial feeding is relatively safe, the mother may be advised not to breastfeed if she is HIV-positive.
- In countries where artificial feeding is a significant cause of infant mortality, exclusive breastfeeding may be the safer option.

WEANING FROM THE BREAST
- When the mother or the baby decides to stop breastfeeding, feeds should be tailed off gradually.
- Breastfeeds may be omitted, one at a time, and spaced further apart.
- Adding supplementary foods should not begin until about 6 months of age.
- If the mother is using solid food to give the baby 'tastes' and the experience of different textures before weaning, these should be given after the breastfeed. Solid foods given before the breastfeed (weaning) will result in the baby taking less milk from the breast and thus less will be produced.

COMPLEMENTARY AND SUPPLEMENTARY FEEDS
Complementary feeds (or 'top-ups') are feeds given *after* a breastfeed. Complementary feeds of breast milk substitutes are not recommended, except for medical indications.
- About 10% of newborns are at risk for hypoglycaemia, and may thus need a higher intake straight from birth than their mothers are able to provide. Where possible, this should be human milk, from a human milk bank.
- Babies who are well but sleepy, jaundiced, unsettled or difficult to attach should, if necessary, be given their mother's own expressed milk in addition to being offered the breast.

If complementary feeds are clinically indicated and the mother is unable to express sufficient milk, donor milk from a human milk bank could be used.

Supplementary feeds are feeds given *in place of* a breastfeed. There can be no justification for their use, except in extreme circumstances (such as severe illness or unconsciousness).

Artificial feeding
Most breast milk substitutes (infant formula) are modified cow's milk. The two main components used are:
- skimmed milk (a by-product of butter manufacture)
- whey (a by-product of cheese manufacture).

Breast milk substitutes may contain fats from any source, animal or vegetable (except from sesame and cotton seeds), provided that they do not contain more than 8% trans-isomers of fatty acids. They may also contain, among other things, soya protein, maltodextrin, dried glucose syrup and gelatinised and precooked starch.

There are two main types of formula:
- whey dominant
- casein dominant.

Whey-dominant formulae

A small amount of skimmed milk is combined with demineralised whey. The ratio of proteins in the formulae approximates to the ratio of whey to casein found in human milk (60:40). Whey-dominant formula feeds only should be used up to 6 months. These feeds are more easily digested than the casein-dominant formulae.

Casein-dominant formulae

Although these are sold as being suitable for use from birth, more of the protein present is in the form of casein (20:80), which forms large relatively indigestible curds in the stomach.

Babies intolerant of standard formulae

- *Hydrolysate formulae*. If breastfeeding is not possible, there are (prescription-only) alternatives that carry less risk of allergy than standard formulae – hydrolysates – some of which are designed to treat an existing allergy. Others are designed for preventative use in bottle-fed babies who are at high risk of developing cow's milk protein allergy.
- *Whey hydrolysates*. These are made from the whey of cow's milk (rather than whole milk) and these are potentially more useful for highly allergenic babies.
- *Amino acid-based formulae or elemental formulae*. This has a completely synthetic protein base providing the essential and non-essential amino acids, together with fat, maltodextrin, vitamins, minerals and trace elements.
- *Soya-based formulae*. These are no longer recommended because of concerns about the possible effects of phyto-oestrogen compounds and the possibility of unavoidably high levels of manganese and aluminium.

Preparation of an artificial feed

All powdered formula available in the UK is now reconstituted using 1 scoop (provided with the powder) to 30 ml water. Many of the major UK manufacturers of formula now produce ready-to-feed cartons. Reconstituted formula should be prepared as required due to the growth of pathogenic bacteria in stored reconstituted formula.

The water supply

It is essential that the water used is free from bacterial, radioactive contamination and any harmful chemicals. It is generally assumed in the UK that boiled tap water will meet these criteria, but from time to time this is shown not to be the case.

If bottled water is used, a still, non-mineralised variety suitable for babies must be chosen and it should be boiled as usual. Softened water is usually unsuitable.

Sterilisation of feeding equipment

The effective cleaning of all utensils should be demonstrated and the method of sterilisation discussed.

- If boiling is to be used, full immersion is essential and the contents of the pan must be boiled for 10 minutes.
- If cold sterilisation using a hypochlorite solution is the method of choice, the utensils must be fully immersed in the solution for the recommended time.
- The manufacturer's advice should be followed with regard to rinsing items that have been removed from the solution. If the item is to be rinsed, previously boiled water should be used, not water direct from the tap.
- Both steam and microwave sterilisation is now possible, but the mother should check that her equipment can withstand it.

Bottle teats

Parents will find it helpful to have several teats with holes of different sizes so that they can be changed throughout the feed as necessary. A useful test for the correct hole size is to turn the bottle upside down; the feed should drip at a rate of about one drop per second.

Feeding the baby with the bottle

Mothers should be warned about the dangers of 'bottle propping', and told that the baby must never be left unattended while feeding from a bottle.

Modern formulae do not, when correctly prepared, cause hypernatraemia. There is therefore no need to give babies extra water. The stools and vomit of a formula-fed baby have an unpleasant sour smell. The stools tend to be more formed than those of a breastfed baby and, unlike a breastfed baby, there is a real risk that an artificially fed baby may become constipated.

THE BABY-FRIENDLY HOSPITAL INITIATIVE

This is an initiative that was launched in 1991 by the World Health Organisation (WHO) and UNICEF to encourage hospitals to promote practices that are supportive of breastfeeding. It was focused around the 'Ten Steps' (Box 29.3), with which all hospitals that wish to achieve 'baby-friendly' status must comply. The evidence for the Ten Steps is contained in the WHO document of the same name, published in 1998.

Box 29.3 The Ten Steps (WHO and UNICEF Baby-Friendly Initiative)

- Have a written breastfeeding policy that is routinely communicated to all healthcare staff
- Train all healthcare staff in the skills necessary to implement this policy
- Inform all pregnant women about the benefits and management of breastfeeding
- Help mothers initiate breastfeeding soon after birth
- Show mothers how to breastfeed and how to maintain lactation, even if they should be separated from their infants
- Give newborn infants no food or drink other than breast milk, unless medically indicated
- Practise rooming-in, allowing mothers and infants to remain together 24 hours a day
- Encourage breastfeeding on demand
- Give no artificial teats or dummies to breastfeeding infants
- Foster the establishment of breastfeeding support groups and refer mothers to them on discharge from hospital or clinic

CHAPTER 30

The Healthy Low-Birth-Weight Baby

CLASSIFICATION OF BABIES BY WEIGHT AND GESTATION

Definitions of low birth weight are based upon weight alone and do not consider the gestational age of the baby. Likewise, definitions of gestational age disregard any considerations of birth weight. It is the *relationship* between these two separate considerations of weight (for assessment of growth) and gestational age (for assessment of maturity) that is of great importance and can be plotted on centile charts (Fig. 30.1). Growth charts should be derived from studies of local populations.

Weight
- Low-birth-weight (LBW) babies are those weighing below 2500 g at birth.
- Very low-birth-weight (VLBW) babies are those weighing below 1500 g at birth.
- Extremely low-birth-weight (ELBW) babies are those who weigh under 1000 g at birth.

Gestational age
A preterm baby is born before completion of the 37th week of gestation, calculated from the first day of the last menstrual period.

Small for gestational age (SGA)
SGA babies are defined as having a birth weight below the 10th centile for gestational age or <2 standard deviations below mean (the 50th centile) for gestational age.

Intrauterine growth restriction (IUGR)
This is failure of normal fetal growth caused by multiple adverse effects on the fetus.

CAUSES OF INTRAUTERINE GROWTH RESTRICTION

Fetal growth is regulated by maternal, placental and fetal factors and represents a mix of genetic mechanisms and environmental influences through which growth potential is expressed. The mechanisms that appear to limit fetal growth

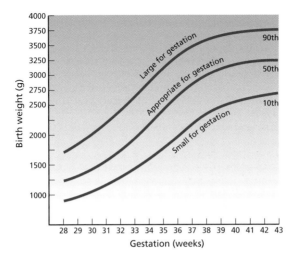

Fig. 30.1: A centile chart, showing weight and gestation. (From Simpson 1997, with permission of Baillière Tindall.)

are multifactorial and can be maternal, fetal or placental, although several factors might be interrelated.

Asymmetric growth (sometimes called acute)

Fetal weight is reduced out of proportion to length and head circumference. This is thought to be caused by extrinsic factors, such as pregnancy-induced hypertension, that adversely affect fetal nutrition.

Appearance
See Box 30.1.

Symmetric growth (chronic)

This is due either to decreased growth potential of the fetus as a result of congenital infection or chromosomal/genetic defects (intrinsic), or to extrinsic factors that are active early in gestational life (e.g. the effects of maternal smoking or poor dietary intake) or a combination of both intrinsic and extrinsic factors.

Appearance
See Box 30.2.

Symmetric growth (genetically small) babies are small normal babies and should be treated in accordance with their gestational age.

THE PRETERM BABY

Birth occurs before the end of the 37th gestational week, regardless of birth weight. Most of these babies are appropriately grown; some are SGA, while a small number are LGA. (These tend to be babies of mothers with diabetes.)

See Box 30.3 for causes of preterm labour.

Box 30.1 Appearance of the baby with asymmetric intrauterine growth restriction

- Head looks disproportionately large compared to the body
- Head circumference is usually within normal parameters
- Bones are within gestational norms for length and density
- Anterior fontanelle may be larger than expected, due to diminished membranous bone formation
- Abdomen looks 'scaphoid', or sunken due to shrinkage of the liver and spleen
- There is decreased subcutaneous fat deposition
- Skin is loose, which can give the baby a wizened, old appearance
- Vernix caseosa is frequently reduced or absent as a result of diminished skin perfusion
- Unless severely affected, these babies appear hyperactive and hungry with a lusty cry

Box 30.2 Appearance of the baby with symmetric intrauterine growth restriction

- Head circumference, length and weight are all proportionately reduced for gestational age
- Babies are diminutive in size
- They do not appear wasted, and have subcutaneous fat appropriate for their size
- Skin is taut
- Babies are generally vigorous and less likely to be hypoglycaemic or polycythaemic
- They may suffer major congenital abnormalities and can be a source of infection to carers, as a result of transplacental infection

CHARACTERISTICS OF THE PRETERM BABY

The appearance at birth of the preterm baby will depend upon gestational age (Box 30.4).

MANAGEMENT AT BIRTH OF THE HEALTHY LOW-BIRTH-WEIGHT BABY

- Current cot availability in the NICU, transitional care unit (as applicable) and postnatal ward should be known.
- The ambient temperature of the birthing room should ideally be between 23°C and 25°C.

Box 30.3 Causes of preterm labour

Spontaneous causes

- 40% unknown
- Multiple gestation
- Hyperpyrexia as a result of viral or bacterial infection
- Premature rupture of the membranes caused by maternal infection
- Maternal short stature
- Maternal age and parity.
- Poor obstetric history; history of preterm labour
- Cervical incompetence
- Poor social circumstances

Elective causes

- Pregnancy-induced hypertension, pre-eclampsia, chronic hypertension
- Maternal disease: renal, cardiac
- Placenta praevia, abruptio placenta
- Rhesus incompatibility
- Congenital abnormality
- IUGR

Box 30.4 Appearance of the preterm baby

- Posture appears flattened with hips abducted, knees and ankles flexed
- Babies are generally hypotonic with a weak and feeble cry
- Head is in proportion to the body
- The skull bones are soft with large fontanelles and wide sutures
- Chest is small and narrow and appears underdeveloped due to minimal lung expansion during fetal life
- Abdomen is prominent because the liver and spleen are large and abdominal muscle tone is poor
- Umbilicus appears low in the abdomen because linear growth is cephalocaudal (more apparent nearer to the head than the feet)
- Subcutaneous fat is laid down from 28 weeks' gestation; therefore its presence and abundance will affect the redness and transparency of the skin
- Vernix caseosa is abundant in the last trimester and tends to accumulate at sites of dense lanugo growth, i.e. face, ears, shoulders, sacral region
- Ear pinna is flat with little curve, the eyes bulge, the orbital ridges are prominent
- Nipple areola is poorly developed and barely visible
- Cord is white, fleshy and glistening
- Plantar creases are absent before 36 weeks
- In girls, the labia majora fail to cover the labia minora; in boys, the testes descend into the scrotal sac in about the 37th gestational week

- The neonatal resuscitaire should be checked and ready for use.
- A second person skilled in resuscitation skills should be present.
- On cutting the cord, leave an extra length, in case access to the umbilical vessels be necessary later.
- The Apgar score is traditionally scored at 1 and 5 minutes.
- Labelling of the LBW baby is particularly important because separation of mother and baby could happen at any time if the baby's condition becomes unstable.
- A detailed but expedient examination of the baby should be carried out.
- Once it is established that the baby is healthy, the midwife may attempt to normalise care by emphasising to the parents the importance of preventing cold stress and promoting skin-to-skin contact for a period of up to 50 minutes.
- Ensure that the baby is thoroughly dried before skin-to-skin contact is attempted.
- The baby's body temperature should be maintained between 36.5°C and 37.3°C.

CARE OF THE HEALTHY LOW-BIRTH-WEIGHT BABY

Many of the care issues relevant to the LBW baby apply to both the preterm and SGA infant.

PRINCIPLES OF THERMOREGULATION

Thermoregulation is the balance between heat production and heat loss. The prevention of cold stress, which may lead to hypothermia (body temperature < 36°C), is critical for the intact survival of the LBW baby. Newborn babies are unable to shiver, move very much or ask for an extra blanket, and therefore rely upon physical adaptations that generate heat by raising their basal metabolic rate and utilising brown fat deposits. As body temperature falls, tissue oxygen consumption rises as the baby attempts to raise its metabolic rate by burning glucose to generate energy and heat. Care measures should aim to provide an environment that supports thermoneutrality.

Thermoregulation and the healthy mature SGA baby
- Rapid heat loss due to the large head to body ratio and large surface area is exaggerated, particularly in the asymmetrically grown SGA baby.
- Wide sutures and large fontanelles add to the heat-losing tendency.
- These babies often have depleted stores of subcutaneous fat, which is used for insulation. Their raised basal metabolic rate helps them to produce heat, but their high energy demands in the presence of poor glycogen stores and minimal fat deposition can soon lead to hypoglycaemia and then hypothermia.
- Once the baby is thoroughly dried, a prewarmed hat will minimise heat loss from the head.

Thermoregulation and the healthy preterm baby

- All preterm babies are prone to heat loss because their ability to produce heat is compromised by their immaturity, so factors like their large surface area to weight ratio, their varying amounts of subcutaneous fat and their ability to mobilise brown fat stores will be affected by their gestational age.
- During cooling, the immature heat-regulating centres in the hypothalamus and medulla oblongata fail, to different degrees, to recognise and marshal adequately coordinated homeostatic controls.
- Preterm babies are often unable to increase their oxygen consumption effectively through normal respiratory function, and their calorific intake is often inadequate to meet increasing metabolic requirements.
- Furthermore, their open resting postures increase their surface area and insensible water losses.
- Babies under 2.0 kg may need incubator care when the baby is not in skin-to-skin contact with either parent. The warm conditions in an incubator can be achieved either by heating the air to 30–32°C (air mode) or by servo-controlling the baby's body temperature at a desired set point (36°C). In servo mode, a thermocouple is taped to the upper abdomen and the incubator heater maintains the skin at that site to a preset constant. Babies are clothed with bedding, in a room temperature of 26°C.
- Most preterm babies between 2.0 and 2.5 kg will be cared for in a cot, in a room temperature of 24°C.

Hypoglycaemia and the healthy LBW baby

- Hypoglycaemia refers to a low blood glucose concentration; it is more likely to occur in conditions where babies become cold or where the initiation of early feeding (within the first hour) is delayed.
- The aim is to maintain the true blood sugar above 2.6 mmol/dl. However, this does not mean that every LBW baby should be *routinely* screened. Well LBW babies who show no clinical signs of hypoglycaemia, are demanding and taking nutritive feeds on a regular basis, and are maintaining their body temperature do not need screening for hypoglycaemia.
- If a baby, despite being fed, presents with clinical signs of hypoglycaemia, a venous sample should be taken by the paediatrician to assess true blood sugar.
- A blood glucose that remains <2.6 mmol/dl, despite the baby's further attempts to feed by breast or to take colostrum by cup, may warrant transfer to the NICU, because glucose by intravenous bolus may be necessary to correct the metabolic disturbance.
- In addition, consideration should be given as to whether there may be some underlying medical condition.

Hypoglycemia and the healthy mature SGA baby

- Asymmetrically grown babies have reduced glycogen stores in liver and skeletal muscles.
- Their greater brain to body mass and a tendency towards polycythaemia increase their energy demands, which in turn increases glucose requirements.
- Mature SGA babies with an asymmetric growth pattern will usually feed within the first half an hour of birth and demand feeds 2–3 hourly thereafter.
- Their susceptibility to hypoglycaemia is relatively short-lived and is limited to the first 48 hours following birth.
- If the baby is taking formula milk, feeds are usually calculated at 90 ml/kg on the first day, with 30 ml increments per day thereafter.

Hypoglycaemia and the preterm baby

- The preterm baby may be sleepier, and attempts to take the first feed may reflect gestational age.
- Total feed requirements (60 ml/kg on the first day, with 30 ml/kg increments per day thereafter) may not be taken directly from the breast and supplementary feeds can be given by cup.

FEEDING THE LOW-BIRTH-WEIGHT BABY

Both preterm and SGA babies benefit from human milk because it contains long-chain polyunsaturated omega 3 fatty acids, which are thought to be essential for the myelination of neural membranes and retinal development. Preterm breast milk has:

- a higher concentration of lipids, protein, sodium, calcium and immunoglobulins
- a low osmolarity
- lipases and enzymes that improve digestion and absorption.

The baby is normally able to co-ordinate breathing with sucking and swallowing reflexes between 32 and 36 weeks. Preterm babies are limited in their ability to suck by their weak musculature and flexor control, which is important for firm lip and jaw closure. Before 32 weeks, most healthy preterm babies will need to be tube-fed on a regular basis, usually on a 3-hourly regime with breast milk, hind-milk or formula milk.

Tube feeding has the advantage that the tube can be left in situ during a cup feed or breastfeed and has been shown to eliminate the need to introduce bottles into a breastfeeding regime. However, several problems have been identified with tube feeding:

- Nasal and oral gastric tubes encourage milk lipid adherence to their inside surfaces and reduce the amount of fat calories available to the baby.
- Babies are preferential nose breathers and the presence of a nasogastric tube will take up part of their available airway.
- Prolonged use has been associated with delay in the development of sucking and swallowing reflexes simply because the mouth is bypassed.

Cup feeding has been used therefore in favour of tube feeding:

- to provide the baby with a positive oral experience
- to stimulate saliva and lingual lipases to aid digestion
- to accelerate the transition from naso/oral gastric feeding to breastfeeding without the introduction of bottles and teats.

Certain behaviours, such as licking and lapping, are well established *before* sucking and swallowing.

- Between 32 and 34 weeks' gestation, cup feeding can act as the main method of feeding, with the baby taking occasional complete breastfeeds.
- From 35 weeks onwards, cup feeding can be gradually replaced by complete breastfeeding.

An unrushed feed can take up to an hour to complete. Feeding frequency can vary between 6 and 10 feeds per day.

THE CARE ENVIRONMENT: PROMOTING HEALTH AND DEVELOPMENT

The ideal environment should provide a cycle of day and night, regular nourishment, rest, stimulation and loving attention. The mother's desire to be involved is seen as an *essential* element in the success of caring for LBW babies on postnatal wards. Parents can be reassured that by paying attention to their baby's behavioural cues, they can work with his or her capabilities.

Handling and touch

Kangaroo care (KC) is used to promote closeness between a baby and mother and involves placing the nappy-clad baby upright between the maternal breasts for skin-to-skin contact. The LBW baby remains beneath the mother's clothing for varying periods of time that suit the mother.

Noise and light hazards

- Noise should be kept to a minimum.
- In dimmed lighting conditions, preterm babies are more able to improve their quality of sleep and alert status.
- Reduced light levels at night will help to promote the development of circadian rhythms and diurnal cycles.
- Screens to shield adjacent babies from phototherapy lights are essential.

Sleeping position

Preterm babies have reduced muscle power and bulk, with flaccid muscle tone; therefore their movements are erratic, weak or flailing. Without support they may, to differing degrees, develop head, shoulder and hip flattening, which in turn can lead to poor mobility.

- Nesting the more immature preterm babies into soft bedding, in addition to the use of close flexible boundaries, helps to keep their limbs in midline flexion.
- However, it is vital that they are nursed in a supine position to prevent asphyxia.

Sudden infant death syndrome (SIDS)

There is a need to remind parents constantly of the risk factors and safety procedures (feet-to-foot sleeping position, smoke-free room) associated with SIDS, alongside teaching them to keep their babies warm. The midwife needs to explain that families should take into consideration time of year, gestational age and postnatal age. Parental training on 'what to do if my baby stops breathing' should be offered to parents but the decision to receive training should be their choice.

The prevention of infection

LBW babies, particularly preterm ones, are especially vulnerable to infections caused by immaturity of their host defence systems.

The provision of neonatal care: the question of venue and facilities

The decision to transfer a healthy LBW baby to a postnatal ward, a transitional unit or a NICU will depend upon the baby's gestational age and weight. In addition, the availability of facilities and level of staffing are also taken into account.

CHAPTER 31

Recognising the Ill Baby

ASSESSMENT OF THE INFANT

Immediately after birth, all infants should be examined for any gross congenital abnormalities or evidence of birth trauma. They should also have their weight and gestational age plotted on a standard growth chart.

HISTORY
Maternal health
Any disease in the mother can have an effect on the pregnancy. Influencing factors include:
- pregnancy-induced hypertension
- history of epilepsy
- maternal diabetes
- history of substance abuse
- history of sexually transmitted diseases.

Fetal wellbeing and health
The following are examples of factors that may have a critical influence on the wellbeing of the infant:
- Small for gestational age (SGA).
- Poor intrauterine growth.
- Evidence of congenital abnormality detected on ultrasound.

Perinatal and birth complications
Labour and birth may also have an effect on the general welfare of the newborn infant in the following ways:
- Prolonged rupture of membranes.
- Abnormal fetal heart rate pattern.
- Meconium staining.
- Difficult or rapid birth.
- Caesarean section and the reason for this.

PHYSICAL ASSESSMENT

THE SKIN

The presence of meconium on the skin, usually seen in the nail beds and around the umbilicus, is frequently associated with infants who have cardiorespiratory problems. The skin of all babies should be examined for:

- pallor
- plethora
- cyanosis
- jaundice
- rashes.

Pallor

A pale, mottled baby is an indication of poor peripheral perfusion. At birth this can be associated with low circulating blood volume or with circulatory adaptation and compensation for perinatal hypoxaemia. The anaemic infant's appearance is usually pale pink, white or in severe cases where there is vascular collapse, grey. Other presenting signs are:

- tachycardia
- tachypnoea
- poor capillary refill.

The most likely causes of anaemia in the newborn period are listed in Box 31.1.

Pallor can also be observed in infants who are hypothermic or hypoglycaemic. Problems associated with pallor include:

- anaemia and shock
- respiratory disorders
- cardiac anomalies
- sepsis (where poor peripheral perfusion might also be observed).

Plethora

The baby's colour may indicate an excess of circulating red blood cells (polycythaemia). This is defined as a venous haematocrit greater than 70%. Newborn infants can become polycythaemic if they are recipients of:

- twin-to-twin transfusion in utero
- a large placental transfusion.

Box 31.1 Common causes of anaemia in the newborn period

- A history in the infant of haemolytic disease of the newborn
- Twin-to-twin transfusions in utero (which can cause one infant to be anaemic and the other polycythaemic)
- Maternal antepartum or intrapartum haemorrhage

Other infants at risk are:
- SGA babies
- infants of diabetic mothers
- chromosomal disorders e.g. Down syndrome
- neonatal hypothyroidism.

Hypoglycaemia is commonly seen in plethoric infants because red blood cells consume glucose. The infant can exhibit a neurological disorder; irritability, jitteriness and convulsions can occur. Other problems that may manifest are:
- apnoea
- respiratory distress
- cardiac failure
- necrotising enterocolitis.

Cyanosis

The mucous membranes are the most reliable indicators of central colour in all babies, and if the tongue and mucous membranes appear blue, this indicates low oxygen saturation levels in the blood, usually of respiratory or cardiac origin. Episodic central cyanotic attacks may be an indication that the infant is having a convulsion. Peripheral cyanosis of the hands and feet is common during the first 24 hours of life; after this time it may be a non-specific sign of illness.

Jaundice (see Ch. 35)

Early-onset jaundice (occurring in the skin and sclera within the first 12 hours of life) is abnormal and needs investigating. If a jaundiced baby is unduly lethargic, is a poor feeder, vomits or has an unstable body temperature, this may indicate infection and action should be taken to exclude this.

Surface lesions and rashes

Rashes (Box 31.2) are quite common in newborn babies but most are benign and self-limiting.

Other factors that affect the appearance of the skin

If the infant is dehydrated, the skin looks dry and pale and is often cool to touch. If gently pinched, it will be slow in retracting. Other signs of dehydration are pallor or mottled skin, sunken fontanelle or eyeball sockets, and tachycardia.

RESPIRATORY SYSTEM

It is important to observe the baby's breathing when he or she is at rest and when active. The midwife should always start by observing skin colour and then carry out a respiratory inspection, taking into account whether the baby is making either an extra effort or insufficient effort to breathe.

Respiratory inspection

The respiration rate should be between 40 and 60 breaths per minute but will vary between levels of activity. Newborn infants are primarily nose breathers and obstructions of the nares may lead to respiratory distress and cyanosis. The chest

Box 31.2 Surface lesions and rashes in the newborn baby

Milia

- White or yellow papules seen over the cheeks, nose and forehead
- Invariably disappear spontaneously over the first few weeks of life

Miliaria

- Clear vesicles on the face, scalp and perineum, caused by retention of sweat in unopened sweat glands
- Appear on the chest and around areas where clothes can cause friction
- Treatment is to care for the infant in a cooler environment or remove excess clothing

Petechiae or purpura rash

- Can occur in neonatal thrombocytopenia, a condition of platelet deficiency that usually presents with a petechial rash over the whole of the body
- There may also be prolonged bleeding from puncture sites and/or the umbilicus and bleeding into the gut
- Thrombocytopenia may be found in infants with:
  ○ Congenital infections, both viral and bacterial
  ○ Maternal idiopathic thrombocytopenia
  ○ Drugs (administered to mother or infant)
  ○ Severe Rhesus haemolytic disease

Bruising

- Can occur extensively following breech extractions, forceps and ventouse deliveries
- Bleeding can cause a decrease in circulating blood volume, predisposing the infant to anaemia or, if the bruising is severe, hypotension

Erythema toxicum

- A rash that consists of white papules on an erythematous base
- Occurs in about 30–70% of infants
- Is benign and should not be confused with a staphylococcal infection, which will require antibiotics
- Diagnosis can be confirmed by examination of a smear of aspirate from a pustule, which will show numerous eosinophils (white cells indicative of an allergic response, rather than infection)

Thrush

- A fungal infection of the mouth and throat
- Very common in neonates, especially if they have been treated with antibiotics
- Presents as white patches seen over the tongue and mucous membranes and as a red rash on the perineum

Herpes simplex virus

- If acquired in the neonatal period, this is a most serious viral infection
- Transmission in utero is rare; the infection usually occurs during birth
- 70% of affected infants will produce a rash, which appears as vesicles or pustules

Box 31.2 Surface lesions and rashes in the newborn baby—cont'd

Umbilical sepsis

- Can be caused by a bacterial infection
- Until its separation, the umbilical cord can be a focus for infection by bacteria that colonise the skin of the newborn
- If periumbilical redness occurs or a discharge is noted, it may be necessary to commence antibiotic therapy in order to prevent an ascending infection

Bullous impetigo

- A condition which makes the skin look as though it has been scalded
- Caused by streptococci or staphylococci
- Presents as widespread tender erythema, followed by blisters that break, leaving raw areas of skin
- Particularly noticeable around the napkin area but may also cause umbilical sepsis, breast abscesses, conjunctivitis and, in deep infections, involvement of the bones and joints

should expand symmetrically. If there is unilateral expansion and breath sounds are diminished on one side, this may indicate that a pneumothorax has occurred. Infants at risk of pneumothorax or other air leaks are:

- preterm infants with respiratory distress
- term infants with meconium-stained amniotic fluid
- infants who require resuscitation at birth.

Increased work of breathing

- Tachypnoea is an abnormal respiratory rate at rest above 60 breaths per minute.
- Note any inspiratory pulling in of the chest wall above and below the sternum or between the ribs (retraction).
- If nasal flaring is also present, this may indicate that there has been a delay in the lung fluid clearance or that a more serious respiratory problem is developing.
- Grunting, heard either with a stethoscope or audibly, is an abnormal expiratory sound. The grunting baby forcibly exhales against a closed glottis in order to prevent the alveoli from collapsing.

These infants may require help with their breathing, either by intubation or continuous positive airway pressure (CPAP) ventilation.

Apnoea

Apnoea is cessation of breathing for 20 seconds or more. It is associated with pallor, bradycardia, cyanosis, oxygen desaturation or a change in the level of consciousness.

Disorders that can cause apnoea, other than the type found in preterm babies, are listed in Box 31.3.

Box 31.3 Causes of apnoea in the newborn baby

- Hypoxia
- Pneumonia
- Aspiration
- Pneumothorax
- Metabolic disorders, e.g. hypoglycaemia, hypocalcaemia, acidosis
- Anaemia
- Maternal drugs
- Neurological problems, e.g. intracranial haemorrhage, convulsions, developmental disorders of the brain
- Congenital anomalies of the upper airway

BODY TEMPERATURE

The normal body temperature range for term infants is 36.5–37.3°C.

Hypothermia

Hypothermia is defined as a core temperature below 36°C. This can cause complications such as:

- increased oxygen consumption
- lactic acid production
- apnoea
- decrease in blood coagulability
- hypoglycaemia (most common).

In preterm infants, cold stress may also cause a decrease in surfactant secretion and synthesis.

When neonates are exposed to cold, they will at first become very restless; then, as their body temperature falls, they adopt a tightly flexed position to try to conserve heat. The sick or preterm infant will tend to lie supine in a frog-like position with all surfaces exposed, which maximises heat loss.

Hypoglycaemia is a common feature of infants with increased energy expenditure associated with thermoregulation and this can cause the infant to have jittery movements of the limbs, even though he or she is quiet and often limp.

Hyperthermia

Hyperthermia is defined as a core temperature above 38°C. The usual cause of hyperthermia is overheating of the environment but it can also be a clinical sign of sepsis, brain injury or drug therapy. If infants are too warm, they become restless and may have bright red cheeks. They will attempt to regulate their temperature by increasing their respiratory rate, and this can lead to an increased fluid loss by evaporation through the airways. Other problems caused by hyperthermia are:

- hypernatraemia
- jaundice
- recurrent apnoea.

CARDIOVASCULAR SYSTEM

The normal heart rate of a newborn baby is 110–160 bpm with an average of 130 bpm. Cardiovascular dysfunction should be suspected in infants who commonly present with lethargy and breathlessness during feeding.

It can be very difficult to identify infants with congenital heart disease because the clinical picture of tachycardia, tachypnoea, pallor or cyanosis may be suggestive of a respiratory problem or sepsis.

Persistent pulmonary hypertension of the newborn is usually seen in term or post-term infants who have a history of hypoxia or asphyxia at birth. The infants are slow to take their first breath or are difficult to ventilate. Respiratory distress and cyanosis are seen before 12 hours of age. Hypoxaemia is usually profound and may suggest cyanotic heart disease. Risk factors include:

- meconium-stained amniotic fluid
- nuchal cord
- placental abruption
- acute blood loss
- maternal sedation.

Cyanosis can be a prominent feature in some cardiac defects but not all. Box 31.4 lists signs that may be indicative of congenital heart disease.

Cardiac shock may resemble early septicaemia, pneumonia or meningitis. The first indication of an underlying cardiac lesion may be the presence of a murmur heard on routine examination. However, a soft localised systolic murmur with no evidence of any symptoms of cardiac disease is usually of no significance.

CENTRAL NERVOUS SYSTEM

Abnormal postures, which include neck retraction, frog-like postures, hyperextension or hyperflexion of the limbs or jittery or abnormal involuntary movements, along with a high-pitched or weak cry, could be indicative of neurological impairment and need investigation.

Box 31.4 Warning signs suggestive of congenital heart disease

- Cyanosis (often out of proportion to the degree of respiratory distress)
- Persistent tachypnoea
- Persistent tachycardia at rest
- Poor feeding: infants may be breathless and sweaty during the feed or after feeding; they may not complete their feeds and subsequently fail to thrive
- A sudden gain in weight leading to clinical signs of oedema; usually noted as the baby having puffy feet or eyelids and, in males, the scrotum being swollen
- A very loud systolic murmur: invariably significant
- Evidence of cardiac enlargement on X-ray, persisting beyond 48 hours of life
- Enlargement of the liver

Neurological disorders

Neurological disorders found at or soon after birth may be either prenatal or perinatal in origin. They include:

- congenital abnormalities: hydrocephaly, microcephaly, encephalocele, chromosomal anomalies
- hypoxic–ischaemic cerebral injuries
- birth traumas: skull fractures, spinal cord and brachial plexus injuries, subdural and subarachnoid haemorrhage
- infections passed on to the fetus: toxoplasmosis, rubella, cytomegalovirus (CMV), syphilis.

Neurological disorders that appear in the neonatal period need to be recognised promptly in order to minimise brain damage. The most common are listed in Box 31.5.

Seizures

Seizures in the newborn period can be extremely difficult to diagnose, as they are often very subtle and easily missed (Table 31.1).

The most common causes of seizure activity are:

- asphyxia
- metabolic disturbance
- intracranial/intraventricular haemorrhage
- infection
- malformation/genetic defect.

Hypotonia (floppy infant)

The term hypotonia describes the loss of body tension and tone. As a result, the infant adopts an abnormal posture which is noticeable on handling.

The causes of hypotonia include:

- maternal sedation
- birth asphyxia
- prematurity
- infection
- Down syndrome

Box 31.5 Neurological disorders recognised In the neonatal period

- *Infection*: meningitis, herpes simplex, viral encephalitis
- *Hypoxia*: birth asphyxia, respiratory distress, apnoeic episodes
- *Metabolic disorders*: acidosis, hypoglycaemia, hyponatraemia, hypernatraemia, hypothermia, hypocalcaemia, hypomagnesaemia
- *Drug withdrawal*: narcotics, barbiturates, general anaesthesia
- *Intracranial haemorrhages/intraventricular haemorrhage (IVH)*
- *Secondary bleeding*: intracranial haemorrhage from thrombocytopenia or disseminated intravascular coagulation

Table 31.1 Neonatal seizure chart	
Type	**Affected infants**
Subtle	
Apnoea usually seen with abnormal eye movements, tonic horizontal deviation, blinking, fluttering eyelids, jerking, drooling, sucking, tonic posturing or unusual movements of limbs (rowing, pedalling or swimming)	Most frequent type and most common in preterm infants
Clonic	
Jerking activity Multifocal or unifocal distinct from jittering	Term infants: hypoxic–ischaemic encephalopathy or inborn errors of metabolism
Focal: movement of one part	Disturbance of the entire cerebrum
Tonic	
Posturing similar to decerebrate posture in adults	Preterm infants with intraventricular haemorrhage
Myoclonic	
Single or multiple jerks of upper or lower extremities	Possible prediction of myoclonic spasms in early infancy

- metabolic problems, e.g. hypoglycaemia, hyponatraemia, inborn errors of metabolism
- neurological problems, e.g. spinal cord injuries (sustained by difficult breech or forceps delivery), myasthenia gravis related to maternal disease, myotonic dystrophy
- endocrine, e.g. hypothyroidism
- neuromuscular disorders.

RENAL/GENITOURINARY SYSTEM

Urinary infections typically present with lethargy, poor feeding, increasing jaundice and vomiting. Urine that only dribbles out, rather than being passed forcefully, may be an indication of a problem with posterior urethral valves. Urine that is cloudy in appearance or smelly may be an indication of a urinary tract infection.

Renal problems may present as a failure to pass urine. The normal infant usually passes urine 4–10 hours after birth. Normal urine output for a term baby in the first day of life should be 2–4 ml/kg/hour. Urine output of less than 1 ml/kg/hour (oliguria) should be investigated.

Common causes of reduced urine output include:
- inadequate fluid intake
- increased fluid loss due to hyperthermia, use of radiant heaters and phototherapy units

- birth asphyxia
- congenital abnormalities
- infection.

GASTROINTESTINAL TRACT

Oesophageal atresia can be diagnosed antenatally because the fetus is unable to swallow the amniotic fluid, giving rise to polyhydramnios in the mother. If, however, the condition is not identified antenatally, the infant usually presents with copious saliva, which causes gagging, choking, pallor or cyanosis. In infants who are inadvertently fed milk this may cause a severe respiratory arrest due to milk aspiration.

Intestinal obstructions may be caused by atresias, malformations or structural damage anywhere below the stomach. In the newborn period, gastrointestinal disorders often present with:

- vomiting
- abdominal distension
- failure to pass stools
- diarrhoea with or without blood in the stools.

However, vomiting in the postnatal period can be caused by factors other than gastrointestinal obstructions. Early vomiting may be caused by the infant swallowing meconium or maternal blood at delivery. This can cause a gastritis, which will eventually settle. Some infants may require a gastric lavage if the symptoms are severe.

All vomit should be checked for the presence of bile or blood. Observe the infant for other signs such as abdominal distension, watery or blood-stained stools and temperature instability.

The infant who has an infection can often display signs of gastrointestinal problems, usually poor feeding, vomiting and/or diarrhoea. Diarrhoea caused by gastroenteritis is usually very watery and may sometimes resemble urine. Loose stools can also be a feature of infants being treated for hyperbilirubinaemia with phototherapy.

Some of the more commonly seen gastrointestinal problems include:

- duodenal atresia
- malrotation of the gut
- volvulus
- meconium ileus
- necrotising enterocolitis (NEC)
- imperforate anus
- rectal fistulas
- Hirschsprung's disease.

Duodenal atresia

Duodenal atresia usually presents with bile-stained vomiting within 24–36 hours of birth. Abdominal distension may not be present. Insertion of a nasogastric tube may reveal a large amount of bile in the stomach and there may be a history of polyhydramnios and a delay in passing meconium.

Malrotation of the gut/volvulus

This is a developmental abnormality where incomplete rotation of the small bowel has taken place, giving rise to signs of obstruction. The infant usually has no problems in the first few days of life, then presents with bilious vomiting and abdominal distension.

Meconium ileus

The infant with meconium ileus often has cystic fibrosis. Clinical signs include marked abdominal distension. Meconium is not passed, but occasionally small pellet-type stools, pale in colour, are mistakenly identified as bowel action. Vomiting gradually increases, mainly gastric secretions and feed, but later becomes bilious.

Necrotising enterocolitis

NEC is an acquired disease of the small and large intestine caused by ischaemia of the intestinal mucosa. It occurs more often in preterm infants, but may also occur in term infants who have been asphyxiated at birth or infants with polycythaemia and hypothermia (commonly found in SGA infants). NEC may present with vomiting or, if gastric emptying is being monitored, the aspirate is large and bile stained. The abdomen becomes distended, while stools are loose and may have blood in them. In the early stages of NEC, the infant can display non-specific signs of temperature instability, unstable glucose levels, lethargy and poor peripheral circulation. As the illness progresses, the infant becomes apnoeic and bradycardic and may need ventilating.

Imperforate anus

All infants should be checked at birth for this.

Rectal fistulas

The midwife should look for the presence of meconium in the urine, or in female infants, meconium being passed per vaginam.

Hirschsprung's disease

Hirschsprung's disease should be suspected in term infants with delayed passage of meconium, certainly beyond the first 24 hours of life. It is caused by an absence of ganglion cells in the distal rectum. The area of aganglionosis varies and may include the lower rectum, colon and small intestine. An incomplete obstruction occurs above the affected segment. Abdominal distension and vomiting are clinical signs, with the vomit becoming bile stained if meconium is not passed.

Metabolic disorders (see Ch. 36)

Metabolic disorders, such as galactosaemia and phenylketonuria, present in the newborn period with vomiting, weight loss, jaundice and lethargy.

CHAPTER 32

Respiratory Problems

ANATOMICAL INFLUENCES

Neonates are susceptible to respiratory compromise resulting from the following:

- Their stage of lung development and contributing lack of maturation in the other body systems.
- An increased work of breathing owing to the high compliance of the neonatal lung, which results from the cartilaginous nature of the rib structure.
- The neonatal diaphragm being more susceptible to fatigue due to the composition and location of the muscle within the neonatal chest.
- Neonatal airways which are smaller; this generates higher resistance to airflow and a smaller area through which perfusion can occur.
- The tendency for pulmonary blood flow to bypass areas of hypoxia, across the alveolar bed, consequently reducing alveolar perfusion.

SIGNS OF RESPIRATORY COMPROMISE

These are listed in Box 32.1.

PNEUMOTHORAX

Pneumothoraces are known to occur spontaneously in 1% of the newborn population either during or after birth; however, only one-tenth of this 1% will be symptomatic. The cause at birth is the result of the large pressures generated by the baby's first breaths. These may range up to 40–80 cm of water. This leads to alveolar distension and rupture, allowing air to leak to a number of sites of which the potential space between the lung pleura is one.

Box 32.1 Signs of respiratory compromise

Grunting
- An audible noise heard on expiration
- Appears when there is the partial closure of the glottis as the breath is expired
- The baby is attempting to preserve some internal lung pressure and prevent the airways from collapsing at the end of the breath

Retractions
- Chest distortions occur due to an increase in the need to create higher inspiratory pressures in a compliant chest
- Appear as intercostal, subcostal or sternal recession across the thorax

Asynchrony
- The breathing appears as a 'see-saw' pattern as the abdominal movements and the diaphragm work out of unison
- A result of increased muscle fatigue and the compliant chest wall

Tachypnoea
- This is a compensatory rise in the respiratory rate (above 60 breaths per minute) initiated from the respiratory centre and aims to remove the hypoxia and hypercarbia

Nasal flaring
- An attempt to minimise the effect of the airways' resistance by maximising the diameter of the upper airways
- The nares are seen to flare open with each breath

Apnoea
- Occurs as the conclusion of increasing respiratory fatigue in the term baby
- The preterm baby may experience apnoea of prematurity due to the immature respiratory centre, as well as apnoea from respiratory fatigue

Babies receiving assisted ventilation also have an increased susceptibility to a pneumothorax due to:
- maldistribution of the ventilated gas in the lungs
- high ventilation settings
- infant–ventilator breathing interactions

Presumptive diagnosis:
- reduced breath sounds on the affected side
- displaced heart sounds
- distorted chest/diaphragm movement with respiration
- distension of the chest on the affected side.

Emergency treatment involves either a needle aspiration or the placement of a chest drain.

Transient tachypnoea of the newborn (TTN)

TTN is frequently seen as a diagnosis of exclusion of other possible respiratory causes. The chest X-ray may show a streaky appearance with fluid apparent in the horizontal fissure, confirming the diagnosis and also accounting for the colloquialism of 'wet lung'.

The most common predisposing factor for TTN is a caesarean section, as the thorax has not been squeezed while the baby descends along the birth canal. This results in lower thoracic pressures after birth. Although these babies require initial care on a neonatal unit, their stay is usually of a short duration with the provision of oxygen and observation.

Infection/pneumonia

Pneumonia in the neonate is difficult to diagnose, as secretions are difficult to obtain and the radiological appearances can be hard to distinguish.

- Pneumonia presenting before 48 hours of age has normally been acquired either at or before birth.
- Presentation after 48 hours indicates infection resulting from hospitalisation.

All infants with infection require antibiotics.

Meconium aspiration syndrome

A baby can develop meconium aspiration syndrome if stimulated to breathe or gasp, either before or after birth, if there is meconium in the airway that could be inhaled.

- The initial respiratory distress may be mild, moderate or severe, with a gradual deterioration over the first 12–24 hours in moderate or severe cases.
- The meconium becomes trapped in the airways and causes a ball-valve effect; the air can get in and the meconium blocks the airway during expiration, causing an accumulation of air behind the blockage.
- This accumulation can then lead to rupture of the alveoli and cause the baby to develop a pneumothorax.
- Where the meconium has contact with the lung tissue, a pneumonitis occurs.
- The surfactant is also broken down in the presence of meconium.

These factors combine with a previously hypoxic infant to produce a severe disease process. These babies will need full intensive care and ventilation to prevent further deterioration.

Respiratory distress syndrome (RDS)

RDS occurs as a result of insufficient production of surfactant, seen most frequently after a premature birth; however, other disorders such as maternal diabetes or meconium aspiration syndrome can also inhibit surfactant production. Surfactant is produced to reduce the surface tension within the alveoli, preventing their collapse at the end of exhalation. It is much harder to inflate collapsed alveoli, in terms of the pressure and exertion required, than to reinflate partially collapsed alveoli.

Diagnosis involves the following:

- Increasing respiratory distress and work of breathing are noted.
- The X-ray shows a ground glass appearance across the lung fields, while severe disease is represented by a 'white-out'.

Treatment includes:

- oxygen therapy
- surfactant administration directly into the lungs
- ventilatory support for the most severely affected.

CARDIAC DISEASE

Cardiac defects (Box 32.2 and Ch. 34), while not a respiratory disease, present with respiratory symptoms.

CARE OF THE RESPIRATORILY COMPROMISED BABY

RESPIRATORY CARE

The following assist in observations of the baby:

- saturation monitors
- transcutaneous monitors
- arterial catheter readings.

Box 32.2 Cardiac lesions

Right-sided lesions

- The most frequently seen lesions are transposition of the great arteries, tetralogy of Fallot and pulmonary atresia or stenosis
- These infants typically present as 'blue' babies. On examination there is little to note other than the presence of cyanosis
- Their respiratory distress, if present, is mild and consists of tachypnoea alone
- These babies will remain cyanotic in the presence of 100% oxygen

Left-sided lesions

- The most frequently seen left-sided lesions are hypoplastic left heart syndrome and coarctation of the aorta
- These frequently present with neonatal heart failure
- Initially, the baby may appear irritable, lethargic, sweaty and uninterested in feeding
- The presence of 'effortless' tachypnoea may be seen, characterised by the lack of any other sign of respiratory compromise; for example, no grunting is heard, there is no head bobbing and recession is minimal
- As the heart failure progresses, the infant shows signs of cardiogenic shock and will go on to require full resuscitative measures if left unsupported

When satisfactory oxygenation is not being achieved, additional oxygen can be delivered:
- via a nasal cannula
- into a headbox
- from high-frequency oscillation (HFOV)
- by conventional mechanical ventilation (CMV)
- with continuous positive airway pressure (CPAP).

Some ventilation techniques, such as extra corporeal membrane oxygenation (ECMO), are available at specialised centres only.

CARDIOVASCULAR SUPPORT

Cardiac failure in a neonate is rare, as the majority of arrests are respiratory in origin. However, neonates may require support to maintain an efficient and effective heart beat. Maintenance of an adequate blood pressure (the mean being equivalent to the gestational age) may need pharmaceutical support. A bradycardia (a heart rate below 80) may be a sign of various influences such as a blocked endotracheal tube or sepsis.

Occasionally, the transition from a fetal to an adult circulation is compromised and the baby develops persistent pulmonary hypertension of the newborn. Nitric oxide is the vasodilator of choice.

NUTRITION AND HYDRATION

A preterm baby has few nutritional reserves and will need supplementation soon after birth to meet the continual demand for glucose from the brain. Oral breast milk feeding is not possible for a sick neonate as the presence of the endotracheal tube or the absence of a suck reflex prevents oral feeding.

The majority of infants will receive a glucose-based intravenous infusion. This allows milk feeds to be given via a nasogastric, orogastric or nasojejunal tube, increasing the volumes as the baby's condition allows. Sick or immature babies need a cautious introduction to milk, whether expressed breast milk or formula feeds, as they are susceptible to necrotising enterocolitis (NEC). When it is expected to take more than 4–5 days before full feeding is established, total parenteral nutrition (TPN) is needed to ensure all nutritional requirements can be met. While some babies may need TPN for many weeks, it can have some undesirable side effects upon the liver, giving rise to a conjugated hyperbilirubinaemia or cholestasis. Prolonged TPN is sometimes needed in very immature babies with gastroschisis and those with NEC.

The causes of NEC are multifactorial:
- Delayed feeding causes a lowered immune response to potential pathogens.
- Administration of antibiotics can alter the dominant gut flora, as can formula milk.

- Bacterial infection can occur following episodes of hypoxia.
- Polycythaemia reduces the arterial blood flow through the mesenteric circulation and causes mucosal ischaemia; reperfusion leads to oedema, haemorrhage, ulceration and necrosis.

Signs and symptoms include:

- a painful distended abdomen
- blood in the stool
- poor feed tolerance
- air within the gut wall, leading to a perforation, hypovolaemic shock or disseminated intravascular coagulation.

Treatment involves:

- antibiotics and medical management initially
- surgery if there is a perforation or a failure to respond to the medical therapy.

The disease can be fatal; long-term problems for those who do recover can include short gut syndrome and gut stenosis.

A SAFE ENVIRONMENT

The respiratorily compromised baby needs all its energy to maintain satisfactory oxygenation and hence particular care is needed to:

- protect from infection
- maintain a thermoneutral environment
- minimise stressors
- detect and treat pain and distress.

THE FAMILY

The midwife and neonatal staff have important roles in assisting parental attachment by maintaining regular, reliable and effective communication about the baby and giving advice on how parents can participate in the baby's care.

CHAPTER 33

Trauma During Birth, Haemorrhage and Convulsions

TRAUMA TO SKIN AND SUPERFICIAL TISSUES

SKIN

Damage to the skin may result from forceps blades, vacuum extractor cups, scalp electrodes and scalpels.

- Abrasions and lacerations should be kept clean and dry.
- If there are signs of infection, antibiotics may be required.
- Deeper lacerations may require closure with butterfly strips or sutures.

SUPERFICIAL TISSUES

Trauma to soft tissue involves oedematous swellings and/or bruising. The oedema consists of serum and blood (serosanguineous fluid).

Caput succedaneum

This is an oedematous swelling under the scalp and above the periosteum (Fig. 33.1 and Box 33.1). A 'false' caput succedaneum can also occur if a vacuum extractor cup is used; the resulting oedematous deformity is known as a 'chignon'.

The baby will usually experience some discomfort.

Other injury

When the face presents, it becomes congested and bruised, and the eyes and lips become oedematous. In a breech presentation the fetus will develop bruised and oedematous genitalia and buttocks.

Uncomplicated oedema and bruising usually resolve within a few days of life. However, if there is significant trauma during a vaginal breech birth, there can be serious complications such as:

- hyperbilirubinaemia
- excessive blood loss, resulting in hypovolaemia, shock, anaemia and disseminated intravascular coagulation
- damage to muscles, resulting in difficulties with micturition and defecation.

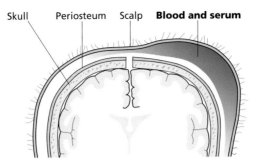

Fig. 33.1: Caput succedaneum.

Box 33.1 Features of a caput succedaneum

- Is present at birth
- Does not usually enlarge
- Can 'pit' on pressure
- Can cross a suture line
- Involves oedema that may move to the dependent area of the scalp
- Usually resolves by 36 hours of life
- Has no longer-term consequences

MUSCLE TRAUMA

Injuries to muscle result from tearing or from disruption of the blood supply.

Torticollis

Excessive traction or twisting can cause tearing to one of the sternomastoid muscles during the birth of the anterior shoulder of a fetus with a cephalic presentation, or during rotation of the shoulders when the fetus is being born by vaginal breech. A small lump can be felt on the affected sternomastoid muscle. It appears painless for the baby. The muscle length is shortened; therefore the neck is twisted on the affected side.

The management of torticollis involves stretching of the affected muscle, achieved under the guidance of a physiotherapist. The swelling will usually resolve over several weeks.

NERVE TRAUMA

Commonly, there is trauma to the facial nerve or to the brachial plexus nerves.

Facial nerve

Damage to the facial nerve usually results from its compression against the ramus of the mandible by a forceps blade, resulting in a unilateral facial palsy.

The eyelid on the affected side remains open and the mouth is drawn over to the normal side. If the baby cannot form an effective seal on the breast or teat, there may be some initial feeding difficulties. Spontaneous resolution usually occurs within 7–10 days.

Brachial plexus

Trauma to this group of nerves usually results from excessive lateral flexion, rotation or traction of the head and neck during vaginal breech birth or when shoulder dystocia occurs. These injuries can be unilateral or bilateral. There are three main types of injury:

- *Erb's palsy*. There is damage to the upper brachial plexus involving the fifth and sixth cervical nerve roots. The baby's affected arm is inwardly rotated, the elbow is extended, the wrist is pronated and flexed, and the hand is partially closed. This is commonly known as the 'waiter's tip position'. The arm is limp, although some movement of the fingers and arm is possible.
- *Klumpke's palsy*. There is damage to the lower brachial plexus involving the seventh and eighth cervical and the first thoracic nerve roots. The upper arm has normal movement but the lower arm, wrist and hand are affected. There is wrist drop and flaccid paralysis of the hand with no grasp reflex.
- *Total brachial plexus palsy*. There is damage to all brachial plexus nerve roots with complete paralysis of the arm and hand, lack of sensation and circulatory problems. If there is bilateral paralysis, spinal injury should be suspected.

All types of brachial plexus trauma will require further investigations such as X-ray and ultrasound scanning (USS), and assessment of the joints. Passive movements of the joints and limb can then be initiated under the direction of a physiotherapist. At approximately 1 month of age, magnetic resonance imaging (MRI) can offer specific data on nerve damage.

Spontaneous recovery within days to weeks is expected for most babies. Follow-up is recommended. Babies with no functional recovery by 6 months of age may require surgical repair.

FRACTURES

Fractures are rare but the most commonly affected bones are:
- clavicle
- humerus
- femur
- skull bones.

HAEMORRHAGE

Haemorrhage can be due to:
- trauma
- disruptions in blood flow

or can be related to:

- coagulopathies
- other causes.

Blood volume in the term baby is approximately 80–100 ml/kg and in the preterm baby 90–105 ml/kg; therefore even a small haemorrhage can be potentially fatal.

HAEMORRHAGE DUE TO TRAUMA

Cephalhaematoma

A cephalhaematoma is an effusion of blood under the periosteum that covers the skull bones (Fig. 33.2 and Box 33.2). During a vaginal birth, if there is friction between the fetal skull and the maternal pelvic bones, such as in cephalopelvic disproportion or precipitate labour, the periosteum is torn from the bone, causing bleeding underneath. Cephalhaematomas can also be caused during vacuum-assisted births. More than one bone may be affected, causing multiple cephalhaematomas to develop (Fig. 33.3).

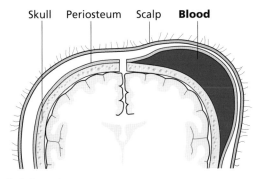

Fig. 33.2: Cephalhaematoma.

Box 33.2 Features of a cephalhaematoma

- Is not present at birth
- Appears after 12 hours
- Involves swelling that grows larger over subsequent days and can persist for weeks
- Is circumscribed and firm
- Does not pit on pressure
- Does not cross a suture and is fixed

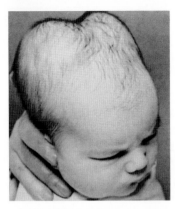

Fig. 33.3 Bilateral cephalhaematoma.

No treatment is necessary and the swelling subsides when the blood is reabsorbed. Erythrocyte breakdown in the extravasated blood may result in hyperbilirubinaemia. A ridge of bone may later be felt round the periphery of the swelling, owing to the accumulation of osteoblasts.

Subaponeurotic and subdural haemorrhage

Less common types of haemorrhage due to trauma are:
- subaponeurotic haemorrhage
- subdural haemorrhage.

These are usually associated with precipitate or difficult births or instrumental deliveries. The most common cause of subdural haemorrhage in a term baby is a tentorial tear.

HAEMORRHAGE DUE TO DISRUPTIONS IN BLOOD FLOW

Subarachnoid haemorrhage

- A primary subarachnoid haemorrhage involves bleeding directly into the subarachnoid space. Preterm babies, those who suffer hypoxia at birth and term babies who suffer traumatic births are vulnerable.
- A secondary haemorrhage involves the leakage of blood into the subarachnoid space from an intraventricular haemorrhage.

The baby may have generalised convulsions from the second day of life and preterm babies may have apnoeic episodes; otherwise they appear normal and some exhibit no signs. If a lumbar puncture is performed, the cerebrospinal fluid will be uniformly blood stained. Management involves control of the consequences of asphyxia and of convulsions. The condition is usually self-limiting.

Germinal matrix/intraventricular haemorrhage (GMH/IVH) and intraparenchymal lesions (IPL)

These haemorrhages/lesions primarily affect babies of less than 32 weeks' gestation and those weighing less than 1500 g, although term babies can be affected.

- A small bleed can have a 'silent' onset and is only detectable on ultrasound scan.
- If the haemorrhage is larger or extends, the clinical features may gradually appear and worsen. These may include apnoeic episodes, which become more frequent and severe, episodes of bradycardia, pallor, falling haematocrit, tense anterior fontanelle, metabolic acidosis and convulsions. The baby may be limp or unresponsive.
- If the GMH/IVH/IPL is large and sudden in onset, the baby may present with apnoea and circulatory collapse.

The care of at-risk babies is focused on prevention: for example, antenatal administration of steroids to the mother, artificial surfactant after birth or antibiotic therapy in the management of preterm premature rupture of the membranes.

The neurological prognosis for babies with small haemorrhages is usually good. Babies who suffer a massive haemorrhage may die within 48 hours of the onset and those who survive are likely to develop significant neurological and intellectual impairment.

HAEMORRHAGE RELATED TO COAGULOPATHIES

These haemorrhages occur because of a disruption in the baby's blood-clotting abilities.

Vitamin K deficiency bleeding

Vitamin K deficiency bleeding (VKDB) can occur up to 12 months of age, although it more commonly occurs between birth and 8 weeks of life. Several proteins require vitamin K to be converted into active clotting factors. A deficiency of vitamin K leads to a deficiency of these clotting factors and resultant bleeding. Neonates are deficient in vitamin K and therefore vulnerable to VKDB.

- Early VKDB (first 24 hours) is rare and principally affects babies born to women who, during pregnancy, have taken warfarin, phenobarbital or phenytoin.
- Classical VKDB (1–7 days) – see Box 33.3.
- Late VKDB (1–12 months) almost exclusively occurs in breastfed babies. However, it may occur in babies who have liver disease or a condition that disrupts the absorption of vitamin K_1 from the bowel – e.g. cystic fibrosis.

Bleeding may be evident superficially as bruising or haemorrhage from the umbilicus, puncture sites, the nose and the scalp. Severe jaundice for more than 1 week and persistent jaundice for more than 2 weeks are warning signs. Gastrointestinal bleeding is manifested as melaena and haematemesis. In early

---

Box 33.3 Babies susceptible to vitamin K deficiency bleeding

- Those who have experienced birth trauma
- Those who have experienced asphyxia
- Those who have experienced postnatal hypoxia
- Those who are preterm
- Those who are of low birth weight
- Those who have been given antibiotic therapy
- Those who cannot maintain enteral feeding or feed poorly

---

and late VKDB, there may be serious extracranial and intracranial bleeding. With severe haemorrhage, circulatory collapse occurs. Diagnosis is confirmed by blood tests.

Babies who have VKDB require careful investigation and monitoring to assess their need for treatment. With all forms of VKDB, the baby will require administration of vitamin K_1, 1–2 mg intramuscularly. VKDB is a potentially fatal condition; therefore prophylactic administration of vitamin K has become the norm in many countries (see Ch. 27).

Thrombocytopenia

Thrombocytopenia is a low count of circulating platelets (<150 000/μl). Babies who are at risk are listed in Box 33.4.

A petechial rash appears soon after birth, presenting in a mild case with a few localised petechiae. In a severe case there is widespread and serious haemorrhage from multiple sites. Diagnosis is based on history, clinical examination and the presence of a reduced platelet count.

- In mild cases, no treatment is required.
- In immune-mediated thrombocytopenia, intravenous immunoglobulin administration is helpful.
- In severe cases, where there is haemorrhage and a very low platelet count, transfusion of platelet concentrate may be required.

Box 33.4 Babies susceptible to thrombocytopenia

- Those who have a severe congenital or acquired infection, e.g. syphilis, cytomegalovirus, rubella, toxoplasmosis or bacterial infection
- Those whose mother has idiopathic thrombocytopenia, purpura, systemic lupus erythematosus or thyrotoxicosis
- Those whose mother takes thiazide diuretics
- Those who have isoimmune thrombocytopenia
- Those who have inherited thrombocytopenia

Disseminated intravascular coagulation (consumptive coagulopathy)

Disseminated intravascular coagulation (DIC) is an acquired coagulation disorder associated with the release of thromboplastin from damaged tissue, stimulating abnormal coagulation and fibrinolysis.

HAEMORRHAGE RELATED TO OTHER CAUSES

Umbilical haemorrhage

This usually occurs as a result of a poorly applied cord ligature. A purse-string suture should always be inserted if umbilical bleeding does not stop after 15 or 20 minutes.

Vaginal bleeding

A small temporary discharge of blood-stained mucus occurring in the first days of life, often referred to as pseudomenstruation, is due to the withdrawal of maternal oestrogen.

Haematemesis and melaena

These signs usually present when the baby has swallowed maternal blood during birth or from cracked nipples during breastfeeding. The diagnosis must be differentiated from other serious causes.

- If the cause is swallowed blood, the condition is self-limiting, requiring no specific treatment.
- However, if the cause is cracked nipples, appropriate treatment for the mother must be implemented.

Haematuria

Haematuria can be associated with coagulopathies, urinary tract infections and structural abnormality of the urinary tract. Birth trauma may cause renal contusion and haematuria. Occasionally, after suprapubic aspiration of urine, transient mild haematuria may be observed. Treatment of the primary cause should resolve the haematuria.

CONVULSIONS

A convulsion is a sign of neurological disturbance, not a disease. It can present quite differently in the neonate and can be difficult to recognise.

Convulsive movement can be differentiated from jitteriness or tremors in that, with the latter two, the movements:

- are rapid, rhythmic and equal
- are often stimulated or made worse by disturbance
- can be stopped by touching or flexing the affected limb
- are normal in an active, hungry baby and are usually of no consequence, although their occurrence should be documented.

Convulsive movements:

- tend to be slower and less equal
- are not necessarily stimulated by disturbance

- cannot be stopped by restraint
- are always pathological.

Subtle convulsions include movements such as:

- blinking or fluttering of the eyelids
- staring
- clonic movements of the chin
- horizontal or downward movements of the eyes
- sucking
- drooling
- sticking the tongue out
- cycling movements of the legs
- apnoea.

Both term and preterm babies can experience subtle convulsions. These movements should be differentiated from the normal ones associated with rapid eye movement sleep.

If the baby has tonic convulsions, there will be:

- extension or flexion of the limbs
- asymmetric postures of body or neck
- altered patterns of breathing
- maintenance of eye deviations.

Tonic convulsions are more common in preterm babies.

Term babies demonstrate multifocal clonic convulsions and the movements include random jerking movements of the extremities.

Term babies also experience focal clonic convulsions in which localised repetitive clonic jerking movements are seen. An extremity, a limb or a localised muscle group can be affected.

Myoclonic convulsions are the least common but affect term and preterm babies. The movements are single or multiple flexion jerks of the feet, legs, hands or arms, which should not be confused with similar movements in a sleeping baby.

During a convulsion the baby may have:

- tachycardia
- hypertension
- raised cerebral blood flow
- raised intracranial pressure.

All of these predispose to serious complications.

There are many conditions that cause newborn convulsions, as shown in Table 33.1.

Immediate treatment of a convulsion involves:

- seeking the assistance of a doctor
- ensuring a clear airway and adequate ventilation
- turning the baby to the semiprone position, with the head neither hyperflexed nor hyperextended.

The prognosis depends on the cause of convulsion, the type of convulsion and the electroencephalograph tracing.

Table 33.1 Selected causes of neonatal convulsions

Category	Selected causes
Central nervous system	Intracranial haemorrhage Intracerebral haemorrhage Hypoxic–ischaemic encephalopathy Kernicterus Congenital abnormalities
Metabolic	Hypo- and hyperglycaemia Hypo- and hypercalcaemia Hypo- and hypernatraemia Inborn errors of metabolism Acquired disorders of metabolism
Other	Hypoxia Congenital infections Severe postnatally acquired infections Neonatal abstinence syndrome Hyperthermia
Idiopathic	Unknown

CHAPTER 34

Congenital Abnormalities

DEFINITION AND CAUSES

By definition, a congenital abnormality is any defect in form, structure or function that is present at birth. Identifiable defects can be categorised in five ways:

- chromosome and gene abnormalities
- mitochondrial DNA disorders
- teratogenic causes
- multifactorial causes
- unknown causes.

Chromosome and gene abnormalities

Each human cell carries 44 chromosomes (autosomes) and two sex chromosomes. Each chromosome comprises a number of genes. The zygote should have 22 autosomes and one sex chromosome from each parent.

Genetic disorders (Mendelian inheritance)

Genes are composed of DNA and each is concerned with the transmission of one specific hereditary factor. Genetically inherited factors may be dominant or recessive.

- *A dominant gene* will produce its effect even if present in only one chromosome of a pair. An autosomal dominant condition can usually be traced through several generations: for example, achondroplasia, osteogenesis imperfecta, adult polycystic kidney disease or Huntington's chorea.
- *A recessive gene* needs to be present in both chromosomes before producing its effect: for example, cystic fibrosis or phenylketonuria.
- *In an X-linked recessive inheritance* the condition affects males almost exclusively, although females can be carriers. X-linked recessive inheritance is responsible for conditions such as haemophilia A and B and Duchenne muscular dystrophy.

Mitochondrial disorders

These are inherited from the mother. Signs and symptoms are diverse but tend to occur in brain and muscles.

Teratogenic causes

A teratogen is any agent that raises the incidence of congenital abnormality. The list of known and suspected teratogens is continually growing (Box 34.1).

Box 34.1 Known and suspected teratogens

- Prescribed drugs, e.g. anticonvulsants, anticoagulants, large amounts of vitamin A
- Drugs used in substance abuse, e.g. heroin, alcohol, nicotine
- Environmental factors, e.g. radiation and chemicals (such as dioxins, pesticides)
- Infective agents, e.g. rubella, cytomegalovirus
- Maternal disease, e.g. diabetes

Multifactorial causes

These stem from a genetic defect in addition to one or more teratogenic influences.

Unknown causes

In spite of a growing body of knowledge, the specific cause of around 80% of abnormalities remains unspecified.

FETAL ALCOHOL SYNDROME/SPECTRUM

The following characteristics are recognisable:
- a growth-restricted infant with microcephaly
- flat facies
- close-set eyes
- epicanthic folds
- small upturned nose
- thin upper lip
- low-set ears.

Being able to establish a direct link between a teratogen and a complex clinical pattern such as this is the exception rather than the rule.

GASTROINTESTINAL MALFORMATIONS

Most of the abnormalities affecting this system call for prompt surgical intervention.

GASTROSCHISIS AND EXOMPHALOS

Gastroschisis (Fig. 34.1) is a paramedian defect of the abdominal wall with extrusion of bowel that is not covered by peritoneum.

Exomphalos or omphalocele is when the bowel or other viscera protrude through the umbilicus. These babies may have other abnormalities, for example heart defects.

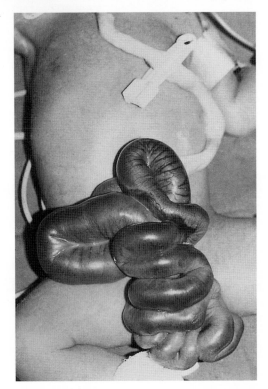

Fig. 34.1: Gastroschisis showing prolapsed intestine to the right of the umbilical cord. (From Rennie & Roberton 1999, with permission of Churchill Livingstone.)

Immediate management of both is as follows:
- Cover the herniated abdominal contents with clean cellophane wrap (Clingfilm) or warm sterile saline swabs.
- Aspirate stomach contents.
- Reduce heat loss.
- Expedite transfer to a surgical unit.

ATRESIAS

Oesophageal atresia

Oesophageal atresia occurs when there is incomplete canalisation of the oesophagus in early intrauterine development. It is commonly associated with tracheo-oesophageal fistula. The most common type of abnormality is where the upper oesophagus terminates in a blind upper pouch and the lower oesophagus connects to the trachea. This abnormality should be suspected in the presence of maternal polyhydramnios. At birth the baby has copious amounts of mucus coming from the mouth.

- The midwife should attempt to pass a wide orogastric tube but it may travel less than 10–12 cm.
- Radiography will confirm the diagnosis.
- The baby must be given no oral fluid but a wide-bore oesophageal tube should be passed into the upper pouch and connected to gentle continuous suction. Usually a double-lumen 10FG (Replogle) tube is used and the baby nursed head up.
- He or she should be transferred immediately to a paediatric surgical unit and continuous suction must be available throughout the transfer.

Duodenal atresia

This is persistent vomiting within 24–36 hours of birth.

A characteristic double bubble of gas may be seen on radiological examination. Prognosis is good if the baby is otherwise healthy, but this abnormality is often associated with other problems, such as Down syndrome.

Rectal atresia and imperforate anus

An imperforate anus should be obvious at birth but a rectal atresia might not become apparent until it is noted that the baby has not passed meconium.

Should a baby fail to pass meconium in the first 24 hours, three other possibilities should be considered:

- malrotation/volvulus
- meconium ileus (cystic fibrosis)
- Hirschsprung's disease.

PYLORIC STENOSIS

Pyloric stenosis arises from a genetic defect which causes hypertrophy of the muscles of the pyloric sphincter. The characteristic clinical presentation is projectile vomiting, usually around 6 weeks of age but possibly earlier.

CLEFT LIP AND CLEFT PALATE

Cleft lip may be unilateral or bilateral and is very often accompanied by cleft palate.

Clefts may affect the hard palate, soft palate, or both. Some defects will include alveolar margins and sometimes the uvula. The palate is examined by means of a good light source rather than by digital palpation.

- If the defect is limited to unilateral cleft lip, breastfeeding is encouraged.
- Where there is the additional problem of cleft palate, arranging for the baby to be fitted with an orthodontic plate may facilitate breastfeeding but will not afford the same stimulus as nipple to palate contact.

- Cup or spoon feeding is an alternative method, and if bottle feeding there is a wide variety of specially shaped teats available to accommodate the different sizes and positions of palate defects.

PIERRE ROBIN SYNDROME

Pierre Robin syndrome is characterised by micrognathia (hypoplasia of the lower jaw), abnormal attachment of muscles controlling the tongue, which allows it to fall backward and occlude the airway, and a central cleft palate. To maintain a clear airway the baby is nursed prone and may require the insertion of an oral airway. Nasal and nasopharyngeal constant positive airways pressure may be necessary for some time after birth. This is one of the few exceptions to the rules given in the 'Back to sleep' campaign aimed at reducing cot deaths. There is a high risk of aspiration occurring when feeding. Suction catheter and oxygen equipment should be ready to hand. An orthodontic plate may be fitted to facilitate feeding.

ABNORMALITIES RELATING TO RESPIRATION

DIAPHRAGMATIC HERNIA

There is a defect in the diaphragm, which allows herniation of abdominal contents into the thoracic cavity. The extent to which lung development is compromised as a result depends on the size of the defect and the gestational age at which herniation first occurred.

At birth:
- the baby is cyanosed
- difficulty is experienced in resuscitation
- heart sounds may be displaced to the right
- the abdomen may have a flat or scaphoid appearance.

Chest X-ray confirms the diagnosis. Continuous gastric suction should be commenced. Prognosis relates to the degree of pulmonary hypoplasia. There is also the possibility of coexistent abnormalities, such as cardiac defects or skeletal anomalies.

CHOANAL ATRESIA (FIG. 34.2)

Choanal atresia describes a unilateral or bilateral narrowing of the nasal passage(s) with a web of tissue or bone occluding the nasopharynx. Tachypnoea and dyspnoea are cardinal features, particularly when a bilateral lesion is present.

Diagnosis rests on the following criteria:
- The baby mouth breathes and finds feeding impossible without cyanosis.
- Nasal catheters cannot be passed into the pharynx.
- If a mirror or cold spoon is held under the nose, no steam will collect.

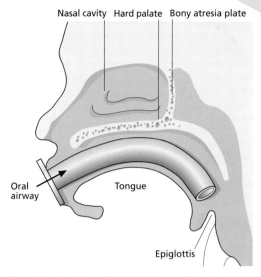

Fig. 34.2: Choanal atresia. A bony plate blocks the nose. (From Rennie & Roberton 1999, with permission of Churchill Livingstone.)

- The baby's colour will improve with crying.
- Maintaining a clear airway is essential; an oral airway may have to be used to effect this.

LARYNGEAL STRIDOR

This is a noise made by the baby, usually on inspiration; it is exacerbated by crying. Most commonly, the cause is laryngomalacia, which is due to laxity of the laryngeal cartilage. The stridor may take up to 2 years to resolve. If it is accompanied by signs of dyspnoea or feeding problems, further investigations such as bronchoscopy or laryngoscopy become necessary to rule out a more sinister cause.

CONGENITAL CARDIAC DEFECTS

POSTNATAL RECOGNITION

Clinically, babies with cardiac anomalies can be divided into two groups: cyanotic and acyanotic congenital heart disease.

...senting with cyanosis

...this group are listed in Box 34.2.

...ice of central cyanosis (that is, cyanosis of the lips and mucous ...), tachypnoea and tachycardia may be the first signs that a cardiac ...present. If there is cyanosis, administration of oxygen to these babies ...be ineffective in improving their colour and oxygen saturation monitoring will show no improvement. Indeed, giving 100% oxygen may encourage closure of the ductus arteriosus, the patency of which is literally a lifeline for some of these babies.

Acyanotic cardiac defects
Anomalies subsumed under this heading are listed in Box 34.2.

SIGNS OF CARDIAC FAILURE

Subtle signs of cardiac failure include:
- tachypnoea
- tachycardia
- incipient cyanosis, especially following the exertion of crying or feeding.

These signs will become more evident, sometimes dramatically so, with the closure of the ductus arteriosus if either coarctation of the aorta or hypoplastic left heart syndrome is present. Detailed examination may disclose heart murmurs and diminution or absence of femoral pulses in both conditions. In this event resuscitation with prostaglandin usually stabilises the baby and allows time for further assessment.

- Coarctation of the aorta is usually amenable to surgical correction, whereas hypoplastic left heart syndrome has a poor long-term outcome.

Box 34.2 Cyanotic and acyanotic congenital heart disease

Conditions presenting with cyanosis
- Transposition of the great vessels
- Pulmonary atresia
- Fallot's tetralogy
- Tricuspid atresia
- Total anomalous pulmonary venous drainage
- Univentricular/complex heart

Conditions presenting without cyanosis
- Persistent ductus arteriosus
- Ventricular or atrial septal defect
- Coarctation of the aorta
- Aortic stenosis
- Hypoplastic left heart syndrome.

- Persistent ductus arteriosus, ventricular septal defects and atrial septal defects seldom entail medical or surgical intervention in early neonatal life, but do require careful follow-up for signs of developing heart failure; surgery or interventional cardiology may be necessary at a later stage.

Not all heart murmurs heard at the first examination are significant.

CENTRAL NERVOUS SYSTEM ABNORMALITIES

ANENCEPHALY

This major abnormality describes the absence of the forebrain and vault of the skull. It is a condition that is incompatible with sustained life, but occasionally such a baby is born alive.

SPINA BIFIDA

Spina bifida results from failure of fusion of the vertebral column.

- There is no skin covering the defect, allowing protrusion of the meninges (meningocele). The meningeal membrane may be flat or appear as a membranous sac with or without cerebrospinal fluid but it does not contain neural tissue (Fig. 34.3).
- *Meningomyelocele* involves the spinal cord (see Fig. 34.3). This lesion may be enclosed or the meningocele may rupture and expose the neural tissue. Meningomyelocele usually gives rise to neural damage, producing paralysis distal to the defect and impaired function of urinary bladder and bowel. The lumbosacral area is the most common site for these to present, but they may appear at any point along the vertebral column.
- An *encephalocele* is at the level of the base of the skull, and may contain brain tissue.

Immediate management involves covering open lesions with a non-adherent dressing.

SPINA BIFIDA OCCULTA

Spina bifida occulta (see Fig. 34.3) is the most minor type of defect where the vertebra is bifid. There is usually no spinal cord involvement. A tuft of hair or sinus at the base of the spine may be noted on first examination of the baby.

HYDROCEPHALUS

This condition arises from a blockage in the circulation and absorption of cerebrospinal fluid, which is produced from the choroid plexuses within the lateral ventricles of the brain. The large lateral ventricles increase in size and eventually compress the surrounding brain tissue. It often accompanies the more severe spina bifida lesions because of a structural

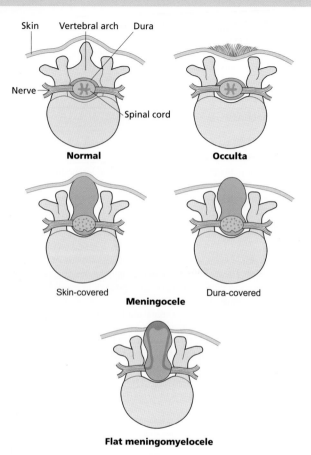

Fig. 34.3: Various forms of spina bifida. (After Wallis S, Harvey D 1979. Copyright Emap Public Sector 1979. Reproduced by permission of *Nursing Times.)*

defect around the area of the foramen magnum known as the Arnold–Chiari malformation. Hydrocephaly may either be present at birth or develop following surgical closure of a myelomeningocele. In the absence of myelomeningocele, aqueduct stenosis is the most common cause of hydrocephalus. The risk of cerebral impairment may be minimised by the insertion of a ventriculoperitoneal shunt. As the baby grows, this will need to be replaced. Signs of increased intracranial pressure include:
- large tense anterior fontanelle
- splayed skull sutures

- inappropriate increase in occipitofrontal circumference
- sun-setting appearance to the eyes
- irritability or abnormal movements.

MICROCEPHALY

The occipitofrontal circumference is more than 2 standard deviations below normal for gestational age. The disproportionately small head may be associated with intrauterine infection, for example rubella, fetal alcohol syndrome or some trisomic disorders. Most babies will be mentally impaired with evidence of cerebral palsy and often seizures.

MUSCULOSKELETAL DEFORMITIES

POLYDACTYLY AND SYNDACTYLY

- In polydactyly the extra digit(s) may be fully formed or may simply be extra tissue attached by a pedicle.
- Syndactyly (webbing) more commonly affects the hands. It can appear as an independent anomaly or as a feature of a syndrome such as Apert syndrome.

LIMB REDUCTION ANOMALIES

Postulated causes include:
- amniotic band syndrome
- environmental teratogens
- iatrogenic trauma, perhaps at the time of chorionic villus sampling
- failure of formation (arrest of development), e.g. thalidomide, an antiemetic.

TALIPES

- Talipes equinovarus (TEV, club foot) is when the ankle is bent downwards (plantarflexed) and the front part of the foot is turned inwards (inverted).
- Talipes calcaneovalgus describes the opposite position where the foot is dorsiflexed and everted.

Possible causes are:
- multiple pregnancy
- macrosomic fetus
- oligohydramnios
- association with spina bifida
- family history
- gender: statistically, more boys than girls are born with talipes.

In the mildest form the foot may easily be turned to the correct position and exercised in this way several times a day. More severe forms will require manipulation, splinting and/or surgical correction.

DEVELOPMENTAL HIP DYSPLASIA

Congenital hip dysplasia is more commonly found where there has been a history of oligohydramnios or breech presentation. It more often occurs in primigravida pregnancies and in a higher percentage of girls. The left hip is more often affected than the right. The dysplastic hip may present in one of three ways:
- dislocated
- dislocatable
- subluxation of the joint.

Examination of the hips is by Ortolani's or Barlow's test. It is usual for the baby to have a splint or harness, such as the Pavlik harness, that will keep the hips in a flexed and abducted position of about 60°.

ACHONDROPLASIA

Achondroplasia is an autosomal dominant condition where the baby is generally small with a disproportionately large head and short limbs.

OSTEOGENESIS IMPERFECTA

This autosomal dominant disorder of collagen production has at least four forms and leads to unduly brittle bones in the affected fetus and infant.

ABNORMALITIES OF THE SKIN

VASCULAR NAEVI

These defects in the development of the skin can be divided into two main types, which commonly overlap.

Capillary malformations

These are due to defects in the dermal capillaries. The most commonly observed are stork marks. These are usually found on the nape of the neck. They are generally small and will fade. No treatment is necessary.

Port wine stain

This is a purple–blue capillary malformation affecting the face. It does not regress with time; laser treatment and the skilful use of cosmetics will help to disguise it.

Should the malformation appear to mimic the distribution of a branch of the trigeminal nerve, further malformations in the meninges may be suspected. This is known as Sturge–Weber syndrome.

Capillary haemangiomata ('strawberry marks')

Capillary haemangiomata are not usually noticeable at birth but appear anywhere as red raised lesions in the first few weeks of life. They are more common in preterm infants and especially in girls. Although the lesion will grow bigger for the first few months, it will then regress and usually disappear completely by the age of 5–6 years. No treatment is normally required.

Pigmented naevi (melanocytic)

These are brown, sometimes hairy, marks on the skin which vary in size and may be flat or raised. A percentage of this type of birthmark may become malignant. Surgical excision may be recommended to preempt this.

GENITOURINARY SYSTEM

At birth the first indications that there is an abnormality of the renal tract may be:

- a single umbilical artery in the umbilical cord
- the abnormal facies associated with Potter syndrome
- no passage of urine within 24 hours
- constant dribbling urine
- poor urine stream.

Dribbling of urine is a sign of nerve damage such as occurs with neural tube defects, while a poor urine stream may indicate lower urinary tract obstruction (posterior urethral valve).

POSTERIOR URETHRAL VALVE(S)

This is an abnormality affecting boys. The presence of valves in the posterior urethra prevents the normal outflow of urine. Back pressure from the distended bladder will ultimately cause hydronephrosis. Treatment normally involves surgical intervention.

POLYCYSTIC KIDNEYS

These are likely to cause problems during the birth due to an increase in abdominal girth. On abdominal examination the kidneys will be palpable. Radiological or ultrasound investigations confirm the diagnosis. The prognosis is poor, with renal failure the likely outcome.

HYPOSPADIAS

The urethral meatus opens onto the undersurface of the penis. The meatus can be placed at any point along the length of the penis and in some cases will open onto the perineum. This abnormality often coexists with chordee, in which the penis is short and bent and the foreskin is only present on the dorsal side. Some babies will require surgery in the neonatal period to 'release' the chordee and enlarge the urethral meatus.

CRYPTORCHIDISM

Undescended testes may be unilateral or bilateral. If on examination of the baby after birth the scrotum is empty, the undescended testes may be found in the inguinal pouch.

AMBIGUOUS GENITALIA

If there is any doubt, a gender must not be assigned to the baby. Examination of the baby may reveal any of the signs listed in Box 34.3.

There are a number of causes of ambiguous genitalia, all of which need expert clarification.

Congenital adrenal hyperplasia

One of the reasons for ambiguous genitalia is an autosomal recessive condition called congenital adrenal hyperplasia. The adrenal gland is stimulated to overproduce androgens because of a deficiency of an enzyme called 21-hydroxylase, which is necessary for normal steroid production from cholesterol. The condition is not always recognised in boys in the neonatal period.

Intersex

This is where the internal reproductive organs are at variance with the external appearance of the genitalia. Ultrasound examination will help identify the nature of internal reproductive organs. True hermaphroditism is extremely rare. Following chromosomal studies to determine genetic make-up, hormone assays and consideration of the potential for cosmetic surgery, the decision of gender attribution is made.

COMMONLY OCCURRING SYNDROMES

TRISOMY 21 OR DOWN SYNDROME

This arises as a non-disjunction process in the majority. Unbalanced translocation occurs in about 2.5% of cases, usually between chromosomes 14 and 21. Mosaic forms also occur. There is no difference in clinical appearance,

---

Box 34.3 Signs of ambiguous genitalia

- Small hypoplastic penis
- Chordee
- Bifid scrotum
- Undescended testes
- Enlarged clitoris
- Incompletely separated or poorly differentiated labia

Box 34.4 Clinical appearance in Down syndrome

- Widely set and obliquely slanted eyes
- Small nose
- Thick rough tongue
- Small head with flat occiput
- Squat broad hands with incurving little finger
- Wide space between thumb and index finger
- Single palmar (simian) crease
- Brushfield spots in the eyes
- Generalised hypotonia

---

the features of which are listed in Box 34.4, Not all of the manifestations listed need be present and any of them can occur alone without implying chromosomal aberration. Babies born with Down syndrome also have a higher incidence of cardiac anomalies, leukaemia and hypothyroidism. The intelligence quotient is below average, at 40–80.

Investigations indicated include karyotyping and echocardiography, because of the increased risk of congenital heart disease. Some centres offer diagnosis within 2 days using fluorescent in-situ hybridisation (FISH) techniques.

TRISOMY 18 (EDWARDS SYNDROME)

This condition is found in about 1 in 5000 births. An extra 18th chromosome is responsible for the characteristic features. The lifespan of these children is short and the majority die during their first year.

- The head is small with a flattened forehead, a receding chin and frequently a cleft palate.
- The ears are low set and maldeveloped.
- The sternum tends to be short.
- The fingers often overlap each other and the feet have a characteristic rocker-bottom appearance.
- Malformations of the cardiovascular and gastrointestinal systems are common.

TRISOMY 13 (PATAU SYNDROME)

An extra copy of the 13th chromosome leads to multiple abnormalities. These children have a short life, only 5% living beyond 3 years.

- Affected infants are small and are microcephalic.
- Midline facial abnormalities, such as cleft lip and palate, are common and limb abnormalities are frequently seen.
- Brain, cardiac and renal abnormalities may coexist with this trisomy.

POTTER SYNDROME

This collection of features is due to the compressive effects of oligohydramnios in renal agenesis or severe hypoplasia.

- The baby's face will have a flattened appearance, with low-set ears, an anti-mongoloid slant to the eyes with deep epicanthic folds and a beaked nose.
- These babies are usually severely asphyxiated at birth because they have lung hypoplasia.
  It is a syndrome incompatible with sustained life.

TURNER SYNDROME (XO)

In this monosomal condition, only one sex chromosome exists: an X.

- The child is a girl with a short, webbed neck, widely spaced nipples and oedematous feet.
- The genitalia tend to be underdeveloped and the internal reproductive organs do not mature.
- The condition may not be diagnosed until puberty fails to occur.
- Congenital cardiac defects may also be found.
- Mental development is usually normal.

KLINEFELTER SYNDROME (XXY)

This is an abnormality that affects boys. It is not normally diagnosed until pubertal changes fail to occur.

CHAPTER 35

Jaundice and Infection

Jaundice is the yellow discoloration of the skin and sclera that results from raised levels of bilirubin in the blood (hyperbilirubinaemia).

CONJUGATION OF BILIRUBIN

Bilirubin is a waste product from the breakdown of haem, most of which is found in red blood cells (RBCs). Ageing, immature or malformed RBCs are removed from the circulation and broken down in the reticuloendothelial system (liver, spleen and macrophages), and haemoglobin becomes the by-products of haem: globin and iron.

- Haem is converted to biliverdin and then to unconjugated bilirubin.
- Globin is broken down into amino acids that are reused by the body to make proteins.
- Iron is stored in the body or used for new red blood cells.

Two main forms of bilirubin are found in the body:

- Unconjugated bilirubin is fat soluble and cannot be excreted easily either in bile or urine.
- Conjugated bilirubin has been made water soluble in the liver and can be excreted in either faeces or urine.

Three stages are involved in the processing of bilirubin:

- transport
- conjugation
- excretion.

Transport
Unconjugated bilirubin is transported in the plasma to the liver, bound to the plasma protein albumin. If not attached to albumin, it can be deposited into extravascular fatty and nerve tissues in the body. The skin and the brain are the two most common sites.

- Staining of the skin is known as *jaundice*.
- Damage to the brain as a result of bilirubin staining and toxicity is known as *kernicterus*.

Conjugation
Once in the liver, bilirubin is combined with glucose and *glucuronic acid*, and conjugation occurs in the presence of oxygen. *Uridine diphosphoglucuronyl*

transferase (UDP-GT or glucuronyl transferase) is the major enzyme involved in bilirubin conjugation. The conjugated bilirubin is now water soluble and available for excretion.

Excretion

The conjugated bilirubin is excreted via the biliary system into the small intestine, where it is catabolised by normal intestinal bacteria to form urobilinogen, then oxidised into orange-coloured urobilin. Most of the conjugated bilirubin is excreted in the faeces but a small amount is excreted in urine.

JAUNDICE

In term neonates, jaundice appears when serum bilirubin concentrations reach 85–120 μmol/l (5–7 mg/dl).

PHYSIOLOGICAL JAUNDICE

This type of jaundice:
- *never* appears before 24 hours of life
- *usually* fades by 1 week of age.
  Bilirubin levels *never* exceed 200–215 μmol/l (12–13 mg/dl).

Causes

Neonatal physiological jaundice is the result of a discrepancy between RBC breakdown and the baby's ability to transport, conjugate and excrete unconjugated bilirubin. Neonates also have increased betaglucuronidase enzyme activity in the gut, which hydrolyses conjugated bilirubin back into the unconjugated state. If feeding is delayed, bowel motility is decreased, further compromising excretion of unconjugated bilirubin.

Exaggerated physiological jaundice in breastfed infants

The exact mechanisms are unknown. A reliable diagnosis can only be made by excluding pathological causes. Cessation of breastfeeding is unnecessary.
- Early-onset jaundice. It is thought that low fluid and calorie intake during colostrum production causes a slower intestinal transit time, which increases exposure to *betaglucuronidase*; this in turn adds more unconjugated bilirubin to the system.
- Prolonged jaundice occurs for unknown reasons in some healthy breastfed babies.

Exaggerated physiological jaundice in preterm babies

This is characterised by bilirubin levels of 165 μmol/l (10 mg/dl) or greater by day 3 or 4, with peak concentrations on days 5–7 that return to normal over several weeks. Preterm babies are more at risk of kernicterus. Contributing factors include:
- a delay in the expression of the enzyme UDP-GT
- shorter red cell life
- complications such as hypoxia, acidosis and hypothermia that can interfere with albumin-binding capacity.

Midwifery practice and physiological jaundice

It is important to distinguish between healthy babies with a normal physiological response who need no active treatment and those who require serum bilirubin testing. Transcutaneous bilirubinometry reduces the number of blood tests. Parents should be advised to report:

- excessive sleepiness
- reluctance to feed
- decrease in the number of wet nappies
- pale stools and yellow or orange urine.

Early, frequent feeding assists newborns to cope with an increased bilirubin load.

PATHOLOGICAL JAUNDICE

Pathological jaundice in newborns usually appears within 24 hours of birth, and is characterised by a *rapid rise* in serum bilirubin. Criteria are listed in Box 35.1.

Causes

The underlying aetiology of pathological jaundice is some type of interference with bilirubin production, transport, conjugation or excretion. Any disease or disorder that increases bilirubin production or that alters the transport or metabolism of bilirubin is superimposed upon normal physiological jaundice.

Production

Factors that increase haemoglobin destruction also increase bilirubin levels. Causes of increased haemolysis include:

- Rhesus anti-D, anti-A, anti-B and anti-Kell and ABO blood group incompatibility
- haemoglobinopathies – sickle cell disease and thalassaemia
- spherocytosis – fragile RBC membrane
- extravasated blood – cephalhaematoma and bruising
- sepsis – can lead to increased haemoglobin breakdown
- polycythaemia – blood contains too many red cells, as in maternofetal or twin-to-twin transfusion.

Box 35.1 Diagnosis of pathological jaundice

- Jaundice within the first 24 hours of life
- A rapid increase in total serum bilirubin >85 µmol/l (5 mg/dl) per day
- Total serum bilirubin >200 µmol/l (12 mg/dl)
- Conjugated (direct-reacting) bilirubin >25–35 µmol/l (1.5–2 mg/dl)
- Persistence of clinical jaundice for 7–10 days in term babies, or 2 weeks in preterm babies

Transport

Factors that lower blood albumin levels or decrease albumin-binding capacity include:

- hypothermia, acidosis or hypoxia (can interfere with albumin-binding capacity)
- drugs that compete with bilirubin for albumin-binding sites, e.g. aspirin, sulphonamides and ampicillin.

Conjugation

As well as immaturity of the neonate's enzyme system, other factors can interfere with bilirubin conjugation in the liver:

- Dehydration, starvation, hypoxia and sepsis (oxygen and glucose are required for conjugation).
- TORCH infections (toxoplasmosis, others, rubella, cytomegalovirus, herpes).
- Other viral infections, e.g. neonatal viral hepatitis.
- Other bacterial infections, particularly those caused by *Escherichia coli*.
- Metabolic and endocrine disorders that alter UDP-GT enzyme activity, e.g. Crigler–Najjar disease and Gilbert syndrome.
- Other metabolic disorders, such as hypothyroidism and galactosaemia.

Excretion

Factors that can interfere with bilirubin excretion include:

- hepatic obstruction caused by congenital anomalies
- obstruction from increased bile viscosity
- saturation of protein carriers needed to excrete conjugated bilirubin into the biliary system
- infection, other congenital disorders and idiopathic neonatal hepatitis (can also cause an excess of conjugated bilirubin).

HAEMOLYTIC JAUNDICE

Rhesus (RhD) isoimmunisation causes haemolytic disease of the newborn (HDN). Few antibodies to blood group antigens other than those in the Rh system cause severe HDN; fetal transfusion is unusual for multiple maternal antibody isoimmunisation without anti-D. ABO incompatibility is possibly the most frequent cause of mild to moderate haemolysis in neonates.

RHESUS D INCOMPATIBILITY

RhD incompatibility can occur when a woman with Rh-negative blood type is pregnant with a fetus with Rh-positive blood type.

- The placenta normally prevents fetal blood entering the maternal circulation. However, during pregnancy or birth, small amounts of fetal Rh-positive blood cross the placenta and enter the circulation of the mother, who has Rh-negative blood.

- The woman's immune system reacts by producing anti-D antibodies that cause sensitisation.
- In subsequent pregnancies these maternal antibodies can cross the placenta and destroy fetal erythrocytes.
- Usually, sensitisation occurs during the first pregnancy or birth, leading to extensive destruction of fetal red blood cells during subsequent pregnancies.

Rh isoimmunisation can result from any procedure or incident where maternal blood leaks across the placenta or from the inadvertent transfusion of Rh-positive blood to the woman.

Prevention of RhD isoimmunisation

This is by routine antenatal anti-D immunoglobulin (Ig) prophylaxis, within 72 hours of birth or after any other sensitising event. Anti-D Ig is a human plasma-based product that prevents the production of anti-D antibodies by the mother.

Administration of anti-D Ig

Anti-D Ig is administered to Rh-negative women who are pregnant with, or have given birth to, an Rh-positive baby. It destroys any fetal cells in the mother's blood before her immune system produces antibodies. The process for non-sensitised women is set out in Box 35.2.

Box 35.2 Administration of anti-D Ig to non-sensitised women

1. Women who are Rh-negative are screened for Rh antibodies (indirect Coombs' test). A negative test shows an *absence* of antibodies or sensitisation

2. Blood is retested at 28 weeks of pregnancy. In countries where antenatal prophylaxis is routine (at 28 and 34 weeks' gestation), the first injection of anti-D Ig is given just after this blood sample is taken

3. Where a policy of routine antenatal anti-D Ig prophylaxis is *not* in place, blood is retested for antibodies at 34 weeks of pregnancy

4. When anti-D Ig prophylaxis is given at 28 weeks, blood is not retested, as it is difficult to distinguish passive anti-D Ig from immune anti-D

5. Following the birth, cord blood is tested for confirmation of Rh type, ABO blood group, haemoglobin and serum bilirubin levels and the presence of maternal antibodies on fetal red cells (direct Coombs' test). Again, a negative test indicates an absence of antibodies or sensitisation. The postnatal dose of anti-D Ig is *still given* if passive anti-D Ig is present

6. A Kleihauer acid elution test is also carried out on an anticoagulated maternal blood sample immediately after birth to estimate the number of fetal cells in a sample of maternal blood

7. Anti-D Ig must always be given as soon as possible, and in any case within 72 hours of any sensitising event and the birth. Anti-D Ig is injected into the deltoid muscle, from which absorption is optimal

Dose of anti-D Ig

Research evidence for the optimal dose is still limited but the doses listed in Box 35.3 are recommended.

Ethical and legal issues

Anti-D Ig is a human plasma-based product. To give informed consent to its use, women need to know the possible consequences of treatment, as opposed to non-treatment, with anti-D Ig.

Management of RhD isoimmunisation

Effects of RhD isoimmunisation

- Destruction of fetal RBCs results in anaemia, possibly oedema and congestive cardiac failure.
- Fetal bilirubin levels also increase as more red cells are destroyed, with possible neurological damage as bilirubin is deposited in the brain.
- Lesser degrees of destruction result in haemolytic anaemia, while extensive haemolysis can cause hydrops fetalis and death in utero.

Antenatal monitoring and treatment of RhD isoimmunisation

Depending on the severity of Rh isoimmunisation, monitoring and treatment can include the following:

- Women who are Rh-negative are screened for Rh antibodies (indirect Coombs' test). A positive test indicates the *presence* of antibodies or sensitisation.
- RBCs obtained by chorionic villus sampling (using an immune rosette technique) can be Rh phenotyped as early as 9–11 weeks' gestation.
- Maternal blood is retested frequently to monitor any increase in antibody titres. Sudden and unexpected rises in serum anti-D levels can result in hydrops fetalis.

Box 35.3 Recommended dosages of anti-D Ig

- 500 IU anti-D Ig at 28 and 34 weeks' gestation for women in their first pregnancy
- At least 500 IU for all non-sensitised Rh-negative woman following the birth of a Rh-positive infant
- 250 IU following sensitising events *up to* 20 weeks' gestation
- At least 500 IU following sensitising events *after* 20 weeks' gestation
- Larger doses for traumatic events and procedures such as caesarean birth, stillbirths and intrauterine deaths, abdominal trauma during the third trimester, or manual removal of the placenta (dose calculated on 500 IU of anti-D Ig suppressing immunisation from 4 ml of RhD-positive red blood cells)
- Larger doses for any other instance of inadvertent transfusion of Rh-positive red blood cells, e.g. from an incorrect blood transfusion of Rh-positive blood platelets

- If antibody titres remain stable, ongoing monitoring is continued.
- If antibody titres increase, Doppler ultrasonography of the middle cerebral artery peak systolic velocity is used rather than amniocentesis to detect fetal anaemia.
- Changes in fetal serum bilirubin levels are observed.
- The fetus is closely monitored by ultrasonography for oedema and hepatosplenomegaly.
- Intravenous immunoglobulin (IVIG) has the potential to maintain the fetus until intrauterine fetal transfusion (IUT) can be performed. IVIG works by blocking Fc-mediated antibody transport across the placenta, blocking fetal red cell destruction and reducing maternal antibody levels.
- IUT can be used from about 20 weeks of gestation to reduce the effects of haemolysis until the fetus is capable of survival outside the uterus.
- Early delivery depends on the ongoing severity of the haemolysis and the condition of the fetus.

Postnatal treatment of RhD isoimmunisation

- Babies with mild to moderate haemolytic anaemia and hyperbilirubinaemia may require careful monitoring but less aggressive management.
- Babies with hydrops fetalis are pale and have oedema and ascites; alternatively, they may be stillborn.
- Management of surviving infants aims to prevent further haemolysis, reduce bilirubin levels, remove maternal Rh antibodies from the baby's circulation and combat anaemia.
- In some cases phototherapy can be effective but exchange transfusion is often required, and packed cell transfusion may be needed to increase Hb levels.
- Infants are at risk of ongoing haemolytic anaemia.

ABO INCOMPATIBILITY

ABO isoimmunisation usually occurs when the mother is blood group O and the baby is group A, or less often group B.

- Type A and B blood has a protein or antigen not present in type O blood.
- Individuals with type O blood develop antibodies throughout life from exposure to antigens in food, Gram-negative bacteria or blood transfusion, and by the first pregnancy may already have high serum anti-A and anti-B antibody titres.
- Some women produce IgG antibodies that can cross the placenta and attach to fetal red cells and destroy them.

First and subsequent babies are at risk; however, the destruction is usually much less severe than with Rh incompatibility. ABO incompatibility is also thought to protect the fetus from Rh incompatibility as the mother's anti-A and anti-B antibodies destroy any fetal cells that leak into the maternal circulation.

Treatment aims to:
- prevent further haemolysis
- reduce bilirubin levels
- combat any anaemia.

As with other causes of haemolysis, if babies require phototherapy it is usually commenced at a lower range of serum bilirubin levels (140–165 µmol/l or 8–10 mg/dl). Babies with a high serum bilirubin level may require exchange transfusion.

MANAGEMENT OF JAUNDICE

PHOTOTHERAPY

Phototherapy is used to prevent the concentration of unconjugated bilirubin in the blood from reaching levels where neurotoxicity may occur. The neonate's skin surface is exposed to high-intensity light, which photochemically converts fat-soluble unconjugated bilirubin into water-soluble bilirubin that can be excreted in bile and urine. Treatment may be intermittent or continuous, with phototherapy interrupted only for essential care.

Indications for phototherapy
The commencement of phototherapy is based on serum bilirubin levels and the individual condition of each baby, particularly when jaundice occurs within the first 12–24 hours.

Side-effects of phototherapy
- Hyperthermia, increased fluid loss and dehydration.
- Damage to the retina from the high-intensity light.
- Lethargy or irritability, decreased eagerness to feed, loose stools.
- Rashes and skin burns.
- Alterations in infant state and neurobehavioural organisation.
- Isolation and lack of usual sensory experiences, including visual deprivation.
- A decrease in calcium levels, leading to hypocalcaemia.
- Low platelet counts and increased red cell osmotic fragility.
- Bronze baby syndrome, riboflavin deficiency and DNA damage.

Care of the baby needing phototherapy
See Box 35.4.

EXCHANGE TRANSFUSION

Excess bilirubin is removed from the baby during a blood exchange transfusion. With HDN, sensitised erythrocytes are replaced with blood compatible with both the mother's and the infant's serum. With the exception of very premature babies and Rh incompatibility, exchange transfusion may now only be used when there is a risk of kernicterus.

Box 35.4 Care of the baby needing phototherapy

Temperature
- Maintain a warm thermoneutral environment
- Observe for hypothermia or hyperthermia

Eyes
- Protect with eye shields, ensuring they do not occlude the nose and are not tight

Skin
- Clean with warm water and observe frequently for rashes, dryness and excoriation
- Creams and lotions are not used

Hydration
- Fluid intake and stool and urine output are monitored

Neurobehavioural status
- Observe sleeping and waking states, feeding behaviours, responsiveness, response to stress, and interaction with parents and other carers

Calcium levels
- Hypocalcaemia may be indicated by jitteriness, irritability, rash, loose stools, fever, dehydration and convulsions

Bilirubin levels
- Levels are usually estimated daily

NEONATAL INFECTION

MODES OF ACQUIRING INFECTION

- Through the placenta (transplacental infection).
- From amniotic fluid.
- From their passage through the birth canal.
- From carers' hands, contaminated objects or droplet infection after birth.

VULNERABILITY TO INFECTION

Newborns are immunodeficient and prone to a higher incidence of infection. Preterm babies are even more vulnerable, as they have less well-developed defence mechanisms at birth (transfer of IgG mainly occurs after 32 weeks' gestation) and are more likely to experience invasive procedures. Full immunocompetence requires both innate (natural) and acquired immune responses.

At birth the baby has some immune protection from the mother but immunoglobulins are deficient. Maternal exposure and transfer of IgG across the placenta limit antibody levels. Breastfeeding increases the baby's immune protection through the transmission of secretory IgA in breast milk. During the early weeks of life the baby also has deficiencies in both the quantity and the quality of neutrophils.

MANAGEMENT OF INFECTION

Individual risk factors for infection

These include:

- a maternal history of prolonged rupture of membranes
- chorioamnionitis
- pyrexia during birth
- offensive amniotic fluid.

Physical assessment

This can include observation of:

- temperature instability
- lethargy or poor feeding, dehydration, starvation, hypothermia, acidosis or hypoxia
- bradycardia or tachycardia, and any apnoea
- urine and stool output and any vomiting
- central nervous system signs that require a complete neurodevelopmental examination.

Investigations

See Box 35.5.

Management

The overall aim of management is to provide prompt and effective treatment that reduces the risk of septicaemia and life-threatening septic shock. Good management includes:

- caring for the baby in a warm thermoneutral environment and observing for temperature instability
- good hydration and the correction of electrolyte imbalance, with demand feeding if possible and intravenous fluids as required

---

Box 35.5 Investigation of neonatal infection

- A complete blood cell count
- Testing of specimens of urine and meconium for specific organisms
- Swabs from the nose, throat and umbilicus, and from any rashes, pustules or vesicles to test for specific organisms
- Magnetic resonance imaging, computed tomography scans and chest X-rays
- A lumbar puncture to enable examination of cerebrospinal fluid (CSF)
- Testing of amniotic fluid, placental tissue and cord blood for specific organisms

- prompt systemic antibiotic or other drug therapy and local treatment of infection
- ongoing monitoring of the baby's neurobehavioural status
- reducing separation of mother and baby
- providing evidence-based information, support and reassurance to parents
- encouraging breastfeeding or expressing of milk, and informing women of the important role of breast milk in fighting infection.

INFECTIONS ACQUIRED BEFORE OR DURING BIRTH

The effects of sexually transmissible and reproductive tract infections are presented in Chapter 15. Others of importance to midwives are discussed below.

Toxoplasmosis

- Toxoplasmosis is caused by *Toxoplasma gondii*, a protozoan parasite found in uncooked meat and cat and dog faeces.
- Infected neonates may be asymptomatic at birth, but can later develop retinal and neurological disease. Maternal–fetal transmission results from poor hygiene.
- Those with subclinical disease at birth can develop seizures, significant cognitive and motor deficits and reduced cognitive function over time.

Varicella zoster

- Varicella zoster virus (VZV) is a highly contagious DNA virus of the herpes family, transmitted by respiratory droplets and contact with vesicle fluid; it causes varicella (chickenpox).
- It has an incubation period of 10–20 days and is infectious for 48 hours before the rash appears until vesicles crust over.

Incidence and effects during pregnancy

Maternal deaths have been associated with varicella infection during pregnancy. Fetal sequelae from primary maternal infection vary with the length of gestation at the time of the infection (Box 35.6).

Rubella

For most immunocompetent children and adults (including pregnant women), the rubella virus causes a mild and insignificant illness that is spread by droplet infection.

Incidence and effects during pregnancy

If primary rubella infection occurs during the first 12 weeks of pregnancy, maternal–fetal transmission rates are high. First-trimester infection can have the results listed in Box 35.7.

Babies with congenital rubella are highly infectious and should be isolated from other infants and pregnant women (but not from their own mothers). Babies should always be followed up for several years, as some problems may not become apparent until they are older.

Box 35.6 Fetal sequelae of maternal infection with varicella zoster

Maternal infection during the first 20 weeks of pregnancy

- 2% risk of fetal varicella syndrome (FVS)
- Symptoms can include skin lesions and scarring in a dermatomal distribution, eye problems such as chorioretinitis and cataracts, and skeletal anomalies, in particular limb hypoplasia
- Severe neurological problems may include encephalitis, microcephaly and significant developmental delay
- About 30% of babies born with skin lesions die in the first months of life

Maternal chickenpox from 20 weeks' gestation up to almost the time of birth (at least)

- A milder form of neonatal varicella that does not result in negative sequelae for the neonate

Maternal infection after 36 weeks and particularly in the week before the birth to 2 days after

- Infection rates of up to 50%
- About 25% of those infected will develop neonatal clinical varicella (or varicella infection of the newborn)
- Newborns are also at risk of contracting varicella from mothers or siblings in the postnatal period
- Most affected babies will develop a vesicular rash and about 30% will die
- Other complications of neonatal varicella include clinical sepsis, pneumonia, pyoderma and hepatitis

Box 35.7 Sequelae of first-trimester infection with rubella

- Spontaneous abortion
- Cataracts
- Sensorineural deafness
- Congenital heart defects
- Microcephaly
- Meningoencephalitis
- Dermal erythropoiesis
- Thrombocytopenia
- Significant developmental delay

Ophthalmia neonatorum

Ophthalmia neonatorum is a notifiable condition. It involves a purulent discharge from the eyes of an infant within 21 days of birth. The condition is usually acquired during vaginal birth and causative organisms include:

- *Staphylococcus aureus*
- *Streptococcus pneumoniae*

- *Haemophilus influenzae*
- *Escherichia coli*
- *Klebsiella*
- *Pseudomonas*
- *Chlamydia trachomatis*
- *Neisseria gonorrhoeae*

A swab must be taken for culture and sensitivity testing, and a doctor notified immediately. Chlamydial and gonococcal infections can cause:

- conjunctival scarring
- corneal infiltration
- blindness
- systemic spread.

Treatment includes:

- local cleaning and care of the eyes with normal saline
- appropriate drug therapy for the baby and also the mother if required.

Candida

- Candida is a Gram-positive yeast fungus that has a number of strains, including *C. albicans*, *C. parapsilosis*, *C. tropicalis* and *C. lusitaniae*.
- *C. albicans* is responsible for most fungal infections, including thrush in infants.
- Infection can affect the mouth (oral candidiasis), skin (cutaneous candidiasis) and other organs (systemic candidiasis).

SOME INFECTIONS ACQUIRED AFTER BIRTH

Eye infections

Mild eye infections are common in babies and can be treated with routine eye care and antibiotics if required. Other more serious conditions must be excluded.

Skin infections

Most neonatal skin infections are caused by *Staph. aureus*. In newborn infants the most likely skin lesions are septic spots or pustules, found either as a solitary lesion or clustered in the umbilical and buttock areas.

- For the well neonate with limited pustules, management includes regular cleansing with an antiseptic solution.
- Antibiotic therapy is given for more extensive pustules.

Meningitis

Neonatal meningitis is an inflammation of the membranes lining the brain and spinal column caused by organisms such as:

- *E. coli*
- group B streptococci
- *Listeria monocytogenes*
- (more unusually) *Candida* and herpes.

Very early signs may be non-specific, followed by those of meningeal irritation and raised intracranial pressure, such as:

- irritability
- bulging fontanelle
- increasing lethargy
- crying
- tremors
- twitching
- severe vomiting
- alterations in consciousness
- diminished muscle tone.

Diagnosis is usually confirmed by examination of CSF. Very ill babies will require intensive care, intravenous fluids and antibiotic therapy. Long-term neurological complications can occur in surviving infants.

Respiratory infections

These may be minor (nasopharyngitis and rhinitis) or more severe (pneumonia).

Gastrointestinal tract infections

In the newborn these can include gastroenteritis or the more severe necrotising enterocolitis. Causative organisms for gastroenteritis include:

- rotavirus
- *Salmonella*
- *Shigella*
- a pathogenic strain of *E. coli*.

The secretory IgA in breast milk offers important protection against these organisms, particularly rotavirus. The correction of fluid and electrolyte imbalance is an urgent priority.

Umbilical infection

Signs can include localised inflammation and an offensive discharge. Untreated infection can spread to the liver via the umbilical vein and cause hepatitis and septicaemia. Treatment may include:

- regular cleansing
- the administration of an antibiotic powder
- appropriate antibiotic therapy.

Urinary tract infections

Urinary tract infections can result from bacteria such as *E. coli*, or less often from a congenital anomaly that obstructs urine flow. The signs are usually those of an early non-specific infection. Diagnosis is usually confirmed through laboratory evaluation of a urine sample.

CHAPTER 36

Metabolic Disturbances, Inborn Errors of Metabolism, Endocrine Disorders and Drug Withdrawal

METABOLIC DISTURBANCES

GLUCOSE HOMEOSTASIS

Following birth there is a fall in glucose concentration. At the same time endocrine changes (decrease in insulin and a surge of catecholamines and release of glucagon) result in an increase in:

- glycogenolysis (breakdown of glycogen stores to provide glucose)
- gluconeogenesis (glucose production from the liver)
- ketogenesis (producing ketones, an alternative fuel)
- lipolysis (release of fatty acids from adipose), bringing about an increase in glucose and other metabolic fuel.

Problems arise in the newborn:

- when there is a lack of glycogen stores to mobilise (preterm and growth-restricted infants), *or*
- when there is excessive insulin production (infants of diabetic mothers), *or*
- when infants are sick and have a poor supply of energy and increased requirements.

Hypoglycaemia

The definition of hypoglycaemia is controversial. Currently a cut-off value in the newborn is 2.6 mmol/l. Signs of hypoglycaemia are listed in Box 36.1.

Box 36.1 Signs of hypoglycaemia

- Lethargy
- Poor feeding
- Seizures
- Decreased consciousness level
- Jitteriness (although this is common in the newborn and on its own is not indicative)

Infants at risk of neurological sequelae of hypoglycaemia

- Preterm babies (of less than 37 weeks).
- Growth-restricted babies (less than third centile for gestation).
- Babies of diabetic mothers.
- Sick term babies, e.g. septic or following perinatal hypoxia–ischaemia.
- Babies with inborn errors of metabolism.

Diagnosis, prevention and treatment of hypoglycaemia

Healthy term babies tolerate low blood glucose concentrations by using alternative fuels such as ketone bodies, lactate or fatty acids. Breastfed babies are a group who are particularly likely to have low blood glucose concentrations, probably because of the low energy content of breast milk in the first few postnatal days. Because of their ability to compensate, clinically well, appropriately grown term babies who are feeding do not require monitoring of their glucose concentration. Doing so would result in many infants being inappropriately treated.

Babies at risk of neurological sequelae should be monitored and hypoglycaemia prevented by:

- adequate temperature control – keep the babies warm
- early feeding (within 1 hour of birth) with 100 ml/kg/day if formula feeding
- frequent feeding (3 hourly or less)
- blood glucose check immediately before the second feed and then 4–6 hourly.

As long as there are no symptoms, there is no advantage to checking the blood glucose concentration earlier than this, as it is likely to be low and the appropriate treatment at that stage is to feed the baby. If there are symptoms, the glucose should be checked and treatment given immediately. Breastfed babies are particularly difficult in this situation because it is important to avoid supplemental feeding with formula to promote successful breastfeeding; the risks associated with significant hypoglycaemia in at-risk infants outweigh this consideration.

- If the blood glucose concentration is <2.6 mmol/l, then feed should be given at an increased volume and decreased frequency (2 hourly or even hourly). This may require supplementary feeding with formula milk in infants who are breastfed, and/or nasogastric tube (NGT) feeding. Breast milk can also be expressed to be given via an NGT.

- If the blood glucose concentration remains low despite these measures and there is an adequate feed volume intake then intravenous treatment with dextrose is required. It is important in this situation that enteral feeding is continued, as feed contains much more energy than 10% glucose and promotes ketone body production and metabolic adaptation.
- If the blood glucose concentration is >2.6 mmol/l before the second and the third feed, then glucose monitoring can be discontinued but feeding should continue at 3-hourly intervals.
- In infants where enteral feeding is contraindicated for some reason, then intravenous 10% dextrose at least 60 ml/kg/day should commence.

Hyperglycaemia

Hyperglycaemia occurs predominantly in preterm and severely growth-restricted babies. It is also seen in term infants in response to stress, especially following perinatal hypoxia. In general, no treatment is required.

ELECTROLYTE IMBALANCES IN THE NEWBORN

Postnatal weight loss, fluid and electrolyte changes

All babies lose weight due to a loss of extracellular fluid. Weighing in the first few days is only needed when babies are unwell or if there are concerns about intake and fluid and electrolyte balance.

Sodium

Sodium is normally excreted via the kidney, controlled by the renin–angiotensin system. This control mechanism is functional in the preterm infant but loss of sodium may occur because of renal tubule unresponsiveness. Term breast milk has relatively little sodium (<1 mmol/kg/day), showing that the normal newborn can preserve sodium via the kidney in order to maintain growth. Normal sodium requirements are 1–2 mmol/kg/day in term infants and 3–4 mmol/kg/day in preterm infants.

The normal serum sodium concentration is 133–146 mmol/l. Changes in serum sodium reflect changes in sodium and water balance. In order to assess changes in sodium concentration it is important to know an infant's weight.

Hyponatraemia

Hyponatraemia is due to either fluid overload or sodium depletion.
- Hyponatraemia in the presence of weight gain represents fluid overload.
- A low sodium with inappropriate weight loss represents sodium depletion. The latter may be due to inadequate intake or excessive losses.

Hypernatraemia

- Hypernatraemia in the presence of a loss of weight suggests dehydration.
- When there is weight gain, hypernatraemia is due to fluid and sodium overload.

Potassium

Potassium is the major intracellular cation. Abnormalities in serum potassium concentration can cause significant arrhythmias. Potassium concentrations can be severely affected by measurement technique and any haemolysis of the blood sample, especially from capillary sampling, is likely to lead to a falsely high value.

Calcium

Calcium metabolism is closely linked to phosphate metabolism. Preterm infants need much higher concentrations of phosphate and calcium. These are given as intravenous supplements, by supplementing breast milk with fortifier or by giving specific preterm milk.

High serum calcium concentrations are unusual but there are rare, important causes of low serum calcium. The normal serum concentration is 2.2–2.7 mmol/l but this must be interpreted with the serum albumin concentration, as serum calcium is bound to albumin; therefore a low albumin concentration will lead to a falsely low serum value.

Calcium concentrations fall within 18–24 hours of birth as the infant's supply of placental calcium ceases, but accretion into bone continues.

INBORN ERRORS OF METABOLISM

Inborn errors of metabolism (IEM) are rare inherited disorders occurring in approximately 1 in 5000 births. They result mainly from enzyme deficiencies in metabolic pathways leading to an accumulation of substrate, which in turn causes toxicity. Early diagnosis and institution of therapy can reduce morbidity. It has been estimated that 20% of infants presenting with sepsis in the absence of risk factors have an IEM.

Inheritance is usually autosomal recessive and the following factors should be explored:
- Affected sibling.
- Previous stillbirth/neonatal death.
- Parental consanguinity.
- Symptoms associated with feeding, fasting or a surgical procedure.
- Improvement when feeds stopped and relapse on restarting.

Clinical examination, however, is usually normal. The features in Box 36.2 indicate that an underlying IEM should be seriously considered.
- Principles of emergency management are to reduce load on affected pathways by removing toxic metabolites and stimulating residual enzyme activity.
- Hypoglycaemia is corrected, adequate ventilatory support and hydration are maintained, convulsions are treated and significant metabolic acidosis is treated with intravenous sodium bicarbonate, and electrolyte abnormalities are corrected.
- Antibiotics are frequently given, as infection may have precipitated metabolic decompensation; dialysis may be required.

Box 36.2 Clinical features of inborn errors of metabolism

- Septicaemia
- Jaundice/liver disease
- Hypoglycaemia
- Severe hypotonia
- Metabolic acidosis
- Unusual body odour
- Convulsions
- Dysmorphic features
- Coma
- Abnormal hair
- Cataracts
- Hydrops fetalis
- Cardiomegaly
- Diarrhoea

PHENYLKETONURIA (PKU)

- An autosomal recessive disorder (1 in 10 000 incidence in the UK).
- Caused by absence or reduction of an enzyme in the liver that converts phenylalanine to tyrosine (phenylalanine hydroxylase).
- Babies are well at birth but begin to be affected during the first few weeks.
- Diagnosed by blood test, 5–8 days after birth, commonly collected on the Neonatal Screening Test Card.
- Untreated, PKU leads to severe mental disability (IQ <30) due to build-up of phenylpyruvic acid.
- It is treated by a diet specifically restricted in phenylalanine. Affected women need to return to a strict diet in pregnancy.

GALACTOSAEMIA

- An autosomal recessive disorder (incidence of 1 in 60 000).
- Caused by an absence or severe deficiency of the enzyme galactose-1-phosphate uridyltransferase (Gal-1-PUT) that converts galactose to glucose.
- As milk's main sugar, lactose, contains glucose and galactose, babies with this condition rapidly become affected.
- Build-up of galactose-1-phosphate is harmful and can quickly cause cataracts and brain injury.
- It is treated with lactose-free formula.

Diagnosis

- Signs of liver failure and renal impairment.
- Considered if babies have unresponsive hypoglycaemia and prolonged/severe jaundice.
- Urine-reducing substances (i.e. galactose) are present but the urine test for glucose is negative.
- Assay is made of the enzyme level (Gal-1-PUT) within red blood cells.

ENDOCRINE DISEASE IN THE NEWBORN

THYROID DISORDERS

The thyroid gland hormones have an effect on the metabolic rate in most tissues. They are also essential for normal neurological development. Thyroid-stimulating hormone (TSH) is produced by the anterior pituitary gland and this stimulates production of T3 and T4 by the thyroid gland with a feedback mechanism to the anterior pituitary.

Hypothyroidism

- Abnormalities in gland formation, defects in hormone synthesis and rarely secondary pituitary causes.
- Babies tend to be large and to have a large posterior fontanelle, coarse features and often an umbilical hernia.
- Untreated babies develop impaired motor development, growth failure, a low IQ, impaired hearing and language problems.
- Screening is by measuring TSH (high) on a blood spot taken along with the screening test for PKU at 5–8 days of age.
- Screening does not detect pituitary causes, as they have a low TSH.

Hyperthyroidism

- Rare and due to maternal Graves' disease.
- Can lead to preterm labour, low birth weight, stillbirth and fetal death.
- Symptoms are uncommon and may be present at birth or delayed till 4–6 weeks.
- Symptoms include irritability, jitteriness, tachycardia, prominent eyes, sweating, excessive appetite and weight loss.
- Babies with symptoms are treated with antithyroid medication.

ADRENAL DISORDERS

The adrenal cortex produces three groups of hormones – glucocorticoids, mineralocorticoids and sex hormones. Glucocorticoids regulate the general metabolism of carbohydrates, proteins and fats on a long-term basis and modify metabolism in times of stress. Mineralocorticoids regulate sodium, potassium and water balance. The sex hormones are responsible for normal development of the genitalia and reproductive organs.

Adrenocortical insufficiency

- Causes are congenital hypoplasia, adrenal haemorrhage, enzyme defects and can be secondary to pituitary problems.
- Diagnosis rests on symptomatic hypoglycaemia, poor feeding, vomiting, poor weight gain and prolonged jaundice.
- Babies may have hyponatraemia, hypoglycaemia, hyperkalaemia and acidosis.
- Treatment is by intravenous therapy with glucose and electrolytes; replacement of corticosteroid and mineralocorticoid hormones is then required.

Adrenocortical hyperfunction

This may occur in the form of congenital adrenal hyperplasia due to deficiency of the enzymes responsible for hormone production within the adrenal gland. The most common enzyme deficiency results in an excess of androgenic hormones, but a deficiency of glucocorticoid and mineralocorticoids often also occurs. These disorders can cause ambiguous genitalia (virilisation of females or inadequate virilisation of males) and symptoms of adrenal insufficiency (vomiting, diarrhoea, vascular collapse, hypoglycaemia and hyponatraemia, hyperkalaemia).

Treatment is by replacement of glucocorticoid and mineralocorticoid hormones. Virilised girls may also require surgical intervention to correct the genital abnormalities.

PITUITARY DISORDERS

Pituitary insufficiency is rare. It may occur in association with other abnormalities, particularly midline developmental defects. Presentation is with signs of glucocorticoid deficiency (hypoglycaemia), prolonged jaundice or signs of hypothyroidism. Growth hormone deficiency generally causes hypoglycaemia but no other signs in the newborn. Treatment is with replacement of the missing hormones.

PARATHYROID DISORDERS

The parathyroid glands are responsible for control of calcium metabolism, but abnormalities of the parathyroids are rare causes of hypocalcaemia or hypercalcaemia in the newborn. When hypoparathyroidism does occur it may be familial or may occur in association with deletions of chromosome 22 (22q11 deletion or DiGeorge syndrome).

EFFECTS OF MATERNAL DRUG ABUSE/USE DURING PREGNANCY ON THE NEWBORN

Opiates and other drugs cross the placenta. Withdrawal may be manifested before birth.

WITHDRAWAL SYMPTOMS

Each drug has a different half-life and this leads to different patterns of withdrawal symptoms. In general, methadone produces symptoms for longer periods than heroin, but benzodiazepines may also contribute to this.

The symptoms most frequently seen are listed in Box 36.3. Infants assessed for signs of drug withdrawal using a scoring system are less likely to be inappropriately treated and may have a shorter hospital stay. It is important not to overtreat infants with drugs but babies who are withdrawing may appear to be in discomfort that needs to be relieved. The long-term effects of withdrawal symptoms are also unclear. The most useful sign is whether infants settle and sleep between feeding. If they do, then pharmacological treatment may be unnecessary.

TREATMENT

Breastfeeding can be encouraged, as long as there is no evidence of HIV or ongoing drug use that precludes this (cocaine, heroin). This includes methadone, as long as the dose is less than 20 mg/day.

- A quiet environment with reduced light and noise is helpful in keeping stimuli to a minimum.
- Swaddling is useful.
- Feeds may need to be given frequently. These infants will often take large volumes of milk; this is acceptable as long as vomiting is not a problem.
- Rocking and cradling are also useful adjuncts to treatment.

Pharmacological treatment

The two most commonly used treatments are:
- oral methadone
- oral morphine.

These appear to control withdrawal seizures much more effectively. They can be given in increasing doses if necessary until symptoms are controlled and then the dose may gradually be reduced.

Box 36.3 Common symptoms of drug withdrawal

- Jitteriness, irritability and constant high-pitched crying
- Often, failure to settle between feeds
- Hyperactivity
- Often, voracious feeding, although some infants have poor sucking
- Vomiting (common)
- Diarrhoea and an irritant nappy rash (common)
- Sneezing and yawning
- Episodes of high temperature in the absence of infection
- In rare circumstances, seizures

If feeding and settling do not improve or profuse watery stools and profuse vomiting continue, other treatment needs to be considered. Alternative medication may sometimes be useful: for example, clonazepam for benzodiazepine use or chloral hydrate as a general sedative.

COCAINE

The effects of cocaine on the newborn are different. It can produce significant withdrawal symptoms but these are often less severe and less troublesome than with other drugs. However, it is associated with many other harmful effects on the fetus (Box 36.4).

Box 36.4 Some harmful effects of cocaine

- Significant fetal growth restriction
- Brain injury due to haemorrhage or infarction
- Abnormalities of brain development
- Limb reduction defects
- Gut atresias
- Small head size and developmental scores

Section 6

Supporting Safe Practice

CHAPTER 37

Supervision of Midwives

The principal function of Supervisors of Midwives is the protection of the public, but the main ethos is support for midwives. Midwives have to notify their intention to practise midwifery each year to the Local Supervising Authority (LSA), and each LSA office maintains a database of all midwives practising within the LSA area. Information from the notifications of intention to practise is added to the details of registration on the Nursing and Midwifery Council (NMC) register.

A Supervisor of Midwives is an experienced practising midwife who has completed an approved programme of preparation and is appointed by the LSA. See Box 37.1 for the activities of a Supervisor of Midwives.

There is always a Supervisor of Midwives on call at any time who can be contacted if there are any practice concerns or if there has been a critical incident.

Box 37.1 Activities of a Supervisor of Midwives

- Supporting best practice and ensuring evidence-based midwifery care
- Being a confident advocate for midwives and mothers
- Acting as an effective agent for change
- Providing leadership and guidance
- Acting as a role model
- Undertaking the role of mentor
- Empowering women and midwives
- Facilitating a supportive partnership with midwives
- Supporting midwives through dilemmas
- Assisting midwives with their personal and professional development
- Facilitating midwives' reflection on critical incidents
- Supporting midwives through supervised practice
- Maintaining an awareness of local, regional and national NHS issues
- Giving advice on ethical issues
- Liaising with clinicians, management and education
- Maintaining records of all supervisory activities
- Investigating allegations of suboptimal care or misconduct
- Accountable to the LSA Midwifery Officer for all supervisory activities.

LOCAL SUPERVISING AUTHORITIES

The LSA has no management responsibility to NHS providers, but it acts as a focus for issues relating to midwifery practice. Its strength lies in its influence on quality in local midwifery services. All LSA officers have to be aware of the wider NHS picture and contemporary issues.

A practising midwife with experience as a Supervisor of Midwives performs the LSA 'Midwifery Officer' role in every LSA.

The duties of the LSA Midwifery Officer are detailed in Box 37.2.

Box 37.2 Duties of the LSA Midwifery Officer

- Provides advice and guidance to Supervisors of Midwives (SoMs)
- Provides a framework of support for supervisory and midwifery practice
- Selects and appoints SoMs and deselects if ever necessary
- Provides education and training for prospective SoMs
- Provides continuing education and training for SoMs
- Ensures appropriate ratios (normally 1:15) of midwives to SoMs in each provider
- Provides advice on midwifery matters to health authorities
- Manages communications within supervisory systems
- Investigates cases of alleged misconduct
- Receives reports of maternal deaths
- Leads the development of standards and audit of supervision
- Determines whether to suspend a midwife from practice, in accordance with the Nursing and Midwifery Council's Midwives Rules and Standards
- Prepares an annual report of supervisory activities within the report year, including audit outcomes and emerging trends affecting maternity services for Health Authorities and providers
- Maintains a list of current supervisors
- Provides a formal link between midwives, their supervisors and the NMC
- Implements the NMC's rules and standards for supervision of midwives
- Ensures midwives meet the statutory requirements for practice
- Works in partnership with other agencies and promotes partnership working with women
- Publishes details of how to contact supervisors
- Publishes details of how the practice of midwives will be supervised
- Receives notifications of intention to practise
- Operates a system that ensures midwives meet statutory requirements for practice
- Conducts regular meetings for supervisors to develop key areas of practice
- Facilitates interprovider activities, such as provision of cover by SoMs from other NHS providers
- Conducts investigations and initiates legal action in cases of practice by persons not qualified to do so under the Nursing and Midwifery Order 2001

CHAPTER 38

Complementary Therapies and Maternity Care

Women may request the presence of a complementary and alternative medicine (CAM) practitioner at the birth. They should ensure that the therapist has a thorough understanding of pregnancy physiopathology, the conventional maternity services and has personal professional indemnity insurance cover.

When a midwife wishes to incorporate some aspect of complementary medicine within her own practice, she must continue to work within the parameters laid down by the Nursing and Midwifery Council (UK).

ACUPUNCTURE

Acupuncture is based on the principle that the body has Qi or 'energy' lines, called meridians, flowing through it from top to hand or toe. Most of these pass through a major organ, after which the meridian is named. There are 12 major meridians, and 365 points on these in total. These points can be stimulated to release and rebalance the energies, either by the insertion of acupuncture needles or by other means. Sometimes thumb pressure is applied to the points (called acupressure, or the similar practice of *shiatsu*, the Japanese equivalent); on other occasions, heat is applied via moxa sticks (e.g. moxibustion for breech presentation). Alternatively, suction can be used if the points are covered with special cups (cupping). Acupuncture needles may also be stimulated by mild electric pulsations; this is similar to transcutaneous nerve stimulation, which is used for pain relief in labour.

Certain acupuncture points are contraindicated during pregnancy as they may trigger contractions. Some antenatal conditions respond well to acupuncture or acupressure, including many of the physiological symptoms of pregnancy. In labour, acupuncture may facilitate progress and ease pain, anxiety and tension.

HOMEOPATHY

Homeopathy uses minute, highly diluted doses of substances that, if given in the full dose, would actually cause the symptoms being treated. Most homeopathic medicines are in tablet form but they do not work pharmacologically and will not interact with prescribed drugs, although certain drugs may inactivate the homeopathic tablet. Homeopathy is not, however, completely harmless.

Only one remedy should normally be taken at a time. Studies into the use of arnica (arnica montana) have been inconclusive but it has been found to be useful in postnatal trauma management.

HERBAL MEDICINE

There is a common misconception that just because herbal remedies are natural they are automatically safe. There are many herbal remedies that should be avoided during pregnancy or breastfeeding because they may induce uterine bleeding or miscarriage, or have other systemic effects on the mother or fetus. Popular herbal remedies such as St John's wort and raspberry leaf tea should be used with caution.

AROMATHERAPY

Aromatherapy is the use of highly concentrated essential oils extracted from plants. Essential oils enter the body by a variety of means, depending on the method of administration. The most frequently used modes of entry are via the skin, usually as massage, and also in the bath or in compresses or creams, via the mucous membranes in pessaries or suppositories and via the respiratory tract in inhalations and vaporisers. All essential oils act in the same way as pharmaceutical drugs, being absorbed, metabolised and excreted via the same pathways; they are therefore likely to interact with prescribed medications.

Safety (see Box 38.1)

Essential oils can be very therapeutic when used appropriately, but also have the potential to be toxic if incorrectly administered or abused. There are many oils that should be avoided during pregnancy, although some may be used in labour.

Box 38.1 'Rules' for the correct administration of essential oils during pregnancy and childbirth

The person administering the essential oil must be adequately and appropriately trained and aware of:
- uses and effects
- precautions and contraindications
- possible complications and side-effects

The correct essential oil should be prescribed and administered:
- to the correct person
- at the correct time
- in the correct dose
- by the correct route
- in the correct frequency
- with an accurate and contemporaneous record in the notes

OSTEOPATHY AND CHIROPRACTIC

Both forms of treatment involve rebalancing of the neuromusculoskeletal system. Disorders, trauma or alterations in the body structure can cause imbalances in the whole system, which in turn can lead to a predisposition to other conditions. Osteopaths are concerned with mobility of joints, whereas chiropractors deal with relative positions of joints. Different manipulative techniques are used and most chiropractors use more X-rays to aid diagnosis (although not for pregnant women). Osteopaths also use more soft tissue massage prior to manipulation.

Craniosacral therapy, or cranial osteopathy, uses gentle manipulation of the bones of the skull, meningeal membranes and nerve endings in the scalp. It has been found to be useful for infants with colic.

REFLEXOLOGY

Reflexology, or reflex zone therapy, involves a precise manipulation of the feet, which are thought to represent a map of the whole body. Every part of the body is reflected on one or both feet and therefore if specific parts of the feet are worked on, other areas of the body can be treated. Reflexology is a powerful therapy that can be very effective when used appropriately, although there are some contraindications, precautions and possible complications of treatment. Reflexology can also be performed on the hands, as well as the tongue, face and back. It is widely thought to work along the meridians used in acupuncture.

Drugs (Medicines)

Class of drug	Drug	Use and risk/contraindications
Anaesthetic	Lidocaine hydrochloride	Local anaesthetic used for perineal infiltration and nerve blocks
	Bupivicaine hydrochloride	Epidural and spinal anaesthesia Contraindicated in hypovolaemia and local sepsis
Analgesia	Non-steroidal anti-inflammatory drugs (NSAIDs) (e.g. ibuprofen, indometacin, voltarol)	Relatively safe in the first trimester but have the potential to cause fetal renal dysfunction, premature closure of the ductus arteriosus, necrotising enterocolitis and intracerebral haemorrhage Safe in breastfeeding
	Opiate analgesics (e.g. pethidine, morphine, diamorphine, codeine, dihydrocodeine)	With long-term use there is a risk of neonatal withdrawal after birth Risk of respiratory depression with large doses in labour
	Paracetamol	Recommended first-line analgesic agent in pregnancy Overdose can be potentially lethal to the mother and/or fetus
	Aspirin	Risk of maternal, fetal and neonatal bleeding with analgesic dose (e.g. 600 mg every 6 hours); therefore contraindicated in pregnancy Low-dose (75 mg daily) aspirin is used for treatment of recurrent miscarriage, thrombophilias (inherited risk of thromboembolism) and prevention of pre-eclampsia and intrauterine growth restriction Causes antiplatelet effect for around 10 days after administration and may prolong the bleeding time; therefore may be discontinued 3–4 weeks prior to expected birth
Antacid drugs	Ranitidine	To reduce the acidity of stomach acid in high-risk labours and prior to caesarean section or general anaesthetic

Class of drug	Drug	Use and risk/contraindications
Antibiotics		To treat infection Caution should be exercised with some drugs during pregnancy
	Aminoglycosides (e.g. gentamicin, netilmicin)	Risk of ototoxicity but often used in serious maternal infection where benefit outweighs risk
	Chloramphenicol	Risk of 'grey baby syndrome' when used in second and third trimesters
	Erythromycin	Used if woman is penicillin sensitive Enhances effect of anticoagulants
	Metronidazole	Used to treat or prevent anaerobic infection Avoid large single doses when breastfeeding
	Nitrofurantoin	Risk of haemolysis in fetus at term – avoid during labour and delivery but safe at other times
	Penicillins	Not known to be harmful, trace amounts in breast milk
	Quinolones (e.g. ciprofloxacin, ofloxacin)	Risk of arthropathy in fetus – most of the evidence for this obtained from animal studies
	Tetracyclines (e.g. tetracycline, oxytetracycline, doxycycline)	Risk of discolouration and dysplasia of fetal bones and teeth, cataracts when used in second and third trimesters
Anticoagulants		History of a previous thromboembolic problem, an acute event, a known thrombophilia or heart valve replacement
	Heparin	Heparin does not cross the placenta and is not excreted into breast milk Given intravenously or subcutaneously Effectiveness is monitored by measuring the activated partial thromboplastin time (APTT) Side effects include bleeding and bruising at the injection site, heparin-induced thrombocytopenia
	Low molecular weight (LMW) preparations (e.g. enoxaparin, dalteparin, tinzaparin)	Have a more predictable anticoagulant response and are usually given by once-daily subcutaneous injection

Continued

Class of drug	Drug	Use and risk/contraindications
	Warfarin	Women on warfarin should be converted to heparin as soon as they become pregnant and will continue on heparin throughout pregnancy Considered safe in breastfeeding The dose required is very variable and is judged by monitoring the INR (international normalised ratio) in the blood
Anticonvulsants	**Carbamazepine Oxcarbazepine Phenytoin Valproate**	Increased risk of teratogenicity, particularly neural tube defects (NTDs) Benefits of treatment should outweigh risks Folic acid 5 mg should be taken daily Risk of neonatal bleeding; prophylactic vitamin K is recommended for mother before birth in addition to the neonatal dose Small amounts in breast milk
	Magnesium sulphate	Treatment of eclampsia Can be given intramuscularly or intravenously Care should be taken to avoid magnesium toxicity; clinical signs are loss of the patellar reflexes, a feeling of flushing, somnolence, slurred speech, respiratory difficulty and, in extreme cases, cardiac arrest The 'antidote' to magnesium sulphate is calcium gluconate
Antiemetics		Non-pharmacological therapies should be tried first
	Metoclopramide	Not known to be harmful but use with caution in pregnancy and breastfeeding
Antihypertensive drugs		Pre-existing hypertension, pregnancy-induced hypertension or pre-eclampsia
	ACE inhibitors (e.g. captopril, enalapril, lisinopril)	Contraindicated in pregnancy
	Beta-blockers (e.g. propranolol, atenolol, labetalol)	May cause intrauterine growth restriction, neonatal hypoglycaemia and bradycardia Considered safe in breastfeeding Contraindicated in women with asthma

Class of drug	Drug	Use and risk/contraindications
	Calcium channel blockers (e.g. nifedipine, nicardipine)	Risk of serious hypotensive reactions, especially in association with magnesium sulphate Slow-release formulations should be used Risk of headache Small amounts in breast milk; avoidance recommended
	Hydralazine	Given by slow bolus injection or by infusion Avoid before third trimester Considered safe in breastfeeding
	Methyldopa	Given in 2–4 divided doses from a starting dose of 250 mg three times daily, up to a total of 3 g daily Considered safe in pregnancy and breastfeeding
Bronchodilators		To treat or prevent an asthma attack
	Inhaled bronchodilators (e.g. salbutamol, salmeterol, ipratropium), **inhaled cromoglicate, inhaled and oral corticosteroids and theophyllines**	Are all considered safe
Corticosteroids	**Prednisolone**	Pre-existing maternal disease such as asthma, rheumatoid arthritis and other inflammatory diseases Crosses the placenta in relatively small quantities; is considered safe for use in pregnancy Women who are on long-term steroid treatment should receive extra corticosteroids in labour, usually given as intravenous hydrocortisone
	Betamethasone and dexamethasone	Fetal lung maturation in actual or threatened preterm delivery Are generally given as intramuscular injections in divided doses over 24–48 hours; the most significant effect is noticed if 48 hours have elapsed between administration of the drug and birth
Diuretics	e.g. furosemide, bendroflumethiazide	Contraindicated in pregnancy

Continued

Class of drug	Drug	Use and risk/contraindications
Drugs for diabetes mellitus		Glycaemic control
	Bovine insulin Metformin Sulphonylureas (oral hypoglycaemic agents) (e.g. glibenclamide, gliclazide)	Avoid in pregnancy
	Synthetic human insulins or pork-derived insulins	May be used in pregnancy
Folic acid		To reduce the risk of NTDs Recommended dose 400 µg daily Women at risk of NTDs and those taking antiepileptic drugs, 5 mg daily
Hypnotics	Benzodiazepines (e.g. temazepam)	Avoid regular use during pregnancy and breastfeeding
Iron preparations		To treat iron deficiency anaemia
	Oral iron (e.g. ferrous gluconate or ferrous sulphate)	May cause gastrointestinal disturbance – constipation, diarrhoea, indigestion, black stools
	Parenteral preparations	Avoid in first trimester
Laxatives	e.g. Lactulose, senna	Considered safe in pregnancy and breastfeeding
Oxytocics		To aid uterine contractility, either in induction of labour or in augmentation of labour, or postpartum for prevention or treatment of uterine atony
	Syntocinon	In labour, generally given by intravenous infusion so the amount given can be titrated against its effect It takes 20–30 minutes for oxytocin to reach a steady state and the rate of infusion should therefore not be increased at time intervals of less than 30 minutes Should not be administered within 6 hours of vaginal prostaglandins For treatment and prevention of postpartum haemorrhage, larger doses can be given either by slow intravenous or intramuscular bolus or by intravenous infusion Can cause water retention and hyponatraemia

Class of drug	Drug	Use and risk/contraindications
	Ergometrine	Treatment and prevention of postpartum haemorrhage Can cause nausea, vomiting and hypertension Contraindicated in women with pre-eclampsia Can be given intramuscularly or intravenously Has a sustained action, up to 2–3 hours
	Syntometrine (oxytocin 5 IU/ml with ergometrine 0.5 mg)	Active management of the third stage of labour Given intramuscularly Has the advantage of the speed of action of oxytocin (within 3 minutes) and the sustained action of ergometrine The disadvantage is the side effect profile of ergometrine
Prostaglandins	**Prostaglandin E$_2$** Dinoprostone	Induction of labour Given by the vaginal route in the form of gel, tablets, slow-release pessary Maximum dose gel = 3 mg (4 mg in primigravida with unfavourable cervix); maximum dose tablets = 6 mg (less in multipara) Propess pessary (10 mg) Oxytocin should not be given within at least 6 hours of prostaglandin because of the risk of uterine hyperstimulation
Tocolytics		To stop uterine activity
	Beta-sympathomimetics (e.g. ritodrine, terbutaline, salbutamol)	Associated with significant maternal side effects, such as tachycardia, palpitations, tremor, nausea, vomiting, headaches, thirst, restlessness, chest pain and breathlessness Blood sugar levels may rise Great care should be taken when administering these drugs and the lowest possible dose should be given
	Calcium channel blockers (e.g. nifedipine)	These have the advantage of oral administration and fewer side effects than some of the other agents Profound maternal hypotension is a risk

Continued

Class of drug	Drug	Use and risk/contraindications
	Magnesium sulphate	Flushing, nausea, vomiting, palpitations and headaches are common maternal side effects Magnesium levels need to be monitored
	NSAIDs (e.g. indometacin)	Maternal side effects include gastrointestinal bleeding, peptic ulceration, thrombocytopenia, allergic reactions and impaired renal function Fetal side effects when used in the long term include oligohydramnios, fetal renal impairment, premature closure of the ductus arteriosus, intraventricular haemorrhage and necrotising enterocolitis
	Oxytocin antagonists (e.g. atosiban)	A new class of drug that appears to have fewer side effects

An Aid to Calculations Used in Midwifery Practice

RELATIONSHIP BETWEEN SI OR METRIC UNITS

All are related by a factor of 1000:

- 1 kilogram (kg) = 1000 grams (g)
- 1 gram = 1000 milligrams (mg)
- 1 milligram = 1000 micrograms (μg)
- 1 litre (l) = 1000 millilitres (ml)

To convert from one unit to another, divide or multiply by 1000.

- Converting from LARGER units, e.g. kilograms to SMALLER units, i.e. grams, multiply by 1000.
- Converting from SMALLER units, e.g. micrograms to LARGER units, i.e. milligrams, divide by 1000.

Example

2 g (larger units) converted to mg (smaller units) =

$$2 \times 1000 = 2000 \, \text{mg}$$

When calculating the quantity of a medicine to be administered, always begin by converting prescription dose and stock volume to the same unit (i.e. grams or milligrams).

Example

To calculate tablets, the formula is:

$$\frac{\text{dose to be given}}{\text{stock strength per tablet}} = \text{quantity of tablets}$$

A prescription requires 1 gram of a medicine to be administered, the stock strength is 500 milligrams per tablet:

$$1 \, \text{gram} = 1000 \, \text{milligrams}$$

$$\frac{1000 \, \text{milligrams}}{500 \, \text{milligrams}} = 2 \, \text{tablets}$$

CONCENTRATION

Expressed as weight of the medicine per volume of solution, e.g. mg/ml, g/l, µg/ml.

This is calculated by dividing the total weight of the medicine by the volume of the solution.

Example

To calculate the concentration of a medicine in an infusion labelled 500 mg in 250 ml glucose 5% concentration:

$$\frac{\text{total weight of medicine}}{\text{total volume of solution}} = \frac{500\,\text{mg}}{250\,\text{ml}} = 2\,\text{mg/ml}$$

PROPORTION

It is often necessary to calculate how much of a mixture you need to administer to give the required dose.

The formula to use is:

$$\frac{\text{dose to be given}}{\text{stock strength}} \times \frac{\text{stock volume}}{1} = \text{amount of mixture to be given}$$

Example

A prescription requires 2 g of a medicine to be given; the stock volume is 500 mg in 10 ml:

$$2\,\text{g} = 2000\,\text{mg}$$

$$\frac{2000}{500} \times \frac{10}{1} = 40\,\text{ml}$$

CALCULATION OF INFUSION RATES

Intravenous (IV) infusion rates may be prescribed as:

a. the volume of fluid to be infused over a specified period of time, *or*
b. the amount of a drug to be administered over a specified period of time

a.

To calculate the volume of fluid to be infused over a specified period of time, the formula is:

$$\frac{\text{total volume of fluid to be given(in ml)}}{\text{time(in hours)}} = \text{ml/hour}$$

Example

1 L of normal saline 0.9% to be given over 8 hours:

$$1L = 1000 \text{ mL}$$

$$\frac{1000}{8} = 125 \text{ ml/hour}$$

To manually calculate the drip rate, the formula is:

$$\frac{\text{volume} \times \text{number of drops per ml}}{\text{time in minutes}}$$

Using the above example and a standard giving set which delivers 20 drops per ml:

$$\frac{125 \times 20}{60} = 41.67 \text{ drops per minute}$$

As drops can only be given as a whole number, 0.49 is rounded down and 0.50 rounded up. The rate is therefore 42 drops per minute.

b.

If a prescription requires a drug in solution to be administered, the formula is:

$$\frac{\text{weight of drug}}{\text{volume of solution}}$$

Example

$$\frac{500 \text{ mg}}{100 \text{ ml}} = 5 \text{ mg/ml}$$

If the prescription requires 15 mg/hour, the drip rate would then be calculated as in the example given in a. above to deliver 3 ml of the solution per hour.

CALCULATING INFANT FEEDING FORMULA

When calculating feeding regimes for babies who require a specified intake, this is based on:
- weight of the baby
- age, i.e. number of days old
- required feeding pattern, i.e. frequency of feeds (e.g. 1, 2, 3 or 4 hourly)

- daily nutritional requirements:
  - day 1: 60 ml/kg
  - day 2: 90 ml/kg
  - day 3: 120 ml/kg
  - day 4: 150 ml/kg, etc.

The formula to calculate volume of milk per feed is:

$$\frac{\text{weight in kg} \times \text{ml/kg/day}}{\text{number of feeds in 24 hours}}$$

Example

A preterm baby weighing 2 kg is 2 days old and he requires 2-hourly feeds:

$$\frac{2 \times 90}{12} = \frac{180}{12} = 15 \text{ ml per feed}$$

Normal Values in Pregnancy

Laboratory or physical measurements are presented as a range representing the average in a particular population. The physiological changes of pregnancy may affect what is considered 'normal' for the non-pregnant population. In addition, 'normal' values in pregnancy might be different at different gestations and hence care must be taken when deciding whether a test result(s) is actually abnormal for the woman/fetus concerned. A large sample of women having a straightforward physiological pregnancy is necessary to produce accurate pregnancy value ranges and hence there can be small variations from book to book.

UNITS OF MEASUREMENT

Care needs to be taken in the interpretation of units of measurement as abbreviations are used and represent very different amounts. In addition, values might be expressed in SI or traditional units. For example:

- g = grams
- mg = milligrams
- mmol = millimoles
- l = litres
- dl = decilitres (N.B. prefix 'd' signifies 10).

WEIGHT GAIN IN PREGNANCY

Average weight gain during pregnancy is about 12.5 kg; however, this varies according to the woman's pre-pregnancy body mass index BMI (weight/height^2). Those women with a low BMI are expected to gain more weight, whereas those women who are obese should gain less.

Category	Pre-pregnant BMI
Low (underweight)	<18.5
Normal	18.5–24.9
High (overweight)	25.0–29.9
Obese	>29.9

BIOCHEMISTRY

Test/units	Non-pregnant Typical range	Pregnant Typical range	Comments
Alanine transaminase (ALT) u/l	6–40	No change	Raised levels indicate liver damage
Alkaline phosphatase IU/l	40–120	Doubled by late pregnancy	Usually elevated in third trimester due to placental production of enzyme
Bile acids μmol/l	<9		Values of total bile acids ≥14 μmol/l are viewed as abnormal, indicating cholestasis
Bilirubin μmol/l	<17		Little change from non-pregnant range
Creatinine μmol/l	50–100	75 approx. is upper limit of normal	Lower in mid-pregnancy but rises towards term
Potassium mmol/l	3.5–5.3	Unchanged	Unchanged in pregnancy
Albumin g/l	30–48	25–35	Total protein and albumin are both lower in pregnancy
Urea mmol/l	2–6.5	Usually ≤4.5	Lower in pregnancy
Uric acid μmol/l	150–350	Lowest values in second trimester, 10 × gestational age in weeks is approx. upper limit of normal	Increases with gestation, although lower levels than non-pregnant

HAEMATOLOGY

Note: pregnancy is a hypercoagulable state and prothrombin, partial thromboplastin and thrombin times are slightly faster than controls.

Test/units	Non-pregnant typical range	Pregnant	Comments
Clotting time	12 min	8 min	Observe whether blood is clotting or oozing from venepuncture sites in high-risk groups
Fibrin degradation products μg/ml	Mean 1.04	High values in third trimester and especially around time of birth	

Test/units	Non-pregnant typical range	Pregnant	Comments
Fibrinogen g/l	1.7–4.1	By term 2.9–6.2	Marked increase in pregnancy, especially in third trimester and around time of birth
Haematocrit l/L	0.35–0.47	0.31–0.35	Lower in pregnancy
Haemoglobin g/dl	11.5–16.5	10.0–12.0 Should be ≤10 in third trimester	Good iron stores needed to maintain pregnancy levels Fall in first trimester whether or not iron and folate taken
Platelets × 10⁹L	150–400	Slight decrease in normal pregnancy Lower limit of 'normal' = 120	No functional significance
White cell count × 10⁹L	4.0–11.0	9.0–15.0 Higher values up to 25.0 around time of birth	Normal increase in pregnancy. Rise in infections

Glossary of Terms and Definitions

NOTIFICATION AND REGISTRATION OF BIRTH

It is the legal duty of the father, or any other person in attendance or present within 6 hours after the birth, to notify the birth. This must be done within 36 hours of birth for any child born after 24 completed weeks of pregnancy, whether alive or dead. It is usual for the midwife to undertake this notification.

The purpose of notification is to enable the primary healthcare team to be aware of a baby's birth. Where appropriate, an entry for the 'at-risk' register is compiled from the details supplied; this is used for providing supervision of care for the children concerned. The birth information is also made available to the Registrar of Births and Deaths of the district in which the birth took place.

REGISTRATION OF BIRTH

Every birth must be registered in the district in which it took place. Births must be registered within 6 weeks (3 weeks in Scotland), although under certain circumstances that time might be extended by the Registrar of Births and Deaths. There is a statutory fine for those who fail to register.

The primary duty to register a birth rests with the mother of the child, although in the case of a married couple the father may attend to register. If a mother is unmarried and wishes the father's name and details to be included, the couple should attend together to give details to the Registrar. If this is not possible, the mother could register the baby with her details only, and then the couple could re-register the birth later, adding the father's particulars. An unmarried father may also attend alone to register if he takes with him a Statutory Declaration made by the mother that he is the father of the child, or certain other court orders. In the event of the parents being unable to register the birth, a number of other people, including the midwife, are qualified to register a birth.

STATISTICS

At the time of registration, the Registrar also collects further information that is not entered in the Register but is used for statistical purposes and passed to the Office for National Statistics.

STILLBIRTHS

DEFINITION OF STILLBIRTH

A 'stillborn baby' means a baby born after the 24th week of pregnancy and which did not at any time after being completely expelled from its mother breathe or show any other signs of life.

REGISTRATION OF STILLBIRTHS

In order to register a stillborn baby, the mother or other informant must have a Medical Certificate of Stillbirth issued by a medical practitioner or midwife who is present at the stillbirth or who examines the body of a stillborn baby. Informants who have responsibility to register a stillbirth are the same as those in the case of a live birth.

The Registrar will record the details in the Stillbirth Register and issue an authority for burial or cremation. If the baby is to be cremated, the Medical Certificate of Stillbirth must be signed by a registered medical practitioner.

The midwife responsible for the care of the woman and her baby must notify the Supervisor of Midwives of the stillbirth.

REGISTRATION OF DEATH OF A BABY

This is the responsibility of the family. They should notify the Registrar of any child who has died after having been born alive.

BIRTH AND DEATH RATES

Vital statistics relate to life and death events, and specifically to the systematic collection of numerical data in order that they may be summarised and studied. In measuring health, there are difficulties in finding objective data to quantify; therefore it is pertinent to study the numbers of deaths occurring at different ages and their causes.

Figure 1 shows the periods relating to different types of death that are of special interest to midwives.

DEFINITION OF 'STILLBIRTH RATE'

To calculate the rate of stillbirths, the number of actual stillbirths in a year is compared with the number of total births (both live and still). This ratio is then related to a group of 1000 of those total births. The mathematical formula is as follows:

$$\frac{\text{number of stillbirths}}{\text{number of total births}} \times 1000 = \text{stillbirth rate per 1000 total births}$$

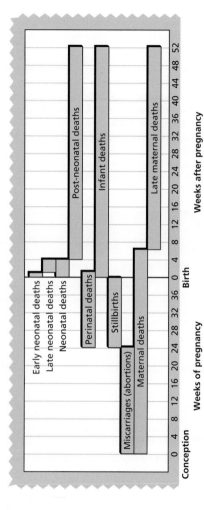

Fig. 1: Subdivision of deaths occurring during pregnancy and within 1 year of birth.

PERINATAL DEATH

- *Perinatal death*: this is either a stillbirth or a death occurring in the 1st week of life (early neonatal death).
- *Perinatal death (or mortality) rate*: This is the number of stillbirths and early neonatal deaths per 1000 total births.

NEONATAL DEATH

- *Neonatal death*: this is a death occurring in the first 28 days of life. Neonatal deaths are divided into early neonatal deaths, which occur during the first 7 days of life, and later neonatal deaths, which occur during the next 21 days. The reason for this is that the causes of early death are more similar to those of stillbirth, whereas the causes of later deaths are different.
- *Neonatal death rate*: this is calculated per 1000 live births.

INFANT DEATH

- *Infant death*: this is a death occurring in the 1st year of life. This includes all neonatal deaths and those termed postneonatal deaths.
- *Infant mortality rate*: this is calculated per 1000 live births. This rate is taken as one of the best measures of a nation's health.

MATERNAL DEATHS

Data on all maternal deaths are collated to produce triennial reports.
- *Maternal death*: this is defined as 'the death of a woman while pregnant or within 42 days of termination of pregnancy, from any cause related to or aggravated by the pregnancy or its management, but not from accidental or incidental causes'.
- *Maternal mortality*: in the UK this is the number of deaths per 100 000 maternities.
- *International maternity mortality rate (MMR)*: this is the number of deaths per 100 000 live births. This figure is useful for international comparisons but care is needed in its interpretation.
- *Direct maternal deaths*: these are classified as those resulting from complications of pregnancy, labour and the puerperium, from interventions, omissions or incorrect treatment, or from a chain of events resulting from any of these (e.g. thromboembolism, haemorrhage, pre-eclampsia and eclampsia, sepsis, anaesthesia, amniotic fluid embolism).
- *Indirect maternal deaths*: these result from previous existing disease or diseases that developed during pregnancy/the puerperium, where death was not due to direct obstetric causes but was aggravated by the physiological effects of pregnancy (e.g. cardiac disease, psychiatric illness).

- *Coincidental deaths* (referred to as fortuitous in the international classification): these are deaths from unrelated causes which happen to occur in pregnancy/the puerperium (e.g. domestic violence, although incidents might first arise in pregnancy).
- *Late deaths*: these occur between 42 days and 1 year after abortion, miscarriage or delivery, and are due to direct or indirect maternal causes of death.

COMMON DEFINITIONS

Abortion
Termination of pregnancy before the fetus is viable, i.e. before 24 weeks' gestation in the UK.

Abruptio placentae
Premature separation of a normally situated placenta. Term normally used from viability (24 weeks).

Acardiac twin
One twin presents without a well-defined cardiac structure and is kept alive through the placental circulation of the viable twin.

Acridine orange
A stain used in fluorescence microscopy that causes bacteria to fluoresce green to red.

Aetiology
The science of the cause of disease.

Amenorrhoea
Absence of menstrual periods.

Amniotic fluid embolism
The escape of amniotic fluid through the wall of the uterus or placental site into the maternal circulation, triggering life-threatening anaphylactic shock in the mother. (The word 'embolism', denoting a clot, is a misnomer.)

Amniotomy
Artificial rupture of the amniotic sac.

Anterior obliquity of the uterus
Altered uterine axis. The uterus leans forward due to poor maternal abdominal muscles and a pendulous abdomen.

Antigen
A substance which stimulates the production of an antibody.

Anuria
Producing no urine.

Atresia
Closure or absence of a usual opening or canal.

Augmentation of labour
Intervention to correct slow progress in labour.

Bandl's ring
An exaggerated retraction ring seen as an oblique ridge above the symphysis pubis between the upper and lower uterine segments, which is a sign of obstructed labour.

Basal body temperature
The temperature of the body when at rest. In natural family planning, it is taken as soon as the woman wakes from sleep and before any activity occurs or after a period of at least 1 hour's rest.

Bicornuate uterus
A structural abnormality of the uterus.

Bishops score
Rating system to assess suitability of the cervix for induction of labour.

Burns Marshall
A method of breech delivery involving traction to prevent the neck from bending backwards.

Calendar calculation
The fertile phase of the menstrual cycle is calculated in accordance

with the length of the woman's 6–12 previous cycles.

Cardiotocograph

Measurement of the fetal heart rate and contractions on a machine that is able to provide a paper print of the information it records.

Central venous pressure line

An intravenous tube that measures the pressure in the right atrium or superior vena cava, indicating the volume of blood returning to the heart and, by implication, hypovolaemia.

Cephalopelvic disproportion

Disparity between the size of the woman's pelvis and the fetal head.

Cerclage

A non-absorbable suture inserted to keep the cervix closed.

Cervical ectropion

Physiological response by cervical cells to hormonal changes in pregnancy. Cells proliferate and cause the cervix to appear eroded.

Cervical intraepithelial neoplasm (CIN)

Progressive and abnormal growth of cervical cells.

Cervical ripening

The process by which the cervix changes and becomes more susceptible to the effect of uterine contractions. Can be physiological or artificially produced.

Cervicitis

Inflammation of the cervix.

Choanal atresia

(Bilateral) membranous or bony obstruction of the nares; the baby is blue when sleeping and pink when crying.

Choroid plexus cyst

Collection of cerebrospinal fluid within the choroid plexi, from where cerebrospinal fluid is derived.

Coloboma

A malformation characterised by the absence of or a defect in the tissue of the eye; the pupil can appear keyhole shaped. It may be associated with other anomalies.

Colposcopy

Visualisation of the cervix using a colposcope.

Commensal

Micro-organisms adapted to grow on the skin or mucous surfaces of the host, forming part of the normal flora.

Conjoined twins

Identical twins in whom separation is incomplete so their bodies are joined together at some point.

Couvelaire uterus (uterine apoplexy)

Bruising and oedema of uterine tissue seen in placental abruption, when leaking blood is forced between muscle fibres because the margins of the placenta are still attached to the uterus.

Cryotherapy

Use of cold or freezing to destroy or remove tissue.

Deoxyribonucleic acid (DNA)

The substance containing genes. DNA can store and transmit information, can copy itself accurately and can occasionally mutate.

Diastasis symphysis pubis
(see Symphysis pubis dysfunction)

Dichorionic twins
Twins who have developed in their own separate chorionic sacs.

Diploid
Containing two sets of chromosomes.

Disseminated intravascular coagulation/coagulopathy
A condition secondary to a primary complication where there is inappropriate blood clotting in the blood vessels, followed by an inability of the blood to clot appropriately when all the clotting factors have been used up.

Dizygotic (dizygous)
Formed from two separate zygotes.

Doering rule
The first fertile day of the cycle is determined by a calculation based upon the earliest previous temperature shift. This is an effective double-check method to identify the onset of the fertile phase.

Dyspareunia
Painful or difficult intercourse experienced by the woman.

Echogenic bowel
Bright appearances of bowel, equivalent to the brightness of bone. Also associated with intra-amniotic bleeding and fetal swallowing of bloodstained liquor.

Echogenic foci in the heart
Bright echoes from calcium deposits in the fetal heart, often the left ventricle. These do not affect cardiac function.

Ectopic pregnancy
An abnormally situated pregnancy, most commonly in a uterine tube.

Embryo reduction
(see Fetal reduction)

Endocervical
Relating to the internal canal of the cervix.

Epicanthic fold
A vertical fold of skin on either side of the nose, which covers the lacrimal caruncle. Can be common in Asian babies, but may indicate Down syndrome in other ethnic groups.

Erb's palsy
Paralysis of the arm due to the damage to cervical nerve roots five and six of the brachial plexus.

Erythema
Reddening of the skin.

Erythropoiesis
The process by which erythrocytes (red blood cells) are formed. After the 10th week of gestation, erythropoiesis rises and seems to be involved in red cell production in the bone marrow during the third trimester.

External cephalic version (ECV)
The use of external manipulation on the pregnant woman's abdomen to convert a breech to a cephalic presentation.

False-negative rate
The proportion of affected pregnancies that would not be identified as high risk. Tests with a high false-negative rate have low sensitivity.

False-positive rate
The proportion of unaffected pregnancies with a high-risk classification. Tests with a high false-positive rate have low specificity.

Ferguson reflex
Surge of oxytocin, resulting in increased contractions, due to stimulation of the cervix and upper portion of the vagina.

Fetal reduction
The reduction in the number of viable fetuses/embryos in a multiple (usually higher multiple) pregnancy by medical intervention.

Fetofetal transfusion syndrome (twin-to-twin transfusion syndrome (TTTS))
Condition in which blood from one monozygotic twin fetus transfuses into the other via blood vessels in the placenta.

Fetus-in-fetu
Parts of a fetus may be lodged within another fetus. This can only happen in monozygotic twins.

Fetus papyraceous
A fetus that dies in the second trimester of the pregnancy and becomes compressed and parchment-like.

Fibroid
Firm, benign tumour of muscular and fibrous tissue.

Fraternal twins
Dizygotic (non-identical) twins.

Fundal height
The distance between the top part of the uterus (the fundus) and the top of the symphysis pubis (the junction between the pubic bones). Measurement of this is undertaken to assess the increasing size of the uterus antenatally and decreasing size postnatally.

Haematuria
Blood in the urine.

Haemostasis
The arrest of bleeding.

Haploid
Containing only one set of chromosomes.

HELLP syndrome
A condition of pregnancy characterised by haemolysis, elevated liver enzymes and low platelets.

Herpes gestationis
An autoimmune disease precipitated by pregnancy and characterised by an erythematous rash and blisters.

Homan's sign
Pain is felt in the calf when the foot is pulled upwards (dorsiflexion). This is indicative of a venous thrombosis and further investigations should be undertaken to exclude or confirm this.

Homeostasis
The condition in which the body's internal environment remains relatively constant within physiological limits.

Hydatidiform mole
A gross malformation of the trophoblast in which the chorionic villi proliferate and become avascular.

Hydropic vesicles
Fluid-filled sacs, or blisters.

Hypercapnia
An abnormal increase in the amount of carbon dioxide in the blood.

Hyperemesis gravidarum
Protracted or excessive vomiting in pregnancy.

Hypertrophy
Overgrowth of tissue.

Hypovolaemia
Reduced circulating blood volume due to external loss of body fluids or to loss of fluid into the tissues.

Hypoxia
Lack of oxygen.

Hysteroscope
An instrument used to access the uterus via the vagina.

Induction of labour
Intervention to stimulate uterine contractions before the onset of spontaneous labour.

Intraepithelial
Within the epithelium, or among epithelial cells.

Intrahepatic cholestasis of pregnancy (ICP)
An idiopathic condition of abnormal liver function.

LAM
A method of contraception based upon an algorithm of lactation, amenorrhoea and a 6-month time period.

Lanugo
Soft downy hair, which covers the fetus in utero and occasionally the neonate. It appears at around 20 weeks' gestation and covers the face and most of the body. It disappears by 40 weeks' gestation.

Løvset manoeuvre
A manoeuvre for the delivery of shoulders and extended arms in a breech.

Macrosomia
Large baby.

Malposition
A cephalic presentation other than normal anterior position of the fetal head, e.g. occipitoposterior.

Malpresentation
A presentation other than the vertex, i.e. face, brow, compound or shoulder. (Breech may be included in this category)

Mauriceau–Smellie–Veit
A manoeuvre to deliver a breech, which involves jaw flexion and shoulder traction.

McRobert's manoeuvre
A manoeuvre to rotate the angle of the symphysis pubis superiorly and release the impaction of the anterior shoulder in shoulder dystocia. The woman brings her knees up to her chest.

Monoamniotic twins
Twins who have developed in the same amniotic sac.

Monochorionic twins
Identical twins who have developed in the same chorionic sac.

Monozygotic (monozygous)
Formed from one zygote (identical twins).

Multifetal reduction
(see Fetal reduction)

Naegele's rule
Method of calculating the expected date of delivery.

Neoplasia
Growth of new tissue.

Neutral thermal environment (NTE)
The range of environmental temperature over which heat production, oxygen consumption and nutritional requirements for growth are minimal, provided the body temperature is normal.

Nuchal fold >5 mm at 20 weeks' gestation
An increased thickness of fetal skin and fat at the back of the fetal neck. Subcutaneous fluid (nuchal translucency) cannot usually be visualised after 14 weeks.

Oedema
The effusion of body fluid into the tissues.

Oligohydramnios
Abnormally low amount of amniotic fluid in pregnancy.

Oliguria
The production of an abnormally small amount of urine.

PaCO$_2$
Measures the partial pressure of dissolved carbon dioxide. This dissolved CO_2 has moved out of the cell and into the bloodstream. The measure of *Pa*CO$_2$ accurately reflects the alveolar ventilation.

PaO$_2$
Measures the partial pressure of oxygen in the arterial blood. It reflects how the lung is functioning but does not measure tissue oxygenation.

Paronychia
An inflamed swelling of the nail folds; acute paronychia is usually caused by infection with *Staphylococcus aureus*.

Pedunculated
Having a stem or stalk.

Pemphigoid gestationis
(see Herpes gestationis)

Perinatal
Surrounding labour and the first 7 days of life.

pH
A solution's acidity or alkalinity is expressed on the pH scale, which runs from 0 to 14. This scale is based on the concentration of hydrogen ions in a solution expressed in chemical units called moles per litre.

Placenta accreta
Abnormally adherent placenta into the muscle layer of the uterus.

Placenta increta
Abnormally adherent placenta into the perimetrium of the uterus.

Placenta percreta
Abnormally adherent placenta through the muscle layer of the uterus.

Placenta praevia
A condition in which some or all of the placenta is attached in the lower segment of the uterus.

Placental abruption
(see Abruptio placentae)

Polyhydramnios
An excessive amount of amniotic fluid in pregnancy.

Polyp
Small growth.

Porphyria
An inherited condition of abnormal red blood cell formation.

Postpartum
After labour.

Pre-eclampsia
A condition peculiar to pregnancy, which is characterised by hypertension, proteinuria and systemic dysfunction.

Primary postpartum haemorrhage
A blood loss in excess of 500 ml or any amount which adversely affects the condition of the mother within the first 24 hours of delivery.

Progestogen
Synthetic progesterone used in hormonal contraception.

Prostaglandins
Locally acting chemical compounds derived from fatty acids within cells. They ripen the cervix and cause the uterus to contract.

Proteinuria
Protein in the urine.

Pruritus
Itching.

Ptyalism
Excessive salivation.

Puerperal fever/pyrexia
A rise in temperature in the puerperium. This is poorly defined in the textbooks but is assumed to be based on the definition of pyrexia, which is a rise above the normal body temperature of 37.2°C. Where pyrexia is used as a clinical sign of importance, the elevation in temperature is generally taken as being 38°C and above.

Puerperal sepsis
Infection of the genital tract following childbirth; a major cause of maternal death.

Puerperium
A period after childbirth where the uterus and other organs and structures that have been affected by the pregnancy are returning to their non-gravid state. Usually described as a period of up to 6–8 weeks.

Quickening
Recognition of fetal movements by the woman in early pregnancy.

Retraction
Process by which the uterine muscle fibres shorten after a contraction. Unique to uterine muscle.

Rubin's manoeuvre
A rotational manoeuvre to relieve shoulder dystocia. Pressure is exerted over the fetal back to adduct and rotate the shoulders.

Sandal gap
Exaggerated gap between the first and second toes.

Secondary postpartum haemorrhage
An 'excessive' or 'prolonged' vaginal blood loss which is usually defined as occurring from 24 hours to 6 weeks after the birth.

Selective fetocide
The medical destruction of an abnormal twin fetus in a continuing pregnancy.

Sheehan syndrome
A condition where sudden or prolonged shock leads to irreversible pituitary necrosis, characterised by amenorrhoea, genital atrophy and premature senility.

Short femur
Shorter than average thigh bone, when compared with other fetal measurements.

Shoulder dystocia
Failure of the shoulders to traverse the pelvis spontaneously after delivery of the head. Incidence is around 0.3% of deliveries.

Siamese twins
Conjoined twins.

Speculum (vaginal)
An instrument used to open the vagina.

Subinvolution
The uterine size appears larger than anticipated for days postpartum, and may feel poorly contracted. Uterine tenderness may be present.

Superfecundation
Conception of twins as a result of sexual intercourse with two different partners in the same menstrual cycle.

Superfetation
Conception of twins as a result of two acts of sexual intercourse in different menstrual cycles.

Surfactant
Complex mixture of phospholipids and lipoproteins, produced by type 2 alveolar cells in the lungs, that decreases surface tension and prevents alveolar collapse at end-expiration.

Symphysiotomy
A surgical incision to separate the symphysis pubis and enlarge the pelvis to aid delivery.

Symphysis pubis dysfunction
A painful condition in which there is an abnormal relaxation of the ligaments supporting the pubic joint.

Talipes
A complex foot deformity, affecting 1 per 1000 live births and more common in males. The affected foot is held in a fixed flexion (equinus) and in-turned (varus) position. It can be differentiated from positional talipes because the deformity in true talipes cannot be passively corrected.

Teratogen
An agent believed to cause congenital abnormalities, e.g. thalidomide.

Torsion
Twisting.

Trizygotic
Formed from three separate zygotes.

Twin-to-twin transfusion syndrome
(see Fetofetal transfusion syndrome)

Uniovular
Monozygotic.

Unstable lie
After 36 weeks' gestation, a lie that varies between longitudinal and oblique or transverse is said to be unstable.

Uterine involution
The physiological process that starts from the end of labour that results in a gradual reduction in the size of the uterus until it returns to its non-pregnant size and location in the pelvis.

Vanishing twin syndrome
The reabsorption of one twin fetus early in pregnancy (usually before 12 weeks).

Vasa praevia
A rare occurrence in which umbilical cord vessels pass through the placental membranes and lie across the cervical os.

Withdrawal bleed
Bleeding due to withdrawal of hormones.

Wood's manoeuvre
A rotational or screw manoeuvre to relieve shoulder dystocia. Pressure is exerted on the fetal chest to rotate and abduct the shoulders.

Zavanelli manoeuvre
Last choice of manoeuvre for shoulder dystocia. The head is returned to its pre-restitution position, then the head is flexed back into the vagina. Delivery is by caesarean section.

Zygosity
Describing the genetic make-up of children in a multiple birth.

INDEX

Note: Page numbers followed by *b* indicate boxes, *f* indicate figures, and *t* indicate tables

D

ROSALIE AND PETE GRIFFIN,

THE LETTERS OF
VINCENT VAN GOGH

AUGUST, 1981

THE LETTERS OF
VINCENT VAN GOGH

Selected, Edited and Introduced by
MARK ROSKILL

FONTANA/COLLINS

The translation from which this selection has been made was
first published by Constable & Co. 1927-29
This edition first issued in Fontana 1963
Ninth Impression August 1980
© In this translation Constable & Co. 1927-1929
© In this selection, introduction and notes
William Collins Sons & Co. Ltd 1963

Made and printed in Great Britain by
William Collins Sons & Co. Ltd Glasgow

EDITORIAL NOTE

The English text of the *Letters* presented here is basically
taken from the three-volume edition published by Constable
in 1927/29; and thanks are due to the proprietors of that
edition and to the Engineer V. W. van Gogh for their co-
operation in permitting its re-use. Thirty years after the first
and only appearance of that edition, it has seemed appropriate to use my editorial licence rather freely in the making
of textual revisions of various kinds, and the recording of
omissions that have since come to light. Similarly I have
included in the form of additional footnotes a certain amount
of explanatory comment on persons, places or situations that
are referred to, together with translations of such quotations
or special phrases as are given in French within the letters
themselves, and a few incidental observations of a broader
sort that may interest the general reader.

Each letter selected for inclusion has been captioned with
its place of origin and a date. Letters that were dated by
van Gogh himself are given with their original headings;
for the most part, however, the artist refrained from dating
his letters, and in all such cases a conjectural date in square
brackets has been given. The sources for these conjectural
dates are threefold. Some of them go back to the earliest
editorial work carried out by Mme. J. van Gogh-Bonger—and
in certain cases are based on evidence or reasoning that can
no longer be reconstructed. Others are owed to a series
of articles recently published in the Dutch periodical *Maatstaf*
by Dr. Jan Hulsker of The Hague; I am personally grateful
to Dr. Hulsker for his permission to make use of his findings
for the present edition, and though I have kept to a rather
broader system of date-brackets than the one he presented
himself, I would like to make warm acknowledgement of
the assistance received from this quarter. The third and final
source has been my own research, independent from that of

Dr. Hulsker; study of the Arles letters in another connection had equipped me with a scheme of dates in this area which indeed largely agrees with his, and I have also, for this edition specifically, re-checked some of Dr. Hulsker's findings and worked over the periods not covered in his articles.

The choice of plates has been made with a view to providing a conspectus of van Gogh's artistic development, and also with a view to illustrating some of the principal subjects or treatments that are referred to in the letters selected.

My thanks are due to Mr. Richard Ollard of Collins for watching over the destiny of this book from first to last, and to my wife for all kinds of help that made progress speedier and more pleasant.

M. R.

NOTE : Apart from a few minor changes of punctuation the Memoir of Vincent by his sister-in-law has been reprinted here exactly as it first appeared.

CONTENTS

PLATES

INTRODUCTION

There are two great works of the nineteenth century which, more than any other writings of the time, give us a sense of what it was like to be a real creator in the visual arts during that marvellously rich and strenuous era. The inner order which they possess is not based on any literary kind of design, but stems from the character and momentum of the painter's life itself. One of them is the Journal of Eugène Delacroix; the other is the correspondence of Vincent van Gogh.

If we want an analogy nearer our own day to van Gogh's total personality—its strength of character, powers of insight, and rough-hewn forcefulness of language—we may find it in the correspondence of D. H. Lawrence. The ways in which the two men suffered and their ideals for art and society were in many ways akin. Despite the laborious and searing character of the struggles of both men to survive materially, to love sincerely and to create, one can equally say of the letters of van Gogh what was written very recently about those of Lawrence: "no-one halfway alive could be untouched by the joy of living that breathes in the slightest of them."[1]

What sort of value and importance do the *Letters to Theo* have for today's reader? The answer is fourfold. First of all they provide a narrative of van Gogh's life. They unfold its main events and disclose in so doing a wealth of passing thoughts and small factual details:

Now I have met Christine [i.e. Sien]. As you know, she was pregnant, ill, out in the cold; I was all by myself ... I took to her, though not immediately with the idea

[1] "Friends and Enemies," *Times Literary Supplement*, 27 April 1962.

of marrying her; but when I got to know her better, it
became plain to me that if I wanted to help her, I had to
do it seriously . . . she said, " I will stay with you, however poor you may be." And this is how it all came
about.

(May, 1882)

Today I saw Dr. Gachet again and I am going to paint
at his house on Tuesday morning, then I shall dine
with him and afterwards he will come to look at my
paintings. He seems very sensible, but he is as discouraged about his job as a country doctor as I am about
my painting. Then I said to him that I would gladly
exchange job for job.

(May, 1890)

Always informative and often most moving from such a point
of view, they speak on this count for themselves (with the
memoir by the artist's sister-in-law, reprinted here, to fill in
the early background and supply necessary strands of continuity). At the same time, too, we learn from them the
influences to which van Gogh was subject at differing times—
what books he read and how he reacted to them, in what
ways the works of other artists appealed to him (especially
the older masters whom he had cause to admire), what
thinkers nourished his own philosophy of art :

I remember quite well having been very much impressed . . . by a drawing by Daumier, an old man under
the chestnut trees in the Champs Elysées (an illustration for Balzac) . . . [there was] something so strong and
manly in Daumier's conception that I thought, it must
be a good thing to think and feel that way, and to over-
look or pass by many things in order to concentrate on
things that provide food for thought, and touch us as
human beings more directly and personally than meadows
or clouds. And so I always feel greatly drawn to the
figures either of the English graphic artists or of the

English authors, because of their Monday-morning-like sobriety and studied simplicity and gravity and analytical candour, as something solid and robust which can give us strength in our times of weakness. The same holds good, among French authors, for Balzac and Zola too. (October, 1882)

I have been re-reading Dickens' *Christmas Books* these days. There are things in them so profound that one must read them over and over; there are tremendously close connections with Carlyle. (April, 1889)

Comments like these tell us not only the kind of man that van Gogh was, but also the way in which his essential ideas grew up and took wing.

Secondly, the letters document the succession of paintings and drawings in a very rich way. Indispensable in this way to the scholar (who uses them in detail for the construction of a full chronology), they have also the more general interest of giving, in many instances, a running commentary upon work in progress:

This week I have done some rather large studies in the woods, and I tried to put into these more vigour and finish than the first ones had. The one which I believe succeeded best is of nothing but a piece of dug-up earth —white, black and brown sand after a downpour of rain. Here and there the clods of earth caught the light and stood out in bold relief. After I had been sitting sketching that patch of ground for quite a while, there was another violent thunderstorm with a tremendous cloudburst, which went on for at least an hour. I was so keen to resume work that I stayed at my post and sheltered myself as well as I could behind a large tree. (August, 1882)

I have a model at last—a Zouave—a lad with a small face, the neck of a bull, the eye of a tiger, and I began with one portrait and made a fresh start with another; the half-length that I did of him was fearfully harsh, in a uniform the colour of saucepans enamelled with blue, with braids of a faded russet-orange, and two stars on his breast, an ordinary blue and really hard to do. His feline and highly bronzed head, with its reddish cap, I focused against a green door and the orange bricks of a wall.   (June, 1888)

Passages like these portray, for one particular canvas or another, the context of the creative process.

Then again the letters are a source of psychological insight. First and foremost they show us the inner workings of van Gogh's relationship with his brother; for example:

I am writing specially in order to tell you how thankful I am for your visit. It was a long time since we had seen each other or corresponded, as we used to do. It is better, all told, to be friends than to be dead to one another . . . The hours that we spent together have at least given us the assurance that we are both still in the land of the living. When I saw you again and walked with you, I had a feeling of the kind which I used once to experience more than I do now—a feeling that life was, so to say, something good and precious which one ought to value; and I felt more cheerful and alive than I had for a long time.   (October, 1879)

And then, over and above this, they illumine such things as the artist's rate of work,

I am always afraid of not working enough; I think I can do so much better still, and that is what I am aiming for, sometimes with a kind of fury.   (May, 1883)

I shall be all in when the " Orchards " are over . . . We would not have too many of them, even if I could bring

off twice as many . . . You will see that the rose-coloured
peach trees were painted with a certain passion. I must
also have a starry night with cypresses, or perhaps surmounting a field of ripe corn . . . I am in a continual
fever of work. (April, 1888)

the ever nervous and broken quality of his pictorial handwriting,

Here is a sketch of an orchard . . . It's absolutely clear
and absolutely straight off the cuff. A frenzy of impastos
faintly tinged with yellow and lilac, worked into a body
of paint that was initially white. (April, 1888)

. . . Nowadays I am putting pressure on myself to find
a brushwork without stippling or anything else, nothing
but the varied stroke. (August, 1888)

The " Olives " . . . are exaggerations from the point of
view of arrangement, their lines are warped like the
ones you find in old forests. (September, 1889)

and the underlying tenor of his imagery :

I have two new drawings now, one of a man reading his
Bible and the other of a man saying grace before his
dinner, which is out on the table . . . My intention in
these two . . . is one and the same; namely to express the
peculiar sentiment of Christmas and the New Year. In
Holland and England alike this is always more or less
religious . . . (December, 1882)

Spring is tender, green young corn and pink apple
blossoms. Autumn is the contrast of the yellow leaves
against violet tones. Winter is the snow with black
silhouettes. (June/July 1884)

Passages such as these make plain how well van Gogh was capable of knowing his desires, and with what control he could set out to realize them.

Lastly one can draw out of the letters revealing parallels to van Gogh's total output of paintings, its constants and its variables. Descriptions of sights in nature that amount to "unpainted pictures" can be compared year by year in their imagery with actual contemporaneous treatments of landscape or figure subjects :

Yesterday . . . in the Noordeinde [part of The Hague] I saw workmen busy pulling down the section opposite the palace, fellows all white with lime dust, with drays and horses. It was cool, windy weather, the sky was grey and the spot was very characteristic.

Then two other larger compositions of labourers in the dunes . . . are the things I should most like to finish. Long rows of diggers—paupers employed by the municipality—before a patch of sandy ground, which has to be dug.

(July, 1883)

This morning I saw the country from my window a long time before sunrise, with nothing but the morning star, which looked very big.

I have two landscapes in hand . . . views taken into the hills, one is the country that I see from the window of my bedroom. In the foreground a field of corn ruined and cast to the ground after a storm. A boundary wall, and beyond the grey foliage of a few olive-trees, some huts and the hills. Finally at the top of the canvas a great white and grey cloud drowned in the azure.

(June, 1889)

Similarly van Gogh's ways of translating the ideas and theories

of others into personal terms can be compared with the
" translations " that he did in line or paint after the works
of earlier masters—Rembrandt, Millet, Delacroix:

> Meanwhile, I have started on copying the Millets. The
> " Sower " is finished, and I have sketched the " Four
> Hours of the Day."

> I told him plainly: " De Bock, . . . if we do not draw
> the figure or draw trees as if they were figures, we are
> people without backbone, or else with a weak one. Do
> you think Millet and Corot, whom we both love so much,
> could draw figures, yes or no? I think those masters
> could do anything.
>
> (May and October, 1881)

> Alone or almost alone amongst painters Rembrandt has
> . . . that heartbroken tenderness, that glimpse into a
> superhuman infinitude that seems so natural there; you
> come upon it in many places in Shakespeare.

> I am perhaps going to try to work from Rembrandt. I
> have especially an idea of doing the " Man at Prayer " in
> the colour-scale that runs from light yellow up to violet.
>
> (June/July, 1889 and May, 1890)

Another most suggestive analogy between the letters and the
paintings involves the interplay of past and present. One can
look for correspondences in the comparative importance of
their roles at different times, and in the ways in which they
were brought into synthesis with one another. For example:

> I think that the town of Arles was infinitely more glori-
> ous once as regards the beauty of its women and the
> beauty of its costumes. Now everything has a worn and

sickly look about it. But when you look at it for long,
the old charm revives.

Do you remember that wonderful page in *Tartarin*
[i.e. *Tartarin de Tarascon* by Alphonse Daudet], the
complaint of the old Tarascon stage-coach? Well, I have
just painted that red and green vehicle in the courtyard
of the inn . . . Here's to the country of good old Tartarin, I am enjoying myself in it more and more, and it
is going to become our second fatherland.

(September and October, 1888)

I shall attack the cypresses and the mountains. I think
that this will be the core of the work that I have done
here and there in Provence . . .

I am thinking of doing a new version of the picture
of peasants at dinner with the lamplight effect [i.e. the
Potato-Eaters of 1885] . . . Then, if you like, I will do
the old tower of Nuenen again and the cottage.

(November, 1889 and April, 1890)

In particular the question of how much his Dutch background
continued to mean to van Gogh during his later years in
France can fruitfully be studied by looking at the two sorts of
record side by side:

Involuntarily—is it the effect of this Ruysdael country?
[Jacob Ruysdael was a Dutch landscapist of the seventeenth century]—I keep thinking of Holland, and across
the twofold remoteness of distance and of time gone by
these memories have a kind of heartbreak in them.

What I learnt in Paris [sc. about painting] *is leaving
me*, and . . . I am returning to the ideas I had in the
country before I knew the impressionists.

(July and August, 1888)

And the answer that comes back from such extracts and others like them is undoubtedly in favour of Holland.

All in all, the *Letters to Theo* are a supremely eloquent record of the ways in which van Gogh's art and life interacted with one another. One particularly telling and wide-ranging example of such interaction is the history told there of van Gogh's appreciation of Japanese art, and its influence on his attitude to the South of France during and after his move to Provence in the spring of 1888. One of van Gogh's reasons for going South came from his discovery of Japanese prints in Antwerp at the end of 1885.[1] During the subsequent two years spent in Paris this original, limited interest widened considerably. In Paris he saw the formal influence of Japanese art extending right across the generation of " impressionist " painters—to use his own blanket term—to which he then attached himself. Out of this, van Gogh developed an inescapable sense of commitment. He saw it as desirable that the " return to nature " of the impressionists be extended still further, and the South, with its natural colouring and bright sunshine, offered a " second Japan." Faced also with his own unhappiness and ill-health, he looked to a climate in which his own modes of feeling would assimilate themselves to those of Japanese painters. He felt it important to investigate what Japanese art would convey, when studied against and within the landscape of this " second Japan "; he was to hang Japanese prints on the walls of his studio just as soon as he took over the Yellow House at Arles, and from the very first he was to see the local countryside (under snow as well as in sunshine) as mirroring the major motifs of Japanese nature-painting. He believed that other artists beside himself could acquire an awareness of how the drawing and colour in Japanese prints were vehicles for the Oriental artists' feelings towards nature. Individuality of expression and technical expansion would then freely bene-

[1] He had known something of Japanese art as far back as his days in Nuenen, but the revelation of Japanese line and colour together came only now.

fit; and European nature-painting as a whole, present and future, would thereby gain immeasurably:

> . . . Other artists will rise up in this lovely country [i.e. Provence] and do for it what the Japanese have done for theirs.

(May, 1888)

Most concrete of all was van Gogh's idea of establishing a colony in the South; a community, that is, to which a whole group of Parisian artists could periodically move—following the path that he had taken himself for the time being—whenever too much exposure to the dank climate of the metropolis and its moral and social hurly-burly put them in need of a change of scene and a refreshment of the sensibility. More than that, once the group arrangement was established, the "studio of the South" would offer an atmosphere that was sunny in its co-operative spirit as well as being warmed by natural sunshine. Under such conditions, the straight-forward, simple values exemplified in Japanese art could be nourished, in place of the spiritually damaging effects of social convention and intellectual over-education; for the "clearer sky" of the South seems to have symbolized for van Gogh a moral order founded upon clarity and simplicity. Besides the practical consequences of companionship and cheaper living, van Gogh envisioned also a further co-operative venture (itself modelled on Japanese precedent) for the exchange of works between artists in different centres. In sum, as the scheme of ideas crystallized that committed van Gogh to his great campaign of work in the South of France, four different sorts of concern drove it along: æsthetic, practical, metaphysical and humane. And the letters show how each and all of these concerns were bound up in van Gogh's urge to live his life to the full.

It was in 1893, only three years after Vincent's suicide, that the first batch of his letters to his brother Theo to appear in print came out in the *Mercure de France*. Emile Bernard,

Vincent's friend and correspondent who had already arranged memorial exhibitions of his work, was responsible for their publication. More letters were subsequently printed in the same magazine, and Theo's widow, Mme. J. van Gogh-Bonger, took on the task of transcribing and editing the whole sequence of letters that, over eighteen years, Theo had so faithfully preserved. The first collected edition was published in 1914, and further letters have come to light since then. In all, some 670 of the letters that Vincent wrote to Theo are known to-day to have survived.

The present edition is the only one to offer a small and representative group of letters, each of which has some special distinction of its own. It is also the only one to give the reader the maximum of editorial help, as he moves along from subject to subject or from one letter to another.

While the earliest of the extant letters dates from 1872, it was not until mid-1880 that the correspondence opened up and acquired a powerful inner rhythm of its own, which only van Gogh's death would interrupt. Before that time, while Vincent was in turn representative for a firm of art-dealers, schoolmaster, bookshop assistant, student preparing for the University and lay preacher, he had written to Theo as the occasion prompted; and the subject of art was mentioned only incidentally, in reference to a picture or print or spectacle of nature that had appealed to him, or in regard to a sketch that he had done. The first letter that dealt explicitly and at length with Vincent's desire and ambition to become an artist was written in July 1880—it appears in this selection :

But you will ask : What is your definite aim? That aim becomes more definite, will stand out slowly and surely, just as the rough draft becomes a sketch, and the sketch becomes a picture . . .

From then on, for almost exactly ten years, Theo loyally continued to provide the financial support which had originally

enabled his brother to commit himself completely to painting.
He did this in the form of regular payments out of his own
salary as a dealer. And throughout the decade in question
Vincent wrote to Theo with an equal regularity; though it is
exceptional for his letters of this period to carry precise dates,
it would seem that in normal circumstances the artist must
have written at least once a week, and sometimes twice
weekly or even twice in a single day (excluding that two-
year period between 1886 and 1888 when the brothers were
sharing rooms in Paris). Concurrently, there were certain
other familiars with whom Vincent communicated regularly—
extended sequences of letters survive that went to his sister
Wil and to his artist friends Anthon van Rappard and Emile
Bernard. But in none of these cases was the correspondence
anywhere nearly as heavy as that with Theo; and almost
invariably, where the subject matter treated is identical, it is
the account to Theo that was more detailed and explicit.

What began, then, as an exchange of personal news between highly affectionate brothers temporarily separated developed into a phenomenon of far broader scope. It is not
simply the fact of sheer quantity. Owing in part to the
power of attraction exerted in our time by the artistic personality as such—a power of attraction extending to every
available private and intimate detail of an artist's thought and
conduct—there is a strong tendency to regard Vincent's letters
to Theo as simply a " confessional " record, a convenient
means for Vincent to unload his immediate feelings. If
indeed the artist is to be looked on as a romantic figure,
standing apart from the everyday world and unfettered by
its conventions, then van Gogh, it may be held, poignantly
epitomizes such a condition. But to accept the above interpretation solely and entirely is to disregard the strong element
of calculation in van Gogh's personality, a very complex
element even more conspicuous in the correspondence with
Theo than in the paintings themselves.

The major clue here is the direct relationship between
what Vincent wrote and what Theo was paying him. It is
scarcely a coincidence that the increase of correspondence after

mid-1880 followed upon Theo's pledge of financial support; that its mood and tempo fluctuated on Vincent's side according as he felt that Theo's attitude gave cause for alarm; or that the first of Vincent's mental breakdowns was closely associated with the news of Theo's imminent marriage and the clear threat this imposed on Theo's capacity to go on providing for him. Enough, moreover, survives of Theo's side of the correspondence—some forty letters, all dating from the last four years of Vincent's life—to make plain that Theo's mind and heart were equally involved. Even where Theo's letters are not preserved, the very ways in which Vincent expressed himself can be seen as contingent upon his brother's reactions. He consistently reported the details of his budget at length, and whenever he ran short of money he would set out in strategically persuasive fashion the reasons why it was desirable that Theo should send him more than usual, or dispatch his regular sum in advance of the customary date. Further, when discussing deeper concerns of his, he characteristically related his hopes and ambitions to the prospect of achieving sales through Theo's agency as a dealer, or to the possibility that his day-to-day living expenses might in some way be reduced.

Vincent expected from his brother both the reassurance that he was doing the right thing in continuing to paint and the faith that the money devoted to his support constituted a sound investment. The very tentativeness with which he phrased his continuous flood of inquiries and suggestions was motivated by the need to draw from this, his most permanent relationship with another human being, self-confidence both in his moral purpose and in his artistic future—so that he could order his doings accordingly and feel sustained by the knowledge that here at least the basic human needs of love and trust were under constant renewal. Because Theo on his part gave his mind to each new problem in turn, offered encouragement, invited clarifications and gave justifications for the best that he could do—because, in other words, his sympathy and solicitude were direct and immediate—the correspondence reflects a psychological relationship to which the nearest parallel in normal experience would be the effect upon a man and woman of years of living together. Far from being a merely one-sided form of emotional release the correspondence took on the function, chiefly under Vincent's impetus, of intensifying a close blood-relationship and common interest in the arts into a form in which two people, spiritually and intellectually, depended on one another in an almost absolute way.

The written word and the painted image are of their nature more deliberate than ordinary speech or action; and the pattern of the letters, side by side with his art, gave Vincent a necessary conviction that a shape and scheme existed in a life which otherwise appeared troubled and lacking in design. It was a shape and scheme which, by its very continuity, implied the possibility of resistance to those forces of psychic disturbance that might otherwise carry the brothers apart and leave Vincent utterly alone—a palpable expression, in fact, of a kinship that prolonged scrutiny of each other's words and actions at close quarters would certainly have destroyed, to judge from the rank disharmony that sprang up during the two-year period when they were living together. When, at last, the same psychic disruptions took their toll on one side, driving the painter to shoot himself, the results on the other side were equally disastrous. Less than three months after Vincent's funeral, Theo himself went mad while straining to organize a commemorative exhibition; he had to be removed from the Paris scene and died immediately afterwards. There, in postscript form, lies the most dramatic of all evidence as to what exactly the dependance between the two brothers entailed.

The relationship by letter with his brother involved van Gogh, as described, in the retailing of every kind of information that was of practical consequence: the state of his health and energies and his consequent rate of work, the amount he was spending on food and rent, the quality of the paints and canvas that could be afforded on his behalf, the current weather conditions and the supply of local people willing to act as models, the disposal of his finished work and the choice

of suitable frames. Again and again the first things that he
had to report ran along lines like these:

As soon as I received your letter I bought 7 guilders'
worth of colour at once, so as to have some provisions
and to replenish my box. Throughout the week we have
had a lot of wind, storm and rain, and I went several
times to Scheveningen to see it. I brought home from
there two small seascapes . . . But another souvenir is
that I caught cold again, with all the outcomes you know,
and this forces me to stay at home for a few days . . .
When you next send money I shall buy some good
marten brushes, which are the real *drawing* brushes, as
I have discovered, for *drawing* a hand or a profile in
colour . . . My painting paper is also almost used up—
towards the first of September I shall have to buy a few
more supplies, but I shall not need more than the usual
allowance.

(August, 1882)

Thank you for your letter, but I've had a poor time of it
these last days; my money ran out on *Thursday,* and
so it proved a *hellishly long time* between then and
Monday noon. During these four days I have lived
mainly off coffee, 23 cups of it, with bread which I still
have to pay for. You are not to blame, if anyone is it's
me. Because I had a furious desire to see my pictures in
frames, and I had ordered rather too many of them for
my budget, seeing that the month's rent and the charwoman had to be paid also. Even now, too, I shall be
drained dry to-day, since I must buy canvas also and prepare it myself . . . I am so much involved in work that
I cannot stop myself short. Rest assured, the bad weather
will stop me only too soon—the way it was today, yesterday and the day before as well.

(October, 1888)

And then too, alongside such prosaic details of an average

week's existence, the correspondence involved van Gogh in the formulation of a theory of art; that is, in statements setting out the nature and direction of his current artistic efforts and the conceptual significance for him of his completed pictures, or in discussions of the artists of the past that he admired most and the future of art as a whole. For example:

> I told you about my plan for a large drawing—well, I started it the very same day that I wrote to you . . . I have worked on it since then . . . I saw it clearly before me and wanted to carry it through. I made the composition simpler still, only one row of diggers. I sketched seven figures in it, five men and two women; the rest are smaller, on the second plane. It is the strongest drawing I have ever made. As to the conception . . . I adopted the manner of certain English artists, without thinking of imitating them—rather, no doubt, because I am attracted by the same kinds of thing in nature; these are taken up by relatively few, so that if one wants to make use of them one must seek a way to express what one feels and venture a little outside the ordinary rules in order to render them exactly as one wants.
>
> (June, 1883)

> Who will be in figure painting what Claude Monet is in landscape? . . . the painter of the future will be *a colourist such as has never yet been* . . . This painter who is to come—I can't imagine him living in little cafés, working away with several false teeth and going to the Zouaves' brothels, as I do. But I think that I am right when I feel that in a later generation it will come, and that as for us we must work as we can towards that end, without doubting and without wavering.
>
> (May, 1888)

Between practical information and pronouncements in the realm of art-theory, two aspects of Vincent's personality and vision revealed themselves as dominant. One of these was his conception of success, and the forms of self-criticism that attended it; the other was his propensity to relate every form of experience to his personal feelings, and instinctively find an identity for it in terms of this kind. For example:

> I think that it would greatly help me in my work if I had an opportunity to see more of printing, for instance ... if I could get work in a printer's office or some such job, it would be a help rather than a hindrance ... I am willing to try my hand at *anything* of that kind, especially if a living may be earned in that way. Indeed, I believe that there will come a time when it will not be necessary for me to earn a living in any other way than by painting.
>
> (November, 1883)

> I wanted to express how those ruins show that *for ages* the peasants have been laid to rest in the very fields which they dug up when alive—I wanted to say what a simple thing death and burial is, just as simple as the falling of an autumn leaf—just a bit of earth dug up—a wooden cross.
>
> (June, 1885)

In fact self-improvement, where his art was concerned, was for van Gogh both a moral and a technical affair. His work, as he saw it, could constantly be bettered by dint of attentive study and practice; to engage in this task in the right spirit and faith would at the same time bring a progressive deepening of his capacities for human understanding. What could be learnt on the technical side from past masters like Rembrandt and Delacroix and from the renewal of self-discipline from work to work merged with what was offered in the theoretical writings of men like Carlyle and Tolstoy, thinkers who believed that art could once more become supremely relevant to the workings of society as a whole. In his invariable optimism about the future, van Gogh set enormous store

by the prospect of his making good—not so much because
success would vindicate his presumed abilities, as because it
would bear witness when it came to the essential "rightness"
of the universe. It was not that the world owed him a debt
and would eventually be compelled to pay it, but rather that
the world would one day receive what he had it in him to
give; and then success would bring repayment to those who
had trusted in him, most especially his brother, and would
increase the expectation at large for the generation of artists
to which he belonged himself, and for other generations to
come.

In the same way van Gogh's absolutely personal way of
translating experience into words or paint merged the concrete and the theoretical as if there was no kind of a gap
between them. The coalescence that he made between the
visible aspects of experience and their internal or philosophic
meaning was supremely intense; so intense, indeed, that it
can almost be compared as a pattern of thought with the idea
of the primitive tribesman that his wooden rain-god *is* the
rain itself. Among many allusions in the letters illustrative
of this point, the most recurrent are van Gogh's admiration
of the works of earlier artists for the reflection he found in
them of his own feelings for the subjects they had depicted,
and, conversely, his use of some familiar pictorial image as a
term of reference for identifying emotions aroused in him by
particular sights and scenes :

Israëls' *An Old Man* . . . is sitting in a corner near the
hearth, on which a small piece of peat is faintly glowing
in the twilight. For it is a dark little cottage where that
old man sits, an old cottage with a small white-curtained
window. His dog, that has grown old with him, sits
beside his chair—those two old friends look at each
other, they look into each other's eyes, the dog and the
man. And meanwhile the old man takes his tobacco
pouch from his pocket and lights his pipe in the twilight; that is all, the twilight, the silence, the loneliness

of those two old friends, the man and the dog, the
understanding between those two . . .

(March, 1882)

One evening recently at Montmajour I saw a red sunset,
shooting its rays on to the trunks and foliage of pines
that were rooted in a conglomeration of rocks, colouring
the trunks and foliage a fiery orange, while other pines on
planes further back in space were silhouetted in Prussian blue against a sky of tender blue-green, cerulean. So
it gave the effect of that Claude Monet, it was superb.

(May, 1888)

Whenever in fact van Gogh linked two categories of experience in order to recreate the newer of them for his own and
his reader's benefit, it was characteristic of him to urge their
complete identity.

Many artists of the past century who have written about
their own work have done so *post facto* and with some kind
of public audience in mind (however indirectly); most often
they have tended to make their case by abstracting from
current literary and æsthetic speculation whatever suited their
individual requirements. Van Gogh's theory of art, on the
other hand, set out to prescribe, not to explain. Indeed, in
view of the inclusiveness of its recommendations, it lays
claim to interpretation as a comprehensive artistic ideology.

Certainly the way of thinking in question here had an
essential solidity, however far and wide it ranged in the promotion of more or less remote possibilities. Van Gogh's
thought was centred always around a nucleus of ideological
belief, and he modified his principles of life and art in the
light of new experiences only to the degree and in the direction permitted by these underlying convictions. This was
true of his visual experiences before both art and nature; of
his experiences of literature—he was an avid reader all his
life, constantly ready to identify himself with the central
character of each book in turn; of his reactions to æsthetic

theories that he read about or heard discussed. He was not
averse to provisional experiment, but in the long run he
always fell back on to fundamentals; the content of the Bible,
for example, was as much of a fundamental to him at the
end of his life as it had been in his youth, even though
specific reference to it came to play a much smaller part in
his letters than it had in the years when religion had offered
him a practical goal. There is, therefore, a good deal of
repetition in his correspondence—even between letters widely
separated in date. There is perhaps also less of an expansion
of ideas between 1880 and 1890 than one might expect a man
of such extraordinary sensitivity to reveal between the ages
of twenty-seven and thirty-seven. It would be wrong, however, to assume on these counts that van Gogh was inflexible
either as a human being or as a thinker. The fact is rather
that, given the way of thinking that he instinctively made his
own, his development was bound to follow a self-extending
pattern; and what this self-extension reached out for was the
finding that in fundamentals lay the true and permanent
source of creative energy.

The solidity of van Gogh's thought has a further and
broader aspect. In terms of the cultural predicament of his
time, this took the form of a passion for wholeness to set
against the fragmentation of artistic sensibility that had
increasingly characterized the nineteenth century. In terms
of his personal life, it expressed a determination to keep his
mind from, literally, going under—because van Gogh knew
in advance what mental breakdown meant, he had the will
and the drive to prescribe preventative measures. As he saw
it, men were the poorer in that art was no longer something
one felt called to, in the way that he did, as a way of transmitting the basic common truths of love and faith and suffering. Instead, the subjects of art had split apart from one
another and so had its technical means (landscape and figure,
for example, colour and modelling). It was above all necessary that art absorb back into its bloodstream the universals
of human existence. Vincent's thought, then, required the
firmness of bulwarks built against an encroaching tide: the

tide of decadence and disorder. It had to command the presence of values, now lost, in works of art and literature transmitted from the past, through which the guide-lines of a continuing tradition were taken to run; and it needed also a wholesome and godly soundness of its own. Other nineteenth century thinkers before van Gogh—notably the proponents of the Gothic Revival—had similarly pleaded for restoration of the values of an earlier age, so that art and society, religion and culture might be re-unified. Certain of these thinkers had carried the Romantic concept of freedom to its logical conclusion, abandoning the present altogether in an advocacy of the past which was tantamount to escapism. But for van Gogh the processes of resistance and re-creation were not inherently divisible.

So finally one comes to the total picture of van Gogh which the *Letters to Theo* proclaim. Precisely where the paintings themselves might most readily tend to mislead, with their dynamic energy and their arbitrariness of colouring, these writings of the artist offer a firm corrective. They show an extraordinarily articulate man—anything but naïve and crazy, as a popular form of myth tends even now to imply. Van Gogh was in fact deeply interested in the contemporary intellectual scene and very much in control of his own destiny for all but a few weeks of his later career—the weeks in which he was actually struck down by his mental disease. Above all he was a man who committed himself to his work and his beliefs to the highest degree. "How difficult life must be," he wrote to Theo in one of his earliest letters, "if it is not strengthened and comforted by faith." And just a few weeks before his death he was able to say: "I still love art and life very much indeed."

M. R.

Cambridge, Mass.
August, 1962

MEMOIR OF VINCENT VAN GOGH

BY HIS SISTER-IN-LAW

The family name, van Gogh, is probably derived from the small town Gogh on the German frontier, but in the 16th century the van Goghs were already established in Holland. According to the "Annales Généalogiques" of Arnold Buchelius, there lived at that time a Jacob van Gogh at Utrecht "In the Owl behind the Town Hall," and Jan Jacob's son, who lived "In the Bible under the flax market," selling wine and books, was Captain of the Civil Guard.

Their coat-of-arms was a bar with three roses, which is still the family crest of the van Goghs.

In the 17th century we find many van Goghs occupying high offices of state in Holland. Johannes van Gogh, magistrate of Zutphen, is appointed High Treasurer of the Union in 1628; Michel van Gogh, at first Consul General in Brazil, afterwards treasurer of Zeeland, belongs to the Embassy that welcomes Charles II of England on his ascent to the throne in 1660. In about the same period, Cornelius van Gogh is a Remonstrant clergyman at Boskoop, and his son Matthias, at first a physician at Gouda, is afterwards clergyman at Moordrecht.

In the beginning of the 18th century the social standing of the family is somewhat lowered. A David van Gogh, who settled at The Hague, is a gold-wire drawer, like his eldest son Jan, who married Maria Stalvius, both belonging to the Walloon Church.

David's second son, Vincent (1729-1802), was a sculptor by profession, and is said to have been in Paris in his youth; in 1749 he was one of the Cent Suisses. With him the practice of art seems to have come into the family, together with fortune; he died single and left some money to his nephew Johannes (1763-1840), the son of his elder brother Jan van Gogh.

This Johannes was at first a gold-wire drawer like his father, but he afterwards became a Bible teacher, and clerk in the Cloister Church at The Hague. He was married to Johanna van der Vin of Malines, and their son Vincent (1789-1874) was enabled, by the legacy of his great uncle Vincent, to study theology at the University of Leiden. This Vincent, the grandfather of our painter, was a man of great intellect and extraordinarily strong sense of duty. At the Latin school he distinguished himself and won all prizes and testimonials; "the diligent and studious youth, Vincent van Gogh, fully deserves to be set up as an example to his fellow students for his good behaviour as well as for his persistent zeal," declares the rector of the school, Mr. de Booy, in 1805. At the University of Leiden he finishes his studies successfully, and graduates in 1811 at the age of twenty-two. He makes friends; his "album amicorum" preserves their memory in many Latin and Greek verses; a little silk embroid-ered wreath of violets and forget-me-nots, signed, E. H. Vry-dag 1810, is wrought by the hand of the girl who became his wife as soon as he got the living of Benschop. They lived long and happily together, first at the parsonage of Benschop, then at Ochten, and from 1822 at Breda, where his wife died in 1857, and where he remained until his death, a deeply respected and honoured man.

Twelve children were born to them, of which one died in infancy; there was a warm cordial family feeling between them, and however far the children might drift apart in the world, they remained deeply attached and took part in each other's weal and woe. Two of the daughters married high placed officers, the Generals Pompe and 's Graeuwen; three remained single.

The six sons all occupied honourable positions in the world. Johannes went to sea and reached the highest rank in the navy, that of Vice-Admiral; at the time that he was command-ant of the Navy Yard at Amsterdam in 1877, his nephew Vincent lived at his house for a time. Three sons became art dealers; the eldest Hendrik Vincent, "Uncle Hein" as he was called in the letters, had his business at first at Rotterdam and afterwards settled at Brussels. Cornelius Marinus became the head of the firm C. M. van Gogh, so well known in Amsterdam. (His nephews often called him by his initials C. M.). The third, who had the greatest influence on the lives of his nephews Vincent and Theo, was Vincent, whose health in his youth had been too weak to enable him to go to college, to the deep regret of his father, who based the greatest expectations on him. He opened a little shop at The Hague, where he sold colours and drawing materials, and which he enlarged in a few years to an art gallery of European renown. He was an extraordinarily gifted, witty, and intelligent man, who had great influence in the world of art at that time; Goupil in Paris offered him the partnership in his firm, which only after van Gogh joined it reached its highest renown. He settled in Paris and Mr. Tersteeg became the head of the firm in The Hague in his place. It was here that Vincent and Theo got their first training in business; Goupil was "the house" that played such a large part in their lives, where Theo remained and made a successful career, where Vincent worked for six years, and to which his heart clung in spite of all, because in his youth it had been to him "the best, the grandest, the most beautiful in the world" (letter 332).

Only one of parson van Gogh's six sons chose the profession of his father. Theodorus (8 Febr. 1822-26 March 1885) studied theology at Utrecht, graduated, and in 1849 got the living of Groot-Zundert, a little village in Brabant on the Belgian frontier, where he was confirmed by his father. Theodorus van Gogh was a man of prepossessing appearance ("the handsome dominie" he was called by some), of a loving nature and fine spiritual qualities, but he was not a gifted preacher, and for twenty years he lived forgotten in the small village of Zundert ere he was called to other places, and even then only to small villages like Etten, Helvoirt and Nuenen. But in his small circle he was warmly loved and respected, and his children idolized him.

In May 1851 he married Anna Cornelia Carbentus, who was born in 1819 at The Hague, where her father Willem

Carbentus was a flourishing bookbinder. He had bound the first Constitution of Holland and thereby earned the title of "bookbinder to the King." His youngest daughter Cornelia was already married to Vincent van Gogh, the art dealer; his eldest daughter was the wife of the well-known clergyman Stricker at Amsterdam. The marriage of Theodorus van Gogh and Anna Carbentus was a very happy one. He found in his wife a helpmate, who shared with all her heart in his work; notwithstanding her own large family that gave her so much work, she visited his parishioners with him, and her cheerful and lively spirit was never quenched by the monotony of the quiet village life. She was a remarkable, lovable woman, who in her old age (she reached her 87th year), when she had lost her husband and three grown-up sons, still retained her energy and spirit and bore her sorrow with rare courage.

One of her qualities, next to her deep love of nature, was the great facility with which she could express her thoughts on paper; her busy hands, that were always working for others, grasped so eagerly not only needle and knitting needle, but also the pen. "I just send you a little word" was one of her favourite expressions, and how many of these "little words" came always just in time to bring comfort and strength to those to whom they were addressed. For almost twenty years they have been to myself a never failing source of hope and courage, and in this book, that is a monument to her sons, a word of grateful remembrance is due to their mother.

On the 30th of March 1852 a dead son was born at the vicarage of Zundert, but a year after on the same date Anna van Gogh gave birth to a healthy boy who was called Vincent Willem after his two grandfathers, and who in qualities and character, as well as in appearance took after his mother more than after his father. The energy and unbroken strength of will which Vincent showed in his life were, in principle, traits of his mother's character; from her also he took the sharp inquisitive glance of the eye from under the protruding eyebrows. The blonde complexion of both the parents turned in Vincent to a reddish hue; he was of medium height, rather broad shouldered, and his appearance made a strong, sturdy impression. This is also confirmed by the words of his mother, that none of the children *except* Vincent was very strong. A weaker constitution than his would certainly have broken down much sooner under the heavy strain Vincent put upon it. As a child he was of difficult temper, often troublesome and self-willed, and his bringing up was not fitted to counterbalance these faults, as the parents were very tender-hearted especially for their eldest. Once grandmother van Gogh, who had come from Breda to visit her children at Zundert, witnessed one of the naughty fits of little Vincent; she who had been taught by experience with her own twelve babies, took the little culprit by the arm and with a sound box on the ears put him out of the room. The tender-hearted mother was so indignant at this that she did not speak to her mother-in-law for a whole day, and only the sweet-tempered character of the young father succeeded in bringing about a reconciliation. In the evening he had a little carriage brought around, and drove the two women to the heath, where under the influence of a beautiful sunset they forgave each other.

Little Vincent had a great love for animals and flowers, and made all kinds of collections; of any extraordinary gift for drawing there was as yet no sign; it is only noted that at the age of eight he once modelled a little elephant of clay, that drew his parents' attention, but he destroyed it at once when according to his notion such a fuss was made about it. The same fate befell a very curious drawing of a cat, which his mother always remembered. For a short time he attended the village school, but his parents found that the intercourse with the peasant boys made him too rough, so a governess was sought for the children of the vicarage, whose number had meanwhile increased to six. Two years after Vincent a little daughter had been born and again two years later on the 1st of May 1857, came a son who was called after his father. After him came two sisters and a little brother. (The younger sister Willemien, who always lived with her mother, was the only one to whom Vincent wrote on rare occasions.) Theo was more tender and kind than his brother, who was four years older; he was more delicately built and finer featured, but of the same reddish fair complexion and he had the same light blue eyes, that sometimes darkened to a greenish blue.

In letter 338 Vincent himself describes the similarity and the difference in their looks, and in 1889 Theo wrote to me the following about Vincent's appearance, referring to Rodin's marble sculpture, the head of John the Baptist. " The sculptor has conceived an image of the precursor of Christ that exactly resembles Vincent. Yet he never saw him. That expression of sorrow, that forehead distorted by deep furrows, which denotes high thinking and iron self discipline, is Vincent's, though his is somewhat more sloping; the form of nose and structure of the head are the same." When I afterwards saw the marble I found in it a perfect resemblance to Theo.

The two brothers were strongly attached to each other from childhood; whereas the eldest sister, recalling youthful memories, speaks of Vincent's teasing ways, Theo only remembers that Vincent could invent such delightful games that once they made him a present of the most beautiful rose bush in their garden, to show their gratitude. Their childhood was full of the poetry of Brabant country life; they grew up among the cornfields, the heath and the pine forests, in that peculiar sphere of a village parsonage, the charms of which remained with them all their lives. It was not perhaps the best training to fit them for the hard struggle that awaited them both; they were still so very young, when they had to go out into the world, and with what bitter melancholy, and with what inexpressible home-sickness did they long during many years for the sweet home in the little village on the heath.

Vincent came back there several times, and remained always in appearance the "country boor," but Theo, who had become quite a refined Parisian, also kept in his heart something of the "Brabant boy" as he laughingly liked to call himself.

Like Vincent once rightly observes: "there will always remain in us something of the Brabant fields and heath," and when their father had died and mother had to leave the parsonage, he complains, "now there is none of us left in Brabant." When afterwards, in the hospital of Arles, the faithful brother visited him and in tender pity laid his head on the pillow beside him, Vincent whispered: "just like Zundert," and shortly after he writes: "during my illness I have seen every room in the house at Zundert, every path, every plant in the garden, the fields around, the neighbours, the churchyard, the church, our kitchen garden behind it— and even the magpie's nest in the high acacia in the church-yard" (letter 573).

So ineffaceable were those first sunny childhood's recollections. When Vincent was twelve years old he was sent to the boarding school of Mr. Provily at Zevenbergen; about this period not a single particular has been found, except that one of the sisters afterwards writes to Theo: "Do you remember how on mother's birthday Vincent used to come from Zevenbergen and what fun we had then?" Of friends in that time nothing is known.

When he was sixteen years old the choice of a profession became urgent and in this Uncle Vincent was consulted.

The latter, who meanwhile had acquired a large fortune as an art dealer, had been obliged by his feeble health to retire early from the strenuous business life in Paris—though still financially connected with the firm—and had settled at Princenhage, near his old father at Breda, and near his favourite brother at Zundert. Generally he passed the winter with his wife at Mentone in the south of France, and on his journey thither he always stayed some time at Paris, so that he remained in touch with the business. His beautiful country house at Princenhage had been enlarged by a gallery for his rare picture collection, and it was here that Vincent and Theo received their first impressions of the world of art. There was a warm cordial intercourse between the Zundert parsonage and the childless home of Princenhage; "the carriage" from there was always loudly cheered by the children at Zundert, for it brought many surprises of flowers, rare fruits and delicacies, while on the other hand the bright, lively presence of the brother and sister from Zundert often cast a cheerful sunbeam on the life of the patient at Princenhage. These brothers, Vincent and Theo too, who differed but one year in age, were thoroughly attached to each other, and the fact of their wives being sisters made the attachment stronger still. What was more natural than that the rich art dealer destined the young nephew who bore his name as his successor in the firm—perhaps even to become his heir?

Thus in 1869 Vincent entered the house of Goupil & Co., at The Hague, as youngest employee under the direction of Mr. Tersteeg, now a bright future seemed to lie in store for him. He boarded with the family Roos on the Beestenmarkt, where Theo afterwards lived also. It was a comfortable home where his material needs were perfectly provided for, but without any intellectual intercourse. This he found at the homes of various relations and friends of his mother, where he often visited, i.e. the Haanebeek's, the van Stockum's and aunt Sophy Carbentus with her three daughters, one of whom married our famous Dutch painter, A. Mauve, a second the less known painter, A. le Comte. Tersteeg sent to the parents good reports about Vincent's zeal and capacities, and like his grandfather in his time, he is " the diligent studious youth " whom everybody likes.

When he had been at The Hague for three years, Theo, who is still at school at Oisterwijk (near Helvoirt, to which village their father has been called), comes to stay with him for a few days. It is after that visit in August 1872 that the correspondence between the two brothers begins, and from this, now faded, yellow, almost childish, little note it is carried on uninterruptedly until Vincent's death, when a half-finished letter to Theo was found on him, of which the desponding " que veux-tu " (what can I say) at the end, seems like a gesture of resignation with which he parted from life.

The principal events of both their lives are mentioned in the letters and are completed in this biographical notice by particulars, either heard from Theo himself, or found in the correspondence of the parents with Theo, also preserved in full. (Vincent's letters to his parents were unfortunately de-

stroyed.) They date from January 1873, when Theo, then
only fifteen years old, went to Brussels to be also brought up
as an art dealer.

These letters, full of the tenderest love and care for the
boy who left home at such a tender age—" well Theo you are
quite a man now at fifteen," says his mother in one of her
letters; the boy to whom they clung so fondly, because he,
more than any of the other children, repays their love with
never failing tenderness and devotion, and grows up to be
" the crowning glory of their old age," as they were so fond
of calling him—these letters tell of all the small events of
daily life at the parsonage; what flowers were growing in the
garden, and how the fruit trees bore, if the nightingale had
been heard yet, what visitors had come, what the little sisters
and brother were doing, what was the text of father's sermon,
and among all this, many particulars about Vincent.

In 1873 the latter has been appointed to the firm in
London. When leaving The Hague he gets a splendid testi-
monial from Mr. Tersteeg, who also writes to the parents
that at the gallery everybody likes to deal with Vincent—
amateurs, clients, as well as painters—and that he certainly
will succeed in his profession. " It is a great satisfaction
that he can close the first period of his career in that way, and
withal he has remained just as simple as he was before,"
writes mother. At first everything goes well with him in
London; Uncle Vincent has given him introductions to some
of his friends and he busies himself with great pleasure in
his work; he earns a salary of £90 a year, and though living
is expensive, he manages to lay by some money to send
home now and then. Like a real business man he buys himself a top hat, " you cannot be in London without one," and
he enjoys his daily trips from the suburbs to the gallery in
Southampton Street in the city.

His first boarding-house is kept by two ladies, who own
two parrots, the place is good but somewhat expensive for
him, therefore he moves in August to the house of Mrs.
Loyer, a curate's widow from the south of France, who with
her daughter Ursula keeps a day school for little children.

Here he spends the happiest year of his life. Ursula makes a deep impression upon him—" I never saw nor dreamt of anything like the love between her and her mother " he writes to one of his sisters, and : " love her for my sake."

He does not mention it to his parents, for he has not even confessed his love to Ursula herself,—but his letters home are radiant with happiness. He writes that he enjoys his life so much—" Oh fulness of rich life, your gift, Oh God."[1]

In September an acquaintance is going over to London and undertook to carry a parcel for Vincent, and it is characteristic to hear that it contains, among other things, a bunch of grass leaves and a wreath of oak leaves, made at home during the holidays by Theo, who has meanwhile been appointed from Brussels to the House Goupil at The Hague. Vincent must have something in his room to remind him of the beloved fields and woods.

He celebrates a happy Christmas with the Loyers, and in those days he sends home now and then a little drawing, from his house and the street and from the interior of his room, " so that we can exactly imagine how it looks, it is so well drawn," writes his mother. In this period he seems to have weighed the possibility of becoming a painter; afterwards from Drenthe he writes to Theo : " how often have I stood drawing on the Thames Embankment, as I went home from Southampton Street in the evening—and the result was nihil; had there been somebody then to tell me what perspective was, how much trouble would have been spared me, how much farther should I be now."

At that time he now and then met Matthew Maris,[2] but was too bashful to speak out freely to him, and shut up all his longings and desires within himself—he had still a long road of sorrow to go ere he could reach his goal.

In January his salary is raised and until spring his letters remain cheerful and happy; he intends to visit Holland in July and before that time seems to have spoken to Ursula of his love. Alas it turns out that she is already engaged to

[1] First line of a well known Dutch poem.
[2] Famous Dutch painter, living in London.

somebody, who boarded with them before Vincent came. He tries all his influence to make her break this engagement but does not succeed, and with this first great sorrow there comes a change in his character; when he comes home for the holidays he is thin, silent, dejected, a changed being. But he *draws* a great deal. Mother writes : " Vincent made many a nice drawing, he drew the bedroom window and the front door, all that part of the house, and also a large sketch of those houses in London upon which their window looks out; it is a delightful talent, that can be of great value to him."

Accompanied by his eldest sister, who wants to find a situation, he returns to London; he takes furnished rooms in Ivy Cottage, 395 Kensington New Road, and there without any family life he grows more and more silent and depressed and also more and more religious.

His parents were glad he left the Loyers—" there were too many secrets and it was not a family like others; but it must have been a great disappointment to him that his illusions were not realized," father writes, and mother complains, " the evenings are so long already and his work finishes early, he must be lonely, if it only does not harm him."

They feel uneasy and worried about his solitary, secluded life. Uncle Vincent also insists upon his mixing more with other people, " that is just as necessary as to learn business "; but the depressed mood continues, letters home grow more and more scarce, and mother begins to think that the London fog depresses him and that even a temporary change might do him good—" poor boy, he means so well, but I believe things are very hard for him just now."

In October 1874, Uncle Vincent effects indeed a short removal to the firm in Paris, but Vincent himself is little pleased by this, in fact he is so angry that he does not write home, to the great grief of his parents. " He is only in a bad temper," his sister says, and Theo comforts, " he is doing all right."

Towards the end of December he returns to London where he takes the same rooms and leads the same retired life. Now for the first time the word *eccentric* is applied to him. His love for drawing has ceased, but he reads much and the quotation from Renan that closes the London period clearly shows what filled his thoughts and how he aimed even then at the high ideal: " to sacrifice all personal desires, to realize great things, to obtain nobleness of mind, to surpass the vulgarity in which the existence of nearly all individuals is spent." He did not know yet which way he had to go to reach that aim.

In May 1875, he is placed permanently in Paris and assigned especially to the picture gallery, where he feels himself quite out of place; he is more at home in his " cabin," the little room at Montmartre where, morning and evening, he reads the Bible with his young friend, Harry Gladwell, than among the mondaine Parisian public.

His parents read from his letters that things are not going well, and when he comes home at Christmas and everything is talked over, father writes to Theo: " I almost think that Vincent had better leave Goupil in two or three months; there is so much that is good in him, but yet it may be necessary for him to change his position, he is certainly not happy." And they love him too well to persuade him to stay in a place where he would be unhappy; he wants to live for others, to be useful, to bring about something great, *how* he does not know as yet, but *not* in an art gallery. On his return from Holland he has the decisive interview with Mr. Boussod (the son-in-law and successor of Mr. Goupil) that ends with his dismissal on the 1st of April, and he accepts it without bringing in any excuses for himself. One of the grievances against him was that he had gone home to Holland for Christmas and New Year, the busiest time for business in Paris.

In his letters he seems to take it rather lightly, but he feels how gloomily and threateningly the clouds begin to gather around him. At the age of twenty-three years he is now thrown out of employment, without any chance of a better career; Uncle Vincent is deeply disappointed in his namesake and washes his hands of him; his parents are well-meaning, but they cannot do much for him having been obliged to touch their capital for the education of their children. (The pastor's salary was about 820 guilders a year.) Vincent has had his share, now others must have theirs. It seems that Theo who becomes so soon the helper and adviser of all, has already at that time suggested Vincent's becoming a painter, but for the moment he will not hear of it. His father speaks of a position in a museum and advises him to open a small art gallery for himself, as Uncle Vincent and Uncle Cor have done before; he would then be able to follow his own ideas about art and be no longer obliged to sell pictures which he considered bad—but his heart again draws him to England and he plans to become a teacher.

Through an advertisement, in April 1876 he gets a position in Ramsgate at Mr. Stokes', who moves his school in July to Isleworth. He received only board and lodging, but no salary, so he soon accepts another position at the somewhat richer school of Mr. Jones, a Methodist preacher, where Vincent acts finally as a kind of curate.

His letters home are gloomy. "It seems as if something were threatening me," he writes, and his parents perceive full well that teaching does not satisfy him. They suggest his studying for a French or German college certificate, but he will not hear of it. " I wish he could find some work in connection with art or nature," writes his mother, who understands what is going on within him. With the force of despair he clings to religion, in which he tries to find satisfaction for his craving for beauty, as well as for his longing to live for others. At times he seems to intoxicate himself with the sweet melodious words of the English texts and hymns, the romantic charm of the little village church, and the lovely, holy atmosphere that envelops the English service. His letters in those days bear an almost morbid sensitiveness. Often and often he speaks about a position related to the church—but when he comes home for Christmas, it is decided that he will not go back to Isleworth, because there is absolutely no prospect for the future. He remains on friendly terms with Mr. Jones, who afterwards comes to stay a few days at the Nuenen parsonage, and whom he later meets in

Belgium. Once more Uncle Vincent uses his influence and procures for him a place in the bookshop of Blussé and Braam at Dordrecht. He accepts it, but without great enthusiasm. Characteristic are the words written to Theo by one of the sisters. "You think that he is something more than an ordinary human being, but I think it would be much better if he thought himself just an ordinary being." Another sister writes, "His religion makes him absolutely dull and unsociable."

To preach the Gospel still seems to him the only desirable thing, and at last an attempt is made to enable him to begin the study of Theology. The uncles in Amsterdam promised to give their aid; he can live with Uncle Jan van Gogh, Commandant of the Navy Yard, which will be a great saving of expenses: Uncle Stricker finds out the best teacher in the classical languages, the well-known Dr. Mendes da Costa, and gives him some lessons himself; in the art gallery at Uncle Cor's he can satisfy his love for pictures and prints and so everybody tries to make it easy for him, all except Uncle Vincent, who is strongly opposed to the plan and will not help to forward it—in which he proved to be right after all. Full of courage Vincent sets to work, he must first prepare himself for a State examination before he can be admitted to the University; it will take him seven years ere he is ready; anxiously the parents ask themselves whether he will have the strength to persevere, and whether he who has never been used to regular study will be able to force himself to it at the age of twenty-four.

That period in Amsterdam from May 1877 to 1878 is one long tale of woe. After the first half-year Vincent begins to lose ardour and courage; the writing of exercises and the study of grammar is not what he wants—he desires to comfort and cheer people by bringing them the Gospel,—and surely he does not need so much learning for that! He actually longs for *practical* work, and when at last his teacher also perceives that Vincent never will succeed, he advises him to give up the study. In the "Handelsblad" of the 30th of November 1910, Dr. Mendes da Costa writes his personal recollections of the afterwards so famous pupil, of whom he tells many characteristic particulars : his nervous, strange appearance, that yet was not without charm, his fervent intention to study well, his peculiar habit of self-discipline, self-chastisement, and finally his total unfitness for regular study. Not along that path was he to reach his goal! Openly he confesses that he is glad things have gone so far and that he can look towards his future with more courage than when he devoted himself hopelessly to Theological study, which period he afterwards called "the worst time of his life."

He will remain "humble" and now wants to become an Evangelist in Belgium; for this no certificates are required, no Latin nor Greek; only three months at the school of Evangelisation at Brussels—where lessons are free and only board and lodging are charged for—and he can get his nomination. In July he travels thither with his father, accompanied by Mr. Jones who on his way to Belgium has spent a few days with them at Etten, and together they visit the different members of the Committee of Evangelization : the Rev. van den Brink from Rousselaere, Rev. Pietersen from Malines, and Rev. de Jong from Brussels. Vincent explained his case clearly and made a very good impression. His father writes : " His stay abroad and that last year at Amsterdam have not been quite fruitless after all, and when he takes the trouble to exert himself he shows that he has learned and observed much in the school of life," and Vincent consequently is accepted as a pupil. But the parents regard this new experiment with fresh anxiety : " I am always so afraid that wherever Vincent may be or whatever he may do, he will spoil everything by his eccentricity, his queer ideas and views on life," his mother writes, and his father adds, " It grieves us so when we see that he literally knows no joy of life, but always walks with bent head, whilst we did all in our power to bring him to an honourable position! It seems as if he deliberately chooses the most difficult path."

In fact that was Vincent's aim—to humble himself, to forget himself, to sacrifice himself, "mourir à soi-même," (to sacrifice every personal desire), that was the ideal he tried to reach as long as he sought his refuge in religion, and he never did a thing by halves. But to follow the paths trodden by others, to submit to the will of other people, that was not in his character, he wanted to work out his own salvation. Towards the end of August he arrives at the school at Brussels, which had only been recently opened and counted but three pupils; in the class of Mr. Bokma he certainly was the most advanced, but he does not feel at home at the school, he is "like a fish out of water" he says, and is ridiculed for his peculiarities in dress and manners. He also misses the talent of extemporizing and is therefore obliged to read his lectures from manuscript; but the greatest objection against him is, "he is not submissive," and when the three months have elapsed he does not get his nomination. Though he writes it (in letter 126) in an off-hand way to Theo, he seems to have been greatly upset by it. His father receives a letter from Brussels, probably from the school, saying that Vincent is weak and thin, does not sleep, and is in a nervous and excited state, so that the best thing will be to come and take him home.

Immediately he travels to Brussels and succeeds in arranging everything for the best. Vincent goes at his own risk to the Borinage where he boards at 30 fr. a month with M. Van der Haegen, Rue de L'Eglise 39, at Paturages near Mons. He teaches the children in the evening, visits the poor and gives lectures from the Bible, and when in January the Committee meets, he will again try to get a nomination. The intercourse with the people there pleases him very well; in his leisure hours he draws large maps of Palestine, of which his father orders four at 10 fr. apiece, and at last, in January 1879, he gets a temporary nomination for six months at Wasmes at 50 fr. a month for which he must give Bible lectures, teach the children and visit the sick—the work of his heart. His first letters from there are very contented and he devotes himself heart and soul to his work, especially the practical part of it; his greatest interest is in nursing the sick and wounded. Soon, however, he falls back to the old exaggerations—he tries to put into practice the doctrines of Jesus, gives away every-

thing, his money, clothes and bed, he leaves the good boarding-house at Denis, in Wasmes, and retires to a miserable hut
where every comfort is wanting. Already they had written to
his parents about it and when, towards the end of February,
the Rev. Rochelieu comes for inspection, the bomb explodes,
for so much zeal is too much for the committee and a person
who neglects himself so cannot be an example to other people.
The Church Council at Wasmes have a meeting and they
agree that if he does not listen to reason he will lose his
position. He himself takes it rather coolly. " What shall we
do now?" he writes, " Jesus was also very calm in the storm,
perhaps it must grow worse before it grows better." Again his
father goes to him, and succeeds in stilling the storm; he
brings him back to the old boarding-house, advises him to be
less exaggerated in his work, and for some time everything is
all right, at least he writes that no reproofs are made. About
that time a heavy mine explosion occurs and a strike breaks
out, so Vincent can devote himself completely to the miners,
and his mother in her naïve religious faith writes, " Vincent's
letters that contain so many interesting things prove that with
all his singularities he yet shows a warm interest in the poor
and that surely will not remain unobserved by God." In that
same time he also writes that he tries to *sketch the dresses
and tools of the miners and will show them when he comes
home.* In July bad tidings come again, " he does not comply
with the wishes of the committee and nothing will change
him. It seems that he is deaf to all remarks that are made to
him," writes his mother, and when the six months of his
temporary nomination are past, he is not appointed again, but
they give him three months to look out for another position.
He leaves Wasmes and travels on foot to Brussels to ask the
Rev. Pietersen, who has moved thither from Malines, for
advice. The latter paints in his leisure hours and has a
studio, which probably was the reason why Vincent went to
him for help. Tired and hot, exhausted and in a nervous
condition he arrives there and so neglected was his appearance that the daughter of the house who opened the door for
him was frightened, called for her father and ran away. The

Rev. Pietersen received him kindly; procured him good lodgings for the night, invited him to his table the next day, showed him the studio, and as Vincent had brought some of his sketches of the miners, they probably talked as much about drawing and painting as about Evangelization.

"Vincent gives me the impression of somebody who stands in his own light," writes the Rev. Pietersen to his parents, and mother adds, "how lucky it is that still he always finds somebody who helps him on, as now the Rev. Pietersen has."

In accordance with the latter's advice, Vincent resolves to stay in the Borinage at his own expense, as he cannot be in the service of the committee, and that he will board with the Evangelist Frank, at Cuesmes. About the middle of August, at his parents' request, he visits them again at Etten. "He looks well, except for his clothes, he reads Dickens all day and speaks only when he is addressed, about his future not a single word," writes his mother. What could he say about his future? Did it ever look more hopeless than it did now? His illusion of bringing through the Gospel comfort and cheer into the miserable lives of the miners had gradually been lost in the bitter strife between doubt and religion, which he had to fight at that time, and which made him lose his former faith in God. (The Bible texts and religious reflections which became more and more rare in his last letters now stop entirely.) No other thing has taken its place yet; he draws much and reads much, among others, Dickens, Beecher Stowe, Victor Hugo, and Michelet, but it is all done without system or aim. Back in the Borinage he wanders about without work, without friends and very often without bread, for though he receives money from home and from Theo, they cannot give him more than is strictly necessary, and as it comes in at very irregular times and Vincent is a very poor financier, there are days and even weeks when he is quite without money.

In October Theo, who has got a permanent position at Goupil's in Paris, comes to visit him on his journey thither and tries in vain to bring him to some fixed plan for the future; he is not yet ripe to take any resolution; before he becomes conscious of his real power he has still to struggle through the awful winter of 1879-80, that saddest, most hopeless time of his never very fortunate life. In these days he undertakes, with ten francs in his pocket, the hopeless expedition to Courrières, the dwelling place of Jules Breton, whose pictures and poems he so much admires, and with whom he secretly hopes to come in contact in some way or other. But the only thing that becomes visible to him is the inhospitable exterior of Breton's newly built studio and he lacks the courage to introduce himself. Disappointed in his hope, he has to undertake the long journey home; his money is all spent, generally he sleeps in the open air or in a hay loft. Sometimes he exchanges a drawing for a piece of bread, and he undergoes so much fatigue and want that his health always suffered from the consequences. In spring he comes once more to the vicarage of Etten and speaks again about going to London. " If he really wants it, I shall enable him to go," writes his father, but finally he returns again to the Borinage and lives that summer of 1880 at the house of the miner Charles Decrucq at Cuesmes. There he writes in July the wonderfully touching letter (133) that tells of what is going on in his innermost self—" My only anxiety is what can I do . . . could I not be of use, and good for something?" It is the old wish, the old longing to serve and comfort humanity, which made him write afterwards, when he had found his calling, " And in a picture I wish to say something that would console me as music does." Now in the days of deepest discouragement and darkness at last the light begins to dawn. Not in books shall he find satisfaction, not in literature find his work, as his letters sometimes suggested; he turns back to his old love, " I said to myself, I'll take up my pencil again, I will take up drawing, and from that moment everything has changed for me." It sounds like a cry of deliverance, and once more, " do not fear for me, if I can continue my work I will succeed." At last he has found his work and herewith the mental equilibrium is restored; he no longer doubts of himself and however difficult or heavy his life may become the inward serenity, the conviction of his own calling never more deserts him.

The little room in the house of the miner Decrucq, which he has to share with the children, is his first studio. There he begins his painter's career with the first original drawing of miners who go to work in the early morning. There he copies with restless activity the large drawings after Millet, and when the room is getting too narrow for him, he takes his work out into the garden.

When the cold autumn weather prevents his doing this, and as his surroundings at Cuesmes are getting too narrow for him, he moves in October to Brussels where he settles in a small hotel on the Bd. du Midi 72. He is longing to see pictures again, but above all he hopes to become acquainted with other artists. Deep in his heart there was such a great longing for sympathy, for kindness and friendship, and though his difficult character generally prevented him from finding this and left him isolated in life, yet he always kept on longing for somebody with whom he could live and work.

Theo, who meanwhile had acquired a good position in Paris, could now assist him in word and deed. He brought Vincent into relation with the young Dutch painter van Rappard, who had worked some time in Paris and now studied at the academy at Brussels. At first the acquaintance did not progress, for the outward difference between the rich young nobleman and the neglected wanderer from the Borinage was too great to ripen the acquaintance at once into friendship; yet the artistic taste and opinions of both were too similar for them not to find each other; a friendship arose—perhaps the only one that Vincent ever had in Holland—it lasted for five years and then was broken through a misunderstanding, which van Rappard always regretted, though he acknowledged that intercourse with Vincent was very difficult.

" I remember as if it happened yesterday the moment of our first meeting at Brussels when he came into my room at nine o'clock in the morning, how at first we did not get on

very well together, but so much the better after we had
worked together a few times," writes van Rappard to Vincent's mother after the latter's death. And again, " whoever
has witnessed this wrestling, struggling and sorrowful existence could not but feel sympathy for the man who demanded
so much of himself, that it ruined body and mind. He belonged to the race that produces the great artists.

" Though Vincent and I had been separated the last years
by a misunderstanding which I have often regretted—I have
never ceased to remember him and the time we spent together
with great sympathy.

" Whenever in the future I shall remember that time, and it
is always a delight for me to recall the past, the characteristic
figure of Vincent will appear to me in such a melancholy but
clear light, the struggling and wrestling, fanatic, gloomy
Vincent, who used to flare up so often and was so irritable, but
who still deserved friendship and admiration for his noble
mind and highly artistic qualities."

Vincent's own opinion of van Rappard is clearly shown in
his letters. A second acquaintance that Vincent made through
Theo, with the painter Roelofs, was of less-during importance.
Roelofs' advice to enter the Academy was not followed by
Vincent, perhaps they did not admit him because he was not
far enough advanced, but probably he had more than enough
of academical institutions and theories, and in painting as well
as in theology he preferred to go his own way; that is the
reason he did not come into contact with other Dutch painters
who were at that same time at the Academy at Brussels, for
instance, Haverman.

He studied anatomy by himself, drew diligently from the
living model, and from a letter to his father it seems that he
took lessons in perspective from a poor painter at 1.50 fr. a
lesson of two hours : it has not been possible to fix the name
of the painter, it may have been Madiol.

At the end of the winter when van Rappard goes away, in
whose studio he has often worked because his own little bedroom was too small, he longs for other surroundings, especially for the country; the expenses in Brussels are also some-

what heavy, and he thinks it will be cheapest to go to his parents at Etten where he has board and lodging free and can use all money he receives for his work.

He stays there for eight months, and this summer of 1881 is again a happy time for him. First, van Rappard comes to stay with him and he too always remembers with pleasure his stay at the vicarage, "And my visit at Etten! I see you still sitting at the window when I came in," he writes to Vincent's mother in the letter quoted above, "I still enjoy that beautiful walk we all took together that first evening, through the fields and along the small path! And our excursions to Seppen, Passievaart, Liesbosch, I often look through my sketch books for them."

In the beginning of August Theo comes over from Paris; shortly after Vincent makes an excursion to The Hague to consult about his work with Mauve, who firmly encourages him, so that he continues with great animation, and finally in those days he meets for the second time a woman who has great influence on his life. Among the guests who spent that summer at the vicarage at Etten was a cousin from Amsterdam—a young widow with her little four-year-old son. Quite absorbed in her grief over the loss of her husband, whom she had loved so tenderly, she was unconscious of the impression which her beauty and touching sorrow made on the cousin, who was a few years her junior. "He was so kind to my little boy," she said when she afterwards remembered that time. Vincent who had great love for children, tried to win the heart of the mother by great devotion to the child. They walked and talked much together, and he has also drawn a portrait of her (which seems to have been lost), but the thought of a more intimate relation did not occur to her, and when Vincent spoke to her at last about his love, a very decided *no* was the immediate reply. She went back to Amsterdam and never saw him again. But Vincent could not abide by her decision, and with his innate tenacity he keeps on persevering and hoping for a change in her feelings for him; when his letters are not answered, he accuses both his and her parents of opposing the match, and only a visit to

Amsterdam, where she refuses to see him, convinces him of the utter hopelessness of his love.

" He fancied that he loved me," she said afterwards, but for him it was sad earnest, and her refusal becomes a turning point in his life. If she had returned his love it would perhaps have been a spur to him to acquire a social position, he would have had to provide for her and her child; as it is he loses all worldly ambition and in the future lives only for his work, without taking one step to make himself independent. He cannot bear to stay in Etten any longer, he has become irritable and nervous, his relations to his parents become strained, and after a violent altercation with his father, in December he leaves suddenly for The Hague.

The two years he spends there are, for his work, a very important period of which his letters give a perfect description. His low spirits rise at first, by the change of surroundings and the intercourse with Mauve, but the feeling of having been slighted and wronged does not leave him and he feels himself utterly abandoned. When he meets in January a poor neglected woman approaching her confinement, he takes her under his protection, partly from pity but also to fill the great void in his life. " I hope there is no harm in his so-called model. Bad connections often arise from a feeling of loneliness, of dissatisfaction," writes his father to Theo, who is always the confidant of both parties and has to listen to all the complaints and worries; father is not far wrong. Vincent could not be alone, he wanted to live for somebody, he wanted a wife and children, and as the woman he loved had rejected him, he took the first unhappy woman who crossed his path, with children that were not his own. At first he feigns to be happy and tries to convince Theo in every letter how wisely and well he has acted, and the touching care and tenderness with which he surrounds the woman when she leaves the hospital after her confinement, strike us painfully when we think on whom that treasure of love was lavished. He prides himself now on having a family of his own, but when their living together has become a fact and he is continually associated with a coarse, uneducated woman, marked by smallpox, who speaks with a low accent and has a spiteful character, who is addicted to liquor and smokes cigars, whose past life has not been irreproachable, and who draws him into all kinds of intrigues with her family,[1] he soon writes no more about his home life; even the posing, by which she won him (she sat for the beautiful drawing, "Sorrow"), and of which he had expected so much, soon ceases altogether. This unfortunate adventure deprives him of the sympathy of all in The Hague who took an interest in him. Neither Mauve nor Tersteeg could approve of his taking upon himself the cares of a family, and such a family! while he was financially dependent on his younger brother. Acquaintances and relatives are shocked to see him walk about with such a slovenly woman; nobody cares to associate with him any longer and his home life is such that nobody comes to visit him. The solitude around him becomes greater and greater and as usual it is only Theo who understands and continues to help him.

When the latter comes to visit Vincent for the second time in The Hague, in the summer of 1883, and witnesses the situation—finds the household neglected, everything in bad condition and Vincent deeply in debt—he too advises to let the woman go her own way as she is not fit for a regulated life. She herself had already felt that things could not continue like that, because Vincent wants too much money for his painting to leave enough for the support of her and the children, and she was already planning with her mother to earn money in another way. Vincent himself feels that Theo is right, and in his heart he longs for a change of surroundings, and liberty to go where his work calls him, but it costs him a bitter struggle to give up what he had taken upon himself, and to leave the poor woman to her fate. Till the last he defends her, and excuses her for her faults with the sublime words, "she has never seen what is good, so how can she be good?"

In those days of inward strife he allows Theo to read deeper than ever into his heart. These last letters from The

[1] This is in fact an exaggerated picture of the woman's character. [Ed.]

Hague (letters 313 to 322) give the key to many things that were incomprehensible until now. For the first time he speaks openly about what has happened at the time of his dismissal from Goupil, for the first time he explains his strange indifference to show his own work or to try to make it productive, when he writes, " it is so painful for me to speak to people. I am not afraid to do so, but I know I make a disagreeable impression; I am so much afraid that my efforts to introduce myself will do me more harm than good," and how naïvely he adds, " human brains cannot bear everything as is shown by van Rappard, who had brain fever and now has gone to Germany to recover." As if he wanted to say : " do not let me make efforts to know strange people, as the same thing might happen to me." Once more he touches the old love story of Etten, " a single word made me feel that nothing is changed in me about it, that it is and remains a wound, which I carry with me, but it lies deep and will never heal, it will remain in after years just what it was the first day." And he expresses openly how different his life would have been without this disappointment in his love.

When at last he starts alone in September for Drenthe, he has made all possible provisions for the woman and the children, and there is a sorrowful parting, especially from the little boy to whom he had become attached as if it were his own child.

The trip to Drenthe proves a failure instead of doing him good. But some of his most beautiful letters date from those days. The season was too far advanced, the country too inhospitable, and what Vincent so ardently desired—to come into contact with some artists, for instance, Lieberman—was not realized.

Bitter loneliness and want of money put a too heavy strain on his nerves. He is afraid of falling ill, and in December 1883 hastens back to the parental vicarage, the only place where he can find a safe shelter.

His father had meanwhile left Etten and been nominated to Nuenen, a village in the neighbourhood of Eindhoven, and the new place and surroundings pleased Vincent so well that instead of paying a short visit, as first was his intention, he stays there for two years.

To paint the Brabant landscape and the Brabant types is now his aim, and to accomplish that aim he overlooks all other difficulties.

To live together with his parents was for him as well as for them a very difficult thing. In a small village vicarage, where nothing can happen without the whole village knowing it, a painter is obviously an anomaly; how much more a painter like Vincent, who had so completely broken with all formalities, conventionalities and with all religion, and who was the last person in the world to conform himself to other people. On both sides there must have been great love and great patience to put up with it so long. When his letters from Drenthe to his parents became more and more melancholy, his father anxiously had written to Theo, " it seems to me that Vincent is again in a wrong mood. He seems to be in a melancholy state of mind; but how can it be otherwise? Whenever he looks back into the past and recalls to his memory how he has broken with all former relations, it must be very painful to him. If he had only the courage to think of the possibility that the cause of much which has resulted from his eccentricity lies in himself. I don't think he ever feels any self-reproach, only soreness against others, especially against the gentlemen at The Hague. We must be very careful with him for he seems to be in a fit of contrariness."

And they *are* so careful. When he comes back to them of his own will, they receive him with so much love and try all in their power to make him comfortable; they are proud too of the progress in his work, of which it must be said they had no great expectations at first. "Do you not like the pen drawings of the tower that Vincent sent you? It seems to come to him so easily," writes his father in the first days of December to Theo, and then on the twentieth of December, "You will be longing to know how things are getting on with Vincent. At first it seemed hopeless, but by and by things have arranged themselves, especially since we approved of his staying here for some time to make studies. He wanted the

inner room fitted up for him; we did not think it a very fit
abode for him, but we had a nice stove put there; as the room
had a stone floor we had it covered with boards, and made it
as comfortable as possible : we put a bed in it on a wooden
stand, that it might not be too damp. Now we will make the
room nicely warm and dry, so that it may turn out better than
we expected. I proposed to have a large window made in it
but he did not want that. In short, with real courage we
undertake this new experiment and we intend to leave him
perfectly free in his peculiarities of dress, etc. The people
here have seen him anyhow, and though it is a pity he is so
reserved in manner, we cannot change the fact of his being
eccentric. . . ." "He seems to occupy himself a great deal
with your plans for the future, but you will be wise enough
not to let yourself be influenced to do things that are not
practical, for alas that certainly is his foible. One thing is
certain, he works hard and finds here lots of subjects, he has
made already several drawings, which we like very much."
Such is the feeling from their side; but Vincent is not satisfied with all that kindness and wants a deeper understanding
of his innermost self than his parents can give, however much
they try. When about the middle of January '84 his mother
meets with an accident and is brought home from Helmond
with a broken leg, the relations become less strained. Vincent,
who has become an expert nurse in the Borinage, helps to
nurse his mother with the greatest devotion, and in every
letter of that time they praise him for his faithful help.
"Vincent is untiring, and the rest of his time he devotes to
his painting and drawing with the greatest zeal." "The
doctor praised Vincent for his ability and care." "Vincent
proves an ideal nurse and at the same time he works with the
greatest ambition." "I fervently hope that his work may find
success for it is edifying to see how much he works," is told
in the letters of February.

Vincent's own letters at that time are gloomy and full of
complaints and unjust reproaches to Theo that he never sells
anything for him and does not even try to, ending at last with
the bitter cry: "A wife you cannot give me, a child you

cannot give me, work you cannot give me—money yes, but what is the use of it when I must miss all the rest!" And Theo, who always understands him, never gives a sharp or angry answer to those reproaches: a light sarcasm is the only reply he sometimes gives to such outbursts. In May Vincent's spirits rise somewhat on his moving into a new, larger studio, two rooms in the house of the sexton of the Catholic church. Shortly after, van Rappard comes to spend some time with him again, and besides, Vincent had during his mother's illness come more in contact with neighbours and friends of the village, who daily came to visit the patient, so that he writes in those days, "I have had a much pleasanter time with the people here than at first, which is worth a great deal to me, for one must have some distraction now and then, and when one feels too lonely the work suffers from it." But with a prophetic glance he continues, "One must keep in mind however that these things do not always last." Indeed, difficult times were approaching for him again. With one of his mother's visitors, the youngest of three sisters who lived next door to the vicarage, he had soon got into a more intimate relation; she was much older than he and neither beautiful nor gifted, but she had an active mind and a kind heart. She often visited the poor with Vincent; they walked much together, and on her part at least the friendship soon changed into love. As to Vincent, though his letters do not give the impression of any passionate feeling for her (the fact is he writes very little about it), yet he seems to have been inclined to marry her, but the family vehemently protested against the plan, and violent scenes took place between the sisters, which were not conducive to keep Vincent in a pleasant mood.

"Vincent works hard but he is not very sociable," writes his mother in July, and it will get worse still, for the young woman, violently excited by the scenes with her sisters, tries to commit suicide, which fails, but shocks her health so much that she had to be nursed at a doctor's in Utrecht. She quite recovered and after half a year she came back to Nuenen,

but their relations were broken for ever and the whole affair
left Vincent in a gloomy, bitter mood.

For his parents the consequences were also painful, because
the neighbours avoided the vicarage from that time, not wishing to meet Vincent, " which is a great privation for me, but it
is not your mother's way to complain," the latter writes in
October of that year. It is in those days that van Rappard
once more comes to stay with them. " He is not a talkative
person, but a hard worker," writes mother, and van Rappard
himself writes in 1890, in the letter to her, quoted above,
" how often do I think of the studies of the weavers which
he made in Nuenen, with what intensity of feeling did he
depict their lives, what deep melancholy pervaded them, however clumsy the execution of his work may have been then.
And what beautiful studies he made of the old church tower
in the churchyard. I always remember a moonlight effect of
it, which particularly struck me at that time. When I think
of those studies in those two rooms near the church, it recalls
to my mind so many memories, and reminds me of the whole
surroundings, the cheerful hospitable vicarage with its beautiful garden, the family Begemann, our visits to the weavers and
peasants, how I did enjoy it all."

After van Rappard's visit Vincent has no other distraction
than a few acquaintances in Eindhoven, with whom he has
come into contact through the house painter, who furnishes
his colours. They are a former goldsmith, Hermans, a tanner,
Kersemakers, and also a telegraphist whose name is not mentioned, all of whom Vincent initiates into the art of painting.
Mr. Kersemakers has recorded his reminiscences of that time
in the weekly " De Amsterdammer " of the 14th and 21st of
April 1912, and gives among others the following description of Vincent's studio, which according to him looked quite
" Bohemian."

" It was quite astonishing to see how crowded the place
was with pictures, with drawings in water-colour and chalk;
heads of men and women whose negro-like turned up noses,
projecting jaw-bones and large ears were strongly accentuated,

the fists callous and furrowed; weavers and weavers' looms, women driving the shuttle, peasants planting potatoes, women busy weaving, innumerable still-lives, at least ten studies in oil of the old church tower at Nuenen, of which he was so fond, and which he had painted in all seasons of the year and in all weathers (afterwards this old tower was demolished by the Nuenen Vandals, as he called them).

Heaps of ashes around the stove, which never had seen brush or polish, a few frayed out rush-bottomed chairs, and a cupboard with at least thirty different birds' nests, all kinds of moss and plants brought from the heath, some stuffed birds, shuttles, spinning-wheel, bed-warmer, all sorts of farmers' tools, old caps and hats, dirty women's bonnets, wooden shoes, etc." He also tells about their trip to Amsterdam (in the autumn of 1885) to see the " Ryksmuseum," how Vincent in his rough ulster and his inseparable fur cap was calmly sitting painting a few small views of the town in the waiting room of the station; how they saw the Rembrandts in the museum, how Vincent could not tear himself away from the " Jewish Bride " and said at last, " Do you know that I would give ten years of my life if I could sit here before this picture a fortnight, with nothing but a crust of dry bread for food."

Dry bread was nothing unusual to him; according to Kersemakers, Vincent never ate it otherwise, in order not to indulge himself too much. His impression of Vincent's work is given as follows : " At my first visit in Nuenen I could not understand it at all, it was so totally different from what I expected, it was so strong, so coarse and unfinished that I could not possibly admire it or see anything in it.

" At my second visit the impression was already much better, though I thought in my ignorance that he could not draw, or totally neglected the drawing of the figures, and I took the liberty of telling him straight out. I did not make him angry, he only laughed and said : ' You will think differently about it later on.' "

Meanwhile the winter days passed on gloomily enough at the vicarage. " For Vincent I should wish that the winter were over, he cannot work out of doors and the long evenings are not profitable for his work. We often think that it would be better for him to be among people of his own profession, but we cannot dictate to him," writes his father in December, and mother complains, "how is it possible to behave so unkindly? If he has wishes for the future, let him exert himself, he is still young enough; it is almost impossible to bear it. I think he wants a change, perhaps he might find something that would give him inspiration, here it is always the same thing and he never speaks to anyone." But still she finds one luminous point to mention : "we saw that Vincent received a book from you, he seems to read it with much pleasure. I heard him say 'that is a fine book,' so you have given him great pleasure. I am glad that we regularly get books from the reading club; the illustrations in the magazines interest him most, and then there is the Nouvelle Revue, etc., every week something new is a great pleasure to him." Incessantly Vincent continues his work in the gloomy cottages of peasants and weavers. " I never began a year of a more gloomy aspect, in a more gloomy mood," he writes on New Year's Day '85. " He seems to become more and more estranged from us," complains his father, whose letters became more and more melancholy, as if he is not equal to the difficulties of living together with his gifted, unmanageable son, and feels himself helpless against his unbridled violence. " This morning I talked things over with Vincent; he was in a kind mood and said there was no particular reason for his being depressed," says the latter, " may he meet with success anyhow," are the last words he writes about Vincent in a letter of the 25th of March. Two days later, coming home from a long walk across the heath, he fell down on the threshold of his home and was carried lifeless into the house. Hard times followed in the vicarage; mother could remain there another year, but for Vincent it brought immediate changes. In consequence of several disagreeable discussions with the other members of the family, he resolved to live no longer at the vicarage, but took up his abode in the studio, where he stayed from May to November. Henceforth there is

not a single thing to distract him from his aim—to paint the
peasant life. He spends those months in the cottages of the
weavers or with the peasants in the field. " It is a fine thing
to be right in the snow in winter, right in the yellow leaves in
autumn, in summer right in the ripe corn, in spring right in
the grass, always with the peasant girls and reapers, in
summer under the open skies, in winter near the open fireplace, and to know that it has always been so and will always
be" (letter 425). He is now in harmony with himself and
his surroundings, and when he sends Theo his first great
picture, " The Potato-Eaters," he can say in good reason that
it is " from the heart of peasant life."

An uninterrupted series of studies follow each other; the
cottages of the old peasants and their witch-like wives, the
old church tower of the cemetery, the autumn landscapes and
the birds' nests, a number of still-lives and the strong drawings of the Brabant peasants. In Nuenen he also writes the
beautiful passages about colour, in reference to Delacroix's
laws of colours. It seems strange to hear him, who was called
afterwards one of the first Impressionists, even Neo-impres-
sionists, declare, " there is a school I think of impressionists,
but I do not know much about it " (letter 402), and in his
usual spirit of contradiction he afterwards adds, " from what
you have told me about impressionism I have learned that it is
different from what I thought it was, but as to me I find
Israëls for instance so enormous that I am little curious about
or desirous of anything different or new. I think I shall
change a great deal in touch and colour but I expect to become rather more dark than lighter." As soon as he came to
France he thought differently of it.

During the last days of his stay in Nuenen difficulties arise
between him and the Catholic priest, who has long since
looked askance at the studio next to his church, and now
forbids his parishioners to pose for Vincent. The latter was
already thinking about a change. He gives notice of leaving
his studio the first of May, but starts for Antwerp, towards
the end of November, leaving all his Brabant work behind.
When in May his mother also leaves Nuenen, everything

belonging to Vincent is packed in cases, left in care of a carpenter in Breda and—forgotten! After several years the carpenter finally sold everything to a junk dealer.

What Theo's opinion about his brother was at that time is shown in the letter to his sister of the 13th of October '85, in which he writes : " Vincent is one of those who has gone through all the experiences of life and has retired from the world, now we must wait and see if he has genius. I think he has. . . . If he succeeds in his work he will be a great man. As to the worldly success, it will perhaps be with him as with Heyerdahl[1] : appreciated by some but not understood by the public at large. Those however who care whether there is really something in the artist, or if it is only outward shine, will respect him, and in my opinion that will be sufficient revenge for the animosity shown him by so many others."

In Antwerp Vincent rents for 25 fr. a month a little room over a small paint-dealer's shop in the " Rue des Images " 194. It is but a very small room but he makes it cosy with Japanese prints on the wall, and when he has rented a stove and a lamp, he feels himself safe and writes with profound satisfaction, " no fear of my being bored I can assure you." On the contrary he spends the three months of his stay in one feverish intoxication of work. The town life which he has missed so long fascinates him; he has not eyes enough to see, nor hands enough to paint : to make portraits of all the interesting types he meets is his delight, and in order to pay the models he sacrifices everything he has. As for food he does not bother. " If I receive money my first hunger is not for food, though I have fasted ever so long, but the desire for painting is ever so much stronger, and I start at once hunting for models till there is nothing left," he writes.

When he sees in January that he cannot go on like that, the expenses being too heavy, he becomes a pupil of the Academy, where the teaching is free and where he finds models every day. Hageman and de Baseleer were there among his fellow pupils and from Holland there was Briët. In the evening he worked again in the drawing class and after that,

[1] Norwegian painter, then in Paris.

often till late at night, at a club where they also draw from life. His health cannot stand such a strain and in the beginning of February he writes that he is literally worn out and exhausted, according to the doctor it is complete prostration. He seems not to think about giving up his work, however, though he begins to make projects for a change, for the course at the Academy is almost finished and he has already had many disagreements with his teachers, for he is much too independent and self-willed to follow their guidance. Something must be done. Theo thinks it better for Vincent to go back to Brabant, but he himself wants to go to Paris. Then Theo proposes to wait at least till June, when he shall have rented a larger apartment, but with his usual impetuosity Vincent cannot wait so long, and one morning in the end of February, Theo receives in his office at the Boulevard a little note written in chalk, that Vincent had arrived and awaits him in the Salon Carré of the Louvre. Probably he left all his work in Antwerp, perhaps his landlord the paint-dealer kept it for the unpaid rent of the room. Certain it is that none of the studies about which he writes, the view of the Park, of the Cathedral, Het Steen, etc., ever has been found again.

The meeting in the Louvre took place, and since then Vincent lived with Theo in the latter's apartment in the Rue de Laval. As there was no room for a studio he worked during the first month at Cormon's studio, which did not satisfy him at all, but when they moved in June to the Rue Lepic 54, on Montmartre, he had there a studio of his own and never went back to Cormon.

The new apartment on the third floor had three rather large rooms, a cabinet and a kitchen. The living room was comfortable and cosy with Theo's beautiful old cabinet, a sofa and a big stove, for both the brothers were very sensitive to the cold. Next to that was Theo's bedroom. Vincent slept in the cabinet and behind that was the studio, an ordinary sized room with one not very large window. Here he first painted his nearest surroundings—the view from the studio window, the Moulin de la Galette viewed from every side, the window of Madame Bataille's small restaurant where he took his meals, little landscapes on Montmartre which was at that time still quite countrified, all painted in a soft tender tone like that of Mauve. Afterwards he painted flowers and still-life and tried to renew his palette under the influence of the French "plein air" painters such as Monet, Sisley, Pisarro, etc., for whom Theo had long since opened the way to the public. The change of surroundings and the easier and more comfortable life, without any material cares, at first greatly improved Vincent's health. In the summer of '86 Theo writes to his mother, "we like the new apartment very much; you would not recognize Vincent, he is so much changed, and it strikes other people more than it does me. He has undergone an important operation in his mouth, for he had lost almost all his teeth through the bad condition of his stomach. The doctor says that he has now quite recovered his health; he makes great progress in his work and has begun to have some success. He is in much better spirits than before and many people here like him . . . he has friends who send him every week a lot of beautiful flowers which he uses for still-life, he paints chiefly flowers, especially to make the colours of his next pictures brighter and clearer. If we can continue to live together like this, I think the most difficult period is past, and he will find his way." To continue living together, that was the great difficulty, and of all that Theo did for his brother, there is perhaps nothing that proved greater sacrifice than his having endured living with him for two years. For when the first excitement of all the attractions in Paris had passed, Vincent soon fell back to his old irritability; perhaps the city life did not agree with him either and overstrained his nerves. Whatever might be the cause, his temper during that winter was worse than ever, and made life very hard for Theo, whose own health was not of the best at that time. Circumstances put too heavy a strain on his strength. His own work was very strenuous and exhausting, he had made the gallery on the Boulevard Montmartre a centre of the Impressionists, there were Monet, Sisley, Pissarro and Raffaelli, Degas who exhibited nowhere else, Seurat, etc. But to introduce that work to the public, which filled the small entresol every afternoon from five until seven, what discussions, what endless debates, had to be held, and on the other hand how he had to defend the rights of the young painters against "ces messieurs," as Vincent always called the heads of the firm. When he came home tired out in the evening he found no rest, but the impetuous, violent Vincent began to expound his own theories about art and art-dealing, which always came to the point that Theo ought to leave Goupil and open a gallery for himself. And this lasted till far into the night, ay sometimes he sat down on a chair before Theo's bed to spin out his last arguments. " Do you feel how hard it sometimes is to have no other conversation than with gentlemen who speak about business, with artists whose life generally is difficult enough, but never to come in contact with women and children of your own sphere? You can have no idea of the loneliness in a big city," writes Theo once to his youngest sister and to her he sometimes opens his heart about Vincent : " my home life is almost unbearable, no one wants to come and see me any more, because it always ends in quarrels, and besides he is so untidy that the room looks far from attractive. I wish he would go and live by himself, he speaks sometimes about it, but if I were to tell him to go away, it would be just a reason for him to stay; as it seems I do him no good. I only ask him one thing, to do me no harm and by his stay—he does so, for I can hardly bear it." " It seems as if he were two persons in one, one marvellously gifted, tender and refined, the other egoistic and hard-hearted. They present themselves in turns, so that one hears him talk first in one way, then in the other, and always with arguments on both sides. It is a pity that he is his own enemy, for he makes life hard not only for others but also for himself." But when his sister advises him to " leave Vincent for God's sake," to himself, Theo answers, " it is such a peculiar case. If he only had another profession I would long ago have done what you advise me, and I have often asked myself if I have not been wrong in helping him continually. I have often been on the point of leaving him to his own devices. After receiving your letter I have thought it over again, but I think in this case I must continue in the same way. He is certainly an artist and if what he makes now is not always beautiful, it will certainly be of use to him afterwards, and then his work will perhaps be sublime, and it would be a shame to keep him from his regular study. However unpractical he may be, if he succeeds in his work there will certainly come a day when he will begin to sell his pictures. . . .

" I am firmly resolved to continue in the same way as till now, but I do hope that he will change his lodgings in some way or other."

However, that separation did not take place. The old love and friendship which bound them together since childhood, did not fail them even now. Theo managed to restrain himself, and in the spring he wrote, " as I feel much stronger than last winter I hope to be able to bring a change for the better in our relations; there will be no other change for the present and I am glad of it. We are already most of us so far from home that it would be no use to bring about still more separation." And full of courage he continues to help Vincent bear the burden of his life.

With spring there came in all respects a better time. Vincent could again work in the open air and painted much at Asnières where he painted the beautiful triptych of " l'Isle de la grande Jatte," the borders of the Seine with their gay, bright restaurants, the little boats on the river, the parks and gardens, all sparkling with light and colour. At that time he saw much of Emile Bernard, a young painter fifteen years younger than himself, whom he had met at Cormon's and who had a little wooden studio in his parents' garden at Asnières, where they sometimes worked together and where Vincent began a portrait of Bernard. But one day he fell into a violent quarrel with old Mr. Bernard about the latter's projects for his son. Vincent could bear no contradiction, he ran away in a passion with the still wet portrait under his arm, and he never set foot again in the house of the Bernards. But the friendship with the young Bernard remained, and in his " Letters of Vincent van Gogh," (published at Vollard's in Paris), are the most beautiful pages written about Vincent.

In the winter of '87-'88, Vincent again paints portraits—the famous self-portrait before the easel, and many other self-portraits, as well as father Tanguy, the old merchant of colours in the Rue Clausel, in whose show-window his customers were allowed to exhibit their pictures by turns, and who unjustly sometimes has been described as a Mæcenas, the qualities for which were absolutely wanting in the poor old man, and even if he had possessed them, his shrewd wife would not have allowed him to use them. He sent, and justly too, very proper bills for the colours he furnished, and did not understand very much about the pictures that were exposed in his window.

From that time dates also the famous picture, "Interior with Lady by a Cradle," and when Theo who has bought that winter a few pictures from young artists, to help them, and wants to do the same for Vincent, the latter paints for him the beautiful "Still Life in Yellow," sparkling and radiant as from an inward glow, and with red letters he graves the dedication "To my brother Theo."

Toward the end of the winter he is tired of Paris, city life is too much for him, the climate too grey and chilly, in February '88 he travels toward the south. "After all these years of care and misfortune his health has not grown stronger and he decidedly wanted to be in a milder climate," Theo writes. "He has first gone to Arles to look around him, and then will probably go to Marseilles.

"Before he went away I went a few times with him to hear a Wagner concert; we both enjoyed it very much. It still seems strange that he is gone. He was so much to me the last time." And Bernard tells how Vincent was busy that last day in Paris arranging the studio, "So that my brother will think me still here."

At Arles, Vincent reaches the summit of his art. After the oppressiveness of Parisian life he, with his innate love of nature, revives in sunny Provence. There follows a happy time of undisturbed and immense productivity. Without paying much attention to the town of Arles itself with its famous remains of Roman architecture, he paints the land-scape, the glorious wealth of blossoms in Spring in a series of orchards in bloom, the cornfields under the burning sun at harvest time, the almost intoxicating richness of colours of the autumn, the glorious beauty of the gardens and parks, " The Poet's Garden," where he sees as in a vision the ghosts of Dante and Petrarch roaming about. He paints " The Sower," " The Sunflowers," " The Starlit Night," the sea at St. Marie : his creative impulse and power are inexhaustible. " I have a terrible lucidity at moments, when nature is so glorious in those days I am hardly conscious of myself and the picture comes to me like in a dream," and rapturously he exclaims, " Life is after all enchanting."

His letters henceforth, written in French, give a complete image of what passes within him. Sometimes when he has written in the morning, he sits down again in the evening to tell his brother how splendid the day has been. " I never had such a chance, nature is extraordinarily beautiful here," and a day later, " I know that I wrote to you yesterday but the day has been again so glorious. My only regret is that you cannot see what I see here."

Completely absorbed in his work as he is, he does not feel the burden of the great loneliness that surrounds him in Arles, for except a short acquaintance with MacKnight, Bock and the Zouave lieutenant Milliet, he has no friends whatever. But when he has rented a little house of his own on the Place Lamartine, and arranges it after his own taste, decorates it with his pictures, makes it a " maison d'artiste," then he feels the old longing again, which he has already uttered at the beginning of his painting career in 1880, to associate himself with another artist, to live together and to work together. Just then he receives a letter from Paul Gauguin from Bretagne, who is in the greatest pecuniary embarrass-ment, and who tries in this roundabout way to ask Theo to try to sell some of his pictures for him : " I wanted to write to your brother but I am afraid to bother him, he being so busy from morning until night. The little I have sold is just enough to pay some urgent debts and in a month I shall have absolutely nothing left. Zero is a negative force . . . I do not want to importune your brother, but a little word from you on this head would set my mind at ease or at least help me to have patience. My God, how terrible are these money questions for an artist."

At once Vincent grasps at the idea of helping Gauguin. He must come to Arles and they will live and work together. Theo will pay the expenses and Gauguin will give him pictures in exchange. Again and again he insists on this plan with his innate perseverance and stubbornness, though Gauguin at first did not seem at all inclined to it. They had made each other's acquaintance in Paris, but it had been no more than a superficial acquaintance, and they were too different in talent and character ever to harmonize in the daily intercourse.

Gauguin, born in Paris in 1848, was the son of a Breton father, a journalist in Paris, and a Creole mother. His youth was full of adventures, he had gone to sea as a cabin boy, had worked in a banker's office and had only painted in his leisure hours. Then after he had married and had a family, he devoted himself wholly to his art. His wife and children returned to her native city Copenhagen, as he was not able to provide for them, and he himself made a journey to Martinique where he painted, among others, his famous picture "The negresses." He was now in Pont Aven in Brittany, without any source of income, so that the great need of money made him accept Vincent's proposition and come to Arles. The whole undertaking was a sad failure and had for Vincent a fatal end.

Notwithstanding the months of superhuman exertion which lay behind him, he strained every nerve in a last manifestation of power before the arrival of Gauguin. "I am conceited enough to want to make a certain impression on Gauguin by my painting. I have finished as far as possible the things I had undertaken, pushed by the great desire to show him something new, and not to undergo his influence before I have shown him indisputably my own originality," writes Vincent in letter 556. When we know that to this last work belongs one of Vincent's most famous pictures, "la chambre à coucher," and the series, "The Poet's Garden," it makes us feel rather sceptical about Gauguin's later assertion that before his arrival Vincent had only been bungling a little, and that he only made progress after Gauguin's lessons. We know then what to think of Gauguin's whole description of the episode at Arles, which is such a mixture of truth and fiction.

The fact is that Vincent was completely exhausted and overstrained, and was no match for the iron Gauguin with his strong nerves and cool arguing. It became a silent struggle between them, and the endless discussions held while smoking in the little yellow house were not fit to calm Vincent. "Your brother is indeed a little agitated and I hope to calm him by and by," Gauguin writes to Theo, shortly after his arrival at Arles. And to Bernard he tells more intimately how little sympathy there really is between Vincent and himself. "Vincent and I generally agree very little, especially about painting. He admires Daudet, Daubigny, Ziem, and the great Rousseau, all people whom I cannot bear. And on the contrary he detests Ingres, Raphaël, Degas, all people whom I admire. I answer, 'Brigadier, you are right,' in order to have peace. He loves my pictures very much, but when I make them he always finds I am wrong in this or that. He is romantic and I rather inclined to the primitive state."[1] And in later years when Gauguin again remembers this period he writes, "between two beings, he and I, he like a Vulcan, and I boiling too, a kind of struggle was preparing itself. . . ."[2] The situation in consequence becomes more and more strained. In the latter half of December Theo receives from Gauguin the following letter: "Dear Mr. van Gogh,—I would be greatly obliged to you for sending me a part of the money for the pictures sold. After all I must go back to Paris, Vincent and I simply cannot live together in peace, in consequence of incompatibility of temper, and he as well as I, we need quiet for our work. He is a man of remarkable intelli-

[1] "Paul Gauguin," by Chas. Morice, "Mercure de France," 1903.
[2] From Gauguin's later narrative of the events at Arles, in his *Avant et Après*, a set of memoirs written in 1903. [Ed.]

gence, whom I highly respect and leave with regret, but I repeat it is necessary. I appreciate all the delicacy in your conduct towards me and I beg you to excuse my decision." Vincent also writes, in letter 565, that Gauguin seems to be tired of Arles, of the yellow house, and of himself. But the quarrel is made up, Gauguin asks Theo to consider his return to Paris as an imaginary thing, and the letter he had written him as a bad dream. But it is only the calm before the storm.

The day before Christmas,—Theo and I were just engaged to be married and intended to go together to Holland—(I was staying in Paris with my brother A. Bonger, the friend of Theo and Vincent)—a telegram arrived from Gauguin which called Theo to Arles. Vincent had on the evening of the 24th of December, in a state of violent excitement, "un accès de fièvre chaude," (an attack of high fever) cut off a piece of his ear and brought it as a gift to a woman in a brothel. A big tumult had been raised. Roulin the postman had seen Vincent home, the police had interfered, had found Vincent bleeding and unconscious in bed, and sent him to the hospital. Theo found him there in a severe crisis, and stayed with him during the Christmas days. The doctor considered his condition very serious. "There were moments while I was with him that he was well, but very soon after he fell back into his worries about philosophy and theology. It was painfully sad to witness, for at times all his suffering overwhelmed him and he tried to weep but he could not; poor fighter and poor, poor sufferer; for the moment nobody can do anything to relieve his sorrow and yet he feels deeply and strongly. If he might have found somebody to whom he could have disclosed his heart, it would perhaps never have gone thus far," Theo wrote to me after he had come back to Paris with Gauguin, and a day later, "there is little hope, but during his life he has done more than many others, and he has suffered and struggled more than most people could have done. If it must be that he dies, be it so, but my heart breaks when I think of it." The anxiety lasted a few more days. Dr. Rey, the house doctor of the hospital, to whose care

Theo had entrusted him so urgently, kept him constantly informed. " I shall always be glad to send you tidings, for I too have a brother, I too have been separated from my family," he writes the 29th of December when the tidings are still very bad. The Protestant clergyman, the Rev. Salles, also visits Vincent and writes to Theo about his condition, and then there is last but not least the postman, Roulin, who is quite dismayed at the accident that befell his friend Vincent, with whom he spent so many pleasant hours at the " Café de la Gare " of Joseph Ginoux, and who has painted such beautiful portraits of him and his whole family! Every day he goes to the hospital for tidings and conveys them faithfully to Paris; as he is not a good penman, his two sons, Armand and Camille, serve him in turn as secretary. His wife too who posed for the " Berceuse " (Mme. Ginoux was the original of the " Arlésienne ") visits her sick friend, and the first sign of recovery is when Vincent asks her about little Marcelle, the handsome baby he had painted such a short time ago. Then there comes a sudden change for the better in his condition. The Rev. Salles writes on the 31st of December that he had found Vincent perfectly calm, and that he is longing to start work again. A day later, Vincent himself writes a short note in pencil to reassure Theo, and on the second of January there comes another note from him, to which Dr. Rey has added a word of reassurance. The 3rd of January an enthusiastic letter of Roulin's, " Vincent has quite recovered. He is better than before that unfortunate accident happened to him," and he, Roulin, will go to the doctor and tell him to allow Vincent to go back to his pictures. The following day they had been out and spent four hours together. " I am very sorry my first letters were so alarming and I beg your pardon; I am glad to say I have been mistaken in this case. He only regrets all the trouble he has given you, and he is sorry for the anxiety he has caused. You may be assured that I will do all I can to give him some distraction," writes Roulin.

On the 7th of January Vincent leaves the hospital, apparently entirely recovered, but, alas, at every great excitement or fatigue, the nervous attacks return . . . they last longer or shorter, but leave him also periods of almost perfect health, during which he goes back to his work with the old vigour. In February he is taken back to the hospital for a short time, but after his return to his little house, the neighbours have grown afraid of him and send a petition to the mayor, saying that it is dangerous to leave him at liberty, in consequence of which he is actually again sent to the hospital on the 27th of February—this time without any cause. Vincent himself for a whole month keeps the deepest silence about this unhappy affair, but the Rev. Salles sends Theo a faithful report. On the 2nd of March he writes, " The neighbours have raised a tumult out of nothing. The acts with which they have re-proached your brother (even if they were exact), do not justify taxing a man with alienation or depriving him of his liberty. Unfortunately, the foolish act which necessitated his first removal to the hospital made people interpret in a quite unfavourable way every singular deed which the poor young man might perform; from anyone else it would remain un-observed, from him, everything takes at once a particular importance. . . . As I told you yesterday, at the hospital he has won everybody's favour and after all it is the doctor and not the chief of police who has to judge in these matters." The whole affair makes a deep impression on Vincent and again causes an attack from which he recovers with astonish-ing rapidity. It is again the Rev. Salles who tells Theo of Vincent's recovery. On the 18th of March he writes, " Your brother has spoken to me with perfect calmness and lucidity of mind about his condition and also about the petition signed by his neighbours. The petition grieves him very much. ' If the police,' he says, ' had protected my liberty by preventing the children and even the grown-ups from crowding around my house and climbing the windows as they have done, (as if I were a curious animal), I should have more easily retained my self-possession, at all events I have done no harm to anyone.' In short, I found your brother transformed, may God maintain this favourable change. His condition has some-thing indescribable, and it is impossible to understand the sudden and complete changes which have taken place in him. It is evident that as long as he is in the condition in which I found him, there can be no question of interning him in an asylum; nobody, as far as I know, would have this sinister courage." A day after this interview with the Rev. Salles, Vincent himself for the first time writes again to Theo and justly complains that such repeated emotions might become the cause of a passing nervous attack changing to a chronic evil. And with quiet resignation, he adds, " to suffer without complaint is the only lesson we have to learn in this life."

He soon recovers his liberty but continues to live in the hospital for a short time, until the Rev. Salles shall have found him new lodgings in a different part of the town. His health is so good that the Rev. Salles writes on the 19th of April, " sometimes even no traces seem left of the disease which has affected him so vividly." But when he was going to arrange with the new landlord, he suddenly avowed to the Rev. Salles that he lacked the courage to start again a new studio, and that he himself thought it best to go to an asylum for a few months. " He is fully conscious of his condition, and speaks with me about his illness, which he fears will come back, with a touching openheartedness and simplicity," writes the Rev. Salles. " I am not fit," he told me the day before yesterday, " to govern myself and my affairs. I feel quite different than I was before." The Rev. Salles had then looked around and advised the asylum of St. Rémy, situated quite near Arles; he adds that the doctors at Arles approve of it, " given the state of isolation in which your brother would find himself upon leaving the hospital."

It was that which troubled Theo mostly. " Yes," he wrote to me, shortly before our marriage, in answer to my question if Vincent would not rather return to Paris, or spend some time with his mother and sisters in Holland, as he was so alone in Arles, " one of the greatest difficulties is, that whether in good or bad health his life is so barren of distraction. But if you knew him you would feel doubly how difficult is the solution of the question what must and can be done for him.

" As you know he has long since broken with what is called

convention. His way of dressing and his manners show directly that he is an unusual personality and people who see him say, ' he is mad.' To me it does not matter, but for mother that is impossible. Then there is something in his way of speaking that makes people either like or dislike him strongly. He has always people around him, who sympathize with him, but also many enemies. It is impossible for him to associate with people in an indifferent way. It is either the one or the other, even to those who are his best friends it is difficult to remain on good terms with him, as he spares nobody's feelings. If I had time for it, I would go to him and, for instance, take a walking tour with him. That is the only thing, I imagine, that would do him good. If I can find somebody among the painters who would like to do it, I will send him. But those with whom he would like to go, are somewhat afraid of him, a circumstance which the visit of Gauguin did not change, on the contrary.

" Then there is another thing which makes me afraid to have him come here. In Paris he saw so many things which he liked to paint, but again and again it was made impossible for him to do so. Models would not pose for him, he was forbidden to paint on the street, and with his irascible temper this caused many unpleasant scenes, which excited him so much that he became unapproachable to everybody and at last he got a great dislike of Paris. If he himself had wanted to come back here, I would not hesitate for a moment . . . but again I think I can do no better than to let him follow his own wishes. A quiet life is impossible for him, except alone with nature or with very simple people like the Roulins, for wherever he passes he leaves the trace of his passing. Whatever he sees that is wrong he must criticize and that often occasions strife.

" I hope that he will find, some time, a wife who will love him so much that she will share his life but it will be difficult to find one who would be fit for that. Do you remember that girl in ' Terre Vierge ' by Tourgenief, who is with the nihilists and brought the compromising papers across the frontiers? I imagine she should be like that, somebody who has gone through life's misery to the bottom. . . . It pains me not to be able to do something for him, but for uncommon people uncommon remedies are necessary and I hope these will be found where ordinary people would not look for them."

When Vincent himself now resolves to go to St. Rémy, Theo's first impression is that this may be a kind of self-sacrifice so as to be in nobody's way, and he writes to him once more asking with emphasis, whether he would not rather go to Pont-Aven or go to Paris.

But as Vincent sticks to his resolution Theo writes to him: " I do not consider your going to St. Rémy a retreat as you call it, but simply as a temporary rest cure which will make you come back with renewed strength. I for my part attribute your illness principally to the fact that your material existence has been too much neglected. In an establishment like that of St. Rémy there is a great regularity in the hours for meals, etc., and I think that regularity will do you no harm, on the contrary." When Theo has arranged everything with the director of the establishment, Dr. Peyron, a free room for Vincent and a room where he can paint, and as much liberty as possible to wander about as he likes, Vincent leaves for St. Rémy on the 8th of May accompanied by the Rev. Salles who writes to Theo the next day: " Our voyage to St. Rémy has been accomplished under the most excellent conditions; Monsieur Vincent was perfectly calm and himself has explained his case to the director as a man who is fully conscious of his condition. He remained with me till my departure and when I took leave of him he thanked me warmly and seemed somewhat moved, thinking of the new life he was going to lead in that house. Monsieur Peyron has assured me that he will show him all the kindness and consideration which his condition demands." How touching sounds that, " somewhat moved," at the departure of the faithful companion! His leave-taking broke the last tie that united Vincent with the outer world and he stayed behind in what was worse than the greatest loneliness; surrounded by neurotics and lunatics, with nobody to whom he could talk, nobody who understood him.

Dr. Peyron was kindly disposed, but he was a reserved silent character, and the monthly letters by which he keeps Theo informed of the situation are not full of the warm sympathy which the doctors in the hospital at Arles showed him.

A full year Vincent spent amid these cheerless surroundings, struggling with unbroken energy against the ever returning attacks of his illness, but continuing his work with the old restless zeal, which alone can keep him living now that everything else has failed him. He paints the desolate landscape which he sees from his window at sunrise and sunset, he undertakes long wanderings to paint the wide fields, bordered by the range of hills of the Alps, he paints the olive orchards with their dismally twisted branches, the gloomy cypresses, the sombre garden of the asylum, and he painted also the "Reaper," "that image of death as the great book of Nature represents it to us."

It is no longer the buoyant, sunny, triumphant work from Arles; there sounds a deeper sadder tone than the piercing clarion sounds of his symphonies in yellow of the last year: his palette has become more sober, the harmonies of his pictures have passed into a minor key.

"To suffer without complaint," well had he learned that lesson; and when in August the treacherous evil attacks him again, just when he had hoped to be cured for good, he only utters a desponding sigh, "I can see no possibility of again having hope or courage."

Having painfully struggled through the winter, in which however he paints some of his most beautiful works, the " Pietà " after Delacroix, the " Resurrection of Lazarus," and the "Good Samaritan" after Rembrandt, the " Quatre heures du jour " after Millet; a few months follow during which he is not able to work, but now he feels that he would lose his energy for ever if he stayed longer in those fatal surroundings, he *must* get away from St. Rémy. For some time Theo had been looking around for a fit opportunity—near Paris and yet in the country—where Vincent could live under the care of a physician, who would at the same time be a friend to him, and when he had found this at last, by the recommendation of

Pissarro at Auvers sur Oise, an hour by train from Paris, where lived Dr. Gachet who had been in his youth a friend of Cézanne, Pissarro and the other Impressionists, then Vincent returns from the south on the 17th of May 1890. First he was going to spend a few days with us in Paris; a telegram from Tarascon informed us that he was going to travel that night and would arrive at ten in the morning. Theo could not sleep that night for anxiety—if anything happened to Vincent on the way, he had but scarcely recovered from a long and serious attack and had refused to be accompanied by anyone. How thankful we were when it was at last time for Theo to go to the station!

From the Cité Pigalle to the Gare de Lyon is a long distance, it seemed an endless time before they came back and I began to be anxious that something had happened, when I saw at last an open fiacre enter the Cité, two merry faces nodded to me, two hands waved—a moment later Vincent stood before me.

I had expected to see a patient and there stood before me a strong, broad-shouldered man, with a healthy colour, a smile on his face and an expression of great resoluteness in his whole appearance; from all the self-portraits the one before the easel is most like him at that period. Apparently there had again come such a sudden puzzling change in his state as the Rev. Salles had already observed to his great surprise at Arles.

" He seems perfectly well, he looks much stronger than Theo," was my first thought.

Then Theo drew him to the room where was the cradle of our little boy, that had been named after Vincent : silently the two brothers looked at the quietly sleeping baby—both had tears in their eyes. Then Vincent turned smilingly to me and said, pointing to the simple crocheted cover on the cradle : " Do not cover him too much with lace, little sister."

He stayed with us three days and was all the time cheerful and lively. St. Rémy was not mentioned. He went out by himself to buy olives which he used to eat every day and which he insisted on our eating too; the first morning he was up very early and was standing in his shirt-sleeves looking at his pictures of which our apartment was full; the walls were covered with them—in the bedroom the "Blooming Orchards," in the dining-room over the mantelpiece the "Potato Eaters," in the sitting-room (salon was too solemn a name for the cosy little room) the great "Landscape from Arles," and the "Night View on the Rhône," besides to the great despair of our *femme de ménage,* there were under the bed, under the sofa, under the cupboards, in the little spare room, huge piles of unframed canvases, that were now spread out on the ground and studied with great attention.

We had also many visitors, but Vincent soon perceived that the bustle of Paris did him no good and he was longing to set to work again. So he started the 21st of May for Auvers, with an introduction to Dr. Gachet, whose faithful friendship was to become his greatest support during the short time he was to spend at Auvers. We promised to come and see him soon, and he also wanted to come back to us in a few weeks to paint our portraits. In Auvers he took up his lodgings at an inn and immediately set to work.

The hilly landscape with the sloping fields and thatched roofs of the village pleased him, but what he enjoyed most was to have models again, and again to paint figures. One of the first portraits he painted was that of Dr. Gachet, who immediately felt great sympathy for Vincent, so that they spent most of their time together and became great friends—a friendship not ended by death, for Dr. Gachet and his children continued to honour Vincent's memory with rare piety, that became a form of worship, touching in its simplicity and sincerity. "The more I think of it the more I think Vincent was a giant. Not a day passes that I do not look at his pictures, I always find there a new idea, something different each day. . . . I think again of the painter and I find him a colossus. Besides he was a philosopher. . . ."

So Gachet wrote to Theo shortly after Vincent's death and speaking of the latter's love for art he says: "The word love of art is not exact, one must call it *faith,* a faith to which

Vincent fell a martyr!" None of his contemporaries had understood him better.

It was curious to note that Dr. Gachet himself somewhat resembled Vincent physically (he was much older) and his son Paul—then a boy of fifteen years—resembled Theo a little.

Their house, built on a hill, was full of pictures and antiques, which received but scanty daylight through the small windows; before the house there was a splendid terraced flower-garden, behind, a large yard where all kinds of ducks, hens, turkeys and peacocks walked about in the company of four or five cats; it was the home of an original, but an original of great taste.

The doctor no longer practised in Auvers, but had an office in Paris where he gave consultations a few days a week, the rest of the time he painted and etched in his room, that looked most like the workshop of an alchemist of the Middle Ages. Soon after, the 10th of June, we received an invitation from him to come with the baby and spend a whole day in Auvers. Vincent came to meet us at the train and he brought a bird's nest as a plaything for his little nephew and namesake. He insisted upon carrying the baby himself and had no rest until he had shown him all the animals in the yard, where a too-loudly crowing cock made the baby red in the face for fear and made him cry, whilst Vincent cried laughingly, " the cock crows cocorico," and was very proud that he had introduced his little namesake to the animal world. We lunched in the open air and after lunch took a long walk; the day was so peacefully quiet, so happy, that nobody would have suspected how tragically a few weeks later our happiness was to be destroyed for ever. In the first days of July, Vincent visited us once more in Paris; we were exhausted by a serious illness of the baby—Theo was again considering the old plan of leaving Goupil and setting up his own business, Vincent was not satisfied with the place where the pictures were kept, and our removal to a larger apartment was talked of; so those were days of much worry and anxiety. Many friends came to visit Vincent, among others, Aurier, who had written recently his famous article about Vincent,[1] and who now came again to look at the pictures with the painter himself, and Toulouse Lautrec who stayed for lunch with us and made many jokes with Vincent about an undertaker they had met on the stairs. Guillaumin was also expected to come, but it became too much for Vincent, so he did not wait for this visit but hurried back to Auvers—overtired and excited, as his last letters and pictures show, in which the threatening catastrophe seems approaching like the ominous black birds that dart through the storm over the cornfields.

" I hope he is not getting melancholy or that a new attack is threatening again, everything has gone so well lately," Theo wrote to me the 20th of July, after he had taken me with the baby to Holland and himself had returned to Paris for a short time, till he also should take his holidays. On the 25th he wrote to me, " there is a letter from Vincent which seems very incomprehensible; when will there come a happy time for him? He is so thoroughly good." That happy time was never to come for Vincent; fear of the again threatening attack or the attack itself, drove him to death.

On the evening of the 27th of July, he tried to kill himself with a revolver. Dr. Gachet wrote that same evening to Theo the following note, " With the greatest regret I must bring you bad tidings. Yet I think it my duty to write to you immediately. At nine o'clock in the evening of to-day, Sunday, I was sent for by your brother Vincent who wanted to see me at once. I went there and found him very ill. He has wounded himself . . . as I did not know your address and he refused to give it to me, this note will reach you through Goupil." The letter reached Theo in consequence only the next morning and he immediately started for Auvers. From there he wrote to me the same day, the 28th of July : " This morning a Dutch painter[2] who also lives in Auvers brought me a letter from Dr. Gachet that contained bad tidings about Vincent and asked me to come. Leaving everything I went

[1] " Les Isolés," " Mercure de France," Janvier 1890.
[2] Hirschig.

and found him somewhat better than I expected. I will not write the particulars, they are too sad, but you must know dearest, that his life may be in danger. . . .

" He was glad that I came and we are together all the time . . . poor fellow, very little happiness fell to his share and no illusions are left him. The burden grows too heavy for him, at times he feels so alone. He often asks for you and the baby, and said that you would not imagine there was so much sorrow in life. Oh! if we could give him some new courage to live. Don't make yourself too anxious, his condition has been so hopeless before, but his strong constitution deceived the doctors." That hope proved idle. Early in the morning of the 29th of July Vincent passed away.

Theo wrote to me, " one of his last words was : ' I wish I could die now,' and his wish was fulfilled. A few moments and all was over. He had found the rest he could not find on earth. . . . The next morning there came from Paris and elsewhere eight friends who decked the room where the coffin stood with his pictures, which came out wonderfully. There were many flowers and wreaths. Dr. Gachet was the first to bring a large bunch of sunflowers, because Vincent was so fond of them. . . .

" He rests in a sunny spot amidst the cornfields. . . ."

From a letter of Theo's to his mother : " One cannot write how grieved one is nor find any comfort. It is a grief that will last and which I certainly shall never forget as long as I live; the only thing one might say is, that he himself has the rest he was longing for . . . life was such a burden to him; but now, as often happens, everybody is full of praise for his talents. . . . Oh! mother he was so my own, own brother."

Theo's frail health was broken. Six months later, on the 25th of January 1891, he had followed his brother.

They rest side by side in the little cemetery between the cornfields of Auvers.

J. VAN GOGH-BONGER

December, 1913

EARLY YEARS

Dear Theo,

I was glad you answered me so soon and that you like Brussels and have found a nice boarding-house. Don't lose heart if it is very difficult at times, everything will come out all right and nobody can in the beginning do as he wishes.

How I pity Uncle Hein, I heartily hope he will recover, but, Theo, I fear he will not. Last summer he was still full of enthusiasm and had so many plans and told me that business was flourishing. It's very sad. Last Sunday I was at Uncle Cor's and spent a very pleasant day there as you can imagine, and saw so many beautiful things. As you know, Uncle has just come back from Paris and brought some beautiful pictures and drawings with him. I remained in Amsterdam till Monday morning and went to see the museums again. Do you know that they are going to build a large new museum in Amsterdam, instead of the Trippenhuis? I think it is right, for the Trippenhuis is small and many pictures are hung so that they can hardly be seen.

How I should have liked to see that picture by Cluysenaer, I have only seen a few pictures of his and those I liked very much. Tell me if that other picture is by " *Alfred* " Stevens, or else what the first name is. I know the photograph after the Rotta[1] and have even seen the picture at the Exhibition in Brussels. Be sure to let me know what pictures you see, I am always glad to know. The album of which you gave me the title is not the one I meant, which is *only* lithographs after Corot. But I thank you for the trouble you have taken. I hope to get a letter from sister Anna soon, she is rather laggard about writing of late. Do surprise her with a letter, that would be such a pleasure to her. I suppose you are very

[1] Italian painter (Venice).

busy, but that is not bad. It is cold here and they are skating already. I walk as much as I can. I wonder if you will have any chance to skate. Enclosed you will find my photograph, but if you write home don't mention it, as you know it is for father's birthday. I have already sent you my congratulations upon that day. My best compliments to Uncle and Aunt, also to Mr. Schmidt and Eduard. Always

Your loving brother,

Vincent

Kind regards from everybody at Haanebeek's, Aunt Fie and Roos.

London, July 31 1874

Dear Theo,

I am glad you have read Michelet[1] and that you understand him so well. Such a book teaches us that there is much more in love than people generally suppose.

That book has been a revelation to me as well as a Gospel at the same time, " no woman is old." (That does not mean that there are no old women, but that a woman is not-old as long as she loves and is loved.) And then such a chapter as " The Aspirations of Autumn," how beautiful it is.

That a woman is quite a different being than a man, and a being that we do not yet know, at least only quite superficially, as you said, yes, I am sure of it. And that man and wife can be one, that is to say one whole and not two halves, yes, I believe that too.

A. keeps well, we take beautiful walks together. It is so beautiful here if one has only an open and simple eye with few beams in it. But if one has that it is beautiful everywhere.

That picture by Thijs Maris which Mr. Teersteg[2] has bought must be beautiful, I have heard about it already and I myself have bought and sold one quite similar.

Since my return to England my love for drawing has

[1] Author of *L'Amour et la Femme*.
[2] Representative of Goupil & Co. in The Hague.

stopped, but perhaps I will take it up again some day or other. I am reading a great deal just now.

Probably we move on the 1st of January, 1875, to another larger house. Mr. Obach is in Paris just now to decide whether we shall take over that other business or not. Don't speak about it for the moment to anybody.

I hope you are all right and will write to us soon. A. begins to enjoy seeing pictures and sees them pretty well, she likes Boughton, Maris and Jacquet, so that is a beginning. *Entre nous*, I think it will be very difficult to find something for her, they say everywhere that she is too young, and generally German is required, but at all events, she has more chances here than in Holland. Adieu.

Vincent

You can imagine how pleasant it is to be here together with A. Tell Mr. Tersteeg the picture arrived in good order and that I will write to him soon.

London, March 6 1875

Dear Theo,

Bravo, Theo. Your appreciation of that girl in "Adam Bede" is very good. That landscape—in which the fallow, sandy path runs over the hill to the village, with its clay or white-washed cottages, with mossgrown roofs, and here and there a black thornbush, on either side of the brown heath, and a gloomy sky over it, with a narrow white streak at the horizon—it is out of Michel.[1]

But there is a still purer and nobler sentiment in it than in Michel. To-day I enclose, in the box we send, the little book containing poetry I spoke of. Also "Jesus" by Renan and "Joan of Arc" by Michelet and also a portrait of Corot from the "London News," which hangs in my room too.

I do not think you have any immediate chance of being transferred to the house in London.

---

[1] The French landscapist of the early nineteenth century, Georges Michel—much influenced by the landscapes of Rembrandt.

Don't regret that your life is too easy, mine is rather easy too; I think that life is pretty long and that the time will arrive soon enough in which " another shall gird thee and carry thee where thou wouldst not."[1]

Adieu, remember me to all the friends. With a firm handshake,

Vincent

Paris, July 24 1875

Dear Theo,

A few days ago we received a picture by de Nittis, a view of London on a rainy day, Westminster Bridge and the Houses of Parliament. I used to pass Westminster Bridge every morning and every evening and know how it looks when the sun sets behind Westminster Abbey and the Houses of Parliament, and how it looks early in the morning, and in winter in snow and fog.

When I saw the picture I felt how much I loved London. Still I think that it is better for me that I left it.

This in answer to your question.

I certainly do not believe that you will be sent to London.

Thanks for the " Springtime of Life." And " At Midnight " by Rückert. The first is very beautiful, the latter reminds me of " September Night " by de Musset. I wish I could send it you, but I do not possess it.

Yesterday we sent a box to The Hague in which you will find what I promised you.

I hear that Anna and Liesbeth are at home, I should like to see them.

Be as happy as you can and write to me soon. With a firm handshake,

Your loving brother,
Vincent

[1] *John* XXI 18.

Paris, September 17 1875

Dear Theo,

A feeling, even a keen one for the beauties of Nature is not the same as a religious feeling, though I think these two stand in close relation to one another.

Almost everybody has a feeling for nature, one more, the other less, but there are a few who feel that God is a spirit and they who worship Him must worship Him in spirit and in truth.[1] Our parents belong to those few; I think Uncle Vincent does too.

You know that there is written: "The world passeth away and the lust thereof."[2] And that there is mention also on the other hand of "a good part that shall not be taken away from us,"[3] and, "a well of water springing up into everlasting life."[4] Let us also pray that we become rich in God; but do not think too deeply about these things, gradually they will become clearer to you, and do as I suggested. Let us ask that our part in life should be to become the poor in the kingdom of God, God's servants. We are still far from it; let us pray that our eye may become single and then our whole body shall be full of light.[5]

Compliments to Roos and to anybody who asks about me.

Your loving brother,

Vincent

It is the same with the feeling for art. Don't give yourself utterly to that. Keep by all means love for your work and respect for Mr. Tersteeg. Later on you will see better than now how much he deserves it.

[1] *John* IV 24.   [2] I *John* II 17.

[3] *Luke* X 42: the closing words of the episode at the house of Martha and Mary—an episode which must have appealed to Vincent in a deep way in terms of the characters involved.

[4] *John* IV 14, describing the meeting with the woman of Samaria —another New Testament character who must have appealed deeply to Vincent, given the close familiarity with the text in point that is indicated by two citations from it in this single short letter.

[5] See *Luke* XI 34, the Biblical metaphor of light was again one of deep significance.

However you need not exaggerate this.

Is your appetite good? Eat especially as much bread as you like. Good night, I must give my boots a shine for to-morrow.

Paris, Sept. 25 1875

Dear Theo,

The path is narrow, therefore we must be careful. You know how others have arrived where we want to go, let us take that simple road too.

*Ora et labora,*1 let us do our daily work, whatever the hand finds to do, with all our strength and let us believe that God will give good gifts, a part that will not be taken away, to those who ask Him for it.

"Therefore if any man be in Christ, he is a new creature : old things are past away; behold all things are become new!" (2 Cor. v. 17.)

I am going to destroy all my books by Michelet, etc. I wish you would do the same.

How I am longing for Christmas, but let us have patience, it will come soon enough.

Courage, lad; my compliments to all the friends, and believe me,

Your loving brother,

Vincent

As soon as possible I will send the money for the frames. When I write to Mr. Tersteeg, I will tell him that for the moment I am rather short of cash; I asked our cashier to hold back every month a part of my salary as I shall want a lot of money around Christmas for my journey, etc., however I hope to send it before long.

Paris, October 14 1875

Dear Theo,

I send you again a few words to cheer myself as well as you. I advised you to destroy your books, and do so now;

___
1 " Pray and work "

yes, do so, it will give you rest; but take care all the same not to become narrow-minded and afraid of reading what is well written; on the contrary doing that is a *comfort* in life. " Whatsoever things are true, whatsoever things are honest, whatsoever things are just, whatsoever things are pure, whatsoever things are lovely, whatsoever things are of good report; if there be any virtue, and if there be any praise, think on these things."[1]

Look for light and freedom and *do not ponder too deeply over the evil in life.*

How I should like to have you here and show you the Luxembourg and the Louvre; but I think you too will come here after a while. Father wrote to me once, " Do not forget the story of Icarus, who wanted to fly to the sun and arrived at a certain height, then lost his wings and dropped into the sea." You will often feel that neither you nor I are what we hope to become some day and that we are still far beneath father and other people; that we are wanting in solidity, simplicity and sincerity; one cannot become simple and true in one day. But let us persevere, *above all let us have patience; those who believe hasten not;* still there is a difference between our longing to become real Christians and that of Icarus to fly to the sun. I think there is no harm in having a relatively strong body, take care to feed yourself well, and if sometimes you are very hungry, or rather have an appetite, eat well then. I assure you that I often do the same, and certainly used to do so. Especially bread, boy, " Bread is the staff of life," is a proverb of the English (though they are very fond of meat too, and in general take too much of it). And now write to me soon and put in the things of everyday life.

Keep good courage and give my compliments to everybody who asks about me; within a month or two I hope we shall see each other.

With a firm handshake, I am always

Your loving brother,

Vincent

[1] *Philippians* IV 8.

Paris, February 19 1876

Dear Theo,

Thanks for your last letter and also for the catalogue sent in the last box.

Have I thanked you already for Andersen's tales, if not I do so now. From home I have heard that this spring you will have to travel on business, you will not be sorry for that I suppose, it is a good exercise and you will see many beautiful things in your travels.

In the next box you will find Longfellow. Yesterday evening Gladwell was with me, he comes every Friday and we read poetry together.

I have not read "Hyperion" yet, but I have heard that it is very beautiful, I have just read a very beautiful book by Eliot, three tales, called "Scenes from Clerical Life"; the last story in particular, "Janet's Repentance," struck me very much.[1] It is the life of a clergyman who lives chiefly among the inhabitants of the dirty streets of a town, his study looks out on the gardens with stumps of cabbage, etc., and on the red roofs and smoking chimneys of poor tenements. For his dinner he usually had nothing but underdone mutton and watery potatoes. He died at the age of thirty-four and during his long illness he was nursed by a woman who was a drunkard, but by his teaching, and leaning as it were on him, she had conquered her weakness and found rest for her soul. At his burial they read the chapter which says, "I am the resurrection and the life, he that believeth in me, though he were dead, yet shall he live."[2] And now it is again Saturday evening, for the days pass so quickly and the time for my

[1] Vincent's paraphrase of the story which follows offers many striking parallels with his own subsequent life; it was characteristic of him to identify himself with fictional heroes, and to pick out from the books he read whatever seemed to have a moral and spiritual application to his own destiny.

[2] *John* XI 25.

departure will soon be here. No answer as yet from Scarborough. Kind greetings and a handshake, always

Your loving brother,

Vincent

Ramsgate, England, April 28 1876

Dear Theo,

Many happy returns, my best wishes for this day, may our mutual love increase with the years.

I am so glad that we have so many things in common, not only memories of childhood but also that you are working in the same business in which I was till now and know so many people and places which I know also, and that you have so much love for nature and art.

Mr. Stokes[1] has told me that he intends to move after the holidays, of course with the whole school, to a little village on the Thames about three hours from London. There he will organize his school somewhat differently and perhaps enlarge it.

Now I am going to tell you about a walk we took yesterday. It was to an inlet of the sea, and the road thither led through fields of young corn and along hedges of hawthorn, etc.

Arriving there, we saw to our left a high steep ridge of sand and stone as tall as a two-storey house. On the top of it were old, gnarled hawthorn bushes, whose black and grey moss-grown stems and branches were all bent to one side by the wind, there were also a few elder bushes.

The ground on which we walked was covered all over with big grey stones, chalk and shells.

To the right lay the sea, as calm as a pond and reflecting the light of the transparent grey sky where the sun was setting.

The tide was out and the water very low.

Thanks for your letter of yesterday, I am very glad that

---

[1] Head of the school; the move was to Isleworth.

Willem Valkis is also an employee of the house. Give him my best regards. I wish I could walk once more with you through my woods, to Scheveningen.

Have a pleasant day to-day and give my love to all who may ask about me and believe me,

Your loving brother,

Vincent

Once more my best wishes, lad, I hope you will begin a happy and prosperous year. These are important years that we are living through now and much depends on them. May everything come out all right.

A hearty handshake. à Dieu.

Ramsgate, England, May 31 1876

Dear Theo,

Bravo, that you got yourself to Etten on the 21st of May, so that four of the six children were at home. Father wrote me in detail how the day was spent.

Thanks also for your last letter.

Did I tell you about the storm I saw lately? The sea was yellowish especially near the shore; at the horizon a streak of light and above it the immense dark grey clouds from which the rain poured down in slanting streaks. The wind blew the dust from the little white path on the rocks into the sea and swayed the blooming hawthorn bushes and wallflowers that grow on the rocks. To the right were fields of young green corn and in the distance the town that looked like the towns that Albrecht Dürer used to etch. A town with its turrets, mills, slate roofs and houses built in Gothic style, and below, the harbour between two dykes, projecting far into the sea. I also saw the sea last Sunday night, everything was dark and grey, but at the horizon the day began to dawn.

It was still very early but a lark was singing already. So were the nightingales in the gardens near the sea. In the distance shone the light from the lighthouse, the guardship, etc.

That same night I looked from the window of my room on the roofs of the houses that can be seen from there and on the tops of the elm trees, dark against the night sky. Over those roofs, one single star, but a beautiful, large, friendly one. And I thought of you all and of my own past years and of our home, and in me arose the words and the feeling : " Keep me from being a son who makes ashamed, give me Thy blessing, not because I deserve it but for my mother's sake. Thou art love, cover all things. Without Thy continued blessings we succeed in nothing."

Enclosed is a little drawing of the view from the window of the school, through which the boys wave good-bye to their parents after a visit when they are going back to the station.

None of us will ever forget the view from the window. *You ought to have seen* it this week when we had rain, especially in the twilight when the lamps were on and their light reflected in the wet street.

Days like that could put Mr. Stokes into a bad temper, and when the boys made more noise than he liked, it sometimes happened that they had to go without their supper.

I wish you could have seen them then looking from the window, it was rather melancholy; they have so little else except their meals to look forward to and to help them pass their days. I also should like you to see them going from the dark stairs and passage to the dining-room, a place of bright sunshine.

Another curious place is the room with the rotten floor, where are six washing basins in which they have to wash themselves and where a dim light flows through the window with its broken panes on the washing stand, this a rather a melancholy sight. I should like to spend a winter with them or have spent a winter with them in the past to know what it is like. The boys made an oil stain on your drawing, please excuse them.

Enclosed a little note for Uncle Jan. And now good night, if anybody should enquire after me give them my kind regards. Do you visit Borchers now and then, if you see him

L.V.G.   D greet him for me, also Willem Valkis and all at Roos'. A handshake from

Your loving brother,

Vincent

Isleworth, England, October 7 1876

Dear Theo,

It is Saturday again and I write once more. How I long to see you again, Oh! my longing is sometimes so strong. Write soon, a little word as to how you are.

Last Wednesday we took a long walk to a village an hour's distance from here. The road led through meadows and fields, along hedges of hawthorn, full of blackberries and clematis, and here and there a large elm tree. It was so beautiful when the sun set behind the grey clouds, and the shadows were long. By chance we met the school of Mr. Stokes, where there are still several of the boys I knew.

The clouds retained their red hue long after the sun had set and the dusk had settled over the fields, and we saw in the distance the lamps lit in the village. While I was writing to you, I was called to Mr. Jones, who asked if I would walk to London to collect some money for him. And when I came home in the evening, hurrah, there was a letter from Father with tidings about you. How I should like to be with you both, my boy. And thank God there is some improvement, though you are still weak. And you will be longing to see Mother, and now that I hear that you are going home with her, I think of the words of Conscience:[1]

" I have been ill, my mind was tired, my soul disillusioned and my body suffering. I whom God has endowed at least with moral energy and a strong instinct of affection, I fell in the abyss of the most bitter discouragement and I felt with horror how a deadly poison penetrated my stifled heart. I spent three months on the moors, you know that beautiful region where the soul retires within itself and enjoys a

[1] A Flemish author.

delicious rest, where everything breathes calm and peace; where the soul in presence of God's immaculate creation throws off the yoke of conventions, forgets society, and loosens its bonds, with the strength of renewed youth; where each thought takes the form of prayer, where everything that is not in harmony with fresh and free nature quits the heart. Oh, there the tired souls find rest, there the exhausted man regains his youthful strength. So I passed my days of illness. . . . And then the evening! To be seated before the big fireplace with one's feet in the ashes, one's eyes fixed on a star that sends its ray through the opening in the chimney as if to call me, or absorbed in vague dreams too much to look at the fire, to see the flames rise, flicker, and supplant one another as if desirous to lick the kettle with their tongues of fire, and to think that such is human life : to be born, to work, to love, to grow and to disappear."

Mr. Jones has promised me that I shall not have to teach so much in future, but that I may work in his parish, visiting the people, talking with them, etc. May God give His blessing to me.

Now I am going to tell you about my walk to London. I left here at twelve o'clock in the morning and reached my destination between five and six. When I came into that part of the town where most of the picture galleries are, around the Strand, I met many acquaintances : it was dinner-time, so many were in the street, leaving the office or going back there. First I met a young clergyman who once preached here, and with whom I then became acquainted, and then the employee of Mr. Wallis, and then one of the Messrs. Wallis himself, whom I used to visit now and then at his house, now he has two children; then I met Mr. Reid and Mr. Richardson,[1] who are already old friends. Last year about this time Mr. Richardson was in Paris and we walked together to Père Lachaise.

After that I went to van Wisselingh, where I saw sketches

[1] Reid was an English art-dealer; Richardson was the travelling representative for Theo's firm.

for two church windows. In the middle of one window stands the portrait of a middle-aged lady, oh, such a noble face, with the words " Thy will be done," over it, and in the other window the portrait of her daughter, with the words, " Faith is the substance of things hoped for, the evidence of things not seen."[1] There, and in the gallery of Messrs. Goupil & Co., I saw beautiful pictures and drawings. It is such an intense delight to be so often reminded of Holland by art.

In the City I went to see Mr. Gladwell and to St. Paul's Church. And from the City to the other end of London, where I visited a boy who had left the school of Mr. Stokes because of illness and I found him quite well, playing in the street. Then to the place where I had to collect the money for Mr. Jones. The suburbs of London have a peculiar charm, between the little houses and gardens are open spots covered with grass and generally with a church or school or workhouse in the middle between the trees and shrubs, and it can be so beautiful there, when the sun is setting red in the thin evening mist.

Yesterday evening it was so, and afterwards I wished you could have seen those London streets when the twilight began to fall and the lamps were lit, and everybody went home; everything showed that it was Saturday night and in all that bustle there was peace, one felt the need of and the excitement at the approaching Sunday. Oh, those Sundays and all that is done and accomplished on those Sundays, it is such a comfort for those poor districts and crowded streets.

In the City it was dark, but it was a beautiful walk along the row of churches one has to pass. Near the Strand I took a bus that took me quite a long way, it was already pretty late. I passed the little church of Mr. Jones and saw in the distance another one, where at that hour a light was still burning; I entered and found it to be a very beautiful little Catholic church, where a few women were praying. Then I came to that dark park about which I have written you already and from there I saw in the distance the lights of Isleworth

[1] *Hebrews* XI 1.

and the church with the ivy, and the churchyard with the weeping willows beside the Thames.

To-morrow I shall get for the second time some small salary for my new work, and with it buy a pair of new boots and a new hat. And then, with God's will, I shall go fitted out afresh.

In the London streets they sell scented violets everywhere, they flower here twice a year. I bought some for Mrs. Jones to make her forget the pipe I smoke now and then, especially late in the evening on the playground, but the tobacco here has a touch of gloom about it.

Well, Theo, try to get well soon and read this letter when Mother is sitting with you, because I should like to be with you both in thought. I cannot tell you how glad I am that Mr. Jones has promised to give me work in his parish, so that I shall find by and by what I want. I am longing so much for you. A handshake for yourself and one for Mother when she is sitting beside you. Many regards to the Roos family and to everyone I know, especially to Mr. Tersteeg. Tell Mother it was delightful to put on a pair of socks knitted by her, after that long walk to London.

This morning the sun rose so beautifully again, I see it every morning when I wake the boys, à Dieu.

> Your loving brother,
>
> Vincent

[Dordrecht, Holland, April 16 1887]

Dear Theo,

Thanks for your letter, be strong and He will strengthen your heart.[1] To-day I received a long letter from home, in which father asked me if we could arrange to go together to Amsterdam next Sunday, to visit Uncle Cor. If you agree I will arrive at The Hague Saturday night at eleven o'clock, and we can go on to Amsterdam by the first train the next morning.

I think we had better do so, Father seems to have set his

---

[1] See *Psalms* XXVII 14.

heart upon it, and it will be nice to spend another Sunday together. Can I stay over night with you—otherwise I could go to a hotel. Write me a postcard if it is all right, let us keep close together.

It is already late, this afternoon I took a long walk, because I felt I needed it, first around the cathedral, then past the New Church, and then along the dyke, where the mills are that one sees in the distance as one walks near the station. There is so much expressed in this peculiar landscape and surrounding, it seems to say : " Be of good courage, fear not."[1]

Oh ! might I be shown the way to devote my life more completely to the service of God and the Gospel. I keep praying for it and I think I shall be heard, I say it in all humility. Humanly speaking, one would say it cannot happen, but when I think seriously about it and penetrate under the surface of what is impossible to man, then my soul is in communion with God, for it is possible to Him, who speaks and it is done; who commands and it stands fast.[2]

Oh ! Theo, Theo boy, if I might only succeed in this, if that heavy depression because everything I undertook failed, that torrent of reproaches which I have heard and felt, if it might be taken from me, and if there might be given to me both the opportunity and the strength needed to come to full development and to persevere in that course for which my father and I would thank the Lord so fervently. A handshake and kind regards to Roos,

Ever your loving brother,

Vincent

Amsterdam, May 30 1877

Dear Theo,

Thanks for your letter that arrived to-day, I am very busy and write in a hurry. I gave your letter to Uncle Jan, he sends you his greetings and thanks for it.

There was a sentence in your letter that struck me, " I wish

[1] See *Deuteronomy* XXXI 6, etc.   [2] See *Psalms* XXXIII 9.

I were far away from everything, I am the cause of all, and bring only sorrow to everybody, I alone have brought all this misery on myself and others." These words struck me because that same feeling, just the same, not more nor less, is also on my conscience.

When I think of the past,—when I think of the future of almost invincible difficulties, of much and difficult work, which I do not like, which I, or rather my evil self, would like to shirk; when I think the eyes of so many are fixed on me,—who will know where the fault is, if I do not succeed, who will not make me trivial reproaches, but as they are well tried and trained in everything that is right and virtuous and fine gold, they will say, as it were by the expression of their faces : we have helped you and have been a light unto you,—we have done for you what we could, have you tried honestly? what is now our reward and the fruit of our labour? See! when I think of all this, and of so many other things like it, too numerous to name them all, of all the difficulties and cares that do not grow less when we advance in life, of sorrow, of disappointment, of the fear of failure, of disgrace,—then I also have the longing—I wish I were far away from everything!

And yet I go on, but prudently and hoping to have strength to resist those things, so that I shall know what to answer to those reproaches that threaten me, and believing that notwithstanding everything that seems against me, I yet shall reach the aim I am striving for, and if God wills it, shall find favour in the eyes of some I love and in the eyes of those that will come after me.

There is written : " Lift up the hands which hang down, and the feeble knees,"[1] and when the disciples had worked all night and had not caught any fish, they were told " go out into the deep and cast your nets again into the sea."[2]

My head is sometimes heavy and often it burns and my thoughts are confused,—I don't see how I shall ever get that difficult and extensive study into it—to get used to and per-

---

[1] A free paraphrase of *Isaiah* xxxv 3.
[2] A free paraphrase of *Luke* v 4.

severe in simple regular study after all those emotional years is not always easy.[1] And yet I go on; if we are tired isn't it then because we have already walked a long way, and if it is true that man has his battle to fight on earth, is not then the feeling of weariness and the burning of the head a sign that we have been struggling? When we are working at a difficult task and strive after a good thing we fight a righteous battle, the direct reward of which is that we are kept from much evil.

And God sees the trouble and the sorrow and He can help in spite of all. The faith in God is firm in me—it is no imagination, no idle faith—but it is so, it is true, there is a God Who is alive and He is with our parents and *His eye is also upon us,* and I am sure He plans our life and we do not quite belong to ourselves as it were—and this God is no other than Christ of Whom we read in our Bible and Whose word and history is also deep in our heart. If I had only given all my strength to it before, yes, I should have been further now,—but even now He will be a strong support, and it is in His power to make our lives bearable, to keep us from evil, to let all things contribute towards a good end, to make our end peaceful.

There is much evil in the world and in ourselves, terrible things, and one does not need to be far advanced in life, to be in fear of much and to feel the need of a firm faith in life hereafter, and to know that without faith in God one cannot live, one cannot bear it.—But with that faith one can go on for a long time.

When I was standing beside the corpse of Aerssen the calmness and dignity and solemn silence of death contrasted with us living people to such an extent, that we all felt the truth of what his daughter said with such simplicity : " he is freed from the burden of life, which we have to go on bearing." And yet we are so much attached to the old life, because next to our despondent moods we have our happy moments when heart and soul rejoice, like the lark that

[1] Vincent had just begun preparing for the State Examination that would admit him to the University to study theology.

cannot keep from singing in the morning, even though the soul sometimes sinks within us and is fearful. And the memories of all we have loved stay and come back to us in the evening of our life. They are not dead but sleep, and it is well to gather a treasure of them.

A handshake and write soon to

Your loving brother,
Vincent

EXTRACTS ONLY

Amsterdam, September 18 1877

Dear Theo,

The time approaches when you will go on your business trip for Messrs. Goupil and Co., and I enjoy beforehand the prospect of seeing you again. I want to ask you one thing: could not you arrange it so that we could be quietly and calmly together for at least one whole day?

This week Mendes is out of town, spending a few days with the Rev. Schröder at Zwolle, a former pupil of his. So having some leisure I could carry out an old plan to go and see the etchings by Rembrandt in the Trippenhuis, I went there this morning and I am glad I did so. While there, I thought, could not Theo and I see them together some day? Think it over, whether you could spare a day or two for such things. How would a man like Father, who so often goes long distances even in the night with a lantern, to visit a sick or dying man, to speak with him about One whose word is light even in the night of suffering and agony, how would he feel about the etchings of Rembrandt, for instance "The Flight to Egypt in the Night" or the "Burial of Jesus"? The collection in the Trippenhuis is splendid, I saw many I had never seen before, they also told me there about drawings by Rembrandt at the Fodor Museum. If you think it possible, speak about it with Mr. Tersteeg and drop me a line when you are coming, then I can finish my work and shall be free and quite at your disposal when you come.

I never see things of that kind, etchings or paintings too, but I think of you and all at home.

But I am up to my ears in my work, for it is becoming clear to me what I really must know, what *they* know and what inspires *those* whom I should like to follow. " Examine the Scriptures " is not written in vain, but that word is a good guide and I should like to become the sort of scribe, who from his treasure brings forth old and new things.

[There follows a section in which Vincent writes of the family life of Kee Vos and her husband as he had experienced it on a recent visit—Vincent was later to fall in love with her as a widow—and of two sermons he had recently heard.]

Father wrote me that you had been to Antwerp, I am longing to hear what you saw there. Long ago I too saw the old pictures in the Museum, and I think I even remember a beautiful portrait by Rembrandt; if one could remember things clearly, that would be fine, but it is like the view on a long road, in the distance things appear smaller and in a haze.

One evening there was a fire here on the river—a boat loaded with arrack, or something like it, was burning : I was with Uncle on the Wassenaar, there was, relatively speaking, no danger as they had removed the burning steamer from between the other ships and had fastened it to the moorings. When the flames rose high one saw the Buitenkant and the black row of people that stood looking there, and the little boats that were hovering around the blaze of the fire looked also black in the water in which the flames were reflected; I do not know if you remember the photographs after the works of Jazet that were in the Galerie Photographique at the time, but have been destroyed since, " Christmas Eve," " The Fire," and others, this was something like them.

Twilight is falling, " blessed twilight," Dickens called it and indeed he was right. Blessed twilight, especially when two or three are together in harmony of mind and like scribes bring forth out of their treasure things old and new.[1]

[1] *Matthew* XIII 52.

Blessed twilight, when two or three are gathered together in His name and He is in the midst of them,[1] and blessed is the man who knows these things and follows them too.

Rembrandt knew that, for from the rich treasure of his heart he brought forth among other things that drawing in sepia, charcoal, ink, etc. which is at the British Museum, representing the house in Bethany. In that room twilight has fallen, the figure of our Lord, noble and impressive, stands out serious and dark against the window through which the evening twilight is shedding itself. At the feet of Jesus sits Mary who has chosen that good part which shall not be taken away from her,[2] and Martha is in the room busy with something or other, if I remember well she stirs the fire or something like it. That drawing I hope never to forget nor what it seems to tell me : " I am the light of the world, he that followeth me shall not walk in darkness, but shall have the light of life."[3]

[A further group of Biblical texts then follows.]

Such things twilight tells to those who have ears to hear and a heart to understand and to believe in God—blessed twilight! And in that picture by Ruyperez, the " Imitation of Jesus Christ," it is also twilight, and also in another etching by Rembrandt : David in Prayer to God.

But it is not always blessed twilight, as you can see from my handwriting, I am sitting upstairs by the lamp, for there are visitors downstairs and I cannot sit there with my books. Uncle Jan sends you his compliments. . . .

Have a good time, write soon and come soon, for it is well to see each other again and to talk things over, perhaps this summer we can go and see the exhibition that will be opened a few days from now. Compliments to the Rooses, à Dieu, a handshake from

Your loving brother,

Vincent

---

[1] See *Matthew* XVIII 20.
[2] See *Luke* X 42.
[3] *John* VIII 12.

Amsterdam, April 3 1878[1]

I have been thinking over what we have been talking about and involuntarily I thought of the saying, "nous sommes aujourd'hui ce que nous étions hier." That does not mean that one must stand still and may not try to develop oneself, on the contrary there is an urgent reason for doing so and succeeding in it. But in order to remain true to that saying one must not slide back and if one has begun to look at things in a free and open way, one must not give it up or deviate from it.

Those who said: "We are the same today as we were yesterday," were "honest men," which is proved by the Constitution they made, which will remain for all time, and which has been said to be written "avec le rayon d'en haut," and "d'un doigt de feu."[2] It is good to be an "honest man" and to try to become so more and more, and he who believes that to be "homme intérieur et spirituel"[3] is part of it also, is right.

The man aware with security and certainty that he belonged to them would always go quietly and calmly on his way, not doubting of the good result in the end.—There was a man who went to church one day and asked: "Can it be that my zeal has deceived me, that I have taken the wrong road, and have not planned it well? Oh! if I might be freed from this uncertainty, and might have the firm conviction that I shall conquer and succeed in the end!" And then a voice answered him: "And if you knew that for certain, what would you do then?—act now as if you knew it for certain, and you will not be confounded." Then the man went forth on his way, believing instead of unbelieving, and he went back to his work, no longer doubting or wavering.

As to being "homme intérieur et spirituel," could not one develop that by the knowledge of history in general and of

[1] In this letter Vincent in his haste omits the "Dear Theo."
[2] "with a ray from on high", "by a finger of fire".
[3] "an inner and spiritual man".

certain persons from all ages, especially from the history of the Bible to that of the Revolution and from the Odyssey to the books of Dickens and Michelet? And could not one learn something from the works of such as Rembrandt and from "Mauvaises Herbes" by Breton, or "The Hours of the Day" by Millet, or "Bénédicité" by de Groux or Brion, or "The Conscript," by de Groux, or the one by Conscience, or "The Large Oaks," by Dupré, or even from "The Mills and Sandy Plains," by Michel?

We have talked a good deal about our duty, and how we could attain the right goal and we came to the conclusion, that in the first place our aim must be to find a steady position and a profession to which we can entirely devote ourselves.

And I believe that we also agreed on this point, that one must especially have the end in mind, and that the victory one would gain after a whole life of work and effort is better than one that is gained sooner. Whoever lives sincerely and encounters much trouble and disappointment, but is not bowed down by them, is worth more than one who has always sailed before the wind and has only known relative prosperity. For who are those that show some sign of higher life? They are those to whom may be applied the words: "Laboureurs, votre vie est triste, laboureurs, vous souffrez dans la vie, laboureurs, vous êtes bien-heureux,"[1] they are those that bear the signs of "toute une vie de lutte et de travail soutenu sans fléchir jamais."[2] It is good to try to become as much. So we go forth on our way, "indefessi favente Deo."[3] As to me I must become a good clergyman, who has something to say that is right and may be of use in the world, and perhaps it is better that I have a relatively long time of preparation, and am strongly confirmed in a staunch conviction before I am called to speak to others about it. . . . If only we try to live sincerely, it will go well with us, even though we are certain to experience real sorrow, and great disappointments,

---

[1] "Labourers, your life is sad, labourers, you suffer in this life, labourers, you are blessed ".

[2] "a full life of struggle and toil borne without ever bowing ".

[3] "unwearied, thanks to the grace of God ".

and also will probably commit great faults and do wrong things, but it certainly is true, that it is better to be high-spirited, even though one makes more mistakes, than to be narrow-minded and all too prudent. It is good to love many things, for therein lies the true strength, and whosoever loves much performs much, and can accomplish much, and what is done in love is well done; if one is struck by some book or other, for instance, by one of Michelet's, like " L'Hirondelle," " L'Alouette," " Le Rossignol," " Les Aspirations d'Aut- omne," " Je vois d'ici une dame," " J'aimais cette petite Ville singulière " it is because it is written from the heart in sim- plicity and meekness of mind. It is better to say few words that have real significance than to say many that are but idle sounds, and are just as useless as they are easy to utter.

If one keeps on loving faithfully what is really worth loving, and does not waste one's love on insignificant and unworthy and meaningless things, one will get more light by and by and grow stronger.

The sooner one tries to master a certain profession and a certain handicraft and adopt a fairly independent way of thinking and acting, and the more one keeps to strict rules, the firmer the character one will acquire, and for all that one need not become narrow-minded.

It is wise to do so, for life is but short, and time passes quickly; if one is master of one thing and understands one thing well, one has at the same time insight into and under- standing of many things into the bargain. Sometimes it is well to go into the world and converse much with people, and at times one is obliged to do so, but whoever would prefer to be quietly alone with his work, and who wants but very few friends, he will go safest through the world and among people. One must never trust the occasion when one is with- out difficulties, or some care or trouble, and one must not take things too easily. And even in the most refined circles and the best surroundings and circumstances one must keep some- thing of the original character of a Robinson Crusoe or anchorite, for otherwise one has no root in oneself, and one must never let the fire go out in one's soul, but keep it burn-

ing. And whoever chooses poverty for himself and loves it,
possesses a great treasure, and will always clearly hear the
voice of his conscience; he who hears and obeys that voice,
which is the best gift of God, finds at last a friend in it, and
is never alone. . . .

So be it with us, boy, and may you have blessings on your
way, and God be with you in all things and make you
succeed, that is the wish, with a hearty handshake on your
departure from[1]

Your so loving brother,
Vincent

Laeken, a suburb of Brussels, November 15, 1878

Dear Theo,

On the evening of the day we spent together, which passed
only too quickly for me, I want to write to you again. It was
a great joy for me to see you again and to talk with you, and
it is a blessing that such a day, that passes in a moment, and
such a joy that is of so short duration, stays in our memory
and will never be forgotten. When we had taken leave I
walked back, not along the shortest way but along the tow-
path. Here are workshops of all kinds that look picturesque,
especially in the evening with the lights, and to us who are
also labourers and workmen, each in his sphere and in the
work to which he is called, they speak in their own way, if
we only listen to them, for they say : Work while it is day,
the night cometh when no man can work.

It was just the moment when the street cleaners came home
with their carts with the old white horses. A long row of
these carts were standing at the so-called Terme des boues, at
the beginning of the tow-path. Some of these old white horses
resemble a certain old aquatint engraving, which you perhaps
know, an engraving that has no great art value, it is true, but
which struck me, and made a deep impression upon me. I
mean the last from that series of prints called " The Life of

[1] Theo had been temporarily transferred to the Goupil house in
Paris.

a Horse."[1] It represents an old white horse, lean and ema-
ciated, and tired to death by a long life of heavy labour, of
too much and too hard work. The poor animal is standing on
a spot utterly lonely and desolate, a plain scantily covered
with withered dry grass, and here and there a gnarled old
tree broken and bent by the storm. On the ground lies a
skull, and at a distance in the background a bleached skeleton
of a horse, lying near a hut where lives a man who skins
horses. Over the whole is a stormy sky, it is a cold, bleak
day, gloomy and dark weather.

It is a sad and very melancholy scene, which must strike
everyone who knows and feels that we also have to pass one
day through the valley of the shadow of death, and " que la
fin de la vie humaine, ce sont des larmes ou des cheveux
blancs."[2] What lies beyond this is a great mystery that only
God knows, but He has revealed absolutely through His word
that there is a resurrection of the dead.

The poor horse, the old faithful servant, is standing there
patiently and meekly, yet bravely and unflinchingly; like the
old guard who said, " la garde meurt mais elle ne se rend
pas,"[3] it awaits its last hour. Involuntarily I was reminded
of that engraving, when I saw tonight those horses of the
ashcarts.

As to the drivers themselves with their filthy dirty clothes,
they seemed sunk and rooted still deeper in poverty than that
long row or rather group of paupers, that Master de Groux
has drawn in his " Bench of the Poor." It always strikes me,
and it is very peculiar, that when we see the image of indescribable and unutterable desolation,—of loneliness, of
poverty and misery, the end of all things, or their extreme,
then rises in our mind the thought of God. At least this is
the case with me and does not Father also say : " There is no
place where I like better to speak than in a churchyard,
for there we are all on equal ground; not only that,

[1] Ten years later, Vincent was to compare the Impressionist artists
he had known in Paris with broken-down old cab-horses.

[2] " that the end of human life partakes of tears or white hairs ".

[3] " the guard accepts death, but never surrender ".

there we always *realize* it." I am glad that we had time to see the museum together and especially the work of de Groux and Leys, and so many other interesting pictures, like that landscape of Cooseman's for instance. I am very pleased with the two prints you gave me, but you ought to have accepted from me that small etching, "The Three Mills." Now you have paid it all yourself, and not allowed me to pay half as I wished to do. But you must keep it for your collection, for it is remarkable, even though the reproduction is not so very good. In my ignorance, I should ascribe it rather to Peasant Breughel than to Velvet Breughel. I enclose the little hasty sketch, " Au Charbonnage."[1]

I should like to begin making rough sketches from some of the many things that I meet on my way, but as it would probably keep me from my real work, it is better not to begin. As soon as I came home I began a sermon about the " barren fig tree," Luke XIII 6-9.

That little drawing " Au Charbonnage " is nothing specially remarkable, but the reason I made it is that one sees here so many people that work in the coal mines, and they are rather a characteristic kind of people. This little house stands not far from the road; it is a small inn attached to the big coal shed, and the workmen come there to eat their bread and drink their glass of beer during the lunch hour.

When I was in England I applied for a position as Evangelist among the miners in the coal mines, but they turned me down, stating that I had to be at least twenty-five years old. You know how one of the roots or foundations, not only of the Gospel, but of the whole Bible is, " Light that rises in the darkness,"[2] *from darkness to light.* Well, who will need this most, who will be open to it? Experience has taught that those who walk in the darkness, in the centre of the earth, like the miners in the black coal mines for instance, are very much impressed by the words of the Gospel, and believe it too. Now there is in the south of Belgium, in

[1] " The Miner's Inn ".

[2] Vincent may have been thinking of *John* I 5, or of *Matthew* IV 16, where *Isaiah* IX 2 is quoted.

Hainault, in the neighbourhood of Mons, up to the French frontiers, aye, even far across it, a district called the Borinage, that has a special population of labourers who work in the numerous coal mines. In a little handbook of geography I found the following about them: " The Borins (inhabitants of the Borinage, situated west of Mons) find their work exclusively in the coal mines. These mines are an imposing sight, 300 metres underground, into which daily descend groups of working men, worthy of our respect and our sympathies. The miner is a special Borinage type, for him daylight does not exist, and except on Sunday he never sees the sunshine. He works laboriously by a lamp whose light is pale and dim, in a narrow tunnel, his body bent double and sometimes he is obliged to crawl along; he works to extract from the bowels of the earth that mineral substance of which we know the great utility; he works in the midst of thousands of ever-recurring dangers; but the Belgium miner has a happy disposition, he is used to that kind of life, and when he descends the shaft, carrying on his hat a little lamp that is destined to guide him in the darkness, he trusts himself to God, Who sees his labour and Who protects him, his wife and his children."

So the Borinage is situated south of Lessines, where one finds the stone quarries.

I should very much like to go there as an Evangelist. The three months' trial demanded of me by the Rev. de Jong and the Rev. Pietersen is almost over. St. Paul was three years in Arabia before he began to preach, and before he started on his great missionary journeys and his real work among the heathen. If I could work quietly for about three years in such a district, always learning and observing, then I should not come back from there without having something to say that was really worth hearing. I say so in all humility and yet with confidence. If God wills, and if He spares my life, I would be ready about my thirtieth year, starting out with a peculiar training and experience, being able to master my work better, and riper for it than now.

I write you this again although we have already spoken about it many a time.

There are already in the Borinage many little Protestant communities and certainly schools also. I wish I could get a position there as Evangelist in the way we spoke about, preaching the Gospel to the poor, that means those who need it most and for whom it is so well suited, and then during the week devoting myself to teaching.

You have certainly visited St. Gilles? I too made a trip there, in the direction of the Ancienne Barrière. Where the road to Mont St. Jean begins there is another hill, the Alsemberg. To the right is the cemetery of St. Gilles, full of cedars and evergreen, from where one has a view over the whole city.

Proceeding further one arrives at Forest. The neighbourhood is very picturesque there, on the slope of the hills are old houses, like those huts in the dunes that Bosboom has sometimes painted. One sees all kinds of field labour performed there, the sowing of corn, the digging of potatoes, the washing of turnips, and everything is picturesque, even the gathering of wood, and it looks much like Montmartre. There are old houses covered with evergreen or vines, and pretty little inns; among the houses I noticed one was that of a mustard manufacturer, a certain Verkisten, his place was just like a picture by Thijs Maris for instance. Here and there are places where stone is found, so they have small quarries, through which hollowed out roads pass, with deeply cut wagon ruts, where one sees the little white horses with red tassels, and the drivers with blue blouses; shepherds are to be found there too, and women in black with white caps, that remind one of those of de Groux. There are some places here, thank God one finds them everywhere, where one feels more at home than anywhere else, where one gets a peculiar pristine feeling like that of homesickness, in which bitter melancholy plays some part; but yet its stimulation strengthens and cheers the mind, and gives us, we do not know how or why, new strength and ardour for our work. That day I walked on past Forest and took a side path leading to a little old ivy-grown church. I saw many linden trees there, still more interwoven, and more Gothic so to say, than those we saw in the Park, and at the side of the hollowed road that leads to the churchyard there were twisted and gnarled stumps and tree roots, fantastical like those Albert Dürer etched in " Ritter, Tod and Teufel."[1] Have you ever seen a picture or rather a photograph of Carlo Dolci's work " The Garden of Olives "? There is something Rembrandtesque in it; I saw it the other day. I suppose you know that large rough etching on the same theme after Rembrandt, it is the pendant of that other, " The Bible Reading," with those two women and a cradle? Since you told me that you had seen the picture by Father Corot on that same subject, I remembered it again; I saw it at the exhibition of his works shortly after his death and it deeply appealed to me.

How rich art is, if one can only remember what one has seen, one is never empty of thoughts or truly lonely, never alone.

A Dieu, Theo, I heartily shake hands with you in thought. Have a good time, have success in your work, and meet many good things on your road, such as stay in our memory and enrich us, though apparently we possess little. When you see Mauve greet him for me and believe me,

Your loving brother,

Vincent

I kept this letter for a few days; the 15th of November is passed, so the three months have elapsed. I spoke with the Rev. de Jong and Master Bokma, they tell me that I cannot attend the school on the same conditions as they allow to the native Flemish pupils; I can follow the lessons free of charge if necessary—but this is the only privilege,—so in order to stay here longer I ought to have more financial means than I have at my disposal, for they are nil. So I shall perhaps soon try that plan involving the Borinage. Once I am in the country I shall not soon go back to a large city.

It would not be easy to live without the Faith in Him and

[1] "The Knight, Death and the Devil."

the old confidence in Him; without it one would lose one's courage.

[Cuesmes, Belgium, July 1880]

My Dear Theo,

It is with a certain reluctance that I write to you, not having done so for so long, for many reasons.

To a certain degree you have become a stranger to me, and I have become the same to you, more than you may think; perhaps it would be better for us not to continue this way. It is likely I would not have written to you even now, if I were not under the obligation and the necessity of doing so, if you yourself had not given me cause. I learned at Etten that you had sent 50 francs for me; well, I have accepted them. Certainly with reluctance, certainly with a rather melancholy feeling, but I am up against a stone wall, and in a sort of mess. How can I do otherwise? So it is to thank you that I write to you.

Perhaps you know I am back in the Borinage; Father would rather have me stay in the neighbourhood of Etten; I refused, and I think I acted in this for the best.

Involuntarily, I have become in the family more or less a kind of impossible and suspect personage, at least somebody whom they do not trust, so how could I in any way be of any use to anybody?

For this reason above all, I think the best and the most reasonable thing for me to do is to go away, and keep at a convenient distance, so that I cease to exist for you all.

As moulting time is for the birds—the time when they change their feathers—so adversity or misfortune is the difficult time for us human beings. One can stay in it, in that time of moulting, one can also come out of it renewed; but anyhow it must not be done in public and it is not at all amusing, therefore the only thing to do is to hide oneself. Well, be it so.

Now, though it is a very difficult and almost impossible thing to regain the confidence of a whole family that is not quite free from prejudices, and other qualities as fashionable and honourable, still I do not quite despair that by and by, slowly but surely, a cordial understanding may be renewed between some of us.

And in the very first place I should like to see that "entente cordiale," not to put it more strongly, re-established between Father and me, and I desire no less to see it re-established between us two.

"Entente cordiale" is infinitely better than misunderstandings. Now I must bore you with certain abstract things, but I hope you will listen patiently to them. I am a man of passions, capable of and subject to doing more or less foolish things, of which I happen to repent, more or less, afterwards. Now and then I speak and act too quickly, when it would have been better to wait patiently. I think other people sometimes commit the same errors. Well, this being the case, what is to be done? Must I consider myself a dangerous man, incapable of anything? I do not think so. But the question is to try by all possible means to put those selfsame passions to a good use. For instance, to name one of the passions : I have a more or less irresistible passion for books, and I continually want to instruct myself, to study if you like, just as much as I want to eat my bread. *You* certainly will be able to understand this. When I was in other surroundings, in the surroundings of pictures and objects of art, you know how I then had a violent passion for them, that reached the highest pitch of enthusiasm. And I do not repent it, for even now, *far from that land, I am often homesick for the land of pictures.*

You remember perhaps that I knew well (and perhaps I know it still) who Rembrandt was, or Millet, or Jules Dupré or Delacroix or Millais or M. Maris. Well, now I do not have those surroundings any more—yet that thing that is called soul, they say it never dies, but lives, and goes on searching always and always and forever. So instead of giving way to this homesickness I said to myself : that land, or the fatherland, is everywhere. So instead of yielding to despair, I chose the part of active melancholy, in so far as I possessed the power of activity, in other words I preferred the melancholy that hopes and aspires and seeks, to that which despairs in stagnation and woe. So I studied fairly seriously the books within my reach, like the Bible, and the "French Revolution" by Michelet, and last winter Shakespeare and a few Victor Hugo and Dickens, and Beecher Stowe, and lately "Æschylus," and then several others, less classical, several great "little masters." You know that among those "little masters" are people like Fabritius or Bida.

Now he who is absorbed in all this is sometimes "choquant," shocking to others, and unwillingly sins on occasion against certain forms and customs and social conventions.

It is a pity however when this is taken in bad part. For instance you know that I have often neglected my appearance; this I admit, and I admit that it is shocking. But look here, poverty and want have their share in the cause, and deep discouragement comes in too for a part, and then it is sometimes a good way to assure oneself the necessary solitude for concentration on some study that preoccupies one.

A very necessary study is that of medicine; there is scarcely anybody who does not try to know a little of it, who does not try to understand what it is about, and you see I do not know as yet one word about it. Yet all this absorbs and preoccupies one, all this gives one something about which to dream, to reflect, to think. Now for more than five years already, I do not know exactly how long, I have been more or less without employment, wandering here and there; you say : since a certain time you have gone downhill, you have deteriorated, you have not done anything. Is this quite true?

It is true that now and then I have earned my crust of bread, now and then a friend has given it to me in charity. I have lived as I could, as luck would have it, haphazardly; it is true that I have lost the confidence of many, it is true that my financial affairs are in a sad state, it is true that the future is only too sombre, it is true that I might have done better, it is true that just from earning my bread I've lost time, it is true that even my studies are in a rather sad and hopeless condition, and that my needs are greater, infinitely greater than my possessions. But is this what you call going downhill, is this what you call doing nothing? You will say, perhaps : but why did you not continue as they wanted you to do, they wanted you to continue through the University? My only answer to this is : the expenses were too heavy, and besides, that future was not much better than the one on the road now before me.

But on the path I have taken now I must keep going; if I don't do anything, if I do not study, if I do not go on seeking any longer, then I am lost. Then woe is me.

That is how I look at it; to continue, to continue, that is what is necessary. But you will ask : What is your definite aim? That aim becomes more definite, will stand out slowly and surely, just as the rough draught becomes a sketch, and the sketch becomes a picture, little by little, by working seriously on it, by pondering over the idea, vague at first, over the thought that was fleeting and passing, till it gets fixed. I must tell you that it is with evangelists as with artists. There is an old academic school, often detestable, tyrannical, the accumulation of horrors, men who wear a cuirass, a steel armour of prejudices and conventions; those people, when they are at the head of affairs, dispose of positions, and by a bureaucratic system they try to keep their protégés in their places, and to exclude the other man. Their God is like the God of Shakespeare's drunken Falstaff, " le dedans d'une église,"[1] indeed some of those evangelical gentlemen find themselves by a curious chance having the same point of view on spiritual things as that drunken type (perhaps they would be somewhat surprised to find it so, if they were capable of human emotions). But there is little fear of their blindness ever changing to clear-sightedness in these matters.

This state of affairs has its bad side for him who does not agree, but protests against it with all his soul and all his heart, and all the indignation of which he is capable. I for my part respect academicians, that are not of this kind, but the respectable ones are more rare than one would believe at first. Now one of the reasons why I am out of employment

[1] "The inside of a church " (see 1 *Hen.* IV, III 3).

now, why I have been out of employment for years, is simply that I have other ideas than the gentlemen who give the places to men who think like they do. It is not merely a question of the dress over which they have hypocritically reproached me, it is a much more serious question, I assure you.

Why do I tell you all this?—not to complain, not to excuse myself for things in which I may more or less have been wrong, but simply to reply to you. During your visit last summer, when we walked together near the abandoned pit which they call "La Sorcière," you reminded me that there had also been a time when we two had walked together near the old canal and mill of Ryswyk, "and then," you said, "we agreed in many things," but you added, "since then you have changed so much, you are not the same any longer." Well, that is not quite true. What has changed is that my life was then less difficult, and my future seemed less dark; but as to the inward state, as to my way of looking at things, and my way of thinking, they have not changed. If there has been any change at all, it is that I think and believe and love more seriously now what I already thought and believed and loved then.

So you would be wrong in persisting in the belief that, for instance, I should now be less enthusiastic for Rembrandt, or Millet, or Delacroix, or whoever it may be, for the contrary is true. But you see, there are many things which one must believe and love. There is something of Rembrandt in Shakespeare, and of Correggio in Michelet, and of Delacroix in Victor Hugo, and then there is something of Rembrandt in the Gospel, or something of the Gospel in Rembrandt, as you like it——it comes to the same, if one only understands the thing in the right way, without misinterpreting it and assuming the equivalence of the comparisons, which do not pretend to lessen the merits of the original personalities. And in Bunyan there is something of Maris or of Millet, and in Beecher Stowe there is something of Ary Scheffer.

If now you can forgive a man for making a thorough study of pictures, admit also that the love of books is as sacred as the love of Rembrandt, and I even think the two complete each other.

I am very fond of the portrait of a man by Fabritius, which one day, when we were walking together, we stood looking at a long while in the museum at Haarlem. Yes, but I am as fond of Sydney Carton, in the "Tale of Two Cities" by Dickens, and I could show you other figures as curiously striking in other books, with a more or less remarkable resemblance. And I think that Kent, a character in Shakespeare's "King Lear," is as noble and distinguished a personage as a figure by Th. de Keyser, though Kent and King Lear had lived in a much earlier period. Not to say more about it. My God, how beautiful Shakespeare is! Who is mysterious like him? His language and style can indeed be compared to an artist's brush, quivering with fever and emotion. But one must learn to read, exactly as one must learn to see, and learn to live.

So you must not think that I disavow things; I am rather faithful in my unfaithfulness, and though changed, I am the same, and my only anxiety is : how can I be of use in the world, cannot I serve some purpose and be of any good, how can I learn more and study certain subjects profoundly? You see, that is what preoccupies me constantly, and then I feel myself imprisoned by poverty, excluded from participating in certain work, and certain necessary things are beyond my reach. That is one reason for not being without melancholy, and then one feels an emptiness where there might be friendship and strong and serious affections, and one feels a terrible discouragement gnawing at one's very moral energy, and fate seems to put a barrier to the instincts of affection, and a flood of disgust rises to choke one. And one exclaims "How long, my God!"

Well, what shall I say; our inward thoughts, do they ever show outwardly? There may be a great fire in our soul, but no one ever comes to warm himself at it, and the passers-by see only a little bit of smoke coming through the chimney, and pass on their way. Now, look here, what must be done, must one tend that inward fire, have salt in oneself, wait patiently yet with how much impatience for the hour when somebody will come and sit down near it,—to stay there maybe? Let him who believes in God wait for the hour that will come sooner or later.

Now for the moment things appear to be going very badly with me, and this has been so for a considerable time already, and may continue so in the future for a while; but after everything has seemed to go wrong, there will perhaps come a time when things will go right. I do not count on it, perhaps it will never happen, but if there should come a change for the better, I would consider it so much gain, I would be contented, I would say: at last! you see *there was something after all!* But you will say: "Yet you are an intolerable being, because you have impossible ideas about religion and childish scruples of conscience." If my ideas are impossible or childish, I hope to get rid of them, I ask no better. But here is a glimpse of what I think on the subject. You will find it in the "Philosophe sous les Toits" by Souvestre how a man of the people, a simple miserable labourer, pictures to himself his own country. "You have perhaps never thought what is really your own country," he said, putting his hand on my shoulder; "it is everything that surrounds you, everything that has brought you up and nourished you, everything you have loved—those fields that you see, those houses, those trees, those young girls that laugh as they pass, that is your country! The laws that protect you, the bread with which your labour is repaid, the words you speak, the joy and the sorrow that come to you from the people and the things among which you live, that is your country! The little room where you used to see your mother, the memories which she has left you, the earth in which she reposes, that is your country! You see it, you breathe it, everywhere! Figure to yourself the rights and the duties, the affections and the needs, the memories and the gratitude, gather all that under one name, and that name will be your country."

Now in the same way I think that everything that is really good and beautiful, of inner moral, spiritual and sublime beauty in men and their works, comes from God, and that all that is bad and wrong in men and in their works is not of God, and God does not approve of it.

But I always think that the best way to know God is to love many things. Love a friend, a wife, something, whatever you like, and you will be on the right way to knowing more about it, that is what I say to myself. But one must love with a lofty and serious intimate sympathy, with strength, with intelligence, and one must always try to know deeper, better and more. That leads to God, that leads to unwavering faith.

To give you an example: someone loves Rembrandt, but seriously,—that man will know that there is a God, he will surely believe it. Someone studies the history of the French Revolution—he will not be unbelieving, he will see that in great things also there is a sovereign power manifesting itself.

Maybe for a short time somebody has followed a free course at the great university of misery, and has paid attention to the things he sees with his eyes and hears with his ears, and has thought them over; he too will end in believing, and he will perhaps have learned more than he can tell. To try to understand the real significance of what the great artists, the serious masters, tell us in their masterpieces, *that* leads to God. One man has written or told it in a book, another in a picture. Then simply read the Gospel and the Bible, that makes you think, and think much, and think all the time. Well, think much and think all the time, that unconsciously raises your thoughts above the ordinary level. We know how to read, well then let us read!

It is true that there may be moments in which one becomes somewhat absent-minded, somewhat visionary; there are those who become too absent-minded, too visionary. This is perhaps the case with me, but it is my own fault; maybe after all there is some excuse, there was some reason for me to be absorbed, preoccupied, troubled but one overcomes this. The dreamer sometimes falls in a well, but he is said to get out of it afterwards. And the absent-minded man has also, in compensation, his lucid intervals. He is sometimes a person who has his reasons for being as he is, but those are not always understood at first, or are unconsciously forgotten most of the time, from lack of interest. A man who has been tossed to and fro for a long time, as if he were tossed on a stormy sea, at last reaches his destination; a man who has seemed good for nothing and incapable of any employment, any function, ends in finding one, and becoming active and capable of action, he shows himself quite different from what he seemed at first. I write somewhat at random whatever comes to my pen. I should be very glad if you could see in me something besides an idle fellow.

Because there are two kinds of idleness, that form a great contrast. There is the man who is idle from laziness, and from lack of character, from the baseness of his nature. You may if you like take me for such an one.

Then there is the other sort of idle man, who is idle in spite of himself, who is inwardly consumed by a great longing for action, yet does nothing because it is impossible for him to do anything, because he seems to be imprisoned in some cage, because he does not possess what he needs to make him productive, because the fatality of circumstances brings him there; such a man does not always know what he could do, but he feels by instinct: all the same I am good for something, my life has an aim after all, I know that I might be quite a different man! How can I then be useful, of what service can I be! There is something inside of me, what can it be?

This is quite a different kind of idle man; you may if you like take me for such an one. A caged bird in spring knows quite well that he might serve some end; he feels well enough that there is something for him to do, but he cannot do it. What is it? He does not remember too well. Then he has some vague ideas and says to himself, " The others make their nests and lay their eggs and bring up their little ones," and so he knocks his head against the bars of the cage. But the cage remains and the bird is maddened by anguish.

" Look at the lazy animal," says another bird that passes by, " he seems to be living at his ease." Yes the prisoner lives, he does not die, there are no outward signs of what passes within him; his health is good, he is more or less gay when the sun shines. But then comes the season of migration, bringing attacks of melancholia. "But he has got everything he wants," say the children that tend him in his cage, while he looks through the bars at the overcast sky, where a thunderstorm is gathering, and he inwardly rebels against his fate. "I am caged, I am caged, and you tell me I do not want anything, fools! You think I have everything I need! Oh! I beseech you, liberty, so that I can be a bird like other birds!"

A certain idle man resembles this idle bird.

And men are often prevented by circumstances from doing things, imprisoned in I do not know what horrible, horrible, most horrible cage. There is also, I know it, the deliverance, the tardy deliverance. A just or unjustly ruined reputation, poverty, inevitable circumstances, adversity, that is what makes men prisoners.

One cannot always tell what it is that keeps us shut in, confines us, seems to bury us, but still one feels certain barriers, certain gates, certain walls. Is all this imagination, fantasy? I do not think so. And then one asks: "My God! is it for long, is it for ever, is it for eternity?" Do you know what frees one from this captivity? it is very deep serious affection. Being friends, being brothers, love, that is what opens the prison by supreme power, by some magic force. But without this one remains in prison.

There where sympathy is renewed, life is restored.

And the prison is also called prejudice, misunderstanding, fatal ignorance of one thing or another, distrust, false shame.

But to speak of other things, if I have come down in the world, you on the contrary have risen. If I have alienated sympathies, you on the contrary have gained them. That makes me very happy, I say it in all sincerity, and it will always do so. If you had only a small degree of seriousness or depth, I would fear that it would not last, but as I think you are very serious and of great depth, I believe that it will. But I should be very glad if it were possible for you to see in me something else than an idle man of the worst type.

If ever then I can do anything for you, be of some use to you, know that I am at your disposal. If I have accepted what you have given me, you might, in the event that I could render you some service, ask it of me; it would make me happy, and I would consider it a proof of confidence. We are rather far apart, and we have perhaps different views on some things, but nevertheless there may come an hour, there may come a day, when we may be of service to one another.

For the present I shake hands with you, thanking you again for the help you have given me.

If sooner or later you wish to write to me, my address is, care of Ch. Decrucq, Rue du Pavillon 3, Cuesmes, near Mons. And know that a letter from you will do me good.

Ever yours,
Vincent

YEARS IN HOLLAND

1881-5

[Etten, Holland, probably November 3 1881]

Dear Theo,

There is something in my heart that I must tell you; perhaps you know about it already and it is not new for you. I want to tell you that this summer a deep love has grown in my heart for Kee;[1] but when I told her this, she answered me that to her, past and future remained one, so she could never return my feelings.

Then there was a terrible indecision within me as to what to do. Should I accept her " no, never never," or considering the question as not finished and decided, should I keep some hope and not give up?

I chose the latter. And up to now I do not repent of that decision, though I am still confronted by that " no, never never." Of course since that time I have met with many " petites misères de la vie humaine,"[2] which written in a book would perhaps serve to amuse some people, but can hardly be termed a pleasant sensation if one has to experience them oneself.

However, I have so far remained glad that I left the resignation of the " how not to do it " system to whoever may like it, and for myself kept some courage.

One of the reasons why I did not write to you about it before is that my position was so vague and undecided that I could not explain it to you. But now we have reached the point where I have spoken about it, besides to her, to Father and Mother, to Uncle and Aunt Stricker, and to Uncle and Aunt at Prinsenhage.

The only one who told me, but very informally and in

[1] Kee Vos, now a widow.   [2] " Small miseries of human life "

128

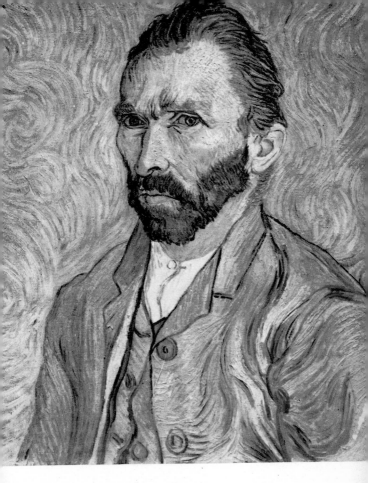

Self-portrait, oil, St.-Rémy, May 1890

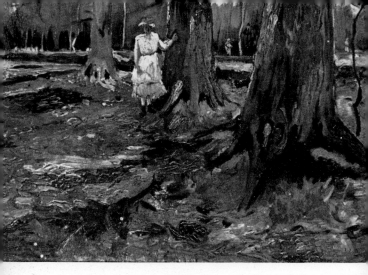

Autumn Wood, oil, The Hague, September 1882
(p. 165)

Miners' Wives Carrying Coal, watercolour,
The Hague, November 1882
(p. 175)

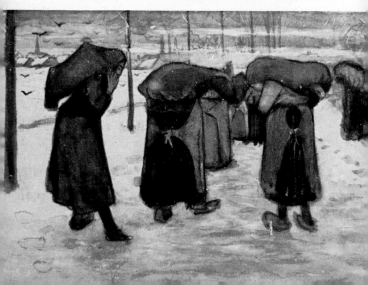

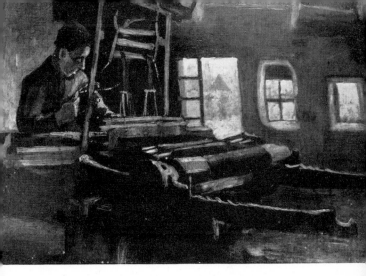

Interior with a Weaver, oil, Nuenen, June/July 1884 (p. 217)

Night Café, oil, Arles, September 1888 (pp. 275, 288-9)

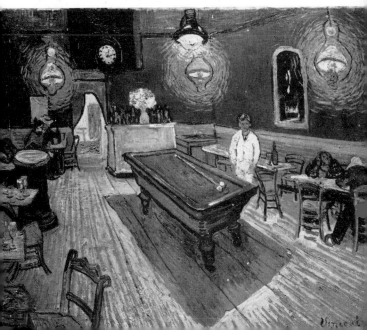

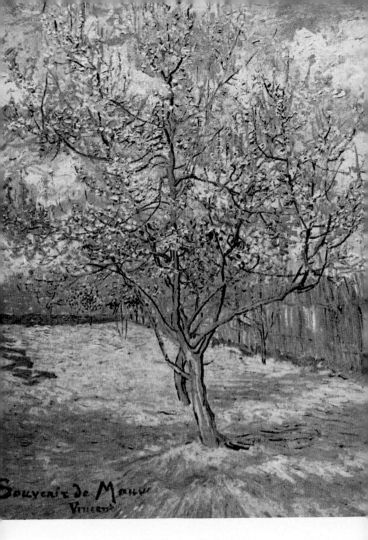

Flowering Tree, 'Souvenir de Mauve', oil, Arles, March 1888
(pp. 263, 265)

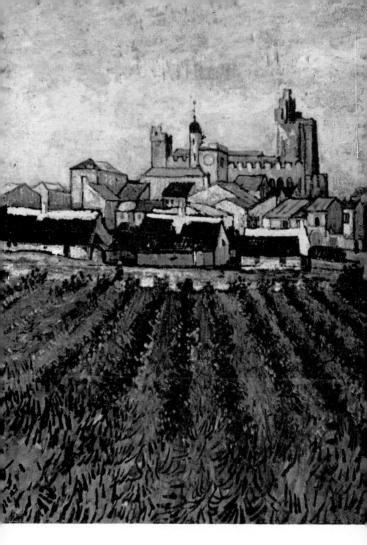

View of Saintes-Maries-sur-Mer, oil, Saintes-Maries, June 1888
(p. 267)

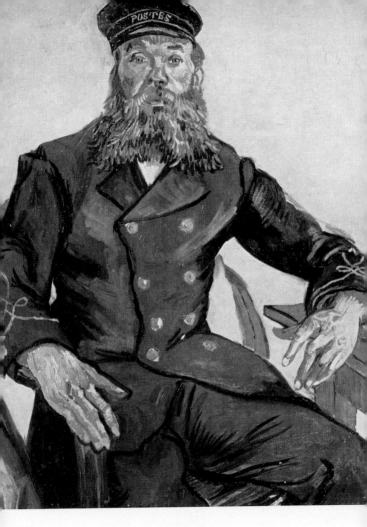

The Postman Roulin, oil, Arles, August 1888
(pp. 274, 278)

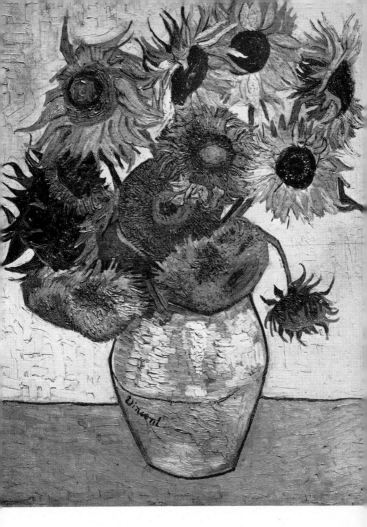

Sunflowers, oil, Arles, August 1888
(p. 284)

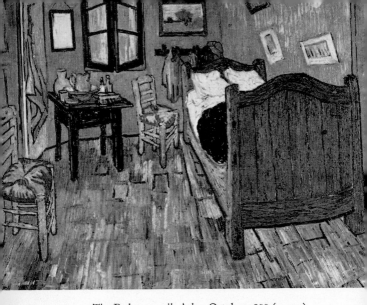

The Bedroom, oil, Arles, October 1888 (p. 297)

Falling Leaves in the Alyscamps Avenue, oil, Arles, November 1888 (p. 30

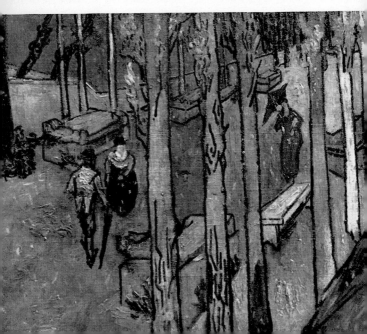

secret, that there really was some chance for me, if I worked hard and had some success, was somebody from whom I did not expect it in the least: Uncle Vincent. He had rather liked the way in which I took Kee's " no, never never "—not taking it too seriously, but rather in a humorous way. Well, I hope to continue to do so, and to keep melancholy and depression far from me, meanwhile working hard; and since I have met her I get on much better with my work.

I told you that my position has become more sharply clarified; I think I shall have the greatest trouble with the older persons, who consider the question as settled and finished, and will try to force me to give it up. For the present I believe they will be very considerate to me, and keep me dangling and put me off with fair promises, until the silver wedding of Uncle and Aunt takes place in December. Then I fear measures will be taken to cut me off.

Pardon me these rather hard expressions, which I use to make the situation clear to you: I admit that the colours are somewhat harsh, and the lines somewhat forcibly drawn, but it will give you a clearer insight into the question than if I beat about the bush. So do not accuse me of disrespect towards the older people. I only believe that they are decidedly *against* it; they will take care that Kee and I cannot see each other or speak to each other or write to each other, because they know perfectly well that if we saw each other or wrote to each other or spoke to each other, there would be a chance of Kee changing her mind.

Kee herself thinks she will never change her mind, and the older people try to convince me that she cannot, yet they are afraid of that change. The older people will only change in this affair, not when Kee changes her mind, but when I have become somebody who earns at least 1000 guilders a year. Again forgive me the harsh outlines in which I draw things. You will perhaps hear it said about me that I try to force the situation, and similar expressions, but who would not understand that forcing is absurd in love. No, that intention is far, very far from me. But it is no unreasonable or unjust

L.V.G.   E desire to wish that Kee and I might see each other, speak to each other and write to each other, in order to become better acquainted, and in this way to get a better insight into whether we are suited to one another or not.

A year of free intercourse with each other would be beneficial for both of us, but the older people are really obdurate on that point.

But now you understand that I hope not to leave a single thing undone that may bring me nearer to her, and it is my intention :

> *To love her so long*
> *That she'll love me in the end.*

Theo, are you perhaps in love too? I wish you were, for believe me, even the little miseries of it have their value. One is sometimes in despair, there are moments when one seems to be in hell, but—there are also other and better things connected with it. There are three stages.

1st. Not to love and not to be loved.

2nd. To love and not to be loved in return.[1]

3rd. To love and to be loved.

Now, I tell you that the second stage is better than the first, —but the third; that is the *best*.

Now, old boy, fall in love too, and then tell me about it. In my case give me your sympathy and take my part.

Rappard has been here; he brought water-colours with him that were very good. Mauve will come here soon, I hope, otherwise I will go to him. I am drawing hard, and believe I am improving; I work more with the brush than before. It is so cold now that I draw exclusively from the figure indoors, a seamstress, a basket-weaver, etc.

A handshake in thought, and write soon, and believe me,

Yours,

Vincent

If ever you should fall in love and get in answer "no, never never," do not resign yourself to it; but you are such a lucky fellow that I trust it will never happen to you.

[1] That is my case.

Dear Theo,   [Etten, second half of December 1881]

I am afraid you sometimes cast aside a book because it is too realistic. Have pity and patience with this letter and read it through, though it may be rather crude.

As I wrote you from the Hague I have some things to talk over with you, now that I am back here. My trip to the Hague is something I cannot remember without emotion. When I came to Mauve[1] my heart palpitated a little, for I said to myself: Will he also try to put me off with fair promises, or shall I be treated differently here? And I found that he helped me in every way, practically and kindly, and encouraged me. Not however by approving of everything I did or said, on the contrary. But if he says to me: " this or that is not right," he adds at the same time: " but try it in this or that way," which is quite another thing than to criticize just for the sake of criticizing. If somebody says to you: " you are ill," that does not help you much, but if he says, " do this or that and you will recover," and his advice is not misguided, that is the thing that will help you.

So when I left him I had a few painted studies and a few water-colours. Of course they are no masterpieces, but still I believe that there is something sound and true in them, at least more than in what I produced before. And so I think this is the beginning of my making serious things. And as I now have a few more technical resources at my disposal, namely paint and brush, all things seem as it were new to me.

But—now we must put that into practice. And then the first thing is that I must find a room large enough to be able to take sufficient distance.

When Mauve saw my studies he said at once: " you are sitting too close to your model." That makes it in many cases almost impossible to take the necessary measurings for the proportion, so that it is certainly one of the first things I must attend to. So I must try to rent a large room somewhere, either a room or a barn. And that will not be so very

[1] Anton Mauve, the artist whom Vincent went to consult about his work.

expensive. A labourer's cottage in these parts costs no more than 30 guilders a year, so I think that a room twice as large as such a cottage would cost 60 guilders. And that is not beyond my reach. I have already seen a barn, but that had too many inconveniences, especially in winter time. But at least when the weather gets somewhat milder I could work there. And then I think, if difficulties should arise here, I could find models not only in Etten, but also in other villages here in Brabant.

However, though I love Brabant very much, I can also appreciate other figures than the Brabant peasant type. I continue, for instance, to find Scheveningen very, very beautiful. But now I am here and can live cheaper here. But I promised Mauve that I would try my best to find a better studio, and besides I must begin to use better paint and better paper now.

However, for studies and sketches the Ingres paper is excellent, and it is much cheaper to make my own sketchbooks in different sizes, than to buy them ready made.

I still have some of that Ingres paper, but when you return that study to me, please enclose some of the same kind; you would greatly oblige me by doing so. But no dead white, rather the colour of unbleached linen, no cold tones.

Theo, what a great thing tone and colour are. And if someone does not learn to have a feeling for them, how far from real life he stands. Mauve has taught me to see many things I did not see before, and what he has told me I will try to tell you sometime, for perhaps there are a few things which you do not see well either. Well, I hope we shall discuss some artistic questions together some day. And you cannot imagine what a feeling of deliverance I begin to have, when I think of what Mauve told me about earning money.

Just think how I have been struggling along for years in a kind of false position. And now, now there comes a dawn of real light. I wish you could see the two water-colours which I brought away with me, for you would see they are water-colours like any other water-colours. There may be many imperfections in them; I would be the first to admit that I am very much dissatisfied with them, but still they are quite different from what I made before, and look more bright and clear. That does not change the fact that others in the future may become brighter and clearer still, but one cannot do right away what one wants. It will come gradually.

I want to keep those two drawings myself for now in order to compare them with those I am going to make here, for I must carry them at least as far as the ones I made at Mauve's.

But though Mauve tells me that after having struggled on for a few more months, coming back to him, say in March, I shall then make salable drawings, still I am now in a very difficult period. The expenses for model, studio, drawing and painting materials increase and I do not earn anything as yet.

It is true Father has said that I need not worry about the necessary expenses, and Father is very happy with what Mauve told him, and also with the studies and drawings that I brought back. But I think it very lamentable indeed that Father will have to pay for it. We hope of course that it will turn out all right, but still it is a heavy load on my mind. For since I have been here Father has not by any means profited from me, and more than once he has for instance bought a coat or a pair of trousers for me, which I would rather not have had, though I needed them, just because I do not want Father to spend money. Particularly since the coat or trousers in question do not fit, and are of little or no use at all. Well, that is again one of the little miseries of human life. Besides, as I told you before, I hate not to be quite free, and though I do not literally have to account to Father for every cent, he always knows exactly how much I spend and on what. And though I have no secrets I do not like to show my hand to everybody, though even my secrets are no secrets for those with whom I am in sympathy. But Father is not a man for whom I can feel what I feel for instance for you or for Mauve. Of course I love Father, but it is quite a different affection from what I have for you or for Mauve. Father cannot sympathize with, or understand me and I cannot be reconciled to Father's system,—it oppresses me, it would choke me. I too read the Bible now and then, just as I read

Michelet or Balzac or Eliot; but in the Bible I see quite different things than Father does, and what Father draws from it in his academic way I cannot find in it at all.

Since the Reverend ten Kate translated Goethe's "Faust" Father and Mother have read that book, for now that a clergyman has translated it, it cannot be so very immoral??? (what does that mean?) But they consider it nothing but the fatal consequences of an ill-timed love. And neither do they understand the Bible. Now take Mauve for instance. When he reads something that is deep, he does not say at once: that man means this or that. For poetry is so deep and intangible that one cannot define everything systematically. But Mauve has a fine sentiment, and, you see, I think that sentiment worth so much more than definitions and criticism. And when I read, and really I do not read so much, only a few authors,—a few men that I discovered by accident—I do this because they look at things in a broader, milder and more affectionate way than I do, and because they know life better, so that I can learn from them; but all that rubbish about good and evil, morality and immorality, I care so very little for it. For indeed it is impossible always to know what is good and what is bad, what is moral and what is immoral. This morality or immorality brings me involuntarily back to Kee.

I have already written to you that it seemed less and less like eating strawberries in spring. Well, that is the truth; if I repeat myself you must forgive me, because I do not know exactly what I wrote to you about what happened in Amsterdam.

I went there thinking: perhaps the "no, never never" is thawing, the weather is so mild.

And on a certain evening I strolled along the Keizersgracht looking for the house, and I found it. I rang the bell and heard that the family were still at dinner. But then I was asked to come in. But they were all there except Kee. And all had a plate before them, but there was not one too many and this little detail struck me. They wanted to make me believe that Kee was out, and had taken away her plate, but I knew that she was there, and I thought this rather like a comedy or a farce. After some time I asked: (after the usual greetings and small talk) "But where is Kee?" Then Uncle repeated my question, saying to his wife: "Mother, where is Kee?" And Mother answered "Kee is out." And for the moment I did not inquire further, and talked a little about the exhibition at Arti, etc. But after dinner the others disappeared and Uncle S. and his wife and the undersigned remained alone and settled down to discuss the case in question. Uncle S. opened the discussion as clergyman and father, and said that he was just about to send a letter to the undersigned, and that he would read that letter aloud. But I asked again: "Where is Kee?" (for I knew that she was in town). Then Uncle S. said "Kee left the house as soon as she heard that you were here." Well, I know her somewhat, but I declare that I did not know then, nor do I know with certainty now, whether her coldness and rudeness was a good or a bad sign. This much I do know, that I never saw her so apparently or really cool, brusque and rude to anyone but me. So I did not say much and remained very calm.

Let me hear that letter, or not hear it, I said, I don't care much about it.

Then came the letter. The document was very reverend and very learned, there was really nothing in it, except that I was requested to stop my correspondence and the advice was given me to make very energetic efforts to put the thing out of my mind. At last the reading of the letter was finished. I merely felt as if I had heard the clergyman in church, after a prance up and down with his voice, say amen; it left me just as cool as an ordinary sermon.

And then I began, and said as calmly and politely as I could: yes, I had heard those opinions before—but now— what further? But then Uncle S. looked up. He seemed full of consternation at my not being fully convinced that the utter limit of human capacity for feeling and thinking had been reached. According to him there was no "further" possible. So we continued, and Aunt M. said a word now and then, and I got somewhat excited and lost my temper. And Uncle S. lost his temper too, as much as a clergyman can do so.

And though he did not exactly say " damn you," any other but a clergyman in Uncle S.'s mood would have said so.

But you know that in my way I love Father and Uncle S., and so I shifted my position a little and I gave in a bit, so that at the end of the evening they told me I could stay the night if I wished. Then I said: " I am very much obliged, but if Kee leaves the house when I come, I do not think it the time to stay overnight; I will go to my lodgings." And then they asked: " Where do you board?" I said, " I do not know where as yet;" and then Uncle and Aunt insisted they should take me to a good and cheap place. And dear me, those two old people went with me through the cold, foggy, muddy streets, and they indeed showed me a very good and cheap inn. I insisted on their not coming, and they insisted on showing me the way.

And, you see, there was something humane in that, and it calmed me. I stayed in Amsterdam for two days and I had another talk with Uncle S., but Kee I did not see once; she kept out of my way whenever I came. And I said that they should know that, though they wished me to consider the question as settled and finished, I for my part could not do so. And then they firmly and steadily answered that I would learn to see that better subsequently.

Lately I read Michelet's " La Femme, la Religion et le Prêtre." Books like that are full of realism, but what is more real than reality itself, and where is more life than in life itself? And we who try our best to live, why do we not live more?

I felt quite lone and lorn during those three days in Amsterdam; I felt absolutely miserable, and that sort of kindness of Uncle and Aunt, and all those discussions, it was all so dismal. Till at last I began to feel quite depressed, and I said to myself: you are not going to become melancholy again, are you?

And then I said to myself: do not let yourself be stunned. And so, on a Sunday morning, I went for the last time to Uncle S. and said: " Just listen, dear Uncle, if Kee were an angel she would be too high for me, and I do not think I could remain in love with an angel. If she were a devil I would not want to have anything to do with her. In the present case I see in her a true woman with a woman's passions and moods, and I love her dearly, and that is the truth and I am glad of it. As long as she does not become an angel or a devil, the case in question is not finished." And Uncle S. had not much to say in reply, and muttered something about a woman's passions—I do not remember well what he said on the subject, and then he went off to church. No wonder one becomes hardened there and turns to stone; I know it from my own experience. And so your brother in question did not want to be stunned, but notwithstanding that he had the feeling of being stunned, a feeling as if he had been standing too long against a cold, hard, whitewashed church wall. And—do you want me to tell you the rest, boy; it is somewhat risky to be a realist, but Theo, Theo, you yourself are also a realist, oh, bear with my realism. I told you that to some my secrets are no secrets. I do not take that back, think of me what you will, and whether or not you approve of what I did, that is of less consequence.

I continue. From Amsterdam I went to Haarlem and spent a few hours pleasantly with our little sister Willemien, and I walked with her, and in the evening I went to The Hague, and at about seven o'clock I arrived at Mauve's.

And I said : listen Mauve, you intended to come to Etten and were to initiate me, more or less, into the mysteries of the palette, but I thought that would not be a matter of a few days only, so I have come to you, and if you agree I will stay four or six weeks, or more or less if you say so, and then we must see what we can do. It is very bold of me to ask so much from you, but you see, *j'ai l'épée dans les reins.*[1] Then Mauve said : did you bring something with you? Yes, here are a few studies; and then he praised them a great deal too much, while at the same time he did criticize, but too little. Well, the next day we put up a still life and he began by telling me : this is the way to keep your palette. And since

[1] " I have a sword in my loins."

then I have made a few painted studies, and then afterwards two water-colours.

So that is the result of the work, but to work with the hands and the brains is not everything in life.

I still felt chilled through and through, to the depths of my soul, by the earlier mentioned real or unreal church wall. And I did not want to be stunned by that feeling. Then I thought : I should like to be with a woman, I cannot live without love, without a woman. I would not set any value on life, if there were not something infinite, something deep, something real. But then I said to myself : you said " she and no other," and you would go to another woman now, that is unreasonable, that is against all logic. And my answer to that was : who is the master, the logic or I, is the logic there for me or am I there for the logic, and is there no reason and no sense in my unreasonableness and lack of sense? And whether I do right or wrong, I cannot act otherwise, that damned wall is too cold for me, I need a woman, I cannot, I may not, I will not live without love. I am but a man, and a man with passions, I must go to a woman, otherwise I freeze or turn to stone, or in short am stunned. But under the circumstances I had a great battle within myself, and in the battle there remained victorious some things which I knew of physic and hygienics, and had learned by bitter experience. One cannot with impunity live too long without a woman. And I do not think that what some people call God and others supreme being, and others nature, is unreasonable and without pity, and in brief I came to the conclusion : I must see whether I can find a woman.

And dear me I had not far to seek. I found a woman,[1] not young, not beautiful, nothing remarkable if you like, but perhaps you are somewhat curious. She was rather tall and strongly built, she did not have a lady's hands like Kee, but the hands of one who works much; she was not coarse or common, and had something very womanly about her. She reminded me of some curious figure by Chardin or Frère, or perhaps Jan Steen. Well, what the French call " une ouv-

[1] Clasina Maria Hoornik, known as Sien.

rière."[1] She had had many cares, one could see that, and life had been hard for her, oh, she was not distinguished, nothing extraordinary, nothing unusual. " Toute femme à tout âge, si elle aime et si elle est bonne, peut donner à l'homme non l'infini du moment, mais le moment de l'infini."[2] Theo, to me there is such a wonderful charm in that slight fadedness, that something over which life has passed. Oh! she had a charm for me, I even saw in her something of Feyen-Perrin or Perugino. You see I am not quite as innocent as a greenhorn or as a baby in the cradle. It is not the first time that I was unable to resist that feeling of affection, yes affection and love for those women, who are so damned and condemned and despised by the clergymen from the pulpit. I do not damn them or condemn them, neither do I despise them. I am almost thirty years old, would you think that I have never felt the need of love? Kee is even older than I am, she has also had experience of love, but just for that reason I love her the better. She is not ignorant, but neither am I. If she wants to live only on that old love and refuses the new, that is her business, and if she continues that and avoids me, I cannot smother all my energy and all my strength of mind for her sake. No, I cannot do that. I love her, but I will not freeze for her sake or unnerve myself. And the stimulus, the spark of fire we want, that is love and not exactly spiritual love.

That woman has not cheated me,—oh, he who regards all those women as cheats, how wrong he is, and how little understanding does he show. That woman has been very good to me, very good, very kind, in what way I shall not tell my brother Theo, because I suspect my brother Theo of having had some such similar experience—so much the better for him. Have we spent much money together? No, for I did not have much, and I said to her : listen, you and I need not make ourselves drunk to feel something for each other, just

[1] " a working woman."
[2] ' Any woman at any age, provided she loves and is good-hearted, can give a man not the timelessness of a moment, but a moment of timelessness."

put in your pocket what I can spare. And I wish I could have spared more, for she was worth it.

And we talked about everything, about her life, about her cares, about her misery, about her health, and with her I had a more interesting conversation than for instance with my very learned, professor-like cousin. Now I tell you these things, hoping that you will see that though I have some sentiment, I do not want to be sentimental in a silly way, that I want to keep some vitality, and to keep my mind clear and my health in good condition, in order to be able to work. In this way I understand my love for Kee, and for her sake I will not be melancholy now that I have started to work, and I will not let myself be upset. The clergymen call us sinners, conceived and born in sin, bah! what dreadful nonsense that is. Is it a *sin* to love, to need love, not to be able to live without love? I think a life without love a sinful and an immoral condition.

If I repent of anything it is of the time when I was induced by mystical and theological notions to lead too secluded a life. Gradually I have thought better of that. When you wake up in the morning and find yourself not alone, but see there in the morning twilight a fellow creature beside you, it makes the world look so much more friendly. Much more friendly than religious diaries and whitewashed church walls, with which the clergymen are in love. It was a modest, simple little room in which she lived, the plain paper on the wall gave it a quiet grey tone, yet warm like a picture by Chardin; a wooden floor with a mat and a piece of old crimson carpet, an ordinary kitchen stove, a chest of drawers, and a large simple bed, in short the interior of a real working woman. She had to stand at the wash-tub the next day. Just so, quite right. In a black petticoat and dark blue camisole she would have been as charming to me as she was now in a brown or reddish-grey dress. And she was no longer young, was perhaps as old as Kee—and she had a child, yes, she had had some experience of life, and her youth was gone, gone?— "il n'y a point de vieille femme."[1] Oh, and she was strong

[1] "there is no such thing as an old woman."

and healthy,—and yet not coarse or common. Those who
care so very much for distinction, are they always able to
discern what is really distinguished? Dear me, people seek it
often in the clouds or under the ground, when it is quite close
at hand sometimes; even I did so now and then.

I am glad I acted as I did, because I think there is no
earthly reason to keep me from my work, or cause me to lose
my good spirits. When I think of Kee I still say, " she and
no other," but those women who are condemned and damned
by the clergymen, it is not just of late that I have a heart for
them, that feeling is even older than my love for Kee. Often
when I walked the streets quite lonely and forlorn, half ill
and in misery, without money in my pocket, I looked after
them and envied the men that could go with them, and I felt
as if those poor girls were my sisters, in circumstances and
experience. And you see that is an old feeling of mine, and
is deeply rooted. Even as a boy I often looked up with
infinite sympathy, and even with respect, into a half-faded
woman's face, on which was written as it were: life in its
reality has left its mark here.

But my love for Kee is something quite new and quite
different. Without realizing it she sits in a kind of prison.
She too is poor and cannot do as she wishes, and she feels a
sort of resignation, and I think that the Jesuitism of clergymen and pious ladies often makes more impression on her
than on me; they have no hold on me any longer, just
because I have learned to detect some of the tricks, but she
believes in them and would not be able to bear it, if the system
of resignation, and sin, and God, and heaven knows what
else proved to be idle.

And she never realizes, I fear, that God perhaps really
begins when we say the word with which Multatuli[1] finishes
his Prayer of an Unbeliever: "O God, there is no God."
That God of the clergymen, he is for me as dead as a door-
nail. But am I an atheist for all that? The clergymen consider me as such,—be it so—but I love, and how could I feel
love if I did not live, and if others did not live; and then if

[1] Dutch author.

we live there is something mysterious in that. Now call that God, or human nature or whatever you like, but there is something which I cannot define systematically, though it is very much alive and very real, and see, that is God, or as good as God.

And dear me, I love Kee for a thousand reasons, but just because I believe in life and reality, I do not become abstract as I used to be, when I had the same thoughts as Kee seems to have now, about God and religion. I do not give her up, but that crisis of soul-anguish in which perhaps she is now must run its course, and I can have patience with it, and nothing that she may do or say makes me angry. But while she clings and holds to the old things, I must work and keep my mind clear for painting and drawing and business. So I have acted as I did from need of vital warmth and for hygienic reasons; I tell you these things also that you shall not think of me afresh as being in a melancholy or abstract, brooding mood. On the contrary I am generally occupied with, and only thinking of, paint, water-colours, finding a studio, etc. etc.

Boy, if only I could find a fitting studio!

Well, my letter has become very long.

I sometimes wish that the three months before I can return to Mauve were up. But they too will bring me some good of their own! Write to me now and then, is there a chance of your coming here this winter? And rest assured I will not take a studio without knowing what Mauve thinks of it; I agreed to send him the plan of the room, and perhaps he will then come and look at it himself. But Father must not meddle with it, Father is not the man to decide any artistic question. And the less Father is mixed up in my affairs the better I can get on with him, for I must be free and independent in many things. That is only natural.

I sometimes shudder when I think of Kee, and see how she buries herself in the past and clings to old dead ideas. There is a kind of fatality in it, and oh, she would not be the worse, if she changed her opinions; I think it rather probable there will come some reaction, there is so much that is healthy and sound in her. And so in March I shall go to The Hague again, and to Amsterdam too. But when I left Amsterdam the last time I said to myself : by no means become melancholy or let yourself be stunned, so that your work suffers from it, just when it is beginning to progress. To eat strawberries in spring, yes, it is possible in life, but only for a short period of the year, and we are now far from it.

And so you envy me for some reason or other. Oh, boy, you must not, for what I am seeking can be found by everyone, perhaps even sooner by you than by me. And oh, in so many things I am very backward and narrow-minded; if I only knew exactly where the fault was and how I could manage to overcome it, but alas we often do not see the beams in our own eye. Write to me soon, and in my letters you must separate the chaff from the grain—if there is some good in them, some truth, so much the better; but of course there is much in them that is not right, more or less exaggerated perhaps, without my always being conscious of it. Indeed I am not a learned man, I am so very ignorant, oh, just like so many others, and even more than others, but I cannot fathom that myself, and much less can I fathom others, and I am often wrong. But in erring we sometimes find the right path, and " il y a du bon en tout mouvement "[1] (à propos I accidentally heard Jules Breton say that, and remembered the comment). Incidentally, did you ever hear Mauve preach? I heard him imitate several clergymen—once he preached about the fishing bark of Peter (the sermon was divided into three parts, 1st had he received or inherited that bark, 2nd had he bought it in instalment or shares, 3rd had he—oh! terrible thought —stolen it?); then he preached on the good intentions of the Lord, and on the " Tigris and Euphrates " and then he imitated Father Bernhard : God—God is Almighty—He has made the sea, He has made the earth, and the sky, and the stars, and the sun, and the moon; He can do everything— everything—everything—no, He is not almighty, there is one thing He cannot do. What is that thing the Almighty cannot do?

[1] " Every shift brings some sort of benefit "

God Almighty cannot cast out a sinner. . . .

Well, adieu, Theo, write to me soon, a handshake in thought, and believe me,

Yours,

Vincent

Dear Theo,   [The Hague, early March 1882]

Perhaps you will find rather harsh what I wrote you about Tersteeg.[1] But I cannot take it back. It must be told him straight out or else it does not penetrate his sheathing. He has considered me for years a kind of dreamer and duffer, he still considers me so, and even says about my drawing: "that is a kind of narcotic which you take in order not to feel the pain it costs you not to be able to make water-colours."

Well, it is all very fine to say this, but thoughtless, superficial and not to the point, the principal reason for my not being able to make water-colours is that I must draw still more seriously, paying more attention to proportion and perspective.

Enough of that, I do not deserve his reproaches and if my drawings do not amuse him, neither then does it amuse me to show them to him.

He condemns my drawings, which have a great deal of good in them, and I did not expect this from him.

If I make serious studies after the model, that is much more practical than his practical talks about what is salable or unsalable, a matter over which I do not need so much instruction as he supposes, having been in the business of selling pictures and drawings myself.

---

[1] Representative of Goupil & Co. in The Hague. He had told Theo the previous month that Vincent could always go to him whenever he wanted anything; Vincent therefore subsequently asked him for 10 francs, and Tersteeg complied, but only to the accompaniment of much unfriendly criticism of what the artist was doing. So Vincent refused to have any contact with him for another six months, and subsequently, on Theo's advice, returned the money.

So I would rather lose his friendship than give in to him in this matter.

Though there are moments when I feel overwhelmed by care, still I am calm, and my calmness is founded on my serious method of work, and on earnest reflection. Though I have moments of passion aggravated by my temperament, yet I am calm, as he who has been acquainted with me so long knows quite well. Even now he said to me: " you have too much patience."

That is not right, in art one cannot have *too much* patience, that word is out of proportion. Perhaps Mr. Tersteeg has in my case *too little* patience.

He must see now, once and for all, that I take things seriously and will not let myself be forced to produce work that does not show my own character. It is especially in my last drawings and studies, which Tersteeg condemned, that my own character is beginning to show.

Perhaps, perhaps I could succeed even now in making a water-colour that would sell if one tried very hard.

That would be forcing water-colours in a hothouse. Tersteeg and you must wait for the natural season, and that has not arrived yet.

He spoke English when he was here because of the model. I said to him: in due time you shall have your water-colours, now you cannot—they are not due as yet—take your time. And that is all I have to say. Enough of it.

Since Tersteeg's visit I have made a drawing of a boy from the Orphanage, blacking shoes. It may be this is done by a hand that does not quite obey my will, but still the type of the boy is there. And though my hand may be unruly, that hand will learn to do what my head wishes. So I have made a sketch of the studio with the stove, the chimney, easel, footstool, table, etc., of course not quite salable as things are, but very useful for practising perspective.

I am longing for your visit, there are so many things for you to see that I have made since you were here last summer. Theo, I count on your judging my work with sympathy and with confidence, and not with hesitation and dissatisfaction.

Because I work so much, Tersteeg thinks it is so easy, in this also he is quite wrong.

For in fact I am a drudge or a slow-going draught ox.

When you come, do not forget the Ingres paper. It is especially the *thick* kind that I like to use and which I think must also be good for studies in water-colour. Believe me, in things of art the saying is true: honesty is the best policy—rather more trouble on a serious study than a kind of chic to flatter the public. Sometimes in moments of worry I have longed for some of that chic, but thinking it over I say: No—let me be true to myself—and in a rough manner express severe, rough, but true things. I shall not run after the amateurs or dealers, let those who want to come to me. In due season we shall reap, if we faint not![1]

Well, I say, Theo, what a big man Millet was.

I borrowed from de Bock the great work by Sensier,[2] it interests me so much that it wakes me up in the night and I light the lamp and sit up to read. For in the day time I must work.

Do send me some money soon, if possible. I wish Tersteeg had to live for a week on what I have to spend, and had to do what I have to do; he would then see that it is not a question of dreaming and brooding, or taking narcotics, but that one must be wideawake to fight against so many difficulties. Neither is it easy to find models and to get them to sit for me. This discourages most painters. Especially when one must save on food, drink, and clothes to pay them.

Well, Tersteeg is Tersteeg, and I am I.

But I must tell you that I am not opposed or hostile to him, but I must make him understand that he judges me too superficially, and—and I believe that he will change his opinion; I fervently hope so, for it grieves and worries me, when there is an unfriendly feeling between us. I hope your letter will

---

[1] *Galatians* VI 9.
[2] A book on the art of Millet, from which Vincent quotes a passage later in the letter; Millet's work was to inspire numerous copies and variations from him at different times throughout his career.

come soon—I spent my last penny on a stamp for this letter. It is true I received only a few days ago the 10 guilders from Tersteeg, but that same day I had to pay 6 of them to the model, to the baker, to the little girl that sweeps the studio.

Adieu, I wish you health and good courage, notwithstanding everything. I myself am not without good courage.

Je te serre la main,[1]

Vincent

I have had a very pleasant visit from Jules Bakhuyzen[2] and I may go to see him whenever I like.

(POSTSCRIPT)

Theo, it is almost miraculous!!!

First comes your registered letter, secondly C. M.[3] asks me to make him 12 small pen drawings, views of The Hague, a propos of some that were ready. (The Paddemoes, the Geest, the Vleersteeg, were finished.) At 2.50 guilders a piece, price fixed by me, with the promise that if they suit him, he will take 12 more at his own price, which will be higher than mine. In the third place I have just met Mauve, happily delivered of his large picture, and he promised to come and see me soon. So, " ça va, ça marche, ça ira encore!"[4]

And another thing affected me—very very deeply—I had told the model not to come to-day,—I did not say why, but nevertheless the poor woman came and I protested. " Yes, but I do not come to pose, I just came to see if you had something for dinner "—she had brought me a dish of beans and potatoes. There are things that make life worth living after all. The following words in Sensier's " Millet " appealed to me, and touched me very much, sayings by Millet :

" L'art c'est un combat—dans l'art il faut y mettre sa peau."

[1] " I shake your hand "
[2] A Dutch artist friend.
[3] Vincent's uncle Cornelius Marinus (C. M. van Gogh), head of the family art-business in Amsterdam. This was to be Vincent's first sale of his work.
[4] " things are moving, things are progressing, they will go on doing so."

" Il s'agit de travailler comme plusieurs nègres : *J'aimerais mieux ne rien dire que de m'exprimer faiblement.*"[1]

It was only yesterday that I read this last saying by Millet, but I had felt the same thing before, that is why I sometimes like to scratch what I want to express, with a hard carpenter's pencil or a pen, instead of with a soft brush. Take care, Tersteeg, take care, you are decidedly in the wrong.

Dear Theo,   [The Hague, early May 1882]

To-day I met Mauve and had a very painful conversation with him, which made it clear to me that Mauve and I are separated forever. Mauve has gone so far that he cannot retract, at least certainly would not want to do so. I had asked him to come and see my work and then talk things over. Mauve refused point-blank : " I will certainly not come to see you, that is all over."

At last he said : "you have a vicious character." Then I turned around, it was on the dunes, and I walked home alone.

Mauve takes offence at my having said, " I am an artist "—which I do not take back, because that word of course included the meaning : always seeking without absolutely finding. It is just the converse of saying, " I know it, I have found it."

As far as I know, that word means : " I am seeking, I am striving, I am in it with all my heart."

I have ears, Theo. If somebody says, " you have a vicious character," what ought I to do then?

I turned around and went back alone, but with a heavy heart, because Mauve had dared to say that to me. I shall not ask him to explain it, nor shall I excuse myself. And still—and still—and still—! I wish Mauve were sorry for it.

They suspect me of something,—it is in the air—I keep

---

[1] " Art is a battle—it costs one the skin off one's back. It is a matter of working like a bunch of negroes : *I would prefer to say nothing rather than express myself poorly.*"

something back. Vincent is hiding something that cannot stand the light.

Well, gentlemen, I will tell you, you who prize good manners and culture, and rightly so if only it be the true kind : which is the more delicate, refined, manly, to desert a woman or to stand by a forsaken woman?

This winter I met a pregnant woman, deserted by the man whose child she bore.[1]

A pregnant woman who had to walk the streets in winter, had to earn her bread, you understand how.

I took that woman for a model, and have worked with her all winter. I could not pay her the full wages of a model, but that did not prevent my paying her rent, and, thank God, I have been able so far to protect her and her child from hunger and cold, by sharing my own bread with her. When I met that woman she attracted my notice because she looked ill. I made her take baths, and as much nourishing food as I could manage, and she has become much stronger. I went with her to Leyden, where there is a maternity hospital in which she will be confined. (No wonder she was ill, the child was not in position, and she had to have an operation, the child had to be turned with forceps. However, there is a good chance of her pulling through. She will be confined in June.)

It seems to me that every man worth a fig would have done the same in a similar case.

What I did was so simple and natural that I thought I could keep it to myself. Posing was very difficult for her, but she has learned, and I have made progress in my drawing because I had a good model. The woman is now attached to me like a tame dove, I for my part can only marry once, and

[1] Sien, first mentioned in the letter of five months earlier included here. Theo's reaction to Vincent's story did not, in fact, lead him to cut off his financial support, as Vincent was afraid it might; but he drew the line at the suggestion that they should marry, and ultimately, exerted moral pressure strong enough to contribute to final break-up of the relationship in September 1883.

how can I do better than marry her, because that is the only way to help her, and otherwise misery would force her back into her old road, that ends in a precipice. She has no money, but she helps me to earn money in my profession.

I am full of ambition and love for my work and profession; when I gave up painting and water-colours for some time it was because I felt so bad about Mauve's deserting me, and if he came back I would begin again with new courage. Now I cannot look at a brush, it makes me nervous.

I have written : Theo can you give me information about Mauve's behaviour, perhaps this letter can give you light. You are my brother, it is natural that I speak to you about private things, but anyone who says to me, "you have a vicious character," to such a person I cannot speak for the time being.

I could not do otherwise, I did what my hand found to do, I worked. I thought I should be understood without words, I had not forgotten another woman for whom my heart was beating,[1] but she was far away and refused to see me, and this one, she walked the street, sick, pregnant, hungry, in winter, I could not do otherwise. Mauve, Theo, Tersteeg, you have my bread in your hands, will you take it from me, or turn your back on me? Now I have spoken, and await what further will be said to me.

Vincent

I send you a few studies because you can see from them that she helps me a great deal by posing.

My drawings are the work " of my model and me." The woman with a white bonnet is her mother.

But I should like to get these three back from you, as in a year, when I shall probably be drawing quite differently, my work will be founded on these studies, which I now make as conscientiously as I can. You see they are made with care. When later on I shall do an interior or a waiting-room or the like, these will be of use to me, because I shall have to consult them for the details. But I thought it would be well perhaps if you could see how I use my time.

[1] Kee Vos.

Those studies require a rather dry technique; had I worked after effect they would be of less use to me subsequently. But I think you will understand this yourself. The paper I should like best is that on which the bent woman's figure is drawn, but if possible the colour of unbleached linen. I have none of it left, *of that thickness,* I think they call it double Ingres, I cannot get it here. When you see how that drawing is carried out, you will understand that it could not be done on thin paper. I wanted to send you with it a small figure in black merino, but I cannot roll it. The chair near the large figure is not finished, because I want there an old oaken chair.

Dear Theo,   [The Hague, mid May 1882]
    To-day I sent you some drawings and sketches; what I want to show you first of all is that what I told you does not keep me from my work, on the contrary I am literally absorbed in my work and enjoy it, and have good courage.
    Now I hope that you will not be angry at my saying so, but I am rather anxious, because you have not answered as yet. I do not believe that you will disapprove of my being with Christine. I do not believe that for that reason, or for the sake of appearances or I do not know what else, you would quite desert me. But can you wonder, after what happened with Mauve and Tersteeg, that I sometimes think with a certain melancholy; perhaps *he* will do the same.
    At least I am eagerly looking out for a letter from you, but I know that undoubtedly you are very busy and that it is not so very long since you wrote. But perhaps you will experience it yourself sooner or later, when you are with a woman who is with child, that a day seems like a week, and a week longer than a month. And that is the reason why I write you so often these days, just as long as I have no answer.
    I wrote to you about my intention of taking the house next door, it being more suitable than this one, which seems so easily blown apart, etc. But you surely know, don't you, that I do not ask imperatively for anything whatever. I only hope

that you will remain to me what you were; I do not think I lowered or dishonoured myself by what I did, though some perhaps will think so. I feel that my work lies in the heart of the people, that I must keep close to the ground, that I must grasp life at its deepest, and make progress through many cares and troubles.

I cannot think of any other way, and I do not ask to be free from trouble or care; I only hope the latter will not become unbearable, and that need not be so as long as I work and can keep the sympathy of people like you. It is in life as in drawing, one must sometimes act quickly and with decision, attack a thing with energy, trace the outlines as quickly as lightning.

This is not the moment for hesitation or doubt, the hand may not tremble, nor may the eye wander, but must remain fixed on what is before one. And one must be so absorbed in it that in a short time something is produced on the paper or the canvas that was not there before, so that afterwards one hardly knows how it got knocked into being. The time of discussing and thinking must precede the decided action. In the *action* itself there is little space for reflection or argument.

To act quickly is the function of a man, and one has to go through a great deal before one is able to do so. The pilot sometimes succeeds in making use of a storm to make headway, instead of being wrecked by it.

What I wanted to say to you again is this: I do not have great plans for the future; if for a moment I feel rising within me the desire for a life without care, for *prosperity,* each time I go fondly back to the trouble and the cares, to a *life full of hardship,* and think: it is better so, I learn more from it, it does not degrade me, this is not the road on which one perishes. I am absorbed in my work and I have confidence enough that with the help of such as you, as Mauve, as Tersteeg, though this winter we disagreed, I will succeed in earning enough to keep myself, not in luxury, but as one who eats his bread in the sweat of his brow. Christine is not a hindrance or a trouble to me, but a help. If she were alone,

he would perhaps succumb; a woman must not be alone in
society and a time like that in which we live, which does
ot spare the weak but treads them under foot, and drives over
weak woman when she has fallen down.

Therefore because I see so many weak ones trodden down,
greatly doubt the sincerity of much that is called progress
nd civilization. I do believe in civilization, even in such a
ime, but only in the kind that is founded on real humanity.
What costs human life I think cruel, and I do not respect it.
Well, enough of this. If it might be that I could rent the
ouse next door and could have regular weekly wages, that
vould be delightful. If it cannot be, I will not lose courage
nd will wait a little longer. But if it can be, I shall be so
appy, and it would save much of my strength for the work,
vhich otherwise is absorbed by cares.

You will see there are all kinds of drawings in the port-
olio.

Keep whatever you think best of what I send, then you can
how them whenever there is a chance. The rest I should like
o get back some time or other. If I thought you would come
oon, I would of course keep these things until you came.
But now it is perhaps good for you to see the things together,
nd I hope you will see from it that I do not live idly on
our money. Considering it superficially you would perhaps
iew the affair with Christine quite differently from what it
eally is.

But when you have read this letter and my earlier one, it
vill be easier for you to understand.

I wish those who mean well by me would understand that
ny actions proceed from a deep feeling and need for love,
hat recklessness and pride and indifference are not the springs
hat move the machine, and this step is a proof of my taking
oot at a low level on life's way. I do not think I should do
vell in aiming at a higher station or in trying to change my
haracter. I must have much more experience, I must learn
till more, before I shall be ripe, but that is a question of time
nd perseverance. Adieu, write soon.

If you can send me something, it will certainly not b
unwelcome. Believe me, with a handshake,

Yours,

Vincent

If I thought my leaving The Hague would please anyone
would do so, and go no matter where, rather than be i
anybody's way.

But I do no harm to anybody, and after what you wrote m
I suppose I must not take too seriously what Tersteeg said.

The house about which I wrote you is to let now, and I an
afraid someone else will take it if I do not do so soon. Tha
is another reason why I am looking out for your letter. Fo
you will understand that after what happened with Mauv
and Tersteeg, and after what I told you about Christine,
must ask you frankly: Theo, do these things make for
change or separation between you and me? If they do not,
would be so happy, and will be twice as glad for your hel
and sympathy as before; if they do, it is better for me t
know the worst than to be kept in suspense.

I like to look things in the face, whether adversity or pros
perity. I have got your answer on the question of Mauve an
Tersteeg, not on the other one. That is something quite apart
there is a barrier between the artistic and the personal matters
but it is well to settle beforehand how we look at thos
things.

And therefore I say to you:

Theo, I intend to marry this woman, to whom I am at
tached and who is attached to me. If unfortunately thi
should bring about a change in your feelings towards me,
hope you will not withdraw your help without giving m
warning some time before, and that you will always tell m
frankly and openly what you think. Of course I hope tha
your help and sympathy will in no way be withdrawn, bu
that we shall continue to grasp hands fraternally, notwith
standing things which the "world" opposes. So, brother, i
you have not written yet when you receive this letter, answe
me by return of post, for after the things I wrote to you,

must be reassured or must know the worst. Adieu, I hope the sky will remain clear between you and me.

Dear brother,   [The Hague, second half of July 1882]

It is already late, but I want to write to you once more. You are not here, but I wish you were, and sometimes it seems to me that we are not far from each other.

To-day I promised myself something, that is to consider my illness, or rather the remains of it, as non-existent.[1] Enough time has been lost, the work must go on. So, well or not well, I shall set to drawing again, regularly from morning until night. I do not want someone to tell me again: "Oh! these are just old drawings."

To-day I made a drawing of the baby's cradle with a few touches of colour in it.

I am also working on a drawing like the one of the meadows I sent you recently. My hands have become too white, but am I to blame?

I will go out and work in the open air, even if it should cause the return of my illness. I cannot keep from working any longer.

Art is jealous, she does not want us to choose illness in preference to her, so I do as she wishes.

Therefore I hope you will again in a short while receive a few rather good new drawings. People like me *may* not be ill, so to speak.

You must understand properly my conception of art. In order to grasp the essence one must work long and hard. What I want and aim at is confoundedly difficult, and yet I do not think I aim too high.

I want to make drawings that *touch* some people. "Sorrow" is a small beginning, perhaps such small landscapes as the "Meerdervoort Avenue," the "Rijswijk Meadows," the "Fish-Drying Barn," are also a small beginning. In those there is at least something directly from my own heart.

[1] He had had to go into hospital with bladder trouble and insomnia.

Either in figure or in landscape I should wish to express, not sentimental melancholy, but serious sorrow.

In short, I want to reach so far that people will say of my work: he feels deeply, he feels tenderly—notwithstanding my so-called roughness, perhaps even because of this.

It seems pretentious now to speak this way, but that is the reason why I want to push on with full strength.

What am I in the eyes of most people?—a nobody, or an eccentric and disagreeable man—somebody who has no position in society and never will have, in short, the lowest of the low. Very well, even if that were true, then I should want to show by my work what there is in the heart of such an eccentric man, of such a nobody.

This is my ambition, which is, notwithstanding everything, founded less on anger than on love, founded more on serenity than on passion. It is true that I am often in the greatest misery, but still there is within me a calm pure harmony and music. In the poorest huts, in the dirtiest corner, I see drawings and pictures. And with irresistible force my mind is drawn towards these things.

More and more other things lose their interest, and the more I get rid of them, the quicker my eye grasps the picturesque things. Art demands persistent work, work in spite of everything, and a continuous observation.

By persistent, I mean in the first place continuous work, but also not giving up your opinion at the bidding of such and such a person. I do hope, brother, that within a few years, perhaps even now, little by little you will see things by me that will give you some satisfaction for your sacrifices.

I have had very little contact with other painters lately. I have not been the worse for it. It is not the language of painters but the language of nature to which one ought to listen. I can now understand better than six months ago why Mauve said: "do not speak to me about Dupré, talk rather about the bank of that ditch, or something of that sort." It sounds rather crude, but it is perfectly true. The feeling for the things themselves, for reality, is more important than the feeling for pictures, at least it is more fertile and more vital.

Because I now have such a broad, ample feeling for art and or life itself, of which art is the essence, it sounds to me so hrill and false when people try to compel me.

I for my part find in many modern pictures a peculiar harm which the old masters lack.

For me one of the highest and noblest expressions of art is lways that of the English, for instance Millais and Herkomer nd Frank Holl.[1] What I mean in regard to the difference etween the old masters and the modern ones is—perhaps the modern ones are deeper thinkers.

There is a great difference in sentiment between the " Chill October " by Millais and the " Bleachery at Overveen " by uysdael, and also between the " Irish Emigrants " by Holl nd the " Bible Reading " by Rembrandt.

Rembrandt and Ruysdael are sublime, for us just as much s for their contemporaries, but there is something in the modern painters that appeals to us more personally and inti-nately.

It is the same with the woodcuts by Swain and those of the ld German masters.

So, I think it was a mistake when a few years ago the modern painters had a phase of imitating the old masters.

Therefore I think Father Millet is right in saying " Il me emble absurde que les hommes veuillent paraître autre chose ue ce qu'ils sont."[2] It seems only a commonplace saying, yet is fathomless, deep as the ocean, and I for my part think me would do well to take it to heart. I just wanted to tell ou that I will set to work regularly again in spite of every-hing, and I want to add that I am longing so very much for letter from you, and now I wish you goodnight. Adieu, ith a handshake,

Yours,
Vincent

Please do not forget the *thick* Ingres if you can get it— enclose a sample. I still have some of the thin kind. On

[1] Vincent knew these as graphic illustrators.
[2] " It seems absurd to me that men should want to appear other an they really are."

the thick Ingres I can wash with water-colours, on the other i
always becomes blurred by no fault of mine.

I hope I shall be able to draw that little cradle *persistently*
a hundred times more, not counting what I did to-day.

Dear Theo,   [The Hague, July 31 1882]
Just a line to welcome you in anticipation of your arrival
Also to let you know of the receipt of your letter and the
enclosed, for which I send my heartiest thanks. It was very
welcome, for I am hard at work and need a few more things

As far as I understand it, we of course agree perfectly
about black in nature. Absolute black does not really exist
But like white, it is present in almost every colour, and forms
the endless variety of greys,—different in tone and strength
So that in nature one really sees nothing else but those tones
or shades.

There are but three fundamental colours—red, yellow and
blue; "composites" are orange, green and purple.

By adding black and some white one gets the endless
varieties of greys—*red*-grey, *yellow*-grey, *blue*-grey, *green*-
grey, *orange*-grey, *violet*-grey. To say, for instance, how many
green-greys there are is impossible, there are endless varieties.

But the whole chemistry of colours is not more complicated than those few simple rules. And to have a clear notion
of this is worth more than seventy different colours of paint,—
since with those three principal colours and black and white,
one can make more than seventy tones and varieties. The
colourist is he who seeing a colour in nature knows at once
how to analyse it, and can say for instance : that green-grey
is yellow with black and blue, etc.

In other words, someone who knows how to find the greys
of nature on his palette. In order to make notes from nature,
or to make little sketches, a strongly developed feeling for
outline is absolutely necessary as well as for strengthening
the composition subsequently.

But I believe one does not acquire this without effort,
rather in the first place by observation, and then especially by

strenuous work and research, and particular study of anatomy and perspective is also needed. Beside me is hanging a landscape study by Roelofs, a pen sketch—but I cannot tell you how expressive that simple outline is, everything is in it.

Another still more striking example is the large woodcut of " The Shepherdess " by Millet, which you showed me last year and which I have remembered ever since. And then, for instance, the pen and ink sketches by Ostade and Peasant Breughel.

When I see such results I feel more strongly the great importance of the outline. And you know for instance from " Sorrow " that I take a great deal of trouble to make progress in that respect.

But you will see when you come to the studio that besides the seeking for the outline I have, just like everyone else, a feeling for the power of colour. And that I do not object to making water-colours; but the foundation of them is the drawing, and then from the drawing many other branches beside the water-colour sprout forth, which will develop in me in time as in everybody who loves his work.

I have attacked that old whopper of a pollard willow, and I think it is the best of the water-colours : a gloomy landscape— that dead tree near a stagnant pool covered with reeds, in the distance a car shed of the Rhine Railroad, where the tracks cross each other; dingy black buildings, then green meadows, a cinder path, and a sky with shifting clouds, grey with a single bright white border, and the depth of blue where the clouds for an instant are parted. In short, I wanted to make it as the signal man in his smock and with his little red flag must see and feel it when he thinks : " it is gloomy weather to-day."

I have worked with great pleasure these last days, though now and then I still feel the effects of my illness.

Of the drawings which I will show you now I think only this : I hope they will prove to you that I am not remaining stationary in my work, but progress in a direction that is reasonable. As to the money value of my work, I do not pretend to anything else than that it would greatly astonish me if my work were not just as salable in time as that of others. Whether that will happen *now* or *later* I cannot of course tell, but I think the surest way, which *cannot* fail, is to work from nature faithfully and energetically. Feeling and love for nature sooner or later find a response from people who are interested in art. It is the painter's duty to be entirely absorbed by nature and to use all his intelligence to express sentiment in his work, so that it becomes intelligible to other people. To work for the market is in my opinion not exactly the right way, but on the contrary involves deceiving the amateurs. And true painters have not done so, rather the sympathy they received sooner or later came because of their sincerity. That is all I know about it, and I do not think I need know more. Of course it is a different thing to try to find people who like your work, and who will love it—that of course is permitted. But it must not become a speculation, that would perhaps turn out wrong and would certainly cause one to lose time that ought to be spent on the work itself.

Of course you will find in my water-colours things that are not correct, but that will improve with time.

But know it well, I am far from clinging to a system or being bound by one. Such a thing exists more in the imagination of Tersteeg, for instance, than in reality. As to Tersteeg, you understand that my opinion of him is quite personal, and that I do not want to thrust upon *you* this opinion that I am forced to have. So long as he thinks about me and says about me the things you know, I cannot regard him as a friend, nor as being of any use to me; quite the opposite. And I am afraid that his opinion of me is too deeply rooted ever to be changed, the more so since, as you say yourself, he will never take the trouble to reconsider some things and to change. When I see how several painters here, whom I know, have problems with their water-colours and paintings, so that they cannot bring them off, I often think : friend, the fault lies in your drawing. I do not regret for one single moment that I did not go on at first with water-colour and oil painting. I am sure I shall make up for that if only I work hard, so that my hand does not falter in drawing and in the perspective; but when I see young painters compose and draw *from memory*—and then haphazardly smear on whatever they like, *also from memory*—then study it at a distance, and put on a very mysterious, gloomy face in the endeavour to find out what in heaven's name it may look like, and finally make something of it, always *from memory*—it sometimes disgusts me, and makes me think it all very tedious and dull.

The whole thing makes me sick!

But those gentlemen go on asking me, not without a certain patronizing air, "if I am not painting as yet?"

Now I too on occasion sit and improvise, so to speak, at random on a piece of paper, but I do not attach any more value to this than to a rag or a cabbage leaf.

And I hope you will understand that when I continue to stick to drawing I do so for two reasons, most of all because I want to get a firm hand for drawing, and secondly because painting and water-colouring cause a great many expenses which bring no immediate recompense, and those expenses double and redouble ten times when one works on a drawing which is not correct enough.

And if I got in debt or surrounded myself with canvases and papers all daubed with paint without being sure of my drawing, then my studio would soon become a sort of hell, as I have seen some studios look. As it is I always enter it with pleasure and work there with animation. But I do not believe that you suspect me of *unwillingness*. It only seems to me that the painters here argue in the following way. They say: you must do this or that; if one does not do it, or not exactly so, or if one says something in reply, there follows a: "so you know better than I?" So that immediately, sometimes in less than five minutes, one is in fierce altercation, and in such a position that neither party can go forward or back. The least hateful result of this is that one of the parties has the presence of mind to keep silent, and in some way or other makes a quick exit through some opening. And one is almost inclined to say: confound it, the painters are almost like a family, namely, a fatal combination of persons with contrary interests, each of whom is opposed to the rest, and two or more are of the same opinion only when it is a question of combining together to obstruct another member. This definition of the word family, my dear brother, is, I hope, not always true, especially not when it concerns painters or our own family. With all my heart I wish peace may reign in our own family, and I remain with a handshake,

Yours,
Vincent

This is nearly enough the effect of the pollard willow,[1] only in the water-colour itself there is no black, except a broken one.

Where in this little sketch the black is darkest, there in the water-colour are the strongest effects, dark green, brown and grey. Well, adieu, and believe me that sometimes I laugh heartily, because people suspect me of all kinds of malignity and absurdities, of which I do not nourish an inkling. (I who am really nothing but a friend of nature, of study, of work, and of people in particular.) Well, hoping to see you soon, with a handshake,

Yours,
Vincent

Dear Theo,   [The Hague, early August 1882]
In my last letter you will have found a little sketch of that perspective frame I mentioned. I just came back from the blacksmith, who made iron points to go on the sticks and iron corners for the frame.

It consists of two long poles; the frame may be attached to them either upright or horizontally with strong wooden pegs.

So on the shore or in the meadows or in the fields one can look through it *as through a window*. The vertical lines and the perpendicular line of the frame and the diagonal lines and the point of intersection, or else the division in squares, certainly give a few basic markers, with the help of which

[1] Vincent included a sketch in the original letter.

one can make a firm drawing, from the indication of the main lines and proportions—at least for those who have some instinct for perspective and some understanding of the reason why and the manner in which perspective gives an apparent change of direction to the lines and a change of size to the planes and to the whole mass. Without this the instrument is of little or no use at all, and it makes one *dizzy* to look through it. I think you can imagine how it is a delightful thing to focus the viewer on the sea, on the green meadows, or in winter on the snowy fields, or in autumn on the fantastic network of thin and thick branches and trunks or on a stormy sky.

With long and continuous practice it enables one to draw quick as lightning,—and once the drawing is established, to paint quick as lightning also.

In fact, *for painting* it is absolutely the thing, for to express sky-earth-sea one needs the brush, or rather in order to express all that in drawing it is necessary to know and to understand the treatment of the brush. I certainly believe that if I paint for some time, it will have great influence on my *drawing*. I already tried it in January, but then I had to stop, the reason for my decision being, aside from a few other things, that I was too hesitant in my drawing. Now six months have passed that have been quite devoted to drawing. Well, it is with new courage that I start to paint again. The perspective frame is really a fine piece of workmanship; I am sorry you did not see it before you left. It cost me quite a bit, but I have had it made so solidly that it will last a long time. So next Monday I begin to make large charcoal studies with it, and begin to *paint* small studies. If I succeed in these two things, then I hope that better painted things will follow soon.

I want my studio to be a real painter's studio by the time you come again. I had to stop in January, as you know, for several different reasons, but after all it may be considered like some defect in a machine, a screw or a bar that was not strong enough and had to be replaced by a stronger one.

I bought a pair of strong and warm trousers, and as I had

bought a pair of strong shoes just before you came, I am now prepared to weather the storm and rain. It is my decided aim to learn from this painting of landscape a few things about *technique* which I feel I need for the *figure,* namely, to express different *materials,* and the *tone* and the *colour.* In one word, to express the bulk—the body—of things. Through your coming it became possible to me, but before you came there was not a day when I did not think in this way about it, only I should have had to keep exclusively to black and white and to the outline a little longer.—But now I have *launched my boat.* Adieu, boy, once more, a hearty handshake and believe me,

Yours,
Vincent

Dear Theo,   [The Hague, early September 1882]
Sunday morning

I have just received your very welcome letter, and as I want to take some rest to-day I answer it at once. Many thanks for it and for the enclosure, and for the things you tell me.

And for your description of that scene with the workmen at Montmartre, which I found very interesting, as you describe the colours too, so that I can see it : many thanks for it. I am glad you are reading the book about Gavarni.[1] I thought it very interesting, and it made me love him twice as much.

Paris and its surroundings may be beautiful, but here we have nothing to complain of either.

This week I painted something which I think would give you the impression of Scheveningen as we saw it when we walked there together : a large study of sand, sea and sky—a big sky of delicate grey and warm white, with one little spot of soft blue gleaming through—the sand and the sea, light— so that the whole becomes blond, but animated by the typically strong and bright-coloured figures and fishing smacks, which are full of tone. The subject of the sketch is a fishing smack with its anchor being raised. The horses are ready to be

[1] French cartoonist and illustrator of the mid nineteenth century.

hitched to it and then to draw the boat into the water. I
enclose a little sketch of it. It was a hard job. I wish I had
painted it on a panel or on canvas. I tried to introduce more
colour into it, namely depth and firmness of colour. How
curious it is that you and I often seem to have the same
thoughts. Yesterday evening, for instance, I came home from
the wood with a study, and for the whole week, and especially
then, I had been deeply absorbed in that question of depth of
colour. And I would have liked to have talked it over with
you, especially as regards the study I made, and, look here,
in your letter of this morning you accidentally speak about
being struck on Montmartre by the strong vivid colours, which
even so remained harmonious.

I do not know if it was exactly the same thing that struck
us both, but I well know that you also would have certainly
felt what struck me so particularly, and probably you too
would have seen it in the same way. I begin by sending you
a little sketch of the subject and will tell you what it was
about.

The wood is becoming quite autumnal—there are effects of
colour which I rarely find painted in Dutch pictures.

Yesterday towards evening I was busy painting a rather
sloping ground in the wood, covered with mouldered and
dry beech leaves. That ground was light and dark reddish
brown, made more so by the shadows of trees which threw
more or less dark streaks over it, sometimes half blotted out.
The question was, and I found it very difficult, to get the
depth of colour, the enormous force and solidity of that
ground—and while painting it I perceived only for the first
time how much light there still was in that dusk—to keep
that light, and to keep at the same time the glow and depth
of that rich colour.

For you cannot imagine any carpet so splendid as that deep
brownish-red, in the glow of an autumn evening sun, tem-
pered by the trees.

From that ground young beech trees spring up which catch
light on one side and are sparkling green there, and the
shadowy side of those stems are a warm deep black-green.

Behind those saplings, behind that brownish-red soil, is a sky very delicate, bluish grey, warm, hardly blue, all aglow— and against it is a hazy border of green and a network of little stems and yellowish leaves. A few figures of wood gatherers are wandering around like dark masses of mysterious shadows. The white cap of a woman, who is bending to reach a dry branch, stands out all of a sudden against the deep red-brown of the ground. A skirt catches the light—a shadow falls—a dark silhouette of a man appears above the underbrush. A white bonnet, a cap, a shoulder, the bust of a woman moulds itself against the sky. Those figures, they are large and full of poetry—in the twilight of that deep shadowy tone they appear as enormous clay figurines being shaped in a studio.

I describe nature to you; how far I rendered the effect in my sketch, I do not know myself; but this I know, that I was struck by the harmony of green, red, black, yellow, blue, brown, grey. It was very de Groux-like, an effect for instance like that sketch of "The Conscript's Departure" formerly in the Ducal Palace.

To paint it was a hard job. I used for the ground one large tube and a half of white—yet that ground is very dark— further red, yellow, brown ochre, black, sienna, bistre, and the result is a reddish-brown, but one that varies from bistre to deep wine-red, and even a pale blond ruddiness. Then there is still the moss on the ground, and a border of fresh grass, which catches light and sparkles brightly, and is very difficult to get. There you have at last a sketch which I maintain has some significance and which expresses something, no matter what may be said about it.

While painting it I said to myself: I must not go away before there is something of an autumn evening air about it, something mysterious, something serious.

But as this effect does not stay, I needed to paint quickly —the figures were painted in at once with a few strong strokes with a firm brush. It struck me how firmly those little stems were rooted in the ground. I began on them with a brush, but because the base was already so clotted, a brush-stroke was lost in it—so I squeezed the roots and trunks in from the tube, and modelled it a little with the brush.

Yes—now they stand there rising from the ground, strongly rooted in it. In a certain way I am glad I have not *learned* painting, because then I might have *learned* to pass by such effects as this. Now I say, no, this is just what I want, if it is impossible, it is impossible; I will try it, though I do not know how it should be done. How I paint it *I do not know myself*. I sit down with a white board before the spot that strikes me, I look at what is before me, I say to myself that that white board must become something; I come back dissatisfied—I put it away, and when I have rested a little, I go to look at it with a kind of fear. Then I am still dissatisfied, because I still have too clearly in my mind that splendid subject, to be satisfied with what I made of it. But after all I find in my work an echo of what struck me. I see that nature has told me something, has spoken to me, and that I have put it down in shorthand. In my shorthand there may be words that cannot be deciphered, there may be mistakes or gaps, but there is something in it of what wood or shore or figure has told me, and it is not a tame or conventional language, proceeding less from nature itself than from a studied manner or a system.

Enclosed another little sketch from the dunes. Small bushes are standing there, the leaves of which are white on one side and dark green on the other and constantly rustle and glitter. Dark trees to the rear.

You see I am absorbed with all my strength in painting; I am absorbed in colour—until now I have restrained myself, and I am not sorry for it. If I had not drawn so much, I would not be able to catch the impression of and get hold of a figure that looks like an unfinished clay figurine. But now I feel myself on the high sea—the painting must be continued with all the strength I can give to it.

When I paint on panel or canvas the expenses increase again. Everything is so expensive, the paint is also expensive, and is so soon gone. Well, those are difficulties all painters have. We must see what can be done. I know for sure that

I have an instinct for colour, and that it will come to me more and more, that painting is in my very bone and marrow. Doubly and twice doubly I appreciate your helping me so faithfully and in such measure. I think so often of you. I want my work to become firm, serious, manly, and that you too will get satisfaction from it as soon as possible.

One thing I want to call your attention to, as being of importance. Might it be possible to get colours, panels, brushes, etc., *wholesale*? Now I have to pay the retail price. Are you connected with Paillard or anyone like that? If so, I think it would be very much cheaper to buy wholesale— white, ochre, sienna, for instance, and we could then arrange about the money. It would of course be much cheaper. Think it over. Good painting does not depend upon using much colour, but in order to paint a ground emphatically, or to keep a sky clear, one must sometimes not spare the tube.

Sometimes the subject requires delicate painting, sometimes the material, the nature of the things themselves requires thick painting. Mauve, who in comparison with J. Maris, and still more in comparison with Millet or Jules Dupré, paints very soberly, has in the corners of his studio cigar boxes full of empty tubes, which are as numerous as the empty bottles in the corners of the rooms after a dinner or soirée, as Zola describes it for instance. Well, if there can be a little extra this month, that will be delightful. If not, it will be all right, too. I shall work as hard as I can. You inquire after my health, but how is yours? I am inclined to believe that my remedy would serve you also—to be in the open air, to paint. I am well, but when I am tired I still feel it. However, it is getting better instead of worse. I think it a good thing that I live as sparingly as possible, but painting is my special remedy. I heartily hope that you are having good luck and that you will find still more. A hearty handshake in thought and believe me,

Yours,
Vincent

You see how in the sketch of the beach there is a blond

tender effect, and in the wood there is a more gloomy serious tone. I am glad both exist in life.

Dear Theo,   [The Hague, beginning of November 1882]

Your letter and its contents were very welcome to me. The question you refer to will perhaps become more and more urgent. People will be obliged to acknowledge that many a new thing in which one at first thought to find progress proves in fact to be less sound than the old ones, and in consequence the need for strong men to redress things will manifest itself. As arguing about this can do little good, I think it rather superfluous to write more about it.

But I can hardly say that I share your thought which you express in the following words: " To me it seems quite natural that the desired change will occur." Just think how many great men are dead or will not be with us for long— Millet, Brion, Troyon, Rousseau, Daubigny, Corot—so many others are no longer among the living; think further back, Leys, Gavarni, de Groux (I name only a few), still further back, Ingres, Delacroix and Géricault, think how old *modern art* already is, add many others as well who have already reached old age.

Up to Millet and Jules Breton, however, there was always in my opinion progress, but to surpass these two—don't even mention it.

Their genius may be equalled in former, present or later times, but to surpass it is not possible. In that high range there is an equality of genius, but higher than the top of the mountain one cannot climb. Israëls, for instance, may equal Millet, but among genii superiority or inferiority is out of the question.

Now in the realm of art the summit has been reached. Certainly we shall still see beautiful things in the years to come, but anything more sublime than we have seen already—no. And I for my part am afraid that perhaps in a few years there will be a kind of *panic* in this regard. Since *Millet* we have greatly deteriorated; the word decadence, now whispered or pronounced in covert terms, (*see* Herkomer[1]) will then sound as an alarm bell. Many an one, for instance I myself, keeps quiet now because one is already labelled as a *mauvais coucheur*,[2] and to speak about it doesn't help. Speaking about it, that is to say, is not what one ought to do, one must work, even if it be with a sorrowful heart; those who will subsequently cry the hardest about decadence will be the most decadent themselves. I repeat—" By these fruits ye shall know them,"[3] by their work, nor will it be the most eloquent who will say the truest things, look at Millet himself, look at Herkomer; they are indeed no orators and they speak almost *à contre cœur*.[4]

Enough of this, I find in you someone who understands many of the great men, and I think it delightful to hear now and then things about them which I did not know; for instance, what you tell me about Daumier. The series of portraits of deputies, etc., the pictures " Third Class Railway Carriage," " The Revolution," I know none of them. It is true that your writing doesn't make me see them myself, but in my imagination Daumier's personality becomes more important as a result of it. I prefer to hear about such men more than, for instance, about the last Salon.[5]

Now what you write about the *Vie Moderne*, or rather about the kind of paper that Buhot promised you,—this is something which interests me very much. Do I understand rightly that this paper is such that when one makes a drawing on it (I suppose with autographic ink) this drawing *just as it is*, without the intermediary of a second draughtsman or engraver or lithographer, can be transferred on to a stone, or a cliché can be made of it, so that an indefinite number of

[1] Vincent's friend, Anthon van Rappard, had sent him a summary of an article by the English illustrator, Herkomer, about modern woodcuts, which had recently come out in an English art periodical.

[2] " an unpleasant customer "

[3] *Matthew* VII 20.

[4] " reluctantly "

[5] The official art-exhibition held annually in Paris.

copies can be pulled?—the latter then being facsimiles of the original drawing. If this is so, be so kind then as to give me all information you can pick up about the way in which one has to work on this paper, and try to get me some of it, so that I can give it a trial.

If I could have a trial before you come, we might on that occasion consult about what we can do with it.

I think it possible that within a relatively short time there will perhaps be a greater demand for illustrators than there is at present.

As for me, if I fill my portfolios with studies from every model I can get hold of, I will have enough of a skill to hope to get employment. *To keep* illustrating, as did for instance Morin, Lançon, Renouard, Jules Ferat, Worms in their times, one needs quite a lot of ammunition, in the form of different studies of all kinds of subjects.

Those I try to get together, as you know, and as you will see when you come.

By the by, I have not so far received the package of studies, which according to your letter you returned to me via the Rue Chaptal. Do you think they have already arrived at the Plaats? If you think so I will send for them, as they will be of use to me in connection with things which I have recently produced.

Do you know whose portrait I drew this morning? Blok, the Jewish book dealer—not David, but the little one who stands on the Binnenhof.

I wish I could draw more members of that family, for they are real good types.

It's awfully difficult to get the types that one likes best; meanwhile I think I'm right in working on *those I can get,* without losing sight of those I would draw if only I could get them.

I am very glad about Blok, he reminds me of things from many years ago. I hope he will come again some Sunday morning.

Of course one always feels, and one must feel, when at

work, a kind of dissatisfaction with oneself, a longing to do it much better; but still it is delightful and comforting little by little to get a collection of all kinds of figures together, though the more one makes the more one wants to make.

One cannot do everything at once, but it will be absolutely necessary for me to make a number of horse studies, not only just scratches made in the street, but to take a model for them. I know an old white horse, just the poorest nag imaginable (at the gas-works); but the man, who lets the poor beast do the hardest possible jobs, and draws from it what he can get, asked me a lot for it, namely, three guilders a morning to come to me and one guilder and a-half at least to come to him, but then it must be on a Sunday.

And when you consider that to get what I need, about thirty large studies for instance, I should have to work many a morning, it would prove to be too expensive. But I shall get a better chance some time.

I can get a horse here and there easily enough for a *very short* time, people are willing enough for that occasionally; but one *cannot* in a very short time do what really must be done, so that does not help me much.

I try to work quickly, for that is necessary, but a study that is of any use requires at least half an hour, on average, so one always falls back on to real posing. At Scheveningen, for instance, on the beach, I have had a boy or man standing for me for a moment, as they call it; the result was always a great longing in me for a longer pose, and the mere standing still of a man or a horse doesn't satisfy me.

If I am properly informed, the draughtsmen for the *Graphic* could always turn by turn find a model at their disposal in a studio at the office. Dickens tells a few good things about the painters of *his* time and their wrong way of working, namely, their following the model servilely, yet only half-way. He says: "Fellows, try to understand that your model is *not* your final aim, but *the means of giving form and strength to your thought and inspiration.* Look at the French (for instance, Ary Scheffer) and see how much better they do it than you do." It seems the English listened to him; *they* continued working with the model, but they have learned to view the model in a broader, stronger way and to use it for healthier, nobler compositions than those of the painters of Dickens's time.

Two things that in my opinion reinforce one another and remain eternally true are : Do not quench your inspiration and your imagination, do not become the slave of your model; and again : Take the model and study it, otherwise your inspiration will never become plastically concrete.

When your letter came, I immediately had many things to pay for. I hope it will not inconvenience you to send again not later than the 10th of November. That question of the process about which Buhot spoke to you seems very important to me, you know. I shall be very happy to learn it and will try my best to do so.

Adieu, with a handshake,

Yours,

Vincent

Do you know what effects one sees here at present early in the morning?—it is splendid—the sort that Brion painted in his picture at the Luxembourg : " The End of the Deluge," namely that streak of red light on the horizon with rain clouds over it. This brings me to the landscape painters. Compare those of the time of Brion with the contemporaries. Is it better now? I doubt it.

I will readily acknowledge that they are more productive now, but though I cannot help admiring what is produced now, the old landscapes done in a more old-fashioned way please me whenever I see them. There was a time for instance when I passed a Schelfout thinking : that's not worth while.

But the modern way, though it has its attraction, doesn't make that strong, deep, durable impression, and when one has been looking for a long time at new things, one sees again with great pleasure a naïve picture like a Schelfout or a Ségé, a Jules Bakhuysen. It is really not intentionally that I feel rather disenchanted about the progress, on the contrary quite against my will; the feeling involuntarily entered my thoughts, because I feel more and more a kind of void, which I cannot fill with the things of to-day.

While looking for an example, I happen to think of some old woodcuts by Jacque, which I saw at least ten years ago at Uncle Cor's; it was a series called " The Months ", done in the manner of those etchings which appeared in yearly series, or even more old-fashioned still. There is less of the local tone in it than in his later work, but the drawing and an element of pithiness remind one of Millet. Look here, in the many sketches in today's magazines, it seems to me that a *not* quite *un*conventional elegance threatens to replace that typical, real rusticity of which the sketches of Jacque, which I mentioned, are an example.

Don't you think the cause of this lies also in the life and personality of the artists? I do not know your experience, but do you find, for instance at present, many people who like to take a lengthy walk in grey weather? You yourself would love it and enjoy it as I do, but for many people it would be unattractive. It also struck me that when one talks with painters, the conversation in most cases is *not* interesting. Mauve has at times the great power of describing a thing in such words that one sees it, and certainly others have that too, when they want to. But that peculiar open-air feeling when you speak to a painter—do you think it is as strong as it used to be?

I read this week in Forster's *Life of Charles Dickens* all kinds of particulars about long walks on Hampstead Heath, etc., outside London, with the object for instance of eating bacon and eggs in a little old inn far away, well out in the country. Those walks were very pleasant and merry, but for all that it was generally in this way that serious plans were made for books, or discussions were held about what changes Dickens should make in this or that figure. There is nowadays a hurry and bustle in everything that doesn't please me, and it seems as if the joy has gone out of most things. I wish your expectation would come true : " that the desired change will come," but to me it doesn't seem " quite natural."

However this may be, it is of very little use to fight back

in words, I think, and the thing for everyone to do who has an interest in the matter is to try in his little circle to make something or to help make something.

I worked again on a water-colour of miners' wives carrying bags of coal through the snow. But especially I drew about twelve studies of figures for it and three heads, and I am not ready yet. In the water-colour I think I found the proper effect, but I do not think it broad enough of character. In reality it is something like " The Reapers " by Millet, severe, so you understand that one mustn't make a snow effect of it, which would be merely an impression and would only then have its raison d'être if it were done by way of a landscape. I think I will start afresh, though I believe the studies that I have at the moment will please you, because they succeeded better than many others. It would really be fit for the *Vie Moderne,* I think. When I get the paper I shall anyhow have *one* of the figures to try out, but it must become a group of women, a small caravan.

[The Hague, end of November 1882]
Dear Theo,   Sunday
    Yesterday I happened to read a book by Murger, namely, " The Water Drinkers." I find something in it of the same charm there is, for instance, in the drawings by Nanteuil, Baron, Roqueplan, Tony Johannot, something witty, something bright.

Still, it is very conventional, at least this book is, I think. I haven't read other books of his as yet, and I think there is the same difference between him and, for instance, Alphonse Karr and Souvestre as there is between a Henri Monnier and a Comte-Calix and the above-mentioned artists. I try to choose the persons I compare all from the same period. It has a fragrance of the era of the Bohemian (though the reality of that time is suppressed in the book), and for that reason it interests me, but in my opinion it lacks originality and sincerity of sentiment. However, perhaps his books in which no artist types occur are better than this one; authors seem to be always unlucky with their types of painters. Balzac, among others (his painters are rather uninteresting), Zola, even though his Claude Lantier is real[1]—there certainly are Claude Lantiers, but, after all, one would like to see another kind of painter depicted by Zola than Lantier, who seems to be drawn from life after somebody who certainly was not the worst example of that school, which I think is called impressionist. And it is not they who form the nucleus of the artistic corps.

On the other hand, I know very few well-drawn or well-painted types of authors; painters on that point generally fall into the conventional and make of an author a man who sits before a table full of papers, that's all, or they do not even go as far as that, and the result is a gentleman with a collar and a face devoid of expression.

There is a painting by Meissonier which I think beautiful, it is a figure seen from behind, stooping over, with his feet I think on the rung of the easel; one sees nothing but a pair of up-drawn knees, a back, a neck, and the back of a head, and just the glimpse of a fist holding a pencil or something similar. But the fellow is there, and one feels the action of strained attention just as in a certain figure by Rembrandt, a little fellow shown reading, who also stoops with his head leaning on his fist, and one feels at once that he is absolutely lost in his book.

Take Bonnat's Victor Hugo, fine, very fine, but I still prefer the Victor Hugo described in words by Victor Hugo himself, nothing but this : " Et moi je me taisais, tel que l'on voit se taire un coq sur la bruyère."[2]

Isn't it splendid, that little figure on the heath? Isn't it just as vivid as a little general of '93 by Meissonier—of about the size of one centimetre.

There is a portrait of Millet by Millet himself which I love, nothing but a head with a kind of shepherd's cap, but the look—from half-closed eyes, the intense look of a painter

[1] Hero of Zola's novel, *L'Œuvre,* first published in 1885/6; the model for Lantier was in principle Cézanne.
[2] " And as for me I was silent, like a cock seen keeping silence on the heath."

—how beautiful it is—also that piercing gleam as in a cock's eye, if I may call it so.

It is Sunday again. This morning I took a walk on the Rijswijk road, the meadows are partly flooded, so that there was an effect of tonal green and silver with the rough black and grey and green trunks and branches of the old trees distorted by the wind in the foreground, a silhouette of the little village with its pointed spire against the clear sky in the background, here and there a gate or a dungheap on which a flock of crows sat pecking. How you would like such a thing, how well you would paint it if you tried.

It was extraordinarily beautiful this morning, and it did me good to take a long walk, for what with drawing and the lithography I had scarcely been outdoors this week.

As to the lithography, I hope to get a proof to-morrow of a little old man. I hope it will turn out well. I made it with a kind of chalk especially patterned for this process, but I am afraid that after all the common lithographic crayon will prove to be the best, and that I shall be sorry I did not use it.

Well, we must see how it turns out.

To-morrow I hope I shall learn several things about printing which the printer will show me. I should love to learn the printer's craft itself. I think it quite possible that this new method will bring new life into the art of lithography. I think there might be a way of combining the advantages of the new with the old way, one cannot tell for certain, but perhaps it may be the cause of new magazines being published.

Monday

I wrote this far last night, this morning I had to go to the printing office with my little old man, now I have witnessed everything, the transfer on to the stone, the preparation of the stone and the printing itself. And I have a better idea now of what changes I can still make by retouching. Enclosed you will find the first print, not counting one spoiled proof. After a time I hope to do better, this doesn't satisfy me at all, but well, the progress must come by work and trying. It seems to me the duty of a painter to try to put an idea into his work. In this print I have tried to express (but I cannot do it well, or so strikingly as it is in reality, of which this is but a weak reflection in a dark mirror) what seems to me one of the strongest proofs of the existence of " quelque chose là-haut "[1] in which Millet believed, namely, the existence of God and eternity—certainly in the infinitely touching expression of such a little old man, of which he himself is perhaps unconscious, when he is sitting quietly in his corner by the fire.

At the same time there is something noble, something great that cannot be destined for the worms. Israëls has painted it so beautifully. In *Uncle Tom's Cabin*, the most beautiful passage is perhaps the one in which the poor slave, knowing that he must die, and sitting for the last time with his wife, remembers the words,

> *Let cares like a wild deluge come,*
> *And storms of sorrow fall,*
> *May I but safely reach my home,*
> *My God, my Heaven, my all.*

This is far from theology, simply a fact that the poorest little wood-cutter or peasant on the heath or miner can have moments of emotion and inspiration which give him a feeling of an eternal home to which he is near.

Returning from the printing office, I find your letter; I think your Montmartre splendid, and I certainly would have shared your emotion, in fact I think that Jules Dupré and Daubigny have often tried to conjure up these thoughts by their work. There is at times something indescribable in those aspects, all nature seems to speak, and on going home one has a feeling of the same sort as when one has finished a book by Victor Hugo, for instance. As for me, I cannot understand that not everybody sees it and feels it, nature or God does it for everyone who has eyes and ears and a heart to understand. For this reason I think a painter is happy because he is in harmony with nature as soon as he can express a little of what he sees.

And that's a great thing, one knows what one has to do,

[1] " something up there "

there are subjects in abundance, and Carlyle rightly says, "Blessed is he who has found his work."

If that work like that of Millet, Dupré, Israëls, etc., strives to bring peace, *sursum corda*, lift up your heart to Heaven, then it is doubly stimulating—one is then less alone also, because one thinks. It's true I'm sitting here lonely, but whilst I am sitting here in silence, my work perhaps speaks to my friend, and whoever sees it will not suspect me of being heartless.

But I tell you that dissatisfaction about bad work, the failure of things, the difficulties of technique can make one dreadfully melancholy. I can assure you that I am sometimes terribly discouraged when I think of Millet, Israëls, Breton, de Groux, so many others, Herkomer for instance; one only knows what these fellows are worth when one is oneself at work. And then to swallow that despair and that melancholy, to bear with oneself as one is, not in order to sit down and rest but to struggle on notwithstanding thousands of shortcomings and faults and the doubtfulness of conquering them, all these things are the reason why a painter is not happy either.

The struggle with oneself, the trying to better oneself, the renewal of one's energy, all this is complicated by material difficulties.

That picture by Daumier must be beautiful. It is a mystery why a thing that speaks as clearly as that picture, for instance, is not understood, at least that the situation is such that you are not sure of finding a buyer for it even at a low price.

This is for many a painter also something unbearable, or at least almost unbearable. One wants to be an honest man, one is so, one works as hard as a slave, but still one cannot make both ends meet; one must give up the work, there is no chance of carrying it out without spending more on it than one gets back for it, one gets a feeling of guilt, of shortcoming, of not keeping one's promises, one is not honest as one would be if the work were paid for at its natural reasonable price. One is afraid of making friends, one is afraid of moving, like one of the old lepers, one would like to call from afar to the people : Don't come too near me, for intercourse with me brings you sorrow and loss; with all that great load of care on one's heart, one must set to work with a calm, everyday face, without moving a muscle, live one's ordinary life, get along with the models, with the man who comes for the rent, with everybody in fact. With a cool head, one must keep one hand on the rudder to continue the work, and with the other hand try to do no harm to others.

And then storms arise, things one had not foreseen, one doesn't know what to do, and one has a feeling that one may strike a rock at any moment.

One cannot present oneself as somebody who comes to propose a good business transaction or who has a plan which will bring great profit. On the contrary, it is clear that it will end with a deficit, and still one feels a power surging within, one has work to do and it must be done.

One would like to speak like the people of '93 : this and that must be done, first these have to die, then those, then the last ones, it is duty, so it is unarguable, and nothing more need be said.

But is it the time to combine and to speak out?

Or is it better, as so many have fallen asleep and do not like to be aroused, to try to stick to things one can do alone, for which one is alone liable and responsible, so that those who sleep may go on sleeping and resting.

Well, you see that for this once I express more intimate thoughts than usual, you yourself are responsible for it as you did the same.

About you I think this, you are certainly one of the watchers, not one of the sleepers—wouldn't you rather watch while painting than while selling pictures? I say this in all coolness without adding what in my opinion would be preferable, and with full confidence in your own insight into things. That there is a great chance of going under in the struggle, that a painter is something like a " lost sentinel ", these and other things need no saying. You must not think of me as so readily scared—for instance, to paint the Borinage would be something so difficult, so relatively dangerous

as to make life a thing far removed from any rest or pleasure.
Yet I would undertake it if I could, that is, if I didn't know
for sure, as I do now, that the expenses would surpass my
means. If I could find people who would interest themselves
in such an enterprise, I would risk it. But just because you
are really the only one for the moment who has a concern
over what I do, the thing has to be put on the shelf for the
present and must remain there, and meanwhile I will find
other things to do. But I do not give it up to spare myself.

I hope you will be able to send the money not later than
the 1st of December. Well, boy, hearty thanks for your
letter and a warm handshake in thought, believe me,

Yours,

Vincent

[The Hague, 1883]

Dear Theo, February 8
My hearty congratulations for Father's birthday, and thanks
for your letter, which I was very glad to receive just now. I
congratulate you especially on the operation being over.[1] Such
things as you describe make one shudder! May the worst be
over now, at least the crisis past! Poor woman! If women
do not always show in their thoughts the energy and elasticity
of men, who are disposed towards reflection and analysis,
we cannot blame them, at least in my opinion, because in
general they have to spend so much more strength than we
in suffering pain. They suffer more and are more sensitive.

And though they do not always understand our thoughts,
they are sometimes truly capable of understanding when one
is good to them. Not always, though, but "the spirit is
willing," and there is in women sometimes a curious kind of
goodness.

There must be a great load off your mind now that the
operation is over.

---

[1] A young woman whom Theo had befriended when she was sick
and alone in Paris—to Vincent's great pleasure, since this paralleled
his own behaviour towards Sien—had had to be operated on for a
tumour of the foot.

What a mystery life is, and love is a mystery within a mystery. It certainly never remains the same in a literal sense, but the changes are like the ebb and flow of the tide and leave the sea unchanged.

Since I wrote to you last, I have given my eyes some rest and it has done me good, though they still ache now and then.

Do you know what has come into my mind, that in the first period of a painter's life one unconsciously makes it very hard for oneself—by a feeling of not being able to master the work—by an uncertainty as to whether one will ever master it—by a great ambition to make progress, by a lack of self-confidence—one cannot banish a certain feeling of agitation, and one hurries oneself though one doesn't like to be hurried.

This cannot be helped, and it is a time which one must go through, and which in my opinion cannot and should not be otherwise.

In the studies, too, one is conscious of a nervousness and a certain dryness which is the exact opposite of the calm, broad touch one strives for, and yet it doesn't work well if one applies oneself too much to acquiring that broadness of touch.

This gives one a feeling of nervous unrest and agitation, and one feels an oppression as on summer days before a thunderstorm. I had that feeling again just now, and when I have it, I change my work, just to make a new start.

That trouble one has at the beginning sometimes gives an awkwardness to the studies.

But I do not take this as a discouragement, because I have noticed it in myself as well as in others, who afterwards just slowly got rid of it.

And I believe that *sometimes* one keeps that *painful* way of working one's whole life, but not always with so little result as in the beginning. What you write about Lhermitte is quite in keeping with the review of the exhibition of Black and White. They, too, speak about the bold touch which can almost be compared only to Rembrandt's. I should like to know such an artist's conception of Judas; you write of his having drawn Judas before the scribes, and I think that Victor Hugo could describe that in detail, *so that one would see it*, but to paint those expressions would be more difficult still.

I found a page by Daumier: " ceux qui ont vu un drame " and " ceux qui ont vu une vaudeville."[1] I have developed a growing longing to see more of Daumier's work. There is pith and a sober depth in him, he is witty and yet full of sentimental passion; sometimes, for instance in " The Drunkards," and possibly also in " The Barricade," which I do not know, I find a passion which can be compared to the white heat of iron.

The same thing occurs in certain heads by Frans Hals, for instance, it is so sober that it seems cold; but when you look at it for a short while you are astonished to see how someone working apparently with so much emotion and so completely wrapped up in nature had at the same time the presence of mind to put it down with such a firm hand. I found the same thing in studies and drawings by de Groux; perhaps Lhermitte operates also at that white heat. And Menzel too.

There are sometimes passages in Balzac or Zola, for instance in *Père Goriot,* where words reach a degree of passion that is white hot.

I sometimes think I will make an experiment, and try to work in quite a different way, that is, to dare more and to risk more, but I am not sure that I should not first do more by way of studying the figure directly from the model.

I am also looking for a way to shut off the light in the studio, or to let it in as I please. It doesn't fall enough from above, I think, and there is too much of it. For the time being I shut it off with cardboard now and then, but I must try and get the landlord to produce some shutters.

What was in the letter I told you I had torn up was quite in keeping with what you say.

But while finding more and more that one is not perfect oneself, and makes mistakes, and that other people do like-

[1] " Spectators who have witnessed a drama " and " spectators who have been present at a vaudeville."

wise, so that difficulties continually arise which are the opposite of illusions, I think that those who do not lose courage and who do not become indifferent, ripen through it, and one must bear hardships in order to ripen.

Sometimes I cannot believe that I am only thirty years old, I feel so much older.

I feel older *only* when I think that most people who know me consider me a failure, and how it really might be so, if some things do not change for the better; and when I think *it might be so,* I feel it so vividly that it quite depresses me and makes me as downhearted as if it were really so. In a calmer and more normal mood I am sometimes glad that thirty years have passed, and not without teaching me something for the future, and I feel strength and energy for the next thirty years, if I should live that long.

And in my imagination I see years of serious work before me, and happier ones than the first thirty.

How it will be in reality doesn't depend *only* on myself, the world and circumstances must also contribute to it.

What concerns me and is a source of responsibility is that I should make the most of the circumstances and try my best to make progress.

The age of thirty is, for the working man, just the beginning of a period of some stability, and as such one feels young and full of energy.

But, at the same time, a phase of life is past. This makes one melancholy, thinking some things will never come back. And it is no silly sentimentalism to feel a certain regret. Well, many things really begin at the age of thirty, and certainly all is not over then. But one doesn't expect out of life what one has already learned that it cannot give, but rather one begins to see more and more clearly that life is only a kind of sowing time, and the harvest is not here.

Perhaps that's the reason that one sometimes feels indifferent toward the opinion of the world, and if that opinion depresses us all too strongly, one may throw it off.

Perhaps I had better tear up this letter as well.

I understand perfectly that you are quite absorbed by the

condition of the woman; that is one of the things which are necessary for her rescue, and also for her recovery.

For one must throw oneself headlong into it, and the English saying is true: "if you want it well done, you must do it yourself, you mustn't leave it to others." That means that one must keep in hand the care in general and the management of the whole.

We had a few real spring days, for instance last Monday, which I enjoyed very much.

The cycle of the seasons is a thing which is strongly felt by the people. For instance, in a neighbourhood like the Geest and in those courts of almshouses or " homes of charity," the winter is always a difficult, anxious and oppressive time, and spring is a deliverance. If one pays attention, one sees that such a first spring day is a kind of Gospel message.

And it is pathetic to see so many grey, withered faces come out of doors on such a day, not to do something special, but as if to convince themselves that spring is there. So, for instance, all kinds of people, of whom one would not expect it, throng the market around the spot where a man sells crocuses, snowdrops, bluebells and other bulbs. Sometimes a dried-up government clerk, apparently a kind of Jusserand in a threadbare black coat with greasy collar—that *he* should be beside the snowdrops is a pretty picture! I think the poor people and the painters have in common that feeling for the weather and the cycle of the seasons. Of course everybody feels it, but for the well-to-do middle-class it is not so important, and it doesn't affect much their frame of mind in general. I thought it a characteristic saying for a navvy: " In winter I suffer as much from the cold as the winter corn does."

Now for your patient too spring will be welcome, may it do her good! How terrible that operation was, at least I was frightened by the description.

Rappard is recovering, did I tell you he had brain fever? It will be some time before he can go to work again, but he is starting to take a walk now and then.

If my eyes do not improve, I'll follow your advice and bathe them with tea. As it is they are getting better, so for the present I'll leave them alone. For they never troubled me before, except once this winter when I had toothache, so I believe it is nothing but strain and overwork.

On the contrary, lately my eyes can stand the fatigue of drawing better than previously.

Write soon again if you can, and believe me, with a hand-shake,

Yours,
Vincent

I do not know whether you know those little almshouses on the Brouwersgracht opposite the hospital. I should like to draw there when the weather permits. This week I made a few scratches there already. They are a few rows of small houses with little gardens which I think belong to the charity board.

Dear Theo,   [The Hague, mid March 1883]
Thanks for your letter of the 9th of March, and for the enclosed. Is your patient improving? I hope in this case " no news is good news."

If it has been as cold in Paris as it was here last week, it cannot have agreed very well with her.

When you say that you sometimes wish we could talk together more, about a variety of things in art, I for my part have that longing continually, and sometimes very strongly.

So often I should like to know your opinion about this or that, about some studies, etc., for instance, if they might be of some use, or if it would be advisable, for some reason or other, to go more deeply into them.

So often I should like to have some more information about things on which you are better informed than I, and I should like to know more about the state of things, I mean what kind of work the painters are producing. One can write about it to some extent, but writing takes time, and one cannot always get to it, nor can one go enough into detail.

And just now, owing to a piling up of studies, it would be worth a great deal to me if we could talk things over together, and I should also like so much to have you see how the studio is improved.

Well, let us hope that it will not be so very, very long before you come to Holland.

Be clear in your mind, dear brother, how strongly and intensely I feel the enormous debt I owe you for your faithful help.

It would be difficult for me to express all my thoughts about it. It constantly remains a source of disappointment to me that my drawings are not yet what I want them to be. The difficulties are indeed numerous and great, and cannot be overcome at once. To make progress is a kind of miner's work; it doesn't advance as quickly as one would like, and as others also expect, but as one stands before such a task, the basic necessities are patience and faithfulness. In fact, I do not think much about the difficulties, because if one thought of them too much one would get stunned or disturbed.

A weaver who has to direct and to interweave a great many little threads has no time to philosophize about it, but rather he is so absorbed in his work that he doesn't think but acts, and he *feels* how things must go more than he can explain it. Even though neither you nor I, in talking together, would come to any definite plans, etc., perhaps we might mutually strengthen that *feeling* that something is ripening within us. And that is what I should like.

This morning I was at Van der Weele's, who was working at a marvellous picture of diggers, horses, and sand wagons, large size. It was beautiful in tone and colour, a grey morning haze, it was virile in drawing and composition, there was style and character in it—in fact it was by far the most beautiful and strongest thing of his I have ever seen. He had also painted three very beautiful serious studies of an old white horse, and also a beautiful little landscape in the dunes.

This week he will probably look in at my studio, which I should like very much indeed.

Last week I met Breitner in the street; his position in Rotterdam frees him from much anxiety; however, Van der Weele had a little note from him just this morning, to the effect that he was ill again. To tell you the truth, the impression I had when I saw him again was not very assuring; he had an air of disappointment, and he spoke in rather a queer way about his work.

Now I still have to tell you about the surprise I have had. I received a letter from Father, very cordial and cheerful, it seemed to me, with twenty-five guilders enclosed. Father wrote he had received some money, on which he had no longer counted, and he wanted me to share in it. Wasn't that nice of him, however it quite embarrasses me.

But, involuntarily, a thought occurred to me. Can it be, perhaps, that Father has heard, from someone or other, that I was very hard up? I hope that this was not his motive, for I think this idea of my circumstances would not be correct. And it might give Father anxieties which would be quite out of place. You will understand my meaning better than Father would if I were to try to explain it to him.

In my opinion, I am often *rich as Crœsus,* not in money, but (though it doesn't happen every day) rich, because I have found in my work something to which I can devote myself heart and soul, and which gives inspiration and significance to life.

Of course my moods vary, but there is an average of serenity. I have a sure *faith* in art, a sure confidence that it is a powerful stream, which bears a man to harbour, though he himself must do his bit too; and at all events I think it such a great blessing, when a man has found his work, that I cannot count myself among the unfortunate. I mean, I may be in certain relatively great difficulties, and there may be gloomy days in my life, but I shouldn't want to be counted among the unfortunate nor would it be correct.

You write in your letter something which I sometimes *feel also* : " Sometimes I do not know how I shall pull through."

Look here, I often feel the same *in more than one respect,* not only in *financial* things, but in art itself, and in *life* in general. But do you think that something exceptional? Don't you think every man with a little pluck and energy has those moments?

Moments of melancholy, of distress, of anguish, I think we all have them, more or less, and it is a condition of every *conscious* human life. It seems that some people have no self-consciousness. But those who have it, they may sometimes be in distress, but for all that they are not unhappy, nor is it something exceptional that happens to them.

And sometimes there comes relief, sometimes there comes new inner energy, and one rises up from it, till at last, some day, one perhaps doesn't rise up any more, *que soit,* but that is nothing extraordinary, and I repeat, *such is the common human fate, in my opinion.*

Father's letter was an answer to a letter of mine, which I remember quite well was very cheerful, for I told him about the changes in the studio, and I did not write anything to Father that could give rise to thoughts of my being in any difficulties, either financial or otherwise. In fact, Father doesn't write anything about it, and his letter is very cheerful and cordial, but the money came so unexpectedly that involuntarily the thought came into my head, can it be that Father is worried about me? If I am mistaken in this, it would be very much out of place to write as if that were the principal impression his kindness has made upon me—the principal impression being that I feel very grateful for having received something which enables me to do several things that otherwise I couldn't have done. But I tell you my thoughts about it, because in case you should perceive that Father is worrying about me, you would be better able to reassure him than I.

At the same time, you see from this that I have had a real stroke of luck. I intend to spend it on getting my water-colour things in good shape. I will pay off Leurs and will be able to arrange for different things in the studio, in order to make it even more practical.

It sometimes seems to me that the prices of the various painting and drawing materials are terribly inflated. So that it thwarts many a person from painting. One of my ideals is that there would be more institutions like the *Graphic,* for instance, where people who want to work can find all the materials, on condition that a certain ability and energy is demonstrated.

Like Cadart, in his day, enabled many a man to etch, who wouldn't have been able to etch, because of the expenses, if he had had to pay them from his own pocket.

I am privileged above many others, but I cannot do everything which I might have the courage and energy to undertake. The expenses are so extensive, beginning with a model and food and housing, and ending with the different colours and brushes.

And that is also like a weaving loom, where the different threads must be kept apart.

But we all have to bear up against the same thing—so just because everyone who paints or draws has to bear it, and if alone would almost sink down under it, why shouldn't more painters join hands, to work together, like soldiers of the rank and file; and why, especially, are those branches of art which are least expensive so much despised?

As to the crayon, I do not know whether the one you gave me came from the Plaats, but I am quite sure that you gave it to me on your visit of last summer, or *perhaps when I was still in Etten*. In a drug store I found a few remnants, perhaps six pieces, but all in small bits. Please keep it in mind. When I again asked Leurs for it, he told me that Jaap Maris had asked him so often for it.

I have made two sketches with it again, a cradle, and one more like the one I sent you already, in which I washed a great deal with sepia. As to what you write about that sketch of those two figures, the one above the other, it is mainly an effect of perspective, and also of the great difference in size between the little child and the woman on the basket.

What I myself dislike more than that line of the composition is something which, in fact, you have noticed, that the two figures are too much of one tone, which is partly the fault of the crayon, which does not express all shades, and one would like to strengthen it with lithographic crayon, for instance. But I think that the principal reason is that I do not always have time enough to work as elaborately as I should like. If one works a long time on a drawing, it is possible to go more into detail, to seek the different tones. But too often I must work in a hurry. I dare not ask too much from my models. If I paid them better, I should have the right to demand longer poses, and could make better progress.

At present, I often think I get more from them than a just return on what I pay them in money.

However, I do not mean to say that there is not a still more important reason, namely, that I must become more skilled than I am before I can be ever so slightly satisfied with myself. And by and by I hope to make better and more elaborate things in the same amount of time that I now spend on them.

Well, brother, my best wishes for your patient, I long sometimes for another description of an aspect of Paris from you, and—rest assured I'll make shift as best I can, with what your faithful help gives me—that I try and try to make an even better use of it, and especially that I blame myself for being unable to manage to do what I want with it. Adieu, with a handshake in thought,

Yours,
Vincent

Dear Theo, ·   [The Hague, end of April 1883]
On your birthday I want you to receive a little word from me too. May it be a happy year for you, and may you have success in your work, and I do hope, especially, that you may have in this year some satisfaction for what you did for your patient; may she recover and start a new life. Do you know it is almost a year since you were here? Yes—I long very much for your coming. It is the work of that whole year that I have to show you, about which we must speak in regard to the future.

Do you think it will be about the same time as last year that you will come? Well, as soon as anything is decided about your coming, let me know.

Some time ago you told me many things about these Swedish painters, Heyerdahl, Edelfelt.

This week I found a reproduction of a picture by Edelfelt: " A Prayer-Meeting on the Beach." There is something in it of Longfellow's poems; it is very beautiful. It shows a sentiment of which I am very fond, and which I think does more good in the world than the Italians and Spaniards with their " Arms Merchants of Cairo," of which I get so tired in the long run.

This week I have been working on the figure of a woman on the heath, who is gathering cuts of peat.

And a kneeling figure of a man.

One must know the structure of the figures so thoroughly, in order to get the expression, at least I cannot see it differently.

The Edelfelt is indeed beautiful in its expression, however the effect lies not only in the expression of the faces, but in the whole position of the figures.

Do you know who has claims to being the cleverest of all these Swedes?

It is perhaps a certain Wilhelm Leibl,[1] an absolutely self-made man.

I have a reproduction of a picture with which he suddenly came out, I think it was at the exhibition in Vienna in '82. It represents three women in a pew, one seated figure of a young woman in a checkered dress (Tyrol), two kneeling old women in black, with kerchiefs round their heads. Its sentiment is beautiful and drawn like Memling or Quinten Matsys. That picture seems to have made a great sensation among the artists at the time, I do not know what became of Leibl since then. I found him very much like Thijs Maris. In England there was also a German of that kind, but less clever—Paul de Gassow, who reminds me a little of Oberländer, whose heads you certainly remember. Well, there still seem to be some good artists in Sweden.

I am longing again for your letter. As to what I wrote you about relations between women and their mothers, I can

[1] A mistake of the author; Wilhelm Leibl was a German.

assure you, in my case nine-tenths of the difficulties which I had with the woman originated directly or indirectly therein.

And yet those mothers are not exactly bad, though they act absolutely wrongly.

But they do not know what they are doing.

Women of about the age of fifty are often distrustful, and perhaps it is that very distrust and cunning that entangles them. If you care to hear them, I can tell you some particulars some day. I do not know whether all women become more serious in getting older, and then want to govern and correct their daughters, which they do in exactly the wrong way.

In some cases their system may have some raison d'être; but they ought not to fix as a principle and accept a priori that all men are deceivers and fools, for which reason women must cheat them and suppose they know everything better. If, by ill chance, the mother-system is applied to a man who is honest and of good faith, he is indeed badly off. . . .

Well, the time has not yet come when *reason*, not only in the sense of *raison*, but also of la conscience, is respected by everyone; to contribute towards bringing about that time is a duty, and in judging characters one of the first things that humanity demands is to take into consideration the circumstances of contemporary society.

How beautiful Zola is—it is especially *L'Assommoir* which I often think of. A propos, how far did you get in reading Balzac? I have quite finished *Les Misérables*. I know very well that Victor Hugo analyses in a different way than do Balzac and Zola, but he probes to the bottom of things just as well.

Do you know what I should prefer in the matter of relations between the woman and her mother—in my case where it has decidedly bad consequences—that the mother came to live with us entirely.

I proposed it this winter, when the mother was very hard up, and I said: If you are so much attached to each other, then come and live together, but I believe they, though worse off themselves, don't think our simple way of living good enough, one which I desire on principle and to which I am forced by circumstances.

Many people care more for the exterior than for the inward life of a family, thinking they act well in doing so. Society is full of that: people who strive to make a show instead of leading a true existence. I repeat: those people are not bad, but they are foolish. . . . A wife's mother is, in some cases, the representative of a meddlesome, slandering, aggravating family, and as such decidedly injurious and hostile, though she may not be so bad herself.

In my case, she would be much better off in my house than in the houses of other members of the family, where she is very often the victim of callous insolence and is incited to intrigues. . . .

Towards your patient you have been absolutely honest and straightforward: that is the principal thing, which keeps the future clear, whatever it may be: but even if one has acted rightly, difficulties may arise. Well, in the year that begins for you to-day, I wish you very few of those—on the contrary may all good be your share. Well, write soon if you have not written already, which I hope will be the case. Adieu, boy, with a hearty handshake,

Yours,

Vincent

Dear Theo,   [The Hague, end of July 1883]

To my surprise, yesterday I received a further letter from you enclosing a banknote. I need not tell you how glad I was, and I thank you heartily for it. But they refused to change the banknote because it was torn too much. However, they gave me ten guilders on it, and it has been forwarded to Paris. If the bank refuses it, I will have to pay back the ten guilders, for which I had to sign a receipt; but if the bank changes it, I will get the rest later.

You write in your letter about the conflict one sometimes feels on the question of whether one is responsible for the unlucky results of a good action, if it would not be better to

act in a way one knows to be wrong, but which at the same
time will bring one out unscathed—I know that conflict too.
If we follow our conscience—conscience is for me the highest
reason—the reason within the reason—we are tempted to
think we have acted wrongly or foolishly; we are especially
upset when more superficial people jeer at us, because they
are so much wiser and have so much more success. Yes, then
it is sometimes difficult, and when circumstances occur which
make difficulties rise to an overflowing tide, one is almost
sorry to be as one is, and would wish to have been less con-
scientious.

I hope you don't think of me in any other way than having
continually that same inward conflict, and often very tired
brains too, and in many cases not knowing how to decide in
questions of right and wrong.

When I am at work, I feel an unlimited faith in art, and
that I shall succeed, but in days of physical prostration, or
when there are financial obstacles, I feel that faith diminishing, and a doubt overwhelms me, which I try to conquer by
setting to work again at once. It is the same thing with the
woman and the children; when I am with them, and the little
chap comes creeping towards me on all fours, crowing for joy,
I have not the slightest doubt that everything is right.

How often has that child comforted me.

When I am at home, he can't leave me alone for a
moment; when I am at work, he pulls at my coat or climbs up
against my leg, till I take him on my lap. In the studio, he
crows at everything, plays quietly with a bit of paper, a bit of
string, or an old brush; the child is always happy. If he
keeps this temperament all his life, he will be cleverer than I
am.

Now what shall we say about the fact that there are times
when one feels there is a certain fatality, that makes the good
turn out wrong, and the bad turn out well.

I think one may consider those thoughts partly as a consequence of overwrought nerves, and if one has them, one
must not think it one's duty to believe that things are really
as gloomy as one supposes; if one did so, it would make one

mad. On the contrary, it is reasonable to strengthen one's physique then, and afterward set to work like a man, and if that does not help, *still one must always continue to use those two means,* and consider that melancholy as fatal. In the long run, one will then feel one's energy increase, and will bear up against the troubles. Mysteries remain, sorrow or melancholy remains, but that everlasting negative is balanced by the positive work which is thus achieved after all. If life were as simple, and things as little complicated as in the tale of Goody-Goody, or the hackneyed sermon of the average clergyman, it would not be so very difficult to make one's way. But it is not so, and things are infinitely more complicated, and right and wrong do not stand separate, any more than black and white do in nature. One must take care not to fall back upon opaque black, that is deliberate wrong; and still more, one has to avoid the whiteness of a white-washed wall, which means hypocrisy and everlasting Pharisaism[1]. He who tries courageously to follow reason, and especially conscience, the very highest reason—the sublime reason—and tries to remain honest, can scarcely altogether lose his way, I think, though he will not get off without mistakes, checks and disheartenments, and will not reach perfection.

And I think it will give him a deep feeling of pity and benevolence, broader than the narrow-mindedness which is the stock-in-trade of clergymen.

One may not be considered by either party as of the least importance, and one may be counted among the mediocrities and feel oneself to be a thoroughly ordinary man among ordinary people—in the end one will after all obtain a rather steady serenity. One will succeed in bringing one's conscience to a state of development such that it becomes the voice of a better and higher self, of which the ordinary self is the servant. And one will not return to scepticism or cynicism, nor belong among the foul mockers. But not at once. I think it a beautiful saying of Michelet's, and that one phrase of Michelet's expresses all I mean : " Socrate naquit un vrai satyre, mais

[1] See *Matthew* XXIII 27 and *Acts* XXIII 3.

par le dévouement, le travail, le renoncement des choses fri-
voles, il se changea si complètement qu'au dernier jour devant
ses juges et devant sa mort il y avait en lui je ne sais quoi
d'un dieu, un rayon d'en haut dont s'illumina le Parthénon."[1]

One sees the same thing in Jesus too, who was first an
ordinary carpenter and then raised himself to something else,
whatever it may have been, a personality so full of pity, love,
goodness, seriousness that one is still attracted by it. Generally a carpenter's apprentice becomes a master carpenter,
narrow-minded, dry, miserly, vain, and whatever may be said
of Jesus, he had another conception of things than my friend
the carpenter of the backyard, who has raised himself to the
level of house owner, and yet is much more vain and thinks
more highly of himself than Jesus did.

But I must not become too abstract. What I first want to
do is to renew my strength, and I think once it has come up
again from below the mark I will get new ideas for my
work, for trying to conquer that dryness.

When you come here we will talk it over. I do not think it
is a question of a few days.

In a few days, when I shall have taken some more nourishing food than of late, I think I shall get rid of my *worst
depression,* but it is *deeper rooted* than that, and I wish I could
get so far that I had plenty of health and strength, which
after all is not impossible when one is much out of doors
and has work that one loves.

For it is a fact that at the moment all my work is *too
meagre and too dry.*

That has become as clear as daylight to me lately, and I
don't doubt in the least that a general thorough change is
necessary. I intend to talk it over with you *after you have
seen the work of this year,* to see whether you agree with me
about certain measures, and if you agree with me, I think we

---

[1] "Socrates was born a real satyr, but through devotion, toil and
the renunciation of frivolous things, he made such a complete change
in himself that when on that last day he stood before his judges and
faced death, some indefinable quality of godhood stood out in him, a
heavenly radiance that lit up the Parthenon."

shall succeed in overcoming the difficulties. We must not hesitate, but have " la foi de charbonnier."[1] I hope they will change the banknote. I am so glad you have managed to send something, for I think it saves me an illness. I will let you know how the story of the banknote ends. And it would be a good thing if you could send again as usual by the first of August. I always think that in looking through the work together it is possible that we shall hit on another plan for the future. I do not know what, as yet—but somewhere there must be work to do, which I can do just as well as anybody else. If London were nearer, I should try there.

Be sure that I should be enormously pleased if I could make something that was salable. I would have less scruples then about the money which comes from you, which after all you need as much as I do. Once more many thanks, goodbye,

Yours,

Vincent

Dear Theo   [The Hague, early August 1883]
As I look forward to your arrival, there is hardly a moment when my thoughts are not with you.

These last days I have gone on to paint several studies, so that you may see them at the same time. And that change of work does me good, for though I cannot do literally as Weissenbruch does, and go and stay in the polders for a few weeks, yet I do do something like it, and to look at the green fields has a calming effect.

Besides, I decidedly hope in this way to make progress in terms of colour. The last painted studies seem to me firmer and more solid in colour. So for instance a few I made recently, in the rain, showing a man on a wet, muddy road, express the sentiment better, I think.

Well, we will see when you come.

Most of them are impressions of landscape, I dare not say as well done as those that sometimes occur in your letters, because still I am often checked by technical difficulties—yet there is something in them, I think—for instance, a silhouette

[1] " the faith of the miner."

of the city in the evening, when the sun is setting, and a towpath with windmills.

For the rest, it is miserable enough that I still feel very faint, when I am not hard at my work, but I believe it is receding. I will decidedly try hard to lay up a reserve of strength, for I shall need it to carry on the painting of the figure with a firm hand.

While painting, I feel of late a certain power of colour awakening in me, stronger and different from what I have felt till now.

It may be that the nervousness of these days is linked up with a kind of revolution in my way of working, for which I have been seeking and of which I have been thinking for a long time already.

I have often tried to work less drily, but it always turned into the same thing over again. But now that a kind of weakness prevents me from working in my usual way, this seems to help, rather than to hinder, and now that I let myself go a little, and look more through the eyelashes, instead of concentrating on the joints and analysing the structure of things, it leads me more directly to seeing things more like adjacent contrasting patches of colour.

I wonder what it will lead to, and how it will develop. I have sometimes wondered why I was not more of a colourist, because my temperament decidedly seems to indicate it—but up till now it developed very little.

I repeat, I wonder how it will develop—but I see clearly that my last painted studies are different.

If I remember rightly, you still have one from last year, of a few tree trunks in the wood.

I do not think that it is really bad, but it is not what one sees in the studies of colourists. Some colours there are correct, but though they are correct they do not have the effect they ought to have, and though the paint is here and there laid on thickly, even so the effect is too meagre. I take this one as an example, and now I think that the last ones which are less thickly laid on are nonetheless becoming more potent in colour, as the colours are more interwoven and the strokes of the brush cover one another, so that it is mellower and more for instance like the downiness of the clouds or of the grass.

At times I have been greatly worried that I made no progress with colour, but now I am hopeful again.

We shall see how it will develop.

Now you will understand that I am very anxious for your coming, for if you also saw that there is a change, I should not doubt that we are on the right track. I dare not quite trust my own eyes as regards my own work. Those two studies, for instance, which I made while it was raining—a muddy road with a little figure—they seem to me exactly the opposite of some other studies. When I look at them I rediscover the sentiment of that dreary rainy day, and in the figure, though it is nothing but a few patches of colour, is a kind of life, that is not called forth by correctness of drawing, for there is in effect no drawing. What I mean to suggest is that in these studies I believe there is something of that mysteriousness one gets by looking at nature through the eyelashes, so that the outlines are simplified to blots of colour.

Time must pass over it, but at present I see in several studies something different in colour and tone.

Recently I often think of a story I read in an English magazine, a tale about a painter, in which there appears a person whose health suffered also in a time of trouble, and who went to a lonely place in the peat fields, and there, in that melancholy setting, found himself again, and began to paint nature as he felt and saw it. It was very well described in the story, evidently by a person who was well up in art, and it struck me when I read it, while now of late I sometimes think of it again.

At any rate I hope we shall soon be able to talk it over and consult together. If you can, write soon, and of course the sooner you can send the money, the better it would be for me.

With a handshake in thought,

Yours,
Vincent

Involuntarily, and without any definite motive, I add a thought that often occurs to me. Not only did I begin drawing relatively late in life, but it may also be that I shall not live for so very many years to come.

If I think of that, calculating coldly, as if I were making an estimate of something, it is in the nature of things that I cannot possibly know anything definite about it.

But in comparison with different people, whose lives one might happen to know, or in comparison with some people with whom one is supposed to have many things in common, one can draw some conclusions which are not altogether without foundation. Therefore, as to the time I have still before me in which I can work, I think I may presume without rashness : that my body will carry on for a certain number of years " quand bien même "[1]—a certain number, say between six and ten for instance. I can assume this the more safely as at the moment there is no immediate " quand bien même."

This is the period on which I count firmly; for the rest, it would be speculating too much at random to dare make a definite pronouncement about myself, because it depends especially on those, let us say, first ten years, whether there will be anything after that time or not.

If one wears oneself out too much in those years, one does not get beyond forty; if one is strong enough to resist certain shocks, which generally attack one then, to solve more or less complicated physical difficulties, then from forty to fifty one is again in a new relatively normal tideway.

But for the present such calculations are out of the question; one can as I said only take into account plans for a period of between five and ten years. I do *not* intend to spare myself, nor to avoid emotion or difficulties—I don't much care whether I live a longer or a shorter time, besides, I am not competent to take care of my physique as for instance a physician can.

Thus I go on like an ignoramus but knowing this one thing : " *in a few years I must finish a certain body of work.*"

[1] " however it be "

I need not overhurry myself, there is no good in that—but I must work on in full calmness and serenity, as regularly and concentratedly as possible, as concisely and economically as possible. The world only concerns me in so far as I feel a certain debt and duty towards it because I have walked that earth for thirty years, and, out of gratitude, want to leave some souvenir in the shape of drawings or pictures—not made to please a certain cult in art, but to express a sincere human feeling. So this work is the aim—and given concentration on that one idea, everything one does is simplified in so far as it is not a chaos, but done in its entirety with one aim in view. Now my work goes slowly—a reason the more to lose no time. Guillaume Régamey was somebody who left little reputation I think (you know there are two Régameys, F. Régamey paints the Japanese, and is his brother), but he was a personality for whom I have a great respect. He died at the age of thirty-eight, and a period of six or seven years had been exclusively devoted to the making of drawings that bear a very distinctive stamp, and were made while he was working under some physical difficulty.

That is one of many, a very good one among the very good.

I do not name him in order to compare myself to him. I cannot be ranked on a level with him—but I mention him as a special example of a certain self-possession and energy clinging to one inspiring idea, of one to whom difficult circumstances showed the way to accomplish good work in full serenity. It is in this way that I regard myself—as having to accomplish in a few years something with heart and love in it, doing this with energy.

If I live longer " tant mieux,"[1] but I do not count on it.

In those few years *something must be done,* that thought controls all my plans about my work. You will now better understand my desire to push on. At the same time, I have a firm resolve to use simple means. And perhaps you will also understand that I do not regard my studies as things apart, but always have in view my work as a whole.

[1] " so much the better "

Dear brother,   [The Hague, mid August 1883]
    I wish you were able to see that in several things I must be
consistent.
    You know what an error in one's point of view represents
in painting, viz. something far different and far worse than a
faulty drawing of such or such a detail. A single point
decides the greater or lesser gradient: the development more
to the right or left of the sideplanes of the objects throughout the whole composition.
    Well, in life there is something like this.
    When I say I am a poor painter and have still years of
struggle ahead—my everyday life I must arrange " à peu
près "[1] like a farm labourer or a factory hand does; then this
is a fixed point, from which many things result, which one
tears from their roots, when one considers them otherwise but
comprehensively. There are painters in other circumstances
who can and must act differently.
    Everyone must decide for himself. If I had had other
chances, had been in different circumstances, and if no decisive things had happened, of course that would have influenced my actions. Now however, and " à plus forte raison,"[2]
if there were even the slightest question of it being considered arrogance on my part to assume a right to which I had
no claim—even if I had this right as a matter of course—the
mere suggestion of the thing would have made me withdraw
of my own accord from any intercourse with people who
occupy a certain rank in life, even my own people.
    So this is the fact: My firm resolve is to be dead to any-
thing except my work. But it is very hard for me to speak
about those things, simple in themselves, but which unfortunately link up with much deeper things.
    There is no anguish greater than the soul's struggle be-
tween duty and love, both in their highest meaning. When I
tell you I choose my duty, you will understand everything.
    A simple word said about it during our walk,[3] made me

----

[1] " approximately "   [2] " a fortiori "
[3] Theo had come on his long-promised visit a few days before.

feel that absolutely nothing is changed in me in that respect, that it is and remains a wound which I carry with me, while it lies deep and cannot be healed. After years it will be the same as it was the first day.

I hope you understand what battle I have had to fight within myself of late.

The upshot was this : ' quoiqu'il en soit "[1] (not taking the *quoi* as interrogative, for I have not the right to consider it so) I will do my utmost to remain an honest man and doubly attentive to *duty*.

I have never suspected her,[2] nor do I now, nor shall I ever suspect her of having had financial motives, more than is honest and just. She went as far as was reasonable, other people exaggerated. But for the rest, you understand that I do not hold any delusive convictions about love for me, and what we talked of on the road remains between us. Since then, things have happened that would not have taken place, if at a certain moment I had not had to face in the first place a decided " no," and secondly a promise that I would not stand in her way. I respected in her a sense of duty—I never have suspected, shall never suspect her of anything mean.

Of myself I know this one thing, that it is of the greatest importance not to deviate from one's duty, and that one should not compromise with duty. Duty is absolute. The consequences? We are not responsible for them, but for the choice of *doing* or *not doing* our duty, we are responsible. This is the direct opposite of the principle : The end justifies the means.

And my own future is a cup that may not pass away from me except I drink it.[3]

So " Fiat voluntas."[4]

Good-bye—good luck on your journey—write soon—but you understand that I trust in the future with serenity, and without one line in my face revealing the struggle in the deepest depth—   Yours,

Vincent

[1] " be that as it may "   [2] Sien.
[3] See *Matthew* XXVI 42.   [4] " Thy will be done."

You will understand, however, that I must avoid everything which might tempt me to hesitate, so that I must avoid
everything and everybody that would remind me of *her*. In
fact that idea has made me this year sometimes more resolute
than I otherwise would have been, and you see that I can do it
in such a way that nobody understands the real motive.

Dear Theo,   [Drenthe, Holland, mid September 1883]
    Now that I have been here a few days, and have strolled
about in different directions, I can tell you more about the
neighbourhood where I have taken up my quarters. I enclose
a little scratch of my first painted study in these parts : a
cottage on the heath. A cottage made only of sods and sticks.
I saw also the interior of about six of that kind, and more
studies of them will follow.

    How the outside of them appears in the twilight, or just
after sunset, I cannot express more directly than by reminding
you of a certain picture by Jules Dupré, which I think belongs
to Mesdag, with two cottages, the moss-covered roofs of which
stand out very deep in tone against a hazy, dusky evening sky.

    So it is here. Inside those cottages, dark as a cave, it is
very beautiful. In drawings of certain English artists who
worked in Ireland on the moors I find shown most realistically what I observe here.

    Alb. Neuhuys gives the same effect, but a little more
poetically than the actual first impression on the eye, but he
never makes a thing that is not fundamentally true.

    I saw splendid figures out of doors—striking in terms of
their sobriety. A woman's breast, for instance, has that
heaving movement which is quite the opposite of voluptuous-
ness, and sometimes, when the creature is old or sickly,
arouses pity or respect. And the melancholy which things in
general have here is of a healthy kind, like in the drawings of
Millet. Fortunately the men here wear short breeches, which
show off the shape of the leg, and make the movements more
expressive.

    In order to give you an idea of one of the many things

which gave me new sensations and feelings on my excursions, I will tell you that one can see here peat barges in the *very middle of the heath*, drawn by men, women, children, white or black horses, just as in Holland, for instance, on the Rijswijk towpath.

The heath is splendid. I saw sheepfolds and shepherds more beautiful than those in Brabant.

The kilns are more or less like the one in Th. Rousseau's "Communal Oven." They stand in the gardens under old apple trees or between cabbages and celery. In many places there are beehives too. One can see on many faces that the people are not in good health; it is not exactly healthy here, I believe; perhaps because of foul drinking water. I have seen a few girls of seventeen, or younger still, perhaps, who look very brisk and beautiful, but generally they look faded very early on. But that does not interfere with the great noble aspect of the figures of some, who, seen from nearby, are already very faded.

In the village there are four or five canals to Meppel, to Dedemsvaart, to Coevorden, to Hollands Veld.

As one sails down them one sees here and there a curious old mill, farmyard, wharf, or lock, and always a bustle of peat barges.

To give you an idea of the character in these parts—while I was painting that cottage, two sheep and a goat came to browse *on the roof* of this house. The goat climbed on the top, and looked down the chimney. Hearing something on the roof, the woman rushed out, and threw her broom at the said goat, which jumped down like a chamois.

The two hamlets on the heath where I have been, and where this incident took place, are called Sanddrift and Blacksheep. I have been in several other places too, and now you can imagine the originality here, as after all Hoogeveen is a town, and yet quite nearby already there are shepherds, those kilns, those peat huts, etc.

I often think with melancholy of the woman and the children,[1] if only they were provided for; oh, it is the woman's

[1] Vincent had parted from Sien on moving to Drenthe.

own fault, one might say, and it would be true, but I am
afraid her misfortunes will prove greater than her offence.
That her character was spoilt I knew from the beginning, but
I hoped she would improve, and now that I do not see her
any more, and ponder over some things I saw in her, it seems
to me more and more that she was too far gone for improvement.

And that just makes my feeling of pity the greater, and it
becomes a melancholy feeling, but it is not in my power to
redress it.

Theo, when I meet on the heath such a poor woman with
a child on her arm, or at her breast, my eyes get moist. It
reminds me of her, her weakness; her untidiness, too, contributes to making the likeness stronger.

I know that she is not good, that I have a complete right
to act as I do, that I *could not* stay with her over there, that I
really could not take her with me, that what I did was even
sensible and wise, whatever you like; but, for all that, it
pierces right through me when I see such a poor little figure
feverish and miserable, and it makes my heart melt within
me. How much sadness there is in life, nevertheless one must
not become melancholy, and one must seek distraction in other
things, and the right thing is to work; but there are moments
when one only finds rest in the conviction : " misfortune will
not spare me either."

Adieu, write soon. Believe me,

Yours,
Vincent

Dear Theo,   [New Amsterdam, end of September 1883]
This once I write to you from the very remotest part of
Drenthe, where I came after an endless long voyage on a
barge through the moors. I see no chance of describing the
country as it ought to be done; words fail me for that, but
imagine the banks of the canal as miles and miles of Michels
or Th. Rousseaus, van Goyens or Ph. de Konincks.

Level planes or strips of different colour, getting narrower and narrower as they approach the horizon. Accentuated here and there by a peat shed or small farm, or a batch of meagre birches, poplars, oaks—heaps of peat everywhere, and one constantly goes past barges with peat or bulrushes from the marshes. Here and there lean cows, delicate in colouring, often sheep—pigs. The figures which now and then appear on the plain are generally of an impressive character; sometimes they have an exquisite charm. I drew, for instance, a woman in the barge with crape over the gold plates on her headdress, because she was in mourning, and afterwards a mother with a baby; the latter had a purple shawl over her head. There are a lot of Ostade types among them : physiognomies which remind one of pigs or crows, but now and then a little figure that is like a lily among thorns.

Well, I am very pleased with this excursion, for I am full of what I have seen. This evening the heath was inexpressibly beautiful. In one of the Boetzel Albums there is a Daubigny which exactly gives that effect. The sky was of an indescribably delicate lilac white, no fleecy clouds, for they were more compact and covered the entire sky, but dashes of more or less glaring lilac, grey, white, a single rent through which the blue gleamed. Then at the horizon a glimmering red streak, under which ran the very dark stretch of brown moor, and standing out against the brilliant red streak a number of low-roofed little huts. In the evening this moor often shows effects which the English call " weird " and " quaint." Don Quixote-like mills, or curious great hulks of drawbridges, stand out in fantastic silhouettes against the vibrating evening sky. Such a village in the evening, with reflections of lighted windows in the water, or in the mud puddles, looks sometimes very cosy.

Before I started out from Hoogeveen, I painted a few studies there, among others a large moss-roofed farm. For I had had paint sent from Furnée, as I thought on the subject like you wrote in your letter, that by absorbing myself in my work, and quite losing myself in it, my mood would change, and it has already greatly improved.

But at times—like those moments when you think of going

to America—I think of enlisting for the East Indies; but those are miserable, gloomy moments, when one is overwhelmed by things, and I could wish you might see those silent moors, which I see here from the window, for such a thing calms one down, and inspires one to more faith, resignation, steady work. In the barge I drew several studies, but I stayed a while here to paint some. I am quite near Zweeloo, where, among others, Liebermann has been; and besides, there is a part here where you still find large, very old turf huts, that have not even a partition between the stable and the living room. I intend first of all to visit that part one of these days.

But what tranquillity, what expanse, what calmness in this landscape; one feels it only when there are miles and miles of Michels between oneself and the ordinary world. I cannot give you a permanent address as yet, as I do not exactly know where I shall be for the next few days, but by 12th October *I shall be at Hoogeveen,* and if you send your letter at the usual time *to the same address,* I shall find it there, on the 12th, at Hoogeveen.

The place where I am now is New Amsterdam.

Father sent me a postal order for ten guilders, which, together with the money from you, makes me able to paint a little now.

I intend to settle for a long time at the inn where I am now, if I can easily reach from there that district with the large old turf huts, as I should have better light and more space there. As to that picture you mention, by that Englishman, with the lean cat and the small coffin, though he got his first inspiration in that dark room, he would hardly have been able to paint it in that same spot, for if one works in too dark a room, the work usually becomes too light, so that when one brings it out to the light, all the shadows are too weak. I just had that experience when I painted from the barn an open door and a glimpse into the little garden.

Well, what I wanted to say is that there will be a chance to remove that obstacle too, for here I can get a room with good light, that can be heated in winter. Well, lad, if you do not think any more about America, nor I of Harderwijk[1] I hope things will work themselves out.

I admit your explanation of C. M.'s[2] silence may be right, but sometimes one can be careless purposely. On the back of the page you will find a few scratches. I write in haste, it is already late.

How I wish we could walk here together, and paint together. I think the country would charm and convince you. Adieu, I hope you are well and are having some luck. During this excursion I have thought of you continually. With a handshake,

Yours,
Vincent

[EXTRACTS ONLY]

Dear brother,   [Drenthe, late October 1883]

My thoughts are always with you, no wonder that I write rather often.

Besides, my impressions have become more fixed, my thoughts are more collected, things adjust themselves, become more tangible. So I can write you about it in all calmness.[3] In the first place, I don't see much probability of your remaining on good terms with Goupil's. It is such an enormous business that it certainly will take a long time before one cannot put up with things any longer, before the corruption has penetrated *everywhere*. But, look here—in my opinion there has already been a very long period of corruption, so I would not be at all astonished if it were far advanced. . . .[4]

But after all, it is not exactly about the condition of the business—about the negative side of things—that I want to

[1] Place where Volunteers enlisted.
[2] His uncle C. M. van Gogh.
[3] Theo was considering leaving his business and becoming a painter himself.
[4] A paragraph is omitted here discussing other employees who had previously left Goupil's.

speak; leaving all that aside, it is about one single positive matter that I have something to say.

A few things have happened to you which I don't think unimportant. You have read in a different and better way than most people do the books of Zola—which I consider among the very best of the present time.

You once said to me " I am like that man in *Pot-Bouille* "; I said : " No. If you were like *that,* you would do well to enter a new business, but you are deeper than he, and I do not know whether you are in fact a man of business, actually deep down I see in you the artist, the true artist."

You have undergone mentally, unsought, deep harrowing emotions; now things are running their course. Why? Whither? To the renewed beginning of a similar career? My decided opinion is—no—there is something deeper than that. Change you must—but it must be a general renewal, not a repetition of the same thing. You were not wrong in the past, no, in the past you had to be as you were; that past was right. Does it follow from that that it was *not* simply a preparation, a basis, nothing but a schooling, and not the definite thing as yet? Why should not that follow? In my opinion it is just that.

I think things speak so much for themselves that it would be impossible for me to tell you anything that is not already quite evident, even to yourself. Besides, it strikes me as rather curious that there is a change in me too of late.

That just *now* I find myself in surroundings which so entirely engross me, which so order, fix, regulate, renew, enlarge my thoughts, that I am quite wrapped up in them. And that I can write you, full of what those silent, desolate moors tell me. Just at this moment, I feel within me the beginning of a change for the better. It isn't there yet, but I see in my work things—which I didn't have a little while ago. Painting comes easier to me. I am eager to try all kinds of things which I left undone till now. I know that circumstances happen to be so unsettled, that it is far from certain that I shall be able to remain here. Perhaps just because of your circumstances it might turn out differently. But

I should be sorry for it, though I would take it quite calmly.

But I cannot help imagining the future, with myself no longer alone, but you and I, painters, and working together as comrades, here in this moorland.

That idea presents itself to me in all its attractiveness. The thing ought to happen without the least fuss, without much disturbance like " une révolution qui est, puisqu'il faut qu'elle soit."[1] That's all—so I only say that I would not be in the least astonished if, after some time, we were *here* together. I feel that it *may* happen, without making any more disturbance than a piece of peat rolling from one place to another. One moment, and it lies perfectly still again, and nobody takes the least notice of it.

But a human being has his roots, transplantation is a painful thing, though the soil may be better in the place to which he is transplanted.

But is that soil better??? What the Puritans were of old, such are the painters in present-day society.

It is no foolish, artificial piety or bigotry; it is something simple and solid. I am speaking now more particularly of the Barbizon School,[2] and that tendency to paint rural life. I see in you, as a man, something that is irreconcilable with Paris. I do not know how many years of Paris have passed over it—yes, a part of your heart is rooted there—I admit it, but a something—a " je ne sais quoi "—is virgin still.

That's the artistic element. It appears to be weak now—but that new shoot bourgeons, and it will bourgeon quickly.

I am afraid the old trunk is split too much, and I say, bourgeon in a quite new direction, otherwise I am afraid the trunk will prove to lack the necessary vitality. It seems so to me—do you think differently?

The more so, because, *if* you became a painter, you would unintentionally have laid the foundation for it yourself, and for the first time, you would have company, friendship, a certain footing. I also think it would bring a change in my own

[1] " a revolution that exists, because it has to exist "
[2] Artists who had worked together in or near the forest of Fontainebleau earlier in the century.

work directly, for what I lack is companionship and encouragement in my work, a certain interchange of opinions with somebody who knows what a picture is. I have been so long quite without it that I think I need that stimulus.

I have so many plans that I hardly dare to undertake them alone—you would soon enough make out what they are, what they mean. Though I wish it were not so, I am extremely sensitive as to what is said of my work, as to what impression I make personally. If I meet with distrust, if I stand alone, I feel a certain void which cripples my initiative. Now, you would be just the person to understand it—I don't want the least flattery, or that people should say "I like it," if they did not; no, what I want is an intelligent sincerity, which is not vexed by failures. Which, if a thing fails six times, just when I begin to lose courage, would say: now you must try again a seventh time. You see, that's the encouragement I need, and cannot do without. And I think you would understand it, and you would be an enormous help to me.

And it is a thing you would be able to do, especially if you were obliged to do likewise. We should help each other, for I, for my part, would be the same to you, and that is of some importance. Two persons must believe in each other, and feel that it *can* be done and *must* be done, in that way they are enormously strong. They must keep up each other's courage. Well, I think you and I would understand each other.

I am not sure you could do it, if you were not a painter. The only obstacle is the doubt, which people generally try to raise: Tersteeg, for instance, who is naturally sceptical, who doesn't know what it is to believe.

Millet, however, is the type of a *believer*. He often used the expression "foi de charbonnier,"[1] and that expression was already a very old one. One must not be a City man, but a Country man, however civilized one may be. I cannot express it exactly. There must be a "je ne sais quoi" in a man, that keeps his mouth shut and makes him active—a certain aloofness even when he speaks—I repeat, an inward silence which leads

[1] "miner's faith"

to action. In that way one achieves great things, why?—because one has a certain feeling of come what may. One works—what next? I do not know——

I will not hurry you, I only want to say: don't thwart nature. What I wish is not foolish, but I have a faint hope that one might begin it in a reasonable way, not absolutely without money, but with only very little, just what is needed for board and lodging. And not wanting to cause an absolute calamity, but in case there is the smallest possibility, I say now:

"Follow that little point, that very slight possibility, there lies the road—follow it—drop all the rest. I do not mean drop all outward relations; you must keep them if you can, but stick to your conviction in saying: *I will become a painter;* so that what Tom, Dick and Harry say is like water on a duck's back."

I don't think you would then feel like a fish out of water, but that it would be like a coming home to your fatherland, that you would feel at once a great serenity—that you would feel surer about becoming a painter than about a new situation, more sure of yourself even than at Goupil's. . . .

[Two paragraphs are omitted here in which Vincent discusses Theo's nervous style and his new signs of trust in his brother.]

How things would go for me, should you *not* decide to become a painter, I cannot tell. If there were a place for me in Paris, I should have to take it, of course, and otherwise I should have to compromise with Father, so that I could live at home, and work in Brabant for a time. But oh, I can tell you that I do not think much about it now for the moment. I think only of my work, and about that plan for you. You are a man with a will, and a good, intelligent, clear head, with an honest heart. I think you may safely become a painter if you can hold out for a time. And I repeat, it would be a definite stimulus for my work.

To-day I have been walking behind the ploughers who were ploughing a potato field, with women trudging behind to pick up a few potatoes that were left.

This was quite a different field from the one I scratched yesterday for you, but it is a curious thing here—always exactly the same, and yet just enough variety, the same subjects like the pictures of artists who work in the same genre and yet are different. Oh, it is so curious here, and *so* quiet, *so* peaceful. I can find no other word for it but peace. Say much about it, say little about it, it is all the same, it does not matter at all. It is a question of wanting an entirely new thing, of undertaking a kind of renovation of yourself, in all simplicity with the fixed idea: ça ira.[1]

I don't mean to say that you will have no cares, things don't run so smoothly, but you must feel " I am doing what seems to me the simplest—I have done with all that is not simple; I don't want the city any longer, I want the country; I don't want an office, I want to paint." That's it. But it must be treated business fashion, though it is deeper, yes, infinitely deeper, but every thought must be fully concentrated on it.

In the future you must look on yourself and me as painters. There may be worries, there may be obstacles, yet *always consider us so—see your own work before you.* Look at a bit of nature and think: *I* will paint *that.* Give yourself up to the fixed idea: to become a painter.

All at once, people, even your best friends, become more or less like strangers. You are preoccupied by other things, exactly. All at once you feel, confound it, am I dreaming? I am on a wrong track, where is my studio, where is my brush? Thoughts like these are very deep; of course one says little or nothing about it, it would be a mistake to ask for advice about it, it wouldn't give you any light. . . .

Now art dealers have certain prejudices, which I think it possible that you have not shaken off yet, particularly the idea that painting is inborn—all right, inborn, but not as is supposed; one must put out one's hand and *grasp* it—that grasping is a difficult thing—one must not wait till it reveals itself. There is something, but not at all what people pretend. Practice makes perfect: by painting, one becomes a painter. If one wants to become a painter, if one delights in it, if one

[1] " It will work."

feels what you feel, one can do it, but it is accompanied by trouble, care, disappointment, periods of melancholy, of help-lessness and all that, that's what I think of it. I think it all such a nuisance that I just had to make a little scratch to forget it.[1] Forgive me, I won't say anything more about it, it is not worth while. . . .

To the world, we would have to show so much courage, so much energy, so much serenity, not taking things too ponder-ously, you know; in spite of serious cares, we would have to be merry, like those Swedes of whom you spoke, like the masters of Barbizon. We would have to take things literally, energetically, thoroughly, not doubting, dreaming or hesitat-ing. This is a plan I should like, for no other plan could I care so much. . . .[2]

It is a great risk, but neither you nor I are afraid to venture something. Just think it over, and, at all events, write soon. Good-bye, lad, with a handshake in thought,

Yours,
Vincent

Dear Theo,   [Nuenen, Holland, June/July 1884]
My hearty thanks for your letter, and the 200 francs en-closed. Thanks for giving the size of the frame, in which I intend to make a little spinner, after the large study.

I was glad to hear some good news about Breitner. The last impressions I had of him were, as you know, rather unfavourable, because of three large canvases which I saw at his studio, and in which I literally did not distinguish any-thing that might be located either in reality or in an imagin-ary world. But a few water-colours which he then had on hand, horses in the dunes, though very sketchy, were much better. And I saw things in it which make me understand quite well that the picture of which you speak must be good. As to the Society of Draughtsmen, firstly, I quite forgot it

---

[1] Here Vincent did a quick sketch on the page.
[2] Several paragraphs are omitted here, which recapitulate the general subject matter of the letter.

because I was busy painting those figures; secondly, now that
your letter reminds me of it, I am not very keen on it, for, as
I told you already last summer, I can only expect a refusal of
my petition for membership, which refusal one can, however,
consider as a kind of necessary evil that can be redressed next
year, and as such the request perhaps has its *raison d'être*.

Besides, as I quite forgot it, I have not one water-colour
on hand, and should have to start new ones in a hurry, if it
were not already too late for this year.

And when I tell you that I am just now quite absorbed
again in two new large studies of interiors of weavers, you
will understand I am in no mood for it. Especially as it might
cause new disagreements if I applied again to the gentlemen
at The Hague.

As to these two treatments of weavers, one shows a part of
the loom, with the figure and a small window.

The other is an interior, with three small windows, looking
out on the yellowish verdure, contrasting with the blue of
the cloth that is being woven on the loom, and the blouse of
the weaver, which is again of another blue.

But what struck me most in nature of late I have not
started on yet, for want of a good model. The half-ripe
cornfields are at present of a dark golden tone, ruddy or gold
bronze. This is raised to a maximum of effect by opposition
to the broken cobalt tone of the sky.

Imagine in such a background women's figures, very rough,
very energetic, with sun-bronzed faces and arms and feet,
with dusty, coarse indigo clothes and a black bonnet in the
form of a barret on their short-cut hair; while on the way
to their work they pass between the corn along a dusty path of
ruddy violet, with some green weeds, carrying hoes on their
shoulders, or a loaf of black bread under the arm—a pitcher
or brass coffee kettle. I have seen that same subject repeatedly
of late, with all kinds of variations. And I assure you that it
was really impressive.

Very rich, and at the same time very sober, delicately artistic.
And I am quite absorbed in it.

But my colour bill has run up so high that I must be wary

of starting new things in a big size, the more so because it will cost me much in models; if I could only get suitable models, just of the type I want (rough, flat faces with low foreheads and thick lips, not sharp, but full and Millet-like) and with those very same clothes.

For it demands great exactness, and one is not at liberty to deviate from the colours of the costume, as the effect lies in the analogy of the broken indigo tone with the broken cobalt tone, intensified by the secret elements of orange in the reddish bronze of the corn.

It would be a thing that gave a good impression of summer. I think summer is not easy to express; generally, at least often, a summer effect is either impossible or ugly, at least I think so, but then, as opposition, there is the twilight.

But I mean to say that it is not easy to find a summer sun effect which is as rich and as simple, and as pleasant to look at as the characteristic effects of the other seasons.

Spring is tender, green young corn and pink apple blossoms.

Autumn is the contrast of the yellow leaves against violet tones.

Winter is the snow with black silhouettes.

But now, if summer is the opposition of blues against an element of orange, in the gold bronze of the corn, one could paint a picture which expressed the mood of the seasons in each of the contrasts of the complementary colours (red and green, blue and orange, yellow and violet, white and black).[1]

Well, I am longing to hear about your journey to London, etc.

Mother is making but little progress in walking. Goodbye, and once more thanks for your letter and the enclosed. Believe me,

Yours,
Vincent

The best thing I know—for the frame—is to take a few stretchers of that size, then we can see which turns out best.

[1] Vincent had been studying at this date the account of Delacroix's colour-theory by Charles Blanc.

Dear Theo,   [Nuenen, September 1884]

I could not phrase my last letter differently than I did.[1]
But I want you to know that it always strikes me as being a
difference between you and me imposed by fate, rather than
one for which we ourselves are to blame.

You tell me that within a short time there will be an
exhibition of the work of Delacroix. All right. You will certainly see there a picture " La Barricade," which I know only
from biographies of Delacroix. I believe it was painted in
1848.[2] You also know a lithograph by De Lemud, I believe;
if it is not by him, then by Daumier, also representing the
barricade of 1848. I wish you could just imagine that you and
I had lived in that year 1848, or some such period, for at the
time of the *coup d'état* by Napoleon there was again something of the kind. I will not make any insinuations—that has
never been my object—I try to make it clear to you to what
degree the difference that has sprung up between us is connected with the general drift of society, and, as such, is something quite different from premeditated reproaches. So take
that period of 1848.

Who were opposed to each other then, that can be taken as
types of all the rest? Guizot, minister of Louis Philippe, on
one side, Michelet and Quinet with the students on the other.

I begin with Guizot and Louis Philippe, were they bad or
tyrannical? Not exactly; in my opinion, they were people,
like for instance Father and Grandfather, like old Goupil.
In short, people with a very venerable appearance, deep—
serious—but if one looks at them a little more closely and
sharply, they have something gloomy, dull, stale, so much that
it makes one sick. Is this saying too much???

Except for a difference of position, they have the same mind,
the same character. Am I mistaken in this?

[1] Vincent had written Theo a very sharp and recalcitrant letter, in
reply to what he took for reproaches from his brother about his
involvement with Margot Begemann.

[2] The reference is to Delacroix's *Liberty at the Barricades,* which
in fact commemorated the rising of July 28th, 1830 and was shown
at the Salon of 1831.

Now Quinet or Michelet, for instance, or Victor Hugo (later), was the difference between them and their opponents very great? Yes, but seen superficially one would not have said so. I myself have formerly admired at one and the same time a book by Guizot and a book by Michelet. But in my case, as I got deeper into it, I found difference and *contrast,* which is stronger still.

In short, that the one comes to a dead end and disappears vaguely, and the other, on the contrary, has something infinite. Since then much has happened. But my opinion is, if you and I had lived *then,* you would have been on the Guizot side, and I on the side of Michelet. And both of us remaining set in our outlooks, with a certain melancholy, we might have stood as direct enemies opposite each other, for instance on such a barricade, you before it as a soldier of the government, I behind it, as revolutionist or rebel.

Now, in 1884, *the digits happen to be the same only just reversed,* we are standing *again* opposite each other, though there are no barricades now. But minds that cannot agree are certainly still to be found.

" Le moulin n'y est plus, mais le vent y est encore."[1]

And in my opinion we are in different camps opposite each other, that cannot be helped. And whether we like it or not, *you* must go on, *I* must go on. But as we are brothers, let us avoid killing each other for instance (in the figurative sense). But we cannot help each other as much as two people who are standing side by side in the same camp. No, if we come in each other's vicinity, we would be within each other's range. *My* sneers are bullets, not aimed at you who are my brother, but in general at the party to which you once and for all belong. Neither do I consider *your* sneers expressly aimed at me, but *you fire* at the barricade and think to gain merit by it, and I happen to be there.

Think this over if you like, for I do not believe you can say much against it; I can only say that I believe things are so. . . .

I hope you will understand that I am speaking figuratively.

[1] " The mill has gone, but the wind remains."

Neither you nor I meddle with politics, but we live in the world, in society, and involuntarily ranks of people group themselves. Can the clouds help whether they belong to one thunder shower or to another? whether they carry positive or negative electricity? now it is also true that men are no clouds. As an individual, one is a part of all humanity. That humanity is divided into parties. How far is it one's own free will, how far is it the fatality of circumstances, that makes one belong to one party or to its opposite?

Well, then it was "'48, now it is '84," "le moulin n'y est plus, mais le vent y est encore." But try to know for yourself where you really belong, as I try to know that for myself. Good-bye,

Vincent[1]

Dear Theo,   [Nuenen, mid December 1884]

I am working very hard on the series of heads from the people, which I have set myself to make. I just enclose a little scratch of the last one; in the evening I generally scratch them from memory on a little scrap of paper, this is one of them.

Perhaps I will make them later on in water-colour too. But first I must paint them. Now just listen—do you remember how in the very beginning I always spoke to you about my great respect and sympathy for the work of Father de Groux ? Of late I think of him *more than ever*. One must not confront him only in his historical pictures, though these are also very good, nor in the first instance in a few pictures with the sentiment of, for instance, the author Conscience. But one must see his " Grace before Meat," " The Pilgrimage," " The Paupers' Bench " and above all, the simple Brabant types. De Groux is appreciated as little as, for instance, Thijs Maris. He is different though, but this they have in common, that they met with violent opposition.

In these days—whether the public is wiser now I can't tell,

[1] A postscript criticising Theo's tactics as a dealer is omitted here.

but this much I know, that it is not at all superfluous to weigh seriously one's thoughts and one's actions.

And at this very moment I could tell you some new names of people that hammer again on the same old anvil on which de Groux hammered. If it had pleased de Groux at that time to dress his Brabant characters in mediæval costumes, he would have run parallel with Leys in genius, and also in fortune.

However, he did not do so, and *now,* years afterwards, there is a considerable reaction against that mediævalism, though Leys always remains Leys and Thijs Maris, Thijs Maris, and Victor Hugo's Notre Dame, Notre Dame.

But the realism *not wanted* then is *in demand* now, and there is more need of it than ever.

The realism that has character and a serious sentiment.

I can tell you that for my part I will try to keep a straight course, and will paint the most simple, the most common things.

For pity's sake, how is it possible that you do not seem able or willing to understand that by having fixed my studio here, and by keeping it here for the present, I have made it possible to have money enough for painting, and if I had done otherwise it would have been a failure for myself as well as for others. If I had not done so I would have had to drudge at least three years more, before I had definitely overcome the difficulties of colour and tone, just because of the expenses. It is now just a year ago since I came here, driven by necessity. It is certainly not for my *pleasure* that I live here at home, but for my painting, and this being so I think it a great mistake of yours if you were to rob me of an opportunity, if I had to leave here *now,* before I had found something else. For my painting I must stay here somewhat longer still, then as soon as I have made more definite progress, I am willing to go anywhere where I shall earn the same money that I have here.

To be put back is not what I need or deserve, nor do I feel the least inclination for it, you see.

And attempt to get rid of you, that I never did, but where you showed me too clearly how little chance there was of our doing real business together, I do accept it for the future, that is true.

Recognize this once and for all, when I ask you for money, I do not ask it for *nothing*; the work which I carry out with it is at your disposal, and if *now* I am in arrears, I am on the right road even to achieving some leeway.

I write this once more, for the same reason as I did the earlier letters; I shall be quite at bay at the end of the month, for I have only enough for two or three days to pay my model.

And I am wretched that I shall again be handicapped for ten or twelve days this month.

And most seriously I repeat, can you not find a way to help me to 20 francs, for instance, to cover those last days? What I mind most, is the time I should otherwise forfeit. Goodbye.

Yours,

Vincent

Dear Theo,   [Nuenen, late January 1885]
You would greatly oblige me by trying to get for me:
Illustration No. 2174, 24th October 1884.

It is already an old number, but at the office you will probably be able to get it. In it there is a drawing by Paul Renouard, a strike of the weavers at Lyons. Also one from a series of Opera sketches (of which he has also published etchings)—called " The Harpist," which I like very much.

Then he has also done just recently, " The World of the Lawcourts," which I got from Rappard, you know it probably from the " Paris Illustré " by Damas.

But I think the drawing of the weavers the most beautiful of all, there is so much life and depth in it that I think this drawing might hold its own beside Millet, Daumier, Lepage.

When I think how he rose to such a height by working from the very beginning from nature, without imitating others, and how he is none the less in harmony with the very clever people, even in technique, though from the very first he had his own style, I find him again a proof that by truly following nature one's work improves every year.

And I am daily more convinced that people who do not in the first place wrestle with nature *never* succeed.

I think that if one has tried to follow attentively the great masters, one finds them all back at certain moments, deep in reality—I mean that their so-called *creations* will be seen by one in reality, if one has the same eyes, the same sentiment as they had. And I do believe that if the critics and connoisseurs were better acquainted with nature their judgment would be more correct than now, when it is the routine to live only among pictures, and to compare them mutually. Which of course, as one side of the question, is good in itself, but it lacks a solid basis if one begins to forget nature and looks only superficially. Can't you understand that I am perhaps not wrong in this, and to say more clearly still what I mean, is it not a pity that you, for instance, seldom or hardly ever enter those cottages, or associate with those people, or see that sentiment in landscape, which is painted in the pictures you like best. I do not say that you *can* do this in your position, just because one must look much and long at nature before one comes to the conviction that the most touching things the great masters have painted still find their origin in life and reality itself. A basis of sound poetry, which exists eternally as a fact, and can be found if one digs and seeks deeply enough.

" Ce qui ne passe pas dans ce qui passe,"[1] it exists.

And what Michelangelo said in a splendid metaphor, I think Millet has said without metaphor, and Millet can perhaps best teach us to see, and get " a faith." If I do better work later on, I certainly shall not work *differently* than now, I mean it will be the same apple, though riper; I shall not change my mind about what I have thought from the beginning. And that is the reason why I say for my part : if I am no good now, I shall be no good later on either, but if later on, then now too. For corn is corn, though people from the city may take it for grass at first, and also the other way round.

In any case, whether people approve or do not approve of what I do and how I do it, I for my part know no other way

[1] " The durable within the transitory "

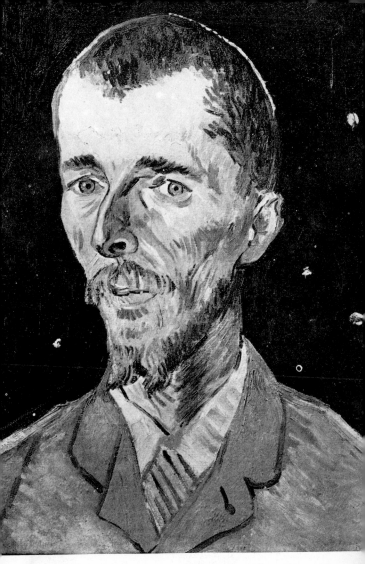

Portrait of an Artist Friend, oil, Arles, September 1888
(pp. 277-8, 285)

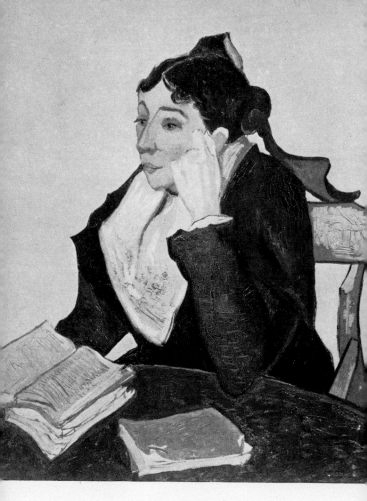

The Arlésienne, portrait of Mme. Ginoux, oil, Arles, November 1888
(pp. 298, 309)

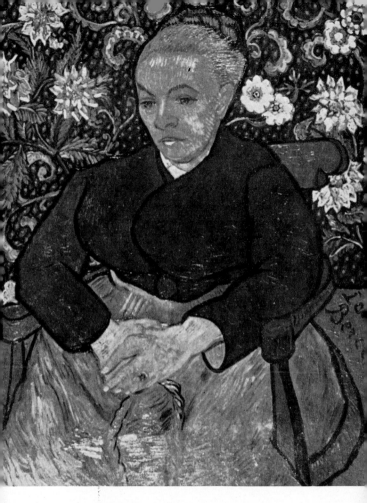

Woman Rocking a Cradle, oil, Arles, December 1888/January 1889
(p. 306)

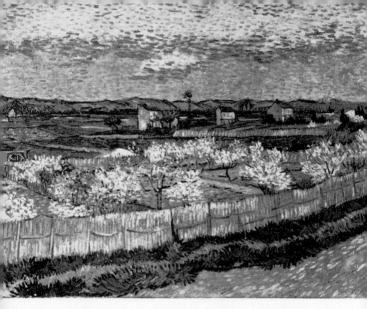

View of an Orchard with Peach Trees (Le Crau), oil, Arles, April 1889 (p. 3

Cypresses and Stars, drawing, St.-Rémy, June 1889 (pp. 265, 319)

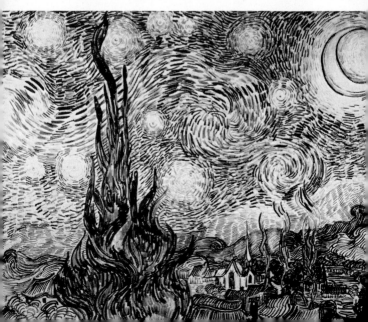

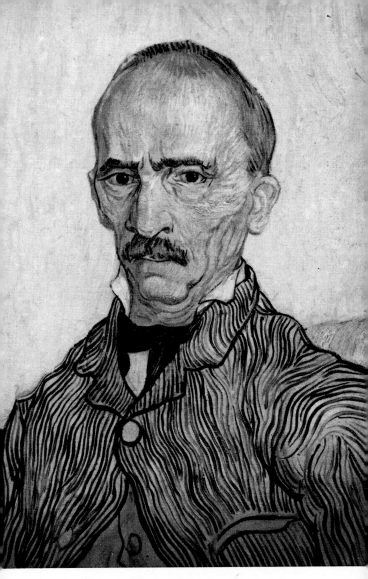

Portrait of the Head Warder at the Saint-Rémy Asylum, oil,
St.-Rémy, September 1889.
(p. 323)

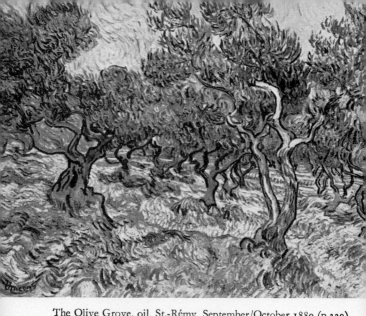

The Olive Grove, oil, St.-Rémy, September/October 1889 (p.329)

Girl with Coffee-Tinted Skin, oil, Arles, August 1888 (p. 283)

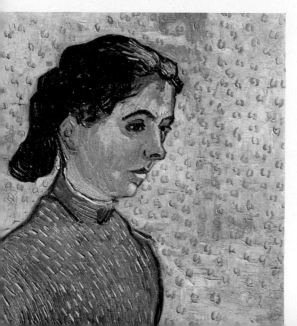

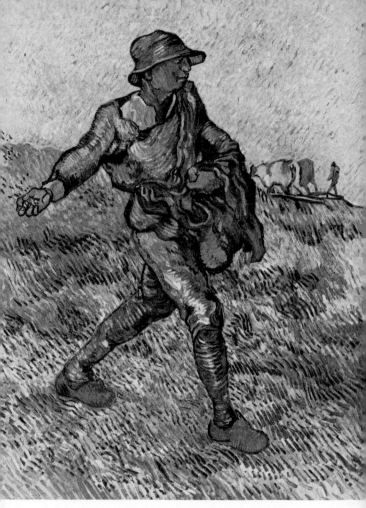

The Sower, after Millet, oil, St.-Rémy, February 1890
(p. 334)

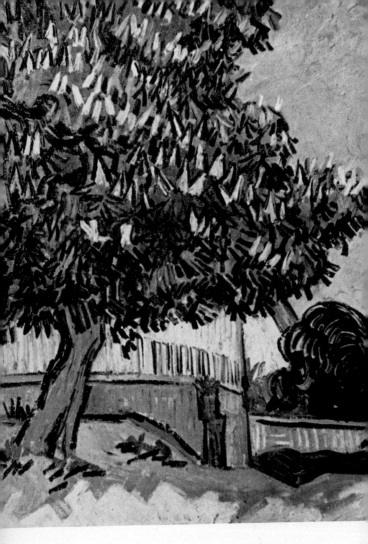

White Chestnuts, oil, Auvers, May, 1890
(p. 337)

than to wrestle so long with nature that she tells me her secret.

All the time I am working at various heads and hands.

I have also drawn some again, perhaps you would find something in them, perhaps not, I can't help it. I repeat, I know no other way.

But I can't understand that you say: perhaps later on we shall admire even the things done now.

If I were you, I should have so much self-confidence and independent opinion that I should know whether I could see *now* what there was or was not in a thing.

Well, you must know those things for yourself.

Though the month is not quite over, my purse is quite empty. I work on as hard as I can, and I for my part think that by constantly studying the model, I shall keep a straight course.

I wish you could send me the money a few days before the 1st for that same reason, that the ends of the month are always hard, because the work brings such heavy expenses, and I don't sell any of it. But this will not go on so for ever, for I work too hard and too much not to arrive eventually at the point of being able to defray my expenses, without being in a dependent position. For the rest, nature outside and the interiors of the cottages, they are splendid in their tone and sentiment just at present; I try hard not to lose time.

Goodbye,

Yours,
Vincent

Dear Theo,   [Nuenen, April 1885]

By the same mail you will receive a number of copies of the lithograph. Please give Mr. Portier as many as he wants. And I enclose a letter for him, which I am afraid you will think rather long, and in consequence unpractical. But I thought that what I had to say couldn't be expressed in more concise terms, and that the chief point is to give him arguments for his own instinctive feelings. And in fact what I write to him I say also to you.

There is a school—I believe—of impressionists. But I know very little about it. But I do know who are the original and most important masters, around whom—as round an axis—the landscape and peasant painters will turn. Delacroix, Corot, Millet and the rest. That is my own opinion, not formulated as it should be.

I mean there are (rather than persons) rules or principles or fundamental truths for *drawing,* as well as for *colour,* upon which *one proves to fall back* when one finds out an actual truth.

In drawing, for instance—that question of drawing the figure beginning with the circle—that is to say taking as one's basis the elliptical planes. A thing which the ancient Greeks already knew, and which will continue to apply till the end of the world. As to colour, those everlasting problems, for instance, that first question Corot addressed to Français, when Français (who already had a reputation) asked Corot (who then had nothing but a negative or rather bad reputation) when he (F.) came to Corot, to get some information: " Qu'est-ce que c'est un ton rompu? Qu'est-ce que c'est un ton neutre?"[1]

Which can be better shown on the palette than expressed in words.

So what I want to tell Portier in this letter is my confirmed belief in Eugène Delacroix and the people of that time.

And at the same time, as the picture which I have in hand is different from lamplights by Dou or Van Schendel, it is perhaps not superfluous to point out how one of the most beautiful things done by the painters of this country has been the painting of *black,* which nevertheless has *light* in it. Well, just read my letter and you will see that it is not unintelligible, and that it treats a subject that just occurred to me while painting.

I hope to have some luck with that picture of the potato-eaters.

[1] "What is a broken tone? What is a neutral tone?"

I also have on hand a red sunset.

In order to paint rural life one must be master of so many things. But on the other hand I don't know anything at which one works with so much calm, in the sense of serenity, however much of a worry one may be having as regards material things.

I am rather worried just now about the moving, that's no easy job, on the contrary. But it had to happen some time, if not now, then later, and in the long run it is better to have a place of one's own, that's a fact.

To change the subject. How typical that saying is about the figures of Millet : *"Son paysan semble peint avec la terre qu'il ensemence!"*[1] How exact and how true. And how important it is to know how to mix on the palette those colours which have no name, and yet are the real foundation of everything. Perhaps, I daresay *for sure,* the questions of *colour,* and more exactly broken and neutral colours, will preoccupy you anew. Art dealers speak so vaguely and arbitrarily about it, I think. So in fact do painters too. Last week I saw at an acquaintance's a decidedly clever, realistic study of an old woman's head, by somebody who is directly, or indirectly, a pupil of the school of The Hague. But in the drawing, as well as in the colour, there was a certain hesitation, a certain narrow-mindedness, much greater, in my opinion, than one sees in an old Blommers or Mauve or Maris. And this symptom threatens to become more and more general. If one takes realism in the sense of *literal* truth, namely *exact* drawing and local colour. There are other things than that. Well, goodbye, with a handshake,

Yours,

Vincent

Dear Theo,   [Nuenen, June 1885]

Thanks for your letter and the enclosure. It was just what

[1] " His peasant appears to be painted with the earth that he is sowing."

I wanted and helped me to work as hard at the end of the month as I did in the beginning.

I am very glad to hear that Serret is a painter, about whom you had already written things which I perfectly well remember, but the name had escaped me. I should like to write to you much more than I shall do in this letter, but of late when I come home, I don't feel like writing, after sitting in the sun all day. As to what Serret says, I quite agree with him—I shall just send him a line, because I should like to become friends with him. As I told you already, I have been busy drawing figures recently; I will send them especially for the sake of Serret, to show him that I am far from indifferent to the unity and the form of a figure.

Do you ever see Wallis, is that water-colour of the auction perhaps something for him; if it were something for Wisselingh,[1] then *he* would certainly be the right one to take it. To Wisselingh I once gave a few heads and recently I have sent him that lithograph. But as he did not answer with a single word, I think if I sent him something more, I should get nothing but an insult.

It has just happened to me that Van Rappard,[2] with whom I have been friends for years, after keeping silent for about three months, writes me a letter, so haughty and so full of insults and so clearly written after he had been in The Hague, that I am almost sure I have lost him for ever as a friend.

Just because I tried it first at The Hague, that is in my own country, I have full right and cause to forget all those worries and to attempt something else outside my own country.

You know Wallis well, perhaps you can broach the subject à propos of that water-colour, but act according to your discretion. If I could earn something with my work, if we had some firm ground, be it ever so little, under our feet for our daily existence, and if then the desire to become an artist took

[1] Wallis and Wisselingh were art-dealers on friendly terms with the two brothers.
[2] Vincent had been corresponding with this artist since 1881, but just recently a radical fissure had developed between them.

or you the form of, let me say, Hennebeau in *Germinal*,[1] discounting all difference in age, etc.—what pictures you could still make then! The future is always different from what one expects, so one never can be sure. The drawback of painting is that, if one does not sell one's pictures, one still needs money for paint and models in order to make progress. And that drawback is a bad thing. But for the rest, painting and, in my opinion, especially the painting of rural life, gives serenity, though one may have all kinds of worries and miseries on the surface of life. I mean painting is a *home* and one does not experience that homesickness, that peculiar feeling Hennebeau had. That passage I copied for you lately had struck me particularly, because at the time I had almost literally the same longing to be something like a grassmower or a navvy.

And I was sick of the *boredom* of civilization. It *is* better, one *is* happier if one carries it out—literally though—one feels at least that one is really alive. And it is a good thing in winter to be deep in the snow, in the autumn deep in the yellow leaves, in summer among the ripe corn, in spring amid the grass; it is a good thing to be always with the mowers and the peasant girls, in summer with a big sky overhead, in winter by the fireside, and to feel that it always has been and always will be so.

One may sleep on straw, eat black bread, well, one will only be the healthier for it.

I should like to write more, but I repeat, I am not in a mood for writing, and I wanted to enclose a note for Serret besides, which you must read also, because I write in it about what I want to send before long, especially because I want to show Serret my complete figure studies. Goodbye,

Yours,

Vincent

Serret may agree with you that to paint good pictures and to sell them are two separate things. But it is not at all true. When at last the public saw Millet, all his work together, then the public both in Paris and in London was enthusiastic.

[1] A famous novel by Zola.

And who were the persons that had suppressed and refused Millet? The art dealers, the so-called *experts*.

Dear Theo,   [Nuenen, July 1885]

I wish the four pictures[1] of which I wrote were gone.

If I keep them here long, I might paint them over again and I think it would be better if you got them just as they come from the heath.

The reason why I do not send them is that I don't want to send them unfranchised at a moment in which you yourself are pinched perhaps, and yet I cannot pay the charge myself.

The little house in which Millet lived, I have never seen it, but I imagine that those four little human nests are of the same kind.

One is the residence of a gentleman, who is known under the name of the " mourning peasant "; the other is inhabited by a " good woman " who, when I came there, did no more mysterious thing than dig her potato pit, but she must also be able to do witchcraft, at any rate she bears the name of " the witch-head."

You remember in the book by Gigoux how it happened to Delacroix that 17 pictures of his were refused at the same time. One sees from this—at least I think so—that he and others of that period—placed before connoisseurs and non-connoisseurs, who none of them either understood or would buy—one sees from this, that those who in the book are rightly called " the valiant," did not call it fighting against hopeless odds, but went on painting. What I wanted to tell you once more, is that if we take that story about Delacroix as a starting-point, we must still paint a lot.

I am compelled into being the most disagreeable of all persons, namely I have to ask for money. And as I do not think things will all at once take a turn for the better in terms of selling, this is bad enough. But I ask you, is it not better after all for both of us to work hard, though it will bring difficulties, than to sit and philosophize at a time like that?

[1] A series depicting peasant huts.

I do not know the future, Theo, but I do know the eternal law that everything changes; go back ten years, and things were different, the conditions, the temperament of the people, well, everything. And ten years hence, things will have shifted again, I am sure.

But the thing one does remains, and one does not easily repent having done a thing. The more activity the better, and I would rather have a failure than sit and do nothing.

Whether Portier may or may not be the man who can do something with my work, we want him now at any rate. And this is what I believe. After having worked for a year or so, we shall have a larger collection than now, and I know for sure that my work will show the better, the more I complete it. People who now have some sympathy for it, who speak of it as he does and show it, they are useful because after my having worked, for instance, another year, they will have collected a few things that will speak for themselves, even if they were totally silent about them. If you happen to see Portier, tell him that, far from giving it up, I intend to send him much more. You must also continue to show the things if you meet likely people.

It won't be so very long before the things we can show will become more important. You will notice yourself, and it is a fact which pleases me enormously, that more and more they begin to arrange exhibitions of one person, or of a very few who belong together.

This is a development in the world of art which I am sure contains more promise for the future than any other undertaking. It is a good thing they begin to understand that a Bougereau does not show off well next to a Jacque, a figure of Beyle or Lhermitte does not do beside a Schelfhout or Koekkoek. Disperse the drawings of Raffaëlli and judge for yourself whether it would be possible to get a good idea of that original artist.

He—Raffaëlli—is different from Régamey, but I think him as impressive a personality.

If I kept my work here, I think I would go on repainting it.

When I send it to you and to Portier just as it comes from the open air or from the cottages, there will now and then be one among them which is no good, but things will be kept together which would not improve if they were often repainted.

Now if you have these four canvases and a few smaller studies of cottages besides, and somebody saw no other work of mine but these, he would of course think that I painted nothing but cottages. And it would be the same for the series of heads. But rural life includes so many different things that when Millet speaks of " travailler comme *plusieurs* nègres "[1] this really must be the case, if one wants to complete the thing.

One may laugh at Courbet's saying " peindre des anges, qui est-ce qui a vu des anges?"[2] but I should like to add, for instance : " des justices au harem, qui est-ce qui a vu des justices au harem?[3] Des combats de taureaux, qui est-ce qui en a vu?" and so many other Moorish, Spanish things, Cardinals, and then all those historical paintings, which they keep on painting and painting, yard after yard. What is the use of it and why do they do it? After a few years it generally gets musty and dull, and becomes more and more uninteresting.

Well! Perhaps they are well painted, they may be; nowadays when critics stand before a picture, like that of Benjamin Constant, like a reception at the Cardinal's by I don't know what Spaniard, it is the custom to speak with a philosophical air about " clever technique." But as soon as those very same critics would come before a picture of rural life, or before a drawing by, for instance, Raffaëlli, they would criticize the technique with the selfsame air.

You think perhaps I am wrong to criticize this, but it strikes me that all those outlandish pictures are painted *in the studio.*

But just go and paint out of doors on the spot itself! then

---

[1] " working like a team of negroes "

[2] " Paint angels, who has ever seen them?"

[3] " Courts of justice in a harem, who has ever seen them? Bull fights, who has ever seen them?" The reference in the first half of this comment is to a painting by Benjamin Constant.

all kinds of things happen; for instance, from the four
paintings which you will receive I had to wipe off at least a
hundred or more flies, not counting the dust and sand, not
counting that when one carries them for some hours across
the heath and through the hedges, some thorns will scratch
them, etc. Not counting that when one arrives on the heath
after some hours' walk in this weather, one is tired and
exhausted from the heat. Not counting that the figures do not
stand still like the professional models, and that the effects
one wants to catch change as the day wears on.

I don't know how it is with you, but as for myself, the
more I work in it, the more I get absorbed with rural life.
And I begin to care less and less either for those Cabanel-like
things among which I count Jacquet also, and Benjamin
Constant as he is to-day, or the so highly praised, but so
inexpressibly dry technique of the Italians and Spaniards.
Imagiers![1] that term of Jacque's is one I often think of. Yet
I have no *parti pris,* I feel for Raffaëlli who paints quite other
things than peasants, I feel for Alfred Stevens, for Tissot, to
name something quite different from peasants; I feel for a
beautiful portrait.

Zola, though in my opinion he makes colossal blunders in
his judgment about pictures, says in " Mes Haines " a beautiful thing about art in general : " dans le tableau (l'œuvre
d'art) je cherche, j'aime l'homme—l'artiste."[2]

Look here, I think this perfectly true; I ask you what kind
of a man, what kind of a prophet, or philosopher, observer,
what kind of a human character is there behind certain paintings, the technique of which is praised; in fact, often *nothing.*
But a Raffaëlli is a personality, Lhermitte is a personality, and
before many pictures by almost unknown artists, one feels
they are made with a *will,* a *feeling,* a passion and love. The
technique of a painting from rural life or—like Raffaëlli—
from the heart of city workmen—brings quite other difficulties

[1] " Image-makers "
[2] " in pictures (works of art) I search after and I love the man—
the artist " (*Mes Haines* contained a collection of Zola's critical
writings.)

than those attached to the smooth painting and pose of a Jacquet or Benjamin Constant. It entails living in those cottages day by day, being in the fields like the peasants, in summer in the heat of the sun, in winter suffering from snow and frost, not indoors but outside, and not during a walk, but day after day like the peasants themselves.

And I ask you, if one considers these things, am I then so far wrong when I criticize the criticism of those critics who these days more than ever talk humbug about this so *often* misused word : technique (it is getting a more and more conventional significance). Considering all the trouble and drudgery needed to paint the " rouwboerke "[1] and his cottage, I dare maintain that this is a longer and more fatiguing journey than many painters of exotic subjects (maybe " Justice in the Harem," or a reception at a Cardinal's) make for their most rarefied eccentric subjects. For in Paris any kind of Arabic or Spanish or Moorish models are to be had if one only pays for them. But he who paints the rag-pickers of Paris in their *own quarter,* like Raffaëlli, has far more difficulties and his work is more serious.

Apparently nothing is more simple than to paint peasants, rag-pickers and labourers of all kinds, but—no subjects in painting are so difficult as these everyday figures!

As far as I know there is not a single academy where one learns to draw and paint a digger, a sower, a woman setting the kettle over the fire, or a seamstress. But in every city of some importance there is an academy with a choice of models for historical, Arabic, Louis XV, in one word *all really non-existent figures.*

When I send to you and Serret some studies of diggers or peasant women who weed, glean, etc., *as the beginning* of a whole series of all kinds of work in the fields, then it may be that either you or Serret will discover faults in them, which will be useful for me to know, and which I shall perhaps admit myself.

But I want to point out something which is perhaps worth while. All academic figures are constructed in the same way

[1] " peasant in mourning "

and let us say *on ne peut mieux*.[1] Irreproachably *faultless*.
You will guess what I am driving at, they do not reveal to us
anything new.

This does not apply to the figures of a Millet, a Lhermitte,
a Régamey, a Daumier; they too are well constructed, but
after all in a different way than the academy teaches.

But I think however correctly academic a figure may be, it
will be superfluous these days, even though it were by Ingres
himself (his " Source "[2] however excepted, because that really
was, and is, and will always remain something new), when it
lacks the essential modern note, the intimate character, the
real *action*.

Perhaps you will ask, when will a figure not be superfluous, though there may be faults, great faults in it in my
opinion?

When the digger digs, when the peasant is a peasant and
the peasant woman a peasant woman.

Is this something new?—yes—even the figures by Ostade,
Terborch[3] are not in action like those painted nowadays.

I should like to say a lot more about this, and I should
like to say how much I myself want to improve my work and
how much I prefer the work of some other artists to my own.

I ask you, do you know in the old Dutch school a single
digger, a single sower??? Did they ever try to paint " a
labourer "? Did Velasquez try it in his water-carrier or types
from the people? No.

The figures in the pictures of the old masters do not *work*.
I am drudging just now on the figure of a woman whom I
saw last winter pulling carrots in the snow.

Look here, Millet has done it, Lhermitte, and in general
the painters of rural life in this century—Israëls for instance
—they find it more attractive than anything else.

But *even* in this century, how relatively few among the in-

---

[1] " incapable of being improved upon "
[2] A famous painting showing a nude female figure fetching water.
[3] Seventeenth century artists of the Low Countries; in fact Terborch
was not one of the painters of " low-life " genre scenes, as Vincent
implies.

numerable painters want the figure—yes, above all—for the sake of the figure, that is to say for the sake of line and modelling, *but cannot imagine* it otherwise than in action, and want to do what the old masters avoided—even the old Dutch masters who clung to many conventional actions—and I repeat—who want *to paint the action for the sake of the action*.

So that the picture or the drawing has to be a drawing of the figure for the sake of the figure and the inexpressibly harmonious form of the human body, but at the same time a pulling of carrots in the snow. Do I express myself clearly? I hope so, and just tell this to Serret. I can say it in a few words : a nude by Cabanel, a lady by Jacquet and a peasant woman, *not by Bastien Lepage himself,* but a peasant woman by a Parisian who has learned drawing at the academy, will always indicate the limbs and the structure of the body in one selfsame way, sometimes charming—correct in proportion and anatomy. But when Israëls, or when Daumier or Lhermitte for instance draw a figure, the shape of the figure will be felt much more, and yet—that is the reason why I like to count in Daumier—the proportions will be sometimes almost *arbitrary,* the anatomy and structure often quite wrong " in the eyes of the academician." But it will *live.* And especially Delacroix too.

It is not yet well expressed. Tell Serret that *I should be desperate if my figures were correct,* tell him that I do not want them to be academically correct, tell him I mean that if one photographs a digger *he certainly would not be digging then.* Tell him that I adore the figures by Michelangelo though the legs are undoubtedly too long, the hips and the backsides too large. Tell him that, for me, Millet and Lhermitte are the real artists, for the very reason that they do not paint things as they are, traced in a dry analytical way, but as *they*—Millet, Lhermitte, Michelangelo—feel them. Tell him that my great longing is to learn to make those very incorrectnesses, those deviations, remodellings, changes of reality, so that they may become, yes, untruth if you like— but more true than the literal truth.

And now I shall have to finish, but I wanted to say once more that those who paint rural life or the life of the people, though they may not belong to the men of the moment, perhaps in the long run they will nonetheless hold out longer than the painters of the exotic harems and Cardinal's receptions, painted in Paris.

I know that it is being very disagreeable to ask for money at inconvenient moments; my excuse, however, is that painting the apparently most common things is sometimes the most difficult and the most expensive.

The expenses which I must afford if I want to work are sometimes very high in proportion to what I have at my disposal. I assure you, if my constitution had not become in all winds and weather like that of a peasant, I should not be able to stand it, as for my own comfort absolutely nothing is left over.

But I don't want comfort for myself, just as little as many peasants want to live differently than they do.

But the amount I ask is for colours, and especially for models.

From what I write about the drawings of the figure, you can perhaps sufficiently judge how passionately I want to carry them out.

You recently wrote to me that Serret had spoken to you " with conviction " about certain faults in the structure of the figures of the potato-eaters.[1]

But you will have seen from my answer that my own criticism also disapproves of them on that point, but I pointed out that this was an impression gained after having seen the cottage in the dim lamplight for many evenings, after having painted forty heads, so it is clear that I started from a different point of view.

But now that we begin to discuss figure drawing, I have a great deal more to say. In Raffaëlli's words I find his opinion about " character "—what he says about this is good,

---

[1] Vincent had painted this subject in April-May 1885, to create his most ambitious canvas to date.

and in its place and it is illustrated by the drawings themselves.

But people who move in artistic, literary circles, like Raffaëlli in Paris, have after all different ideas than mine, for instance, here in the heart of peasant life.

I mean they want one word to encompass all their ideas; he uses for the figures of the future the word " character." I agree with it, with the *meaning* I think, but in the correctness of the word I believe as little as in the correctness of other words; as little as in the correctness or cogency of my own expressions.

Rather than say there must be character in a digger, I circumscribe it by saying: that peasant *must* be a peasant, that digger *must* dig, and then there will be something essentially modern in them. But I feel myself that from these very words conclusions may be drawn that I do not endorse, and would be even if I were to go on a great deal further.

Instead of diminishing the expenses for models, now already so heavy for me, I would think it better, much better, to spend a little more on them, for what I aim at is quite a different thing than being able to do a little figure drawing. To draw *a peasant's figure in action,* I repeat, that's an essentially modern image, the very heart of modern art, something neither the Greeks nor the Renaissance nor the old Dutch school have done.

This is a question which occupies me daily. But this difference between the great as well as the little masters of to-day (the great ones, like, for instance, Millet, Lhermitte, Breton, Herkomer: the little ones such as Raffaëlli and Régamey) and the old masters, I have not often found it openly expressed in the articles about art.

Just think over whether you don't find this to be true. They started a peasant's and a labourer's figure as a " genre," but at present, with Millet the great master as leader, this is the very heart of modern art, and will remain so.

People like Daumier, we must respect them, for they are among the pioneers. The simple *nude* but *modern* figure, like Henner and Lefèvre have renewed it, ranks high.

Baudry and especially the sculptors, like, for instance, Mercier, Dalou, that too is serious work.

But peasants and labourers are after all not nude, and it is improper to imagine them nude. The more painters begin to paint labourers' and peasants' figures, the better I shall like it. And I myself know nothing I like so well. This is a long letter and I do not know whether I have expressed clearly enough what I mean. I shall perhaps write a little word to Serret, if I do so I shall send you the letter for you to read, for I should like to make it very clear how high I rate that question of figure drawing.

Dear Theo,   [Nuenen, late October 1885]

I read your letter about black with great pleasure, and it convinces me that you have no prejudice against black.

Your description of Manet's study, "The Dead Toreador," was well analysed. And the whole letter proves the same as your sketch of Paris suggested to me at the time, that if you put yourself to it, you can paint a thing in words.

It is a fact that by studying the laws of the colours, one can move from instinctive belief in the great masters to the analysis of why one admires—what one admires—and that indeed is necessary nowadays, when one realizes how terribly arbitrary and superficially people criticize.

You must just let me maintain my pessimism about the art trade as it is these days, for it does *not* at all include discouragement. This is my way of reasoning. Supposing I am right in considering that curious haggling about prices of pictures to be more and more like the bulb trade. I repeat, supposing that like the bulb trade at the end of the last century, so the art trade, along with other branches of speculation at the end of this century, will disappear as they came, namely rather quickly. The bulb trade may disappear—the *flower-growing* remains. And I for myself am contented, for better or for worse, to be a small gardener, who loves his plants.

Just now my palette is thawing and the frigidness of the first beginning has disappeared.

It is true, I often blunder still when I undertake a thing, but the colours follow of their own accord, and taking one colour as a starting-point, I have clearly before my mind what must follow, and how to get life into it.

Jules Dupré is in landscape rather like Delacroix, for what enormous variety of mood did he express in symphonies of colour.

Now a marine, with the most delicate blue-greens and broken blue and all kinds of pearly tones, then again an autumn landscape, with a foliage from deep wine-red to vivid green, from bright orange to dark havana, with other colours again in the sky, in greys, lilacs, blues, whites, forming a further contrast with the yellow leaves.

Then again a sunset in black, in violet, in fiery red.

Then again, more fantastic, what I once saw, a corner of a garden by him, which I have never forgotten : black in the shadow, white in the sun, vivid green, a fiery red and then again a dark blue, a bituminous greenish brown, and a light brown-yellow. Colours that indeed have something to say for themselves.

I have always been very fond of Jules Dupré, and he will become still more appreciated than he is. For he is a real colourist, always interesting, and so powerful and dramatic.

Yes, he is indeed a brother to Delacroix.

As I told you, I think your letter about black very good, and what you say about not painting local colour is also quite correct. But it doesn't satisfy me. In my opinion there is much more behind that not painting local colour.

" Les vrais peintres sont ceux qui ne font pas la couleur locale "[1]—that was what Blanc and Delacroix discussed once.

May I not boldly take it to mean that a painter does better to start from the colours on his palette than from the colours in nature? I mean, when one wants to paint, for instance, a head, and sharply observes the reality one has before one, then one may think : that head is a harmony of red-brown, violet,

[1] " The true painters are those who do not render local colour "

yellow, all of them broken—I will put a violet and a yellow
and a red-brown on my palette and these will break each other.

I retain from nature a certain sequence and a certain correctness in placing the tones, I study nature, so as not to do
foolish things, to remain reasonable—however, I don't mind
so much whether my colour corresponds exactly, as long as
it looks beautiful on my canvas, as beautiful as it looks in
nature.

Far more true is a portrait by Courbet, manly, free, painted
in all kinds of beautiful deep tones of red-brown, of gold, of
colder violet in the shadow with black as repoussoir, with a
little bit of tinted white linen as a repose to the eye—finer
than a portrait by whomever you like, who has imitated the
colour of the face with horribly close precision.

A man's head or a woman's head, well contemplated and at
leisure, is divinely beautiful, isn't it? Well, that *general harmony* of tones in nature, one loses it by painfully exact imitation, one keeps it by recreating in an equivalent colour range,
that may be not exactly or far from exactly like the model.

Always and intelligently to make use of the beautiful tones
which the colours form of their own accord, when one breaks
them on the palette, I repeat—to start from one's palette, from
one's knowledge of colour-harmony, is quite different from
following nature mechanically and obsequiously.

Here is another example : suppose I have to paint an
autumn landscape, trees with yellow leaves. All right—when
I conceive it as a symphony in yellow, what does it matter
whether the fundamental colour of yellow is the same as that
of the leaves or not? It matters *very little*.

Much, everything depends on my perception of the infinite
variety of tones of one and the *same family*.

Do you call this a dangerous inclination towards romanticism, an infidelity to " realism," a " peindre de chic,"[1] a
caring more for the palette of the colourist than for nature?
Well, que soit. Delacroix, Millet, Corot, Dupré, Daubigny,
Breton, thirty names more, are they not the heart and soul of

[1] " painting without copying reality "

the art of painting of this century, and are they not all rooted in romanticism, though they *surpassed* romanticism?

Romance and romanticism are of our time, and painters must have imagination and sentiment. Luckily realism and naturalism are not free from it. Zola creates, but does not hold up a *mirror* to things, he creates *wonderfully,* but *creates, poetises,* that is why it is so beautiful. So much for naturalism and realism, which nonetheless stand in connection to romanticism.

And I repeat that I am touched when I see a picture of about the years '30-'48, a Paul Huet, an old Israëls, like the "Fisherman of Zandvoort," a Cabat, an Isabey.

But I find so much truth in that saying: "ne pas peindre le ton local,"[1] that I far prefer a picture in a lower tonal scale than nature to one which is exactly like nature.

Rather a water-colour that is somewhat vague and unfinished than one which is worked up to simulate reality.

That saying: "ne pas peindre le ton local," has a broad meaning, and it leaves the painter free to seek for colours which form a whole and harmonize, which stand out the more in contrast to another combination.

What do I care whether the portrait of an honourable citizen tells me exactly the milk-and-watery bluish, insipid colour of that pious man's face—which I would never have noticed. But the citizens of the small town, where the above-mentioned individual has rendered himself so meritorious that he thought himself obliged to impress his physiognomy on posterity, are highly edified by the correct exactness.

Colour expresses something by itself, one cannot do without this, one must use it; that which is beautiful, really beautiful—is also correct; when Veronese had painted the portraits of his beau-monde in the "Marriage at Cana," he had spent on it all the richness of his palette in sombre violets, in splendid golden tones. Then—he thought still of a faint azure and a pearly-white—which does not appear in the foreground. He detonated it on in the background—and it was right, spontaneously it changes into the ambience of marble palaces and

[1] "do not paint local tone"

sky, which characteristically consummates the ordering of
the figures.

So beautiful is that background that it arose spontaneously
from a calculation of colours.

Am I wrong in this?

Is it not painted *differently* than somebody would do it
who had thought at the same time of the palace *and* of the
figures as one whole?

All that architecture and sky is conventional and subordin-
ate to the figures, it is calculated to make the figures stand
out beautifully.

Surely *that is* real painting, and the result is more beautiful
than the exact imitation of the things themselves. To think
of one thing and to let the surroundings belong to it and
proceed from it.

To study from nature, to wrestle with reality—I don't want
to do away with it, for years and years I myself have been so
engaged, almost fruitlessly and with all kinds of sad results.

I should not like to have missed that *error*.

I mean that it would be foolish and stupid always to go on
in that same way, but *not* that all the pains I took should be
absolutely dismissed.

" On commence par tuer, on finit par guérir,"[1] is a doctor's
saying. One starts with a hopeless struggle to follow nature,
and everything goes wrong; one ends by calmly creating
from one's palette, and nature agrees with it, and follows.
But these two contrasts are not separable from one another.
The drudging, though it may seem in vain, gives an intimacy
with nature, a sounder knowledge of things. And a beautiful
saying by Doré (who sometimes is so clever!) is: *je me
souviens.*[2] Though I believe that the best pictures are more
or less freely painted by heart, still I *cannot* divorce the
principle that one can never study and toil too much from
nature. The greatest, most powerful imaginations have at
the same time made things directly from nature which strike
one dumb.

[1] " One begins by killing, one ends by healing "
[2] " I remember "

In answer to your description of the study by Manet, I send you a still-life of an open—so a broken white—Bible bound in leather, against a black background, with a yellow-brown foreground, with a touch of citron yellow.

I painted that in *one rush,* during a single day.

This to show you that when I say that I have perhaps not plodded completely in vain, I dare say this, because at present it comes quite easily to me to paint a given subject unhesitatingly, whatever its form or colour may be. Recently I painted a few studies out of doors, of the autumn landscape. I shall write again soon, and send this letter in haste to tell you that I was quite pleased with what you say about black.

Goodbye,

Yours,
Vincent

[Antwerp, end of November 1885]
Dear Theo,   Saturday evening

I want to write you a few more impressions of Antwerp.

This morning I had a fruitful walk in the pouring rain, the object of this trudge was to fetch my things from the custom house; the various dockyards and warehouses on the quays are very fine.

I have walked along the docks and the quays several times already, in all directions. Especially when one comes from the sand and the heath and the quiet of a peasant village, and has for a long time been in none but quiet surroundings, the contrast is curious. It is an unfathomable mêlée. One of de Goncourt's sayings was " Japonaiserie for ever." Well, those docks are a famous Japonaiserie, fantastic, peculiar, unheard of—at least one can take it in that way.

I should like to walk there with you, just to know whether we see alike. One could undertake everything there, town views—figures of most varied character—the ships as the principal thing, with water and sky a delicate grey—but most of all—Japonaiserie. I mean, the figures are always in action, one sees them in the queerest surroundings, everything fantastic, and at all instants interesting contrasts present themselves.

A white horse in the mud, in a corner where heaps of merchandise are lying covered with oilcloth—against the old black smoky walls of the warehouse. Quite simple, but an effect of Black and White.

Through the window of a very elegant English bar, one will look out on the dirtiest mire, and on a ship from which, for instance, dainty merchandise like hides and buffalo horns is being unloaded by huge dock hands or exotic sailors; a very dainty and fair young English girl is standing at the window looking at it, or at something else. The interior with the figure altogether in tone, and for light—the silvery sky above that mud, and the buffalo horns, again a series of rather sharp contrasts. There will be Flemish sailors, with almost too healthy faces, with broad shoulders, strong and full, and thoroughly Antwerpian folk, eating mussels or drinking beer, and it will happen with a lot of noise and movement, while in contrast a tiny figure in black with her little hands against her body comes stealing noiselessly along the grey walls. Framed by raven-black hair—a small oval face, brown? orange-yellow? I don't know. For a moment she lifts her eyelids, and looks with a sideways glance from a pair of jet black eyes.

It is a Chinese girl, mysterious, quiet as a mouse—small, bug-like in character. What a contrast to that group of Flemish mussel eaters.

Another contrast—one passes through a very narrow street, between tremendously high houses, warehouses, and sheds. But down below in the street pubs of all nationalities with attending male and female individuals, shops with eatables, seamen's clothes, motley and crowded.

That street is long, every minute one sees something compelling. Now and again there is a row, when a quarrel is going on, intenser than elsewhere; for instance, there you are walking, looking about, and suddenly there arises a burst of cheering, and all kinds of shouting. In broad daylight a sailor is being thrown out of a bordello by the girls, and followed by a furious fellow and a bunch of girls, of whom he seems rather afraid—at least I saw him scramble over a heap of sacks and disappear through a warehouse window.

Now, when one has had enough of all this tumult—at the end of the piers where the Harwich and Havre steamers lie at anchor, with the city to one's rear, one sees in front nothing, absolutely nothing but an infinite expanse of flat, half-inundated fields, awfully dreary and wet, waving dry rushes, mud, the river with a single little black boat, the water in the foreground grey, the sky, foggy and cold, grey—quiet as a desert.

As to the panorama of the harbour or a dock—at one moment it is more tangled and fantastic than a thorn hedge, so confused that one finds no rest for the eye and gets giddy, is forced by the whirling of colours and lines to look first here, then there, without it being possible, even by looking for a long time at one point, to distinguish one thing from another. But when one stands on a spot where one has a vague plot as foreground, then one sees the most beautiful quiet lines, and the effects which Mols, for instance, often paints.

Now one sees a girl who is of splendid health, and who looks on the face of it loyal, simple and jolly, then again a face so sly and false, that it makes one afraid, like a hyena's. Not to forget the faces damaged by smallpox, which wear the colour of boiled shrimps, with pale grey eyes, without eyebrows, and a little sleek thin hair, the colour of real pigs' bristles or somewhat more yellow; Swedish or Danish types. It would be fine to work there, but how and where?

For one would very soon get into a scrape.

However I have traversed quite a number of streets and back alleys without meeting with adventures, and I have sat and talked quite jovially to various girls that seemed to take me for a sailor.

I don't think it improbable that by painting portraits I shall get hold of good models.

To-day I got my things and drawing materials, for which I was longing very much. And so my studio is all fixed. If I could get good models for almost nothing, I should not be afraid of anything.

I do not think it so very bad either that I have not got so much money as to be able to force things by paying for them.

Perhaps the idea of making portraits, and having them paid for by posing, is the safer way, because in a city it is not the same as with peasants. Well, one thing is sure, that Antwerp is very curious and fine for a painter.

My studio is not bad, especially as I have pinned a lot of little Japanese prints on the wall, which amuse me very much. You know those little women's figures in gardens, or on the beach, horsemen, flowers, knotty thorn branches.

I am glad I made the move, and hope not to sit still this winter. Well, I feel safe now that I have a little den, where I can sit and work when the weather is bad.

But of course I shall not exactly live in immense luxury these days.

Try and send your letter off on the 1st, because I have provided myself with bread till then, but after that I should be in rather a fix.

My little room is better than I expected, and it certainly doesn't look dull. Now that I have here the three studies I took with me, I shall try and go to the picture dealers, who seem however to live in private houses, with no show window on the street.

The park is nice too, I sat and drew there one morning.

Well, so far I have had no ill luck, as to my lodgings I am well off, since by spending a few francs more I have got a stove and a lamp.

I shall not easily get bored, I assure you. I have also found the " October " of Lhermitte, women in a potato field in the evening, beautiful. But I have not seen " November," did you get it perhaps? I have also noticed that there is a *Figaro* illustrated with a fine drawing by Raffaëlli.

My address you know is 194, Rue des Images, so please

forward your letter there, and the second part of de Goncourt[1] when you have finished it.

Goodbye,

Yours,
Vincent

It is curious that my painted studies seem darker in town than in the country. Is that because the light everywhere in town is less bright? I don't know, but it may make a greater difference than one would superficially say, so it struck me, and I could understand that things you have look darker than I in the country thought they were. However, the ones I have with me now don't come out badly for all that, the mill, the avenue with autumn trees and a still-life and a few little ones.

Dear Theo,   [Antwerp, end of December 1885]

It is high time for me to thank you for the 50 francs you sent which helped me to get through the month, though as from today it will be pretty much the same.

But—there are a few more studies made, and the more I paint the more progress I think I make. As soon as I received the money I took a beautiful model and painted her head life-size.

It is quite light except for the black, you know. Yet the head itself stands out simply against a background in which I tried to put a golden shimmer of light.

Here follows the colour scheme—a well-toned flesh-colour, in the neck rather bronze-like, jet black hair—black which I had to make with carmine and Prussian blue, reduced white for the little jacket, light yellow, much lighter than the white, for the background. A touch of scarlet in the jet black hair and a second scarlet bow in the reduced white.

This is a girl from a café chantant, and yet the expression which I sought was rather Ecce Homo-like.[2]

---

[1] The collection of essays on French painting by the de Goncourt brothers.

[2] viz, like the expression on the face of Christ when he was shown to the people by Pilate.

But as I want to remain *real*, especially in the expression, though I can let my fancy go, this is what I wanted to express in it.

When the model came, she had apparently been very busy the last few nights, and she said something that was rather characteristic: "Pour moi le champagne ne m'égaye pas, il me rend tout triste."[1]

Then I understood, and I tried to express something voluptuous and at the same time grievously afflicted.

From the same model, I began a second study in profile.

Then I made that portrait which I spoke about, the one that was promised to me, and I painted a study of that head for myself, and now these last days of the month I hope to paint another head of a man.

I feel quite cheerful, especially about the work, and it is good for me to be here.

I fancy that whatever those whores are like, one can make a profit from them more readily than in any other way. There is no denying that they are sometimes damned beautiful and that it is the spirit of the time that that kind of picture is on the way up more and more.

And even from the highest artistic point of view, nothing can be said against it; *to paint human beings,* that was the old Italian art, that was what Millet did and what Breton does.

The question is only whether one starts from the soul or from the clothes, and whether the form serves as a clothes-peg for ribbons and bows, or if one considers the form as the means of depicting impression and sentiment, or if one models for the sake of modelling, because it is so infinitely beautiful in itself.

Only the first is transitory, and the latter two are both high art.

What rather pleased me was that the girl who posed for me wanted me to paint a portrait for her to keep, on the same lines as the ones I did for myself.

[1] "Personally I am not cheered up by champagne, it makes me all sad."

And she has promised to let me paint as soon as possible a study of her in her room, in a dancer's dress.

She cannot do this now, because the owner of the café where she operates objects to her posing, but as she is going to live in rooms with another girl, both she and the other girl would like to have their portraits painted. And I fervently hope that she will come back, for she has an imposing face and is witty.

But I must train myself, given that it all depends on skilfulness and speed; for they have not much time or patience, although in any case the work need not be less well done for being done quickly, and one must be able to work even if the model does not sit rigidly still. Well, you see that I am at work with full vitality. If I sold something so that I earned a little more, I should work more vigorously still.

As to Portier, I do not lose courage yet, but poverty is at my back, and at present the dealers all rather suffer from the same evil, that of being more or less a " lost tribe," that is in eclipse. They have too much spleen, and how can one be expected to feel inclined to dip into all that indifference and dullness; besides, this complaint is catching.

For it is all nonsense that no business can be done, but one must work in any case, with conviction and with enthusiasm, in short with a certain warmth.

As to Portier, you wrote me yourself that he was the first to exhibit the impressionists, and that his thunder was completely stolen by Durand-Ruel.

Well, one might conclude from this that he is a man of initiative, not only saying things but doing them. Perhaps it is the fault of his sixty years, and for the rest his is perhaps one of the many cases in which, at the time when pictures were the fashion and business prospered, a lot of intelligent persons were wantonly put aside, as if they were of no importance and without talent, only because they could not bring themselves to believe in the stability of that sudden craze for pictures, and the enormous lift in prices.

Now that business is slack, one sees those very same dealers who were so very enterprising, let us say ten years ago, pass into complete eclipse. And we are not yet at the end.

Personal initiative with little or no capital is perhaps the germ for the future. It remains to be seen.

Yesterday I saw a large photograph of a Rembrandt which I did not know, and which struck me tremendously; it was a woman's head, the light fell on the bust, neck, chin and the nostrils—the lower jaw.

The forehead and eyes under the shadow of a large hat, probably with red feathers. Probably also red or yellow in the low-cut jacket. A dark background. The expression, a mysterious smile like that of Rembrandt himself in his self-portrait, where Saskia is sitting on his knee and he has a glass of wine in his hand.

My thoughts are all the time full of Rembrandt and Hals these days, not because I see so many of their pictures, but because I see among the people here so many types that remind me of that time.

I still often go to those popular balls, to see the heads of the women, and the heads of the sailors and soldiers. One pays the entrance fee of 20 or 30 centimes, and drinks a glass of beer, for they drink very little spirits, and one can amuse oneself a whole evening, at least I do, by observing how these people enjoy themselves.

To paint much from the model—that is what I have to do, and it is the only thing that seriously helps to make progress.

I notice that I have been underfed too long, and when I received your money my stomach could not digest the food; but I will try to remedy that.

And it does not prevent my having all my energy and capacity when at work.

But when I am out of doors, the work in the open air is too much for me, and I feel too faint.

Well, painting is a thing that wears one out. But Dr. Van der Loo[1] told me, when I went to see him shortly before I came here, that I am after all fairly strong. That I need not despair of reaching the age which is necessary for producing a life's

[1] The physician at Eindhoven.

work. I told him that I knew of several painters who, not-withstanding all their nervousness etc., reached the age of sixty or even seventy, luckily for themselves, and that I should like to do the same.

Then I think that if one keeps one's serenity and good spirits, the mood in which one is acts as a great help. In that respect I have gained by coming here, for I have got new ideas and I have new means of expressing what I want, because better brushes will help me, and I am crazy about those two colours, carmine and cobalt.

Cobalt is a divine colour, and there is nothing so beautiful for putting atmosphere around things. Carmine is the red of wine, and it is warm and lively like wine.

The same with emerald-green. It is bad economy not to use these colours, the same with cadmium.

Something about my constitution which made me very glad was what a doctor in Amsterdam told me, whom I consulted once about a few things which sometimes made me fear that I was not going to last out for long, and whose opinion I did not ask straight out, but just to know the first impression of somebody who absolutely did not know me. This was the way of it, profiting from a small complaint I had then, in the course of conversation I alluded to my constitution in general—how glad I was that this doctor took me for an ordinary working man and said: " I suppose you are an iron-worker." This is just what I have tried to change in myself; when I was younger, I looked like one who was intellectually overwrought, and now I look like a bargee or an ironworker.

And to change one's constitution so that one gets " tough-skinned " is no easy matter.

But I must be careful nonetheless, and try to keep what I have, and gain in strength.

I want you above all to write me if the idea seems so absurd to you that one would gain in courage if one planted the germ of a business of one's own?

As to my work at present, I feel that I can do better; however, I need some more space and air, I mean—I ought to

be able to spend a little more. Above all, above all I cannot
take in sufficient models. I could produce work of a better
quality, but my expenses would be heavier. But is it not true
that one needs to aim at something lofty, something true, of
some distinction?

The women's figures which I see here among the people
give me a tremendous urge, much more to paint them than to
possess them, though indeed I should like both.

I read over again the book by de Goncourt. It is excellent.
The preface to " Chérie ", which you will read, tells the story
of what the de Goncourts went through, and how at the end
of their lives they were melancholy, yes, but felt sure of
themselves, knowing that they had *accomplished* something,
that their work would remain. What fellows they were. If
we thought more alike than we do now, if we could agree
absolutely, why should not we *do the same*?

By the way, because I shall have in any case at the end of
this year four or five days of absolute fast in everything, do
send your letter on the first of January and not later. Perhaps you will not be able to understand, but it is true that
when I receive the money my greatest appetite is not for
food, though I have fasted, but the appetite for painting is
stronger still, and I set out at once to hunt for models, and
continue until all the money is gone. While all I have to
live on is my breakfast from the people with whom I lodge,
and in the evening for supper a cup of coffee and bread in
the dairy, or else a loaf of rye that I have in my trunk.

As long as I am painting it is more than sufficient, but
when the models have left there comes a feeling of weakness.

I am attached to the models here, because they are so different from the models in the country. And especially because their character is so entirely different, and the contrast
gives me new ideas, especially for the flesh-colours. And
what I have now arrived at in the last head I painted, though
it is not yet such that I am satisfied with it, remains different
from the former heads.

I know that you are convinced enough of the importance
of being *true,* so that I can speak out freely to you.

If I paint peasant women I want them to be peasant women; for the same reason, if I paint harlots I want a harlot-like expression.

That was why a harlot's head by Rembrandt struck me so enormously. Because he had caught so infinitely beautifully that mysterious smile, with a gravity such as only he possesses, the magician of magicians.

This for me is a new thing, and it is essentially what I want. Manet has done it, and Courbet, damn it, I have the same ambition; besides, I have felt too strongly in bone and marrow the infinite beauty of the analyses of women by the very great men in literature, a Zola, Daudet, de Goncourt, Balzac.

Even Stevens does not satisfy me, because his women are not those I know personally. And those he chooses are not the most interesting, I think. Well, however that may be—I want to get on at all costs—and I want to be myself.

I feel quite obstinate, and I do not care any more what people say about me or about my work.

It seems very difficult here to get models for the nude, at least the girl I painted refused.

Of course that "refused" is perhaps merely relative, but at least it would not be easy, though I must say she would be splendid. From a business point of view I can only say that we are already in what is beginning to be termed the "end of a century," that women have a charm of the same kind as in a time of revolution—in fact have as much prestige—and one would be outside the trend if one kept them outside one's work.

It is everywhere the same, in the country as well as in the city; one must take the women into account if one wants to be up-to-date.

Goodbye, good wishes for the New Year. With a handshake,

Yours,

Vincent

Dear Theo,   [Antwerp, January 1886]
   I decidedly want to tell you that it would greatly alleviate
me if you would approve of my coming to Paris much earlier
than June or July. The more I think about it the more
anxious I am to do so.
   Just think that if all goes well, and if I had good food,
etc., all that time, which will certainly leave something to be
desired, even in that case it will take about six months before
I shall have fully recovered.
   But it would certainly take much longer still, if in
Brabant from March to July I had to go through the same
things as I have undergone these last months, and probably
it would not be any different.
   Now, at this moment, I feel terribly weak, even worse than
that, from reaction after overwork, but that is the natural
course of things and nothing extraordinary; as however it is
a question of taking better nourishment, etc., you see that in
Brabant I shall drain myself of money again by taking models;
the same story will begin all over again, and I do not think
that will be right. In that way we stray from our path. So
please allow me to come sooner, I should almost say at once.
   If I rent a garret in Paris, and bring my paint box and
drawing materials with me, then I can finish at once what is
most pressing—those studies from the antique, which will
certainly help me a great deal when I go to Cormon's.[1] I can
go and draw either at the Louvre or at the École des Beaux
Arts.
   For the rest, before settling in a new place, we could plan
and arrange matters so much better. If it must be, I am
willing to go to Nuenen for the month of March, to see how
things are there and how the people are and whether or not
I can get models there. But if there is no such need, as I presume, I should come straight to Paris after March, and begin
to draw at the Louvre, for instance.
   I have thought over well what you wrote about taking a
studio, but I think it would be a good thing if we looked for it

[1] The artist in whose studio in Paris Vincent was to take lessons.

together, and if before we went to live together definitely, we did so temporarily, and if I began by renting a garret, from April for instance, till June.

I shall then feel at home again in Paris by the time I go to Cormon's.

And in this way I shall keep up my spirits better.

I must also tell you that, although I keep going there, it is often almost unbearable, that nagging of the people at the academy, for they remain decidedly spiteful.

But I try systematically to avoid all quarrels, and go my own way. And I fancy I am on the track of what I am seeking, and perhaps I should find it the sooner if I could go my own way over the drawing from plaster casts.

I am glad after all that I went to the academy, for the very reason that I have abundant opportunity to observe the results of *prendre par le contour*.[1]

For that is what they do systematically, and that is why they nag at me. "Faites d'abord un contour, votre contour n'est pas juste, je ne corrigerai pas ça, si vous modelez avant d'avoir sérieusement arrêté votre contour."[2]

You see how it always ends in the same fashion. And now you ought to see how flat, how lifeless and how insipid the results of that system are; oh, I can tell you I am very glad just to see it once at close quarters. Like David, or worse still, like Pieneman in full vigour. I wanted at least twenty-five times to say, "Votre contour est un truc, etc.,"[3] but I have not thought it worth while to quarrel. Yet though I do not say anything, I irritate them, and they me.

But this does not matter so much, the task is to go on trying to find a better working-system. So—patience and perseverance.

They go so far as to say, "La couleur et le modelé c'est peu

[1] "proceeding from the contour"
[2] "First make a contour, your contour is not correct, I will not correct your work, if you insist on modelling before you have seriously determined your contour."
[3] "To hell with your contour"

de chose, cela s'apprend très vite, c'est le contour qui est l'essentiel et le plus difficile."[1]

You see, one can learn something new at the academy. I never knew before that colour and modelling came so easily.

I finished just yesterday the drawing which I made for the competition of the evening class. It is the figure of Germanicus[2] which you know. Well, I am sure I shall come out bottom, because all the drawings of the others are utterly alike, and mine is absolutely different. But that drawing which they will think the best, I have seen how it was done. I was sitting just behind it and it is correct, it is whatever you like, but it is *dead*, and that is what all the drawings are which I saw.

Enough of this, but let it irritate us so much that it makes us enthusiastic for something nobler, and that we hasten to reach this.

You, too, need more vitality in your life, and if we might succeed in joining up, together we would know more than each apart, and would be able to do more.

Tell me, did you notice that subtle saying of Paul Mantz's: "Dans la vie les femmes sont peut-être la difficulté suprême."[3] It was in an article on Baudry.

We shall experience our share of it, besides the experience we may already have acquired.

It struck me in a chapter from "L'Œuvre," by Zola, printed in the Gil Blas, that the painter, Manet of course, had a scene with a woman who had posed for him, and afterwards he had become indifferent to her, oh—curiously well described. What one can learn in this respect from the academy here is never in that light to paint women.

They hardly ever use nude women models. At least not at all in the class, and only most exceptionally in private.

---

[1] "Colour and modelling matter very little, they can be picked up very fast; it is the contour that is essential and most difficult."
[2] The task was to make a drawing after a plaster cast of this famous Roman statue.
[3] "In life women probably present the supreme difficulty."
L.V.G.

I

Even in the antiquities class there are ten men's figures to one woman's figure. That is easy enough.

In Paris, of course, this will be better, and it seems to me that, in fact, one learns so much from the constant comparing of the masculine figure with the feminine, which are always and in everything so totally different. It may be " supremely " difficult, but what would art and what would life be without it?

Goodbye, write to me soon. With a handshake,

Yours,

Vincent

My being in Nuenen at least for the month of March would only be for the sake of the moving, and I have to be there anyhow for my change of domicile. But as to myself, I am quite willing not to go back there at all.

PARIS

Dear old boy,   [Paris, summer 1887)][1]
   Thank you for your letter and what it contained. It
depresses me to think that even when it's a success, painting
never pays back what it costs.

   I was touched by what you wrote about home—" They
are fairly well but still it is sad to see them." A dozen years
ago one would have sworn that at any rate the family would
always prosper and get on. It would give great pleasure to
Mother if your marriage came off, and for the sake of your
health and your work you ought not to remain single.

   As for me—I feel I am losing the desire for marriage and
children, and now and then it saddens me that I should be
feeling like that at thirty-five just when it should be the
opposite. And sometimes I have a grudge against this rotten
painting. It was Richepin who said somewhere:
   " The love of art means loss of real love "
      (*L'amour de l'art fait perdre l'amour vrai.*)
   I think that is terribly true, but on the other hand real
love makes you disgusted with art.

   And at times I feel already old and broken, and yet still
enough of a lover not to be a real enthusiast for painting. To
succeed one must have ambition, and ambition seems to me
absurd. What will come of it I don't know; I would like
above all things to be less of a burden to you—and that is not
impossible in the future—for I hope to make such progress
that you will be able to show my stuff boldly without compromising yourself.

[1] Vincent was in Paris for almost two years—March 1886 to
February 1888—but the fact that he was living with Theo there
meant that he wrote very few letters to his brother at this period.
Indeed, it is for this very reason that the Paris period is the phase
in Vincent's career about which least is known by way of exact detail.

And then I will take myself off somewhere down south,[1] to get away from the sight of so many painters that disgust me as men.

You can be sure of one thing, that I will not try to do any more work for the Tambourin.[2] I think besides that it is going into other hands, and I certainly shall not try to stop it.

As for the Segatori, that's very different. I still have some affection for her and I hope she still has some for me.

But just now she is in a bad way; she is neither a free agent nor mistress in her own house, and worst of all she is ill and in pain.

Although I would not say this openly, my own conviction is that she has procured an abortion (unless indeed she has had a miscarriage), but anyway in her position I should not blame her. In two months' time she will be better, I hope, and then perhaps she will be grateful that I did not bother her. Once she is well, mind you, if she refuses in cold blood to give me what belongs to me, or does me any wrong I shall not spare her—but that will not be necessary. I know her well enough to trust her still. And mind you, if she manages to keep her place going, from the point of view of business I should not blame her for choosing to be top dog, and not underdog. If in order to get on she tramples on my toes a bit, well, she has my leave. When I saw her again she did not trample on my heart, which she would have done if she had been as bad as people said.

I saw Tanguy[3] yesterday, and he has put a canvas I've just done in his window. I have done four since you left, and I have a big one on hand.

I know that these big long canvases are difficult to sell, but

[1] This idea would finally be put into effect some eight months later, when Vincent left for Arles.

[2] A café in Montmartre where Vincent had exhibited some of his work; he had also done some pictures for the decoration of the interior and these the concern had refused to give back after it went bankrupt. La Segatori was the proprietress.

[3] The owner of a shop which dealt in colours and also in pictures and Japanese prints; it was a great meeting-place for artists.

later on people will see that there is open air in them and
that they are good-humoured.

So now the whole lot would do for decorations for a dining-
room, or a country house.

And if you fall very much in love, and then get married, it
doesn't seem to me out of the question that you will rise to a
country house yourself some day, like so many other picture
dealers. If you live well you spend more, but you gain
more ground that way, and perhaps one gets on better these
days by looking rich than by looking shabby. It's better to
have a gay life of it than commit suicide. Remember me to
all at home.

Yours,
Vincent

ARLES

My dear Theo,   [Arles, early March 1888]

This morning, at long last, the weather changed and turned milder—and likewise I have already had an opportunity for learning what a mistral is: I have been for several walks in the country round here but in this wind it is impossible ever to do anything. The sky is a hard blue with a great bright sun, which has melted almost the whole bulk of the snow, but the wind is cold and so dry that it gives you goose-flesh.

But all the same I have seen lots of beautiful things—a ruined abbey on a hill covered with holly, pines, and grey olives.[1]

We'll have a try at that soon, I hope.

I have just finished a study like the one Lucien Pissarro has of mine, but this time it is oranges. That makes eight studies so far. But this doesn't really count, because I haven't yet been able to work in any comfort or warmth. The letter from Gauguin which I meant to send you, and which I thought for the moment had got burnt with other papers, I have since found, and send it you enclosed.[2] But I have already written direct to him, and sent him Russell's address, also that of Gauguin to Russell, so that if they like they can deal with each other direct.

But how difficult for many of us—and assuredly we ourselves are among the number—the future still is! I firmly believe in victory at the last, but will the artists themselves obtain any advantage from it, and will they see less troubled days?

I have bought some coarse canvas here, and had it pre-

[1] The abbey of Montmajour, a few miles outside Arles.

[2] Gauguin had written from Brittany that he was ill and in desperate financial straits; he wanted Vincent to try and get help for him from Theo, who was his dealer at the time. John Russell was an Australian artist-friend who might, in Vincent's view, be able to help Gauguin.

pared for mat effects. I can get everything now almost at the same prices as in Paris. Saturday evening I had a visit from two amateur artists, a grocer who sells painting materials as well, and a magistrate who seems a nice fellow, and intelligent.

Worse luck, I can hardly manage to live any cheaper than in Paris, I must reckon on 5 fr. per day.

I have not yet found any sort of small place where I could have private board and lodging, but all the same something of the kind must exist.

If the weather is milder in Paris too, it will do you good. What a winter! I dare not roll up my studies yet because they are hardly dry and there are some bits of impasto which will take some time to dry.

I have just been reading "Tartarin on the Alps"[1] which amused me hugely. Has that confounded Tersteeg written to you yet? All to the good if he has. If he doesn't answer he will hear of us all the same, and we shall see to it that he can find no fault with our actions. For instance we will send a picture to Mme. Mauve in memory of Mauve,[2] with a letter from both of us, in which, supposing Tersteeg does not reply, we shall not say a word against him, but we will manage to convey that we do not deserve to be treated as if we were dead.

But indeed it is not likely that Tersteeg will have any prejudice against us on the whole. Poor Gauguin has no luck. I am very much afraid that in his case convalescence will last even longer than the fortnight which he has had to spend in bed.

My God! Will we ever see a generation of artists with healthy bodies! Sometimes I am perfectly furious with myself, for it isn't good enough to be neither more nor less ill than the rest; the ideal would be a constitution tough enough

---

[1] The sequel by Alphonse Daudet to "Tartarin de Tarascon." Arles was in fact right in the Tartarin country.

[2] The artist who had given Vincent lessons in The Hague had just died; Vincent sent one of his *Orchards in Blossom* to the widow.

to live till eighty, and besides that blood in one's veins that would be right good blood.

It would be some comfort, however, if one could think that a generation of more fortunate artists was to come.

I wanted to write to you at once that I am in hopes the winter is really over, and I hope that it is the same in Paris.

With a handshake,

Yours,
Vincent

My dear Theo, [Arles, first half of April 1888]

Thank you for your letter and the 100 franc note enclosed. I have sent you sketches of the pictures which are to go to Holland. Of course the painted studies are more brilliant in colour. I'm once again hard at it, still orchards in blossom.

The air here certainly does me good. I wish you could fill your lungs with it; one effect it has on me is comical enough; one small glass of brandy makes me tipsy here, so that as I don't have to fall back on stimulants to make my blood circulate, there will be less strain on my constitution. The only thing is that my stomach has been terribly weak since I came here, but after all that's probably only a matter of time. I hope to make progress this year, and indeed I greatly need to.

I have a fresh orchard, as good as the rose-coloured peach trees, apricot trees of a very pale rose. At the moment I am working on some plum trees, yellowish-white, with thousands of black branches. I am using a tremendous lot of colours and canvases, but I hope it isn't a waste of money all the same. Out of four canvases perhaps one at the most will make a *picture,* like the one for Tersteeg or Mauve, but the studies, I hope, will come in useful for exchanges.

When can I send you anything? I have a great mind to do a second version like Tersteeg's, because it is better than the Asnières[1] studies.

Yesterday I saw another bull fight, where five men played

[1] A locale where Vincent had painted while in Paris.

the bull with darts and cockades. One toreador crushed a
testicle jumping the barricade. He was a fair man with grey
eyes and plenty of sang-froid; people said he'll be ill long
enough. He was dressed in sky blue and gold, just like the
little horseman in our Monticelli, the three figures in a wood.
The arenas are a fine sight when there's sunshine and a crowd.

Bravo for Pissarro, I think he is right. I hope he will make
an exchange with us some day.

And Seurat the same. It would be a good thing to have a
study painted by him.

Well, I'm working hard, hoping that we can do something
with things of this kind.

This month will come hard on both you and me, but if
you can manage it will be to our advantage to make the most
we can of the orchards in bloom. I am well started now, and
I think I must have ten more, the same subject. You know I
am changeable in my work, and this craze for painting
orchards will not last for ever. After this it may be the
arenas. Then I must do a *tremendous* lot of drawing, because
I want to make some drawings in the manner of Japanese
prints. I can only go on striking for as long as the iron is
hot.

I shall be all in when the orchards are over, for they are
canvases of sizes 25 and 30 and 20. We would not have
too many of them, even if I could bring off twice as many.
It seems to me that this might really break the ice in Holland.
Mauve's death was a terrible blow to me. You will see that
the rose-coloured peach trees were painted with a certain
passion.

I must also have a starry night with cypresses,[1] or perhaps surmounting a field of ripe corn; there are some wonderful nights here. I am in a continual fever of work.

I'm very curious to know what the result will be at the end

[1] Vincent was not in fact to paint this subject until he was at
Saint-Rémy in June 1889, but meanwhile in September 1888 he
painted the Rhône under a starry night sky. Such a sky symbolised for
him God's beneficent and eternal surveillance of the universe—probably under the inspiration of the poetry of Walt Whitman; the
cypresses, as graveyard trees, were a symbol of death.

of a year. I hope that by that time I shall be less bothered with sick turns. At present I am pretty bad some days, but I don't worry about it in the least, as it is nothing but the reaction after last winter which was out of the ordinary. And my blood is coming right, that is the great thing.

I must reach the point when my pictures will cover what I spend, and even more than that, taking into account so much spent in the past. Well, it will come. I don't make a success of everything, I admit, but I'm getting on. So far you have not complained of my expenses here, but I warn you that if I continue to work on the same scale, I shall have real trouble ahead of me. But the work is really heavy.

If there should happen to be a month or a fortnight in which you were hard pressed, let me know and I will set to work on some drawings, which will cost us less. I mean you must not put yourself out unnecessarily, there is so much to do here, all sorts of studies, not the way it is in Paris, where you can't sit down wherever you want.

If you can support a rather heavy month so much the better, since orchards in bloom are the kind of thing one has some chance of selling or exchanging.

But it came to my mind that you have to pay your rent, so you must tell me if things are too steep.

I am still going about all the time with the Danish painter,[1] but he is soon going home. He's an intelligent lad, and all right as far as fidelity and manner goes, but his painting is still rather flabby. You will probably see him when he passes through Paris.

You did well to go and see Bernard. If he goes to serve in Algiers, who knows but that I might go there too to keep him company.

Is it at long last really over, this winter in Paris?. I think what Kahn[2] said is very true, that I have not sufficiently considered values, but they'll be saying very different things in a little while—and no less true.

[1] Mourier Petersen.
[2] Gustave Kahn, an art-critic writing for some of the independent Parisian reviews.

It isn't possible to get values and colour.

Th. Rousseau did it better than anyone else, and with the mixing of his colours, the darkening caused by time has increased and his pictures are now unrecognizable.

You can't be at the pole and the equator at the same time.

You must choose your line, as I hope to do, and it will probably be colour. Goodbye for the present. A handshake to you, Koning[1] and the crowd.

Vincent

[Saintes-Maries-sur-Mer, second half of June 1888]
My dear Theo,

I am writing to you from Stes. Maries on the shore of the Mediterranean at last. The Mediterranean has the colouring of mackerel, changeable I mean. You don't always know if it is green or violet, you can't even say it's blue, because the next moment the changing reflection has taken on a tinge of rose or grey.

A family is a queer thing—quite involuntarily and in spite of myself I have been thinking here between whiles of our sailor uncle, who must many a time have seen the shores of this sea.

I brought along canvases and have covered them—two sea-scapes, a view of the village, and then some drawings which I will send you by post, when I return to-morrow to Arles.

I have board and lodging for 4 francs a day, although they began by asking 6.

As soon as I can I shall probably come back here again to make some more studies.

The shore here is sandy, no cliffs nor rocks—like Holland without the dunes, and bluer.

You get better fried fish here than on the Seine. Only there is not fish to be had every day, as the fishermen go off to sell it at Marseilles. But when there is some it is frightfully good.

If there isn't—the butcher is not much more appetising

[1] A Dutch artist-friend whom Theo had staying.

than the butcher fellah of M. Gérôme—if there is no fish it is pretty difficult to get anything to eat, as far as I can see.

I do not think there are 100 houses in the village, or town. The chief building, after the old church and an ancient fortress, is the barracks. And the houses—like the ones on our heaths and peat-mosses at Drenthe; you will see some specimens of them in the drawings.

I am forced to leave my three painted studies here, for they are naturally not dry enough to be submitted with safety to five hours' jolting in the carriage.

But I expect to come back here again.

Next week I would like to go to Tarascon to do two or three studies.

If you have not written yet I shall naturally expect the letter at Arles. A very fine gendarme came to interview me here, and the curé too—the people can't be very bad here, because even the curé looked almost like a decent fellow.

Next month it will be the season for open air bathing here. The number of bathers varies from 20 to 50. I am staying till to-morrow afternoon, I've still some drawings to make.

One night I went for a walk by the sea along the empty shore. It was not gay, but neither was it sad—it was—beautiful. The deep blue sky was flecked with clouds of a blue deeper than the fundamental blue of intense cobalt, and others of a clearer blue, like the blue whiteness of the Milky Way. In the blue depth the stars were sparkling, greenish, yellow, white, rose, brighter, flashing more like jewels, than they do at home—even in Paris : opals you might call them, emeralds, lapis, rubies, sapphires.

The sea was very deep ultramarine—the shore a sort of violet and faint russet as I saw it, and on the dunes (about seventeen feet high they are) some bushes of Prussian blue. Besides half-page drawings I have a big drawing, the companion to the last one.

Goodbye for the present only, I hope, with a handshake,

Yours,

Vincent

My dear Theo,   [Arles, mid July 1888]

I have come back from a day at Mont Majour, and my friend the second lieutenant was with me. We explored the old garden together and stole some excellent figs. If it had been bigger it would have made me think of Zola's Paradou, great reeds, vines, ivy, fig trees, olives, pomegranates with lusty flowers of the brightest orange, hundred-year-old cypresses, ash trees and willows, rock oaks, half-broken flights of steps, ogive windows in ruins, blocks of white rock covered with lichen, and scattered fragments of crumbling walls here and there among the greenery. I brought back another big drawing, but not of the garden. That makes three drawings. When I have half a dozen I shall send them along.

Yesterday I went to Fontvieilles to visit Bock and McKnight,[1] only these gentlemen had gone on a little trip to Switzerland for a week.

I think the heat is still doing me good, in spite of the mosquitoes and flies.

The grasshoppers—not like ours at home, but of this sort,[2] like those you see in Japanese albums, and Spanish flies, gold and green in swarms on the olives. The grasshoppers (I think they are called cicadas) sing as loud as a frog.

I have been thinking too that when you remember that I painted old Tanguy's portrait, and that he also had the portrait of his old lady (which they have sold), and of their friend (it is true that I got 20 francs from him for this latter portrait), and that I have bought without discount 250 francs' worth of paints from Tanguy, on which naturally he made something, and finally that I have been his friend no less than he has been mine, I have very serious reason to doubt his right to claim money from me; and it really is squared by the study he still has of mine, all the more so because there was an express arrangement that he should pay himself by the sale of a picture.

[1] Two artist friends, one Belgian and the other American.
[2] A sketch was included here.

Xantippe,[1] Mother Tanguy, and some other good ladies have by some queer freak of Nature heads of silex or flint. Certainly these ladies are a good deal more dangerous in the civilized world they go about in than the poor souls bitten by mad dogs who live in the Pasteur Institute. And old Tanguy would be right a hundred times over to kill his lady . . . but he won't do it, any more than Socrates.

And for this reason old Tanguy has more in common—in resignation and long suffering anyhow—with the ancient Christians, martyrs and slaves, than with the present day rotters of Paris.

That does not mean that there is any reason to pay him 80 francs, but it is a reason for never losing your temper with him, even if he loses his, when, as you may do in this instance, you chuck him out, or at least send him packing.

I am writing to Russell at the same time. I think we know, don't we, that the English, the Yankees, etc. have this much in common with the Dutch, that their charity . . . is very Christian. Now, the rest of us not being very good Christians. . . . That's what I can't put out of my head writing again like this.

This Bock has a head rather like a Flemish gentleman of the time of the Compromise of the Nobles, William the Silent's time and Marnix's. I shouldn't wonder if he's a decent fellow.

I have written to Russell that I would send him my parcel in a roll direct to him, for our exchange, if I knew that he was in Paris.

That means he must in any case answer me soon. Now I shall *soon* need some more canvas and paints. But I have not yet got the address of that canvas at 40 francs for 20 metres.

I think it is well to work especially at drawing just now, and to arrange to have paints and canvas in reserve for when Gauguin comes.[2] I wish paint was as little of a worry to

---

[1] The wife of Socrates.

[2] The plan had now been mooted that Gauguin should join Vincent at Arles.

work with as pen and paper. I often pass up a painted study
for fear of squandering the colour.

With paper, whether it's a letter I'm writing, or a drawing
I'm working on, there's never a misfire—so many pages of
Whitman, so many drawings. I think that if I were rich I
should spend less than I do now.

Well, old Martin would say, then it's up to you to get
rich, and he is right, as he is about the masterpiece.

Do you remember in Guy de Maupassant the gentleman
who hunted rabbits and other game, and who had hunted so
hard for ten years, and was so exhausted by running after the
game that when he wanted to get married he found he was
impotent, which caused the greatest embarrassment and consternation. Without being in the same state as this gentleman
as to its being either my duty or my desire to get married, I
begin to resemble him in physique. According to the worthy
Ziem, man becomes ambitious as soon as he becomes impotent. Now though it's pretty much all one to me whether I
am impotent or not, I'm damned if that's going to drive me to
ambition. It is only the greatest philosopher of his place and
time, and consequently of all places and all times, good old
master Pangloss,[1] who could—if he were here—give me
advice and steady my soul.

There—Russell's letter is in its envelope, and I have
written as I intended.

I asked him if he had any news of Reid, and I ask you the
same question.

I told Russell I left him free to take what he liked, and
from the first lot I sent as well. And that I was only waiting
for his explicit answer, to know whether he preferred to make
his choice at his or your place; that if, in the former circumstance, he wanted to see them at his own house, you would
send him along some orchards as well, and fetch the lot back
again when he had made his choice. So he cannot quarrel
with that. If he takes nothing from Gauguin it is because he
cannot. If he can I am inclined to anticipate that he will;
I told him that if I ventured to press him to buy, it was *not*

[1] The optimist in Voltaire's *Candide*.

because nobody else would if he didn't, but because Gauguin having been ill, and with the further complication of his having been laid up in bed and having to pay his doctor, it all fell rather heavily on us, and we were all the more anxious to find a purchaser for a picture.

I am thinking a lot about Gauguin, and I would have plenty of ideas for pictures, and about work in general.

I have a charwoman now for one franc, who sweeps and scrubs the house[1] for me twice a week. I am banking very much on her, reckoning that she will make our beds if we decide to sleep in the house. Otherwise we could make some arrangement with the fellow where I am staying now. Anyhow we'll try to manage so that it would work out as an economy instead of more expense. How are you now? Are you still going to Gruby?[2] What you tell me of the conversation at the Nouvelle Athènes is interesting. You know the little portrait by Desboutin that Portier has?

It certainly is a strange phenomenon that all the artists, poets, musicians, painters, are unfortunate in material things —the happy ones as well—what you said lately about Guy de Maupassant is a fresh proof of it. That brings up again the eternal question : is the whole of life visible to us, or isn't it rather that this side death we see one hemisphere only?

Painters—to take them only—dead and buried, speak to the next generation or to several succeeding generations through their work.

Is that all, or is there more besides? In a painter's life death is not perhaps the hardest thing there is.

For my own part, I declare I know nothing whatever about it, but to look at the stars always makes me dream, *as simply* as I dream over the black dots of a map representing towns and villages. Why, I ask myself, should the shining dots of the sky not be as accessible as the black dots on the map of

---

[1] Vincent had moved to the " Yellow House " in Place Lamartine in May, first using it for a studio where he also slept, and later starting to furnish it as the living- and working-quarters for himself and a companion.

[2] Theo's physician.

France? If we take the train to get to Tarascon or Rouen, we take death to reach a star. One thing undoubtedly true in this reasoning is this, that while we are *alive* we *cannot* get to a star, any more than when we are dead we can take the train.

So it seems to me possible that cholera, gravel, phthisis and cancer are the celestial means of locomotion, just as steam-boats, omnibuses and railways are the terrestrial means. To die quietly of old age would be to go there on foot.

Now I am going to bed, because it is late, and I wish you good night and good luck.

A handshake.

Yours,
Vincent

My dear Theo,   [Arles, early August 1888]
I think you were right to go to our uncle's funeral, since Mother seemed to be expecting you. The best way to tackle a death is to swallow the image of the illustrious dead, whatever he was, as the best man in the best of all possible worlds, where everything is always for the best. Which not being contested, and consequently incontestable, it is doubtless allowable for us to return afterwards to our own affairs. I am glad that our brother Cor has grown bigger and stronger than the rest of us. And he must be stupid if he does not get married, for he has nothing but that and his hands. With that and his hands, and that and what he knows of machinery, I for one would like to be in his shoes, if I had any desire at all to be anyone else.

And meanwhile I am in my own hide, and my hide within the cog-wheels of the Fine Arts, like corn between the mill-stones.

Did I tell you that I had sent the drawings to friend Russell? At the moment I am doing practically the same ones again for you, there will be twelve likewise. You will then see better what there is in the painted studies in the way of drawing. I have already told you that I always have to fight against the mistral, which makes it absolutely impossible to be master of your stroke. That accounts for the "haggard" look of the studies. You will tell me that instead of drawing them, I ought to paint them again on fresh canvases at home. I think so myself now and then, for it is not my fault in this case that the execution lacks a livelier touch. What would Gauguin say about it if he were here, would he advise seeking a more sheltered place?

I now have another unpleasant thing to tell you about the money, which is that I shall *not* manage this week, because this very day I am paying out 25 frs.; I shall have money for five days, but *not* for seven. This is Monday; if I get your next letter on Saturday morning there will be no need to increase the enclosure. Last week I did not one only but two portraits of my postman,[1] a half-length with the hands, and a head, life size. The good fellow, as he would not accept money, *cost more* eating and drinking with me, and I gave him besides the "Lantern" of Rochefort. But that is a trifling and immaterial evil, considering that he posed very well, and that I expect to paint his baby very shortly, for his wife has just been brought to bed.

I will send you, at the same time as the drawings that I have in hand, two lithographs by de Lemud, "Wine" and "The Café"; in "Wine" there is a sort of Mephistopheles, rather reminiscent of C.M.[2] when younger, and in "The Café . . ." it is Raoul exactly, you know that old Bohemian student type, whom I knew last year. What a talent that de Lemud had, like Hoffman or Edgar Poe.

And yet he is one who is little talked of. Perhaps you will not care tremendously for these lithographs at first, but it is just when you look at them for a long time that they grow on you. I have come to the end both of paints and canvas and I have already had to buy some here. And I must go back for still more.

So please do send the letter so that I'll have it on Saturday

[1] Roulin; in December Vincent would do portraits of the whole family.
[2] Vincent's uncle Cornelius.

morning. Today I am probably going to begin the interior of the Café where I eat, by gas light, in the evening.

It is what they call here a Café de Nuit (they are fairly frequent here), staying open all night. "Night prowlers" can take refuge there when they have no money to pay for a lodging, or are too tight to be taken in. All those things— family, native land—are perhaps more attractive in the imaginations of such people as us, who pretty well do without native land or family either, than they are in reality. I always feel I am a traveller, going somewhere and to some destination.

If I tell myself that the somewhere and the destination do not exist, that seems to me very reasonable and likely enough.

The brothel keeper, when he kicks anyone out, has similar logic, argues as well, and is always right, I know. So at the end of my course I shall find my mistake. Be it so. I shall find then that not only the Arts, but everything else as well, were only dreams, that one's self was nothing at all. If we are as *flimsy as that,* so much the better for us, for then there is nothing against the unlimited possibility of future existence. Whence comes it that, in the present instance of our uncle's death, the face of the dead was calm, peaceful, and grave, while it is a fact that while living he was scarcely like that, either in youth or age. I have often observed a like effect as I looked at the dead as though to question them. And that for me is *one* proof, though not the most serious, of a life beyond the grave.

And in the same way a child in the cradle, if you watch it at leisure, has the infinite in its eyes. In short, I know nothing about it, but it is just this feeling of *not knowing* that makes the real life we are actually living now like a one-way journey in a train. You go fast, but cannot distinguish any object very close up, and above all you do not see the engine.

It is rather curious that Uncle as well as Father believed in the future life. Not to mention Father, I have several times heard Uncle arguing about it.

Ah—but then, they were more assured than us, and were affirmers who got angry if you dared to go deeper.

Of the *future* life of artists *through their works* I do not think much. Yes, artists perpetuate themselves by handing on the torch, Delacroix to the impressionists, etc. But is that all?

If the kind old mother of a family, with ideas that are pretty well limited and tortured by the Christian system, is to be immortal as she believes, and seriously too—and I for one do not gainsay it—why should a consumptive or neurotic cab horse like Delacroix and de Goncourt, with broad ideas, be any less immortal?

Granted that it seems just that the most destitute should feel the most the springing of this unaccountable hope.

Enough. What is the good of worrying about it? But living in the full tide of civilization, of Paris, of the Arts, why should not one keep this "I" of the old women, if women themselves without their instinctive belief that "*so it is*," would not find strength to create or to act?

Then the doctors will tell us that not only Moses, Mahomet, Christ, Luther, Bunyan and others were mad, but also Frans Hals, Rembrandt, Delacroix, and also all the dear narrow old women like our mother.

Ah—that's a serious matter—one might ask these doctors; where then are the sane people?

Are they the brothel keepers who are always right? Probably. Then what to choose? Fortunately there is no choice.

With a handshake.

Yours,
Vincent

My dear Theo,   [Arles, mid August 1888]

You are shortly to make the acquaintance of Master Patience Escalier, a sort of "man with a hoe," formerly cowherd of the Camargue, now gardener at a house in the Crau. This very day I am sending you the drawing I have done after this painting, and also the drawing after the portrait of Roulin the postman. The colouring of this peasant portrait is not so black as in the "Potato Eaters" of Nuenen, but our highly civilized Parisian *Portier*—probably so called because he chucks pictures out[1]—will find himself blocked by the same old thing. You have changed since then, but you will see that he has not, and it really is a pity that there are not more *sabot* pictures[2] in Paris. I do not think it would be an affront to the Lautrec you have to put my peasant beside it, and I even am bold enough to hope that the Lautrec would show up still more distinguished in the simultaneous contrast, and that mine would gain by the odd juxtaposition, because that sun-steeped, sun-burnt quality, tanned and swept with air, would show up more beside that rice powder and elegance.

What a mistake that Parisians have not acquired a palate for crude things, for Monticellis, for earthenware. But there, one must not lose heart because Utopia is not coming true. It is only that what I learnt in Paris *is leaving me*, and that I am returning to the ideas I had in the country before I knew the impressionists. And I should not be surprised if the impressionists soon find fault with my way of working, for it has been fertilized by the ideas of Delacroix rather than by theirs. Because, instead of trying to reproduce exactly what I have before my eyes, I use colour more arbitrarily so as to express myself forcibly. Well, let that be as a matter of theory, but I am going to give you an example of what I mean.

I should like to paint the portrait of an artist friend,[3] a man who dreams great dreams, who works as the nightingale sings, because it is his nature. He'll be a fair man. I want to put into the picture my appreciation, the love that I have for him. So I paint him as he is, as faithfully as I can, to begin with.

But the picture is not finished yet. To finish it I am now going to be the arbitrary colourist. I exaggerate the fairness of the hair, I get to orange tones, chromes and pale lemon yellow.

Beyond the head, instead of painting the ordinary wall of

---

[1] The pun is based on the fact that *portier* means *doorman*.

[2] i.e. pictures of peasants in their working attire.

[3] This idea was to produce the *Poet* of early September, for which Bock served as the model.

the mean room, I paint infinity, a plain background of the richest, intensest blue that I can contrive, and by this simple combination the bright head illuminated against a rich blue background acquires a mysterious effect, like a star in the depths of an azure sky.

In the portrait of the peasant I again worked in this way, but without wishing in this case to evoke the mysterious brightness of a pale star in the infinite. Instead, I think of the man I have to paint, terrible in the furnace of the full ardours of harvest, at the heart of the south. Hence the orange shades like storm flashes, vivid as red hot iron, and hence the luminous tones of old gold in the shadows.

Oh, my dear boy . . . and the nice people will only see the exaggeration as caricature.

But what has that to do with us, we have read *La Terre* and *Germinal*,[1] and if we are painting a peasant we would like to show that what we have read has come in the end very near to being part of us.

I do not know if I can paint the postman *as I feel him,* this man is like old Tanguy in so far as he is revolutionary, he is probably thought a good republican because he wholeheartedly detests the republic which we now enjoy, and because by and large he begins to doubt, to be a little disillusioned, as to the republican principle itself.

But I once watched him sing the *Marseillaise,* and I thought I was watching '89, not next year, but that of 99 years ago. It was a Delacroix, a Daumier, a straight old Dutchman.

Unfortunately he is unable to pose, and yet to make a picture you must have an intelligent model.

And now I must tell you that these days, as far as material things go, are cruelly hard. Living, no matter what I do, is pretty dear here, almost like Paris, where you can spend 5 or 6 francs a day and have very little to show for it.

If I have models, I suffer for it a good deal. But it does not matter, and I am going to continue. And I can assure you that if you happened to send me a little extra money sometimes, it would benefit the pictures, but not me. The only

[1] Works by Zola.

choice I have is between being a good painter and a bad one.
I choose the first. But the needs of painting are like those of
a ruinous mistress, you can do nothing without money, and
you never have enough of it. That is why painting ought to
be done at the public expense, instead of the artists being
overburdened with it.

But there, we had better hold our tongues, because *no one
is forcing us to work,* indifference to painting being on fate's
decree widespread, and by way of being eternal.

Fortunately my digestion is so nearly all right again that I
have lived for three weeks in the month on ship's biscuits with
milk and eggs. It is the blessed warmth that is bringing back
my strength, and I was certainly right in going *at once* to the
south, instead of waiting until the evil was impossible to
remedy. Yes, really, I am as well as other men now, which
I have never been except momentarily at Nuenen for instance,
and it is rather pleasant. By other men I mean something like
the navvies, old Tanguy, old Millet, the peasants. If you are
well you must be able to live on a bit of bread while you are
working all day, and have enough strength to smoke and to
drink your whack at night, that's a necessary part of the thing.
And all the same to feel the stars and the infinite high and
clear above you. Then life is after all almost enchanted. Oh!
those who don't believe in this sun here are real infidels.

Unfortunately along with the good god sun three quarters
of the time there is this devil of a *mistral.*

Saturday's post has gone, damn it, and I never doubted but
I should get your letter. However you see I am not fretting
about it.

With a handshake.

Yours,
Vincent

My dear Theo,   [Arles, mid August 1888]
Thank you very much for sending me the canvas and
paints which have just arrived. This time there was 9.80 fr.
carriage to pay, so I shan't go and get them out till I get your

next letter, not having the cash at the moment. But we must make sure that Tasset, who generally pays the bill in advance and does not fail to note the prepayment on his account, has refrained this time. In the same way I paid on the *last but one* consignment 5.60 fr., so if cost of transport was put down on the last bill but one it would be an overcharge. If he had made two separate parcels (usually the cost of carriage is about 3 francs) we should only have had to pay 5.60 fr.

Now if on the 10 metres of canvas I paint only master-pieces half a metre in size and sell them cash down and at an exorbitant price to distinguished connoisseurs of the Rue de la Paix, nothing will be easier than to make a fortune on this consignment.

I think it is likely that we are going to have great heat now without wind, since the wind has been blowing for six weeks. If so, it is a very good thing that I have a supply of paints and canvas, because already I have my eye on half a dozen subjects, especially that little cottage garden I sent you the drawing of yesterday.

I am thinking about Gauguin a lot, and I am sure that in one way or another, whether it is he who comes here, or I who go to him, he and I will like practically the same subjects, and I have no doubt that I could work at Pont-Aven,[1] and on the other hand I am convinced that he would tremendously like the country down here. Well, at the end of a year, sup-posing he gives you one canvas a month, which would make altogether a dozen per year, he will have made money on it, assuming that during the year he has not incurred any debts and has worked steadily without interruption; certainly he won't have been the loser, while the money which he will have had from us would be largely made good by the economies that will be possible if we set up house in the studio instead of both of us living in cafés. Besides that, provided we keep on good terms and are determined not to quarrel, we shall be in a stronger position as far as reputation goes.

If we each live alone it means living like madmen or criminals, in appearance at any rate, and also a little in reality.

[1] The locale in Brittany where Gauguin was based at the time.

I am happier to feel my old strength returning than I ever thought I could be. I owe this largely to the people of the restaurant where I have my meals at the moment, who really are extraordinary. Certainly I have to pay for it, but it is something you don't find in Paris, that you really do get something to eat for your money.

And I would very much like to see Gauguin here for a good long time.

What Gruby says about the benefit of doing without women and eating well is true, for if your very brain and marrow are going into your work, it is pretty logical not to expend yourself more than you must in love-making. But it is easier to put into practice in the country than in Paris.

The desire for women that you catch in Paris, isn't it somewhat the effect of that very enervation of which Gruby is the sworn enemy, rather than a sign of vigour? So one feels this desire disappearing just at the moment that one is one's self again. The root of the evil lies in the constitution itself, in the fatal weakening of families from generation to generation, and besides that, in one's unwholesome job and the dreary life of Paris. The root of the evil certainly lies there, and there's no cure for it.

I think that when the day comes that you get free of those futile accounts and the absurdly complicated management at Goupil's, you would gain enormously in influence with the collectors; these complicated systems of management are the very devil, and I think that no brain exists, no temperament, whoever the man on the job is, but loses 50% over it. Our uncle was quite right in what he said about it; a big concern with a few men in on it, and not a little concern with a lot in on it. Unluckily for him he was himself caught in the wheels.

This job of working among people so as to make sales is a job that needs observation and coolness. But if you are forced to give too much attention to the books, you lose some of your poise.

I do want to know exactly how you are. Anyway, provided the impressionists produce good stuff and make friends, there

is always the chance and the possibility of a more independent
position for you later on. It's a pity that it cannot be from
now on.

No letter from Russell yet, but now that he must have got
the drawings he is bound to reply.

This restaurant where I am is very queer; it is completely
grey; the floor is of grey bitumen like a street pavement,
grey paper on the walls, green blinds always drawn, a big
green curtain in front of the door which is always open, to
stop the dust coming in. Just as it is it is a Velasquez grey—
like in the *Spinning Women*—and the very narrow, very
fierce ray of sunlight through a blind, like the one that
crosses Velasquez's picture, even that is not wanting. Little
tables, of course, with white cloths. And behind this room,
in Velasquez grey you see the old kitchen, as clean as a
Dutch kitchen, with floor of bright red bricks, green vegetables, oak chest, the kitchen range with shining brass things
and blue and white tiles, and the big fire a clear orange.
And then there are two women who wait, both in grey, a little
like that picture of Prévost's you have in your place—you
could compare it point for point.

In the kitchen, an old woman and a short, fat servant also
in grey, black, white. I don't know if I describe it clearly
enough to you, but it's here, and it's pure Velasquez.

In front of the restaurant there is a covered court, paved
with red brick, and on the walls wild vine, convolvulus and
creepers.

It is the real old Provençal still, while the other restaurants
are so much modelled on Paris that *even when they have no
kind of concierge whatever,* there's his booth just the same and
the notice " Apply to the Concierge ! "

It isn't always all vibrant here. Thus I saw a stable with
four coffee-coloured cows, and a calf of the same colour. The
stable bluish white hung with spiders' webs, the cows very
clean and very beautiful, and a great green curtain in the
doorway to keep out flies and dust.

Grey again—Velasquez's grey.

There was such quiet in it—the café au lait and tobacco

colour of the cows' hides, with the soft bluish grey white of the walls, the green hanging and the sparkling sunny golden-green outside to make a startling contrast. So you see there's something still to be done, quite different from anything I have done up to now.

I must go and work. I saw another very quiet and lovely thing the other day, a girl with a coffee-tinted skin if I remember rightly, ash blond hair, grey eyes, a print bodice of pale rose under which you could see the breasts, shapely, firm and small. This against the emerald leaves of some fig trees. A woman of the real country sort, every line of her virgin.

It isn't altogether impossible that I shall get her to pose in the open air, and her mother too—a gardener's wife—earth coloured, dressed just then in soiled yellow and faded blue.

The girl's coffee-tinted complexion was darker than the rose of her bodice.

The mother was stunning, the figure in dirty yellow and faded blue thrown up in strong sunlight against a square of brilliant flowers, snow white and lemon-yellow. A perfect Van der Meer[1] of Delft, you see.

It's not a bad place, the south. A handshake.

Yours,
Vincent

My dear Theo,   [Arles, late August 1888]

I write in great haste, to tell you that I have had a note from Gauguin to say that he has not written much, but that he is quite ready to come south as soon as the opportunity occurs.

They are enjoying themselves very much painting, arguing, and fighting with the worthy English; he speaks well of Bernard's work, and B. speaks well of Gauguin's.

I am hard at it, painting with the enthusiasm of a Marseillais eating bouillabaisse, which won't surprise you when you know that what I'm at is the painting of some great sunflowers.

[1] More correctly Vermeer.

I have three canvases in hand—1st, three huge flowers in a green vase, with a light background, a canvas of size 15; 2nd, three flowers, one gone to seed, stripped of its petals, and another in bud against a royal blue background, canvas of size 25; 3rd, twelve flowers and buds in a yellow vase (canvas of size 30). The last is therefore light on light, and I hope will be the best. I probably shall not stop at that.[1] Now that I hope to live with Gauguin in a studio of our own, I want to make a decoration for the studio. Nothing but big sunflowers. Next door to your shop, in the restaurant, you know there is a lovely decoration of flowers; I always remember the big sunflower in the window there.

If I carry out this idea there will be a dozen panels. So the whole thing will be a symphony in blue and yellow. I am working at it every morning from sunrise, for the flowers fade so soon, and the thing is to do the whole at one go.

You were quite right to tell Tasset that he must give us some tubes of colour for the 15 francs carriage not prepaid on the two parcels. When I have finished these sunflowers I may need yellow and blue perhaps. If so I will send a small order to that effect. I very much like the ordinary canvas from Tasset which was 50 centimes dearer than Bourgeois's, it is very well prepared.

I am very glad that G. is well.

I am beginning to like the south more and more.

I have another study of dusty thistles on hand, with an innumerable swarm of white and yellow butterflies.

I have again missed some models which I had hoped to have over the last few days. Koning has written saying that he is going to live in The Hague, and that he means to send you some studies.

I have heaps of ideas for new canvases. I saw again to-day the same coal boat with the workmen unloading it that I told you about before, at the same place as the boats carrying sand of which I sent you the drawing. It would be a splendid subject. Only I am beginning more and more to try for a simple technique which is not perhaps impressionist. I would like

[1] In fact he was to do two more.

to paint in such a way that everybody, at least if they had eyes, would see it. I am writing in a hurry, but I wanted to send a line enclosed to our sister.

A handshake, I must get back to work.

Yours,

Vincent

Gauguin said that Bernard had made an album of my sketches and had shown it to him.

My dear Theo,   [Arles, early September 1888]

I spent yesterday with the Belgian[1] again, who also has a sister among the " Vingtistes."[2] It was not fine, but a very good day for talking; we went for a walk and anyway saw some very fine things at the bull fight and outside the town. We talked more seriously about the plan, that if I keep a place in the south, he ought to set up a sort of post among the collieries. Then Gauguin and I and he, if the importance of a picture made it worth the journey, could change places—and so be sometimes in the north, but in familiar country with a friend in it, and sometimes in the south.

You will soon see him, this young man with the look of Dante, because he is going to Paris, and if you put him up—if the room is free—you will be doing him a good turn; he is very distinguished in appearance, and will become so, I think, in his painting.

He likes Delacroix, and we talked a lot about Delacroix yesterday. He even knew the violent study for the " Bark of Christ."[3] Well, thanks to him I have at last a first sketch of that picture which I have dreamt of for so long—the poet. He posed for me. His fine head with that keen gaze stands out in my portrait against a starry sky of deep ultramarine; for clothes, a short yellow coat, a collar of unbleached linen, and spotted tie. He gave me two sittings in one day.

Yesterday I had a letter from our sister, who has seen a

[1] Bock.
[2] A group of artists which organised exhibitions in Brussels.
[3] " Christ on the Lake of Gennaseret."

great deal. Ah, if she could marry an artist it would not be so bad. Well, we must go on inducing her to develop her personality rather than her artistic abilities.

I have finished *L'Immortel* by Daudet. I rather like the saying of the sculptor Védrine, that to achieve *fame* is something like ramming the lighted end of your cigar into your mouth when you are smoking. But I certainly like *L'Immortel* less, far less than *Tartarin*.

You know, it seems to me that *L'Immortel* is not so fine in colour as *Tartarin*, because it reminds me with its mass of true and subtle observations of the dreary pictures of Jean Bérend which are so dry and cold. Now *Tartarin* is *really great*, with the greatness of a masterpiece, just like *Candide*.

I do strongly ask you to keep my studies of this place as open to the air as possible, because they are not yet thoroughly dry. If they remain shut up or in the dark the colours will get devalued. So the portrait of "The Young Girl," "The Harvest" (a wide landscape with the ruin in the background and the line of the Alpilles), the little "Seascape," the "Garden" with the weeping tree and clumps of conifers, if you could put these on stretchers it would be well. I am rather keen on those. You will easily see by the *drawing* of the little seascape that it is the most thought out.

I am having two oak frames made for my new peasant's head and for my Poet study. Oh, my dear boy, sometimes I know so well what I want. I can very well do without God both in my life and in my painting, but I cannot, ill as I am, do without something which is greater than I, which is my life—the power to create.

And if, defrauded of the power to create physically, a man tries to create thoughts in place of children, he is still very much part of humanity.

And in a picture I want to say something comforting as music is comforting. I want to paint men and women with that something of the eternal which the halo used to symbolize, and which we seek to confer by the actual radiance and vibration of our colourings.

Portraiture so understood does not become like an Ary

Scheffer, just because there is a blue sky behind as in the " St. Augustine." For Ary Scheffer is so little of a colourist.

But it would be more in harmony with what Eug. Delacroix attempted and brought off in his " Tasso in Prison,"[1] and many other pictures, representing a *real* man. Ah! portraiture, portraiture with the thought, the soul of the model in it, that is what I think must come.

The Belgian and I talked a lot yesterday about the advantages and disadvantages of this place. We quite agree regarding both. And on the great advantage it would be to us if we could *move* now north, now south.

He is going to stay with McKnight again so as to live more cheaply. That, however, has I think one disadvantage, because living with a slacker makes one slack.

I think you would enjoy meeting him, he is still young. I think he will ask your advice about buying Japanese prints and Daumier lithographs. As to these—the Daumiers—it would be well to get some more of them, because later there will be none to be got.

The Belgian was saying that he paid 80 francs for board and lodging with McKnight. So what a difference there is in living together, since I have to pay 45 a month for nothing but lodging. And so I always come back to the same reckoning, that with Gauguin I should not spend more than I do alone, and be no worse off. But we must consider that they were very badly housed, not for sleeping, but for the possibility of work at home.

So I am always between two currents of thought, first the material difficulties, turning round and round to make a living; and second, the study of colour. I am always in hope of making a discovery there, to express the love of two lovers by a marriage of two complementary colours, their mingling and their opposition, the mysterious vibrations of kindred tones. To express the thought of a brow by the radiance of a light tone against a sombre background.

To express hope by some star, the eagerness of a soul by

[1] " Tasso in the Madhouse " is the normal title.

a sunset radiance. Certainly there is nothing in that of trompe l'œil realism, but is it not something that actually exists?

Goodbye for the present. I will tell you another time when the Belgian may be going through, because I shall see him again tomorrow.

With a handshake,

Yours,

Vincent

The Belgian says that his people at home have a de Groux, the study for the "Benedicité" in the Brussels Museum.

The portrait of the Belgian is something like the portrait of Reid which you have, in execution.

My dear Theo,   [Arles, September 8 1888]

Thank you a thousand times for your kind letter and the 300 francs it contained; after some worrying weeks I have just had a much better one. And just as worries do not come singly, neither do the joys. For just because I am always bowed down under this difficulty of paying my landlords, I made up my mind to take it gaily. I swore at the said landlord, who after all isn't a bad fellow, and told him that to revenge myself for paying him so much money for nothing, I would paint the whole of his rotten shanty so as to repay myself. Then to the great joy of the landlord, of the postman whom I had already painted, of the visiting night prowlers, and of myself, for three nights running I sat up to paint and went to bed during the day. I often think that the night is more alive and more richly coloured than the day. Now, as for getting back the money I have paid to the landlord by my painting, I do not dwell on that, for the picture[1] is one of the ugliest I have done. It is the equivalent, though different, of the "Potato Eaters."

I have tried to express the terrible passions of humanity by means of red and green.

The room is blood red and dark yellow with a green

[1] The *Night Café*.

billiard table in the middle; there are four lemon-yellow lamps
with a glow of orange and green. Everywhere there is a clash
and contrast of the most alien reds and greens, in the figures
of little sleeping hooligans, in the empty dreary room, in
violet and blue. The blood-red and the yellow-green of the
billiard table, for instance, contrast with the soft tender Louis
XV green of the counter, on which there is a rose nosegay.
The white clothes of the landlord, on vigil in a corner of this
furnace, turn lemon-yellow, or pale luminous green.

I am making a drawing of it with the tones in water-
colour to send to you to-morrow, to give you some idea of it.

I wrote this week to Gauguin and Bernard, but I did not
talk about anything but pictures, just so as not to quarrel when
there is probably nothing to quarrel about.

But whether Gauguin comes or not, if I were to get some
furniture, henceforth I should have, whether in a good spot
or a bad one is another matter, a pied à terre, a home of my
own, which frees the mind from the dismalness of finding
oneself in the streets. That is nothing when you are an
adventurer of 20, but it is bad when you have turned 35.

To-day in the *Intransigeant* I noticed the suicide of M.
Bing Levy. It can't be the Levy, Bing's manager, can it?[1] I
think it must be someone else.

I am greatly pleased that Pissarro thought something of
the " Young Girl." Did Pissarro say anything about the
" Sower "? Afterwards, when I have gone further in these
experiments, the " Sower " will still be the first attempt in
that style. The " Night Café " carries on from the " Sower,"
and so also do the head of the old peasant and of the poet, if
I manage to do this latter picture.[2]

It is colour not locally true from the point of view of the
trompe l'œil realist, but colour to suggest some emotion of an
ardent temperament.

[1] Bing managed a gallery in Paris specialising in Oriental art,
which Vincent had much frequented.
[2] What Vincent had completed so far was only the study, and
not the final version; he did make an attempt at the latter, but subsequently destroyed the result.

L.V.G.   K

When Paul Mantz saw at the exhibition the violent an inspired sketch by Delacroix that we saw at the Champ Elysées—the "Bark of Christ"—he turned away from i exclaiming in his article: "I did not know that one could b so terrible with a little blue and green."

Hokusai wrings the same cry from you, but he does it b his *line*, his *drawing*; as you say in your letter—"the wave are *claws* and the ship is caught in them, you feel it."

Well, if you make the colour exact or the drawing exac it won't give you sensations like that.

Anyhow, very soon, to-morrow or next day, I will write t you again about this and answer your letter, and send you th sketch of the "Night Café."

Tasset's parcel has arrived. I will write to-morrow on th' question of the coarse grained colour. Milliet[1] is coming to se you and pay his respects to you one of these days, he writes t me that he is coming back. Thank you again for the mone you sent. If I went first to look for another place, would not very likely mean fresh expense, equal at least to th expense of a removal? And then should I find anythin better all at once? I am so very glad to be able to do th furnishing, and it can't but help me on. Many thanks ther and a good handshake, till tomorrow.

Yours,

Vincent

My dear Theo,   [Arles, end of September 1888

The fine weather of the last few days has gone and instea we have mud and rain, but it will certainly come back agai before the winter.

Only the thing will be to make use of it, because the fin days are short. Especially for painting. This winter I inten to draw a great deal. If only I could manage to draw figure from memory, I should always have something to do. But i you take the cleverest figure of all the artists who sketch o

[1] The lieutenant of the Zouave regiment who had been quartere at Arles.

he spur of the moment, Hokusai, Daumier, in my opinion
hat figure will never come up to the figure painted from the
1odel by those same masters, or other portrait painters.

And in the end, if models, especially intelligent models,
re doomed to fail us too often, we must not despair for this
eason or grow weary in the struggle.

I have arranged in the studio all the Japanese prints and
he Daumiers, and the Delacroixs and the Géricaults. If you
nd the " Pietà " by Delacroix again or the Géricault I
trongly advise you to get as many of them as you can. What
should love to have in the studio as well is Millet's " Work
1 the Fields," and Lerat's etching of his " Sower " which
Durand-Ruel sells at 1.25 francs. And lastly the little etching
y Jacquemart after Meissonier, the " Man Reading," a
Meissonier that I have always admired. I cannot help liking
Meissonier's things.

I am reading an article in the *Revue des deux Mondes* on
Tolstoi. It appears that Tolstoi is enormously interested in
he religion of his race, like George Eliot in England.

There must be a book of Tolstoi's about religion. I think it
s called *My Religion,* it must be very fine. In it he is trying
o find, so I understand from this article, what remains etern-
lly true in the religion of Christ, and what all religions have
n common. It appears that he does not admit the resurrec-
ion of the body, or even of the soul, but says, like the
iihilists, that after death there is nothing more, yet with the
nan dead, and thoroughly dead, humanity, living humanity
bides.

Anyway, not having read the book itself, I cannot say
1ow exactly he understands the matter, but I think that his
eligion cannot be a cruel one which would increase our
ufferings, but that on the contrary it must be very comfort-
ng, and would inspire serenity and energy and courage to
ive and heaps of things.

I think the drawing of the " Blade of Grass " and the
arnations and the Hokusai in Bing's reproductions are *admir-
ble.*

But whatever you say, the most common prints coloured

with a flat wash are admirable to me for the same reaso
as Rubens and Veronese. I know perfectly well that the
are not true primitive art. But because the primitives[1] a
admirable, that is no reason whatever for me to say, as it
becoming the fashion to do, " When I go to the Louvre,
cannot get beyond the primitives."

If one said to a *serious* collector of Japanese prints,
Levy himself, " My dear sir, I cannot help admiring the
prints at 5 sous," he would more than likely be rather shocke
and would pity one for one's ignorance and bad taste. Ju
as formerly it appeared bad taste to like Rubens, Jordaen
and Veronese.

I think I shall end by not feeling lonesome in the hous
and that during the bad days in the winter for instanc
and the long evenings, I shall find some occupation that wi
take all my attention. Weavers and basket makers ofte
spend whole seasons alone or almost alone, with their occupa
tion for their only distraction.

But what makes these people stay in one place is precise
the feeling of domesticity, the *reassuring familiar look*
things. I should certainly like company, but if I have not g
it, I shall not be unhappy because of that, and then too th
time will come when I shall have someone. I have litt
doubt of it. I think that if you were willing to put peopl
up in your house too, you would find plenty among th
artists for whom the question of lodgings is a very seriov
problem. For my part I think that it is absolutely my dut
to try to make money by my work, and so I see my wor
very clear before me.

Oh, if only every artist had something to live on, and t
work on, but as that is not so, I want to produce, to produc
a lot and with a consuming drive. And perhaps the tim
will come when we can extend our business and be mor
help to the others.

[1] At the period this was a blanket term for the earlier Italia
schools, prior to Raphael, and for Flemish art of the fifteent
century.

But that is a long way off and there is a lot of work to get through first.

If you lived in time of war, you might possibly have to fight, you would regret it, you would lament that you weren't living in times of peace, but after all the necessity would be here and you would fight.

And in the same way we certainly have the right to wish for a state of things in which money would not be necessary in order to live. However, as everything is done by money now, one has got to think about making it so long as one spends it, but I have more chance of making it by painting than by drawing.

On the whole there are a good many more people who can do clever sketches than there are who can paint readily and can get at nature through colour. That will always be rarer, and whether the pictures are a long time in being appreciated or not, they will find a collector some day.

But about those pictures in rather thick impasto, I think they must be left longer *here* to dry. I have read that the Rubenses in Spain have remained infinitely richer in colour than those in the North. Ruins exposed to the open air remain white here, while in the north they become grey, dirty, black, etc. You may be sure that if the Monticellis had dried in Paris they would now be much duller. I am beginning now to see the beauty of the women here better, and then again and again I think afresh of Monticelli. Colour plays such a tremendous part in the beauty of the women here. I do not say that their shape is not beautiful, but it is not there that the special charm is found. That lies in the grand lines of the costume, vivid in colour and admirably carried, the *tone* of the flesh rather than the shape. But I shall have some trouble before I can do them as I begin to see them. Yet what I am sure of is that to stay here is to go forward. And to make a picture which will be really of the south, it's not enough to have a certain dexterity. It is looking at things for a long time that ripens you and gives you a deeper understanding. I did not think when I left Paris that I should ever find Monticelli and Delacroix so *true*. It is only now

after months and months that I begin to realize that the
did not imagine any of it. And I think that next year yo
are going to see the same subjects over again, orchards, an
harvest, but with a different colouring, and above all
change in the workmanship.

And these shifts and variations will always go on.

I feel that while going on working I must not hurr
After all, how would it be to put in practice the old saying—
you must study for ten years, and then produce a few figure
That is what Monticelli did, however, not counting some
his pictures as studies.

But then figures such as the woman in yellow, and th
woman with the parasol—the little one you have, and th
lovers that Reid had, those are complete figure studies
which as far as the drawing goes there is nothing left but
praise. For in them Monticelli achieves a sweeping, magn
ficent drawing like Daumier and Delacroix. Certainly co
sidering the price Monticellis are at, it would be an excelle
speculation to buy some. The time will come when h
beautifully *drawn* figures will be considered very great art.

I think that the town of Arles was infinitely more glorio
once as regards the beauty of its women and the beauty of i
costumes. Now everything has a worn and sickly look abo
it.

But when you look at it for long, the old charm revives.

And that is why I see that I lose absolutely nothing l
staying where I am and being content to watch things pass,
a spider waits in its web for the flies. I cannot force an
thing, and now that I am settled in I can profit by all the fir
days, and every opportunity for snatching a good picture fro
time to time.

Milliet has luck, he has as many Arlésiennes as he want
but then he cannot paint them, and if he were a painter h
would not get them. I must bide my time without rushin
things.

I have read another article on Wagner—" Love in Music
—I think by the same author who wrote the book on Wagne
How one needs the same thing in painting.

It seems that in the book, *My Religion,* Tolstoi implies that whatever happens in the way of violent revolution there will also be a private and secret revolution in men, from which a new religion will be reborn, or rather something altogether new, which will have no name, but which will have the same effect of consoling, of making life possible, which the Christian religion used to have.

It seems to me that the book ought to be very interesting. We shall end by having had enough cynicism and scepticism and humbug, and we shall want to live more musically. How will that come to pass, and what will we really find? It would be interesting to be able to predict, but it is better still to be able to feel that kind of foreshadowing, instead of seeing absolutely nothing in the future beyond the disasters that are all the same bound to fall like terrible lightning on the modern world and on civilization, through a revolution or war, or the bankruptcy of worm-eaten states. If we study Japanese art, we see a man who is undoubtedly wise, philosophic and intelligent, who spends his time how? In studying the distance between the earth and the moon? No. In studying the policy of Bismarck? No. He studies a single blade of grass.

But this blade of grass leads him to draw every plant and then the seasons, the wide aspects of the countryside, then animals, then the human figure. So he passes his life, and life is too short to do the whole.

Come now, isn't it almost an actual religion which these simple Japanese teach us, who live in nature as though they themselves were flowers?

And you cannot study Japanese art, it seems to me, without becoming much gayer and happier, and we must return to nature in spite of our education and our work in a world of convention.

Isn't it sad that the Monticellis have never yet been reproduced in good lithographs or vivid etchings? I would very much like to see what artists would say if an engraver like the man who engraved the Velasquez made a fine etching from them. Never mind, I think it is more our job to try to admire and know things for ourselves, than to teach them other people. But the two can go together.

I envy the Japanese the extreme clearness which everythir has in their work. It is never wearisome, and never seems be done too hurriedly. Their work is as simple as breathin, and they do a figure in a few sure strokes with the same ea as if it were as simple as buttoning your waistcoat.

Oh! I must manage somehow to do a figure in a fe strokes. That will keep me busy all the winter. Once I can that, I shall be able to do people walking the boulevards, alor the streets, and heaps of new subjects. While I have bee writing this letter I have drawn about a dozen. I am on th track of it, but it is very complicated because what I am afte is that in a few strokes the figure of a man, a woman, youngster, a horse, a dog, shall have head, body, legs, arm all in keeping.

Good-bye for the present and a good handshake from

Yours,

Vincent

Mme. de Lareby Laroquette said to me once—" But Mont celli, Monticelli, why he was a man who ought to have bee at the head of a great studio in the south."

I wrote to our sister and to you the other day, yo remember, that sometimes I thought that I was the continua tion of Monticelli here. Well, you see it happening now, tha studio in question, we are founding it. What Gauguin doe what I do, will be in line with that fine work of Monticelli' and we will try to prove to the good folk that Monticelli di not wholly die sprawled over the café tables of the Canne bière, but the good old chap's still alive. And the thing won even end with us, we shall set it going on a pretty solid basi

My dear Theo,   [Arles, mid October 1888

At last I am sending you a small sketch to give you at leas an idea of the form which the work is taking. For today am all right again. My eyes are still tired, but then I had new idea in my head and here is the sketch of it. Another canvas of size 30. This time it's just simply my bedroom, only here colour is to do everything, and giving by its simplification a grander style to things, is to be suggestive here of *rest* or of sleep in general. In a word, to look at the picture ought to rest the brain or rather the imagination.

The walls are pale violet. The floor is of red tiles.

The wood of the bed and chairs is the yellow of fresh butter, the sheet and pillows very light lemon-green.

The coverlet scarlet. The window green.

The toilet table orange, the basin blue.

The doors lilac.

And that is all—there is nothing in this room with closed shutters.

The broad lines of the furniture must again express inviolable rest. Portraits on the walls, and a mirror and a towel and some clothes.

The frame—as there is no white in the picture—will be white.

This by way of revenge for the enforced rest I have been obliged to take.

I shall work at it again all day tomorrow, but you see how simple the conception is. The shadows and the thrown shadows are suppressed, it is coloured in free flat tones like Japanese prints. It is going to be a contrast with, for instance, the Tarascon diligence and the night café.

I am not writing you a long letter, because tomorrow very early I am going to begin in the cool morning light, so as to finish my canvas.

How are the pains? Do not forget to tell me about them.

I hope that you will write one of these days.

I will make you sketches of the other rooms too some day. With a good handshake,

Yours,
Vincent

My dear Theo,   [Arles, early November 1888]
   Gauguin and I[1] thank you very much for the 100 fr. you
sent and also for your letter.

   Gauguin is very pleased that you like what he sent from
Brittany, and that other people who have seen them like them
too.

   Just now he has in hand some women in a vineyard,
altogether from memory, but if he does not spoil it or leave it
unfinished it will be very fine and very unusual. Also a picture of the same night café that I painted too.[2]

   I have done two canvases of falling leaves, which Gauguin
liked, I think, and I'm working now on a vineyard all purple
and yellow.[3]

   Then I have an Arlésienne at last, a figure (size 30 canvas)
slashed on in an hour, background pale lemon, the face grey,
the clothes black, deep black, with perfectly raw Prussian
blue. She is leaning on a green table and seated in an arm-
chair of orange wood.[4]

   Gauguin has bought a chest of drawers for the house, and
various household utensils, also 20 metres of very strong
canvas, and a lot of things that we needed, and that at any
rate it was more convenient to have. Only we have kept an
account of all he has paid out, which comes almost to 100
francs, so that either at the New Year or say in March we
can pay him back, and then the chest of drawers etc. will
naturally be ours.

   I think this is right on the whole, since he intends to put

   [1] Gauguin had finally arrived at Arles on October 23rd; he had
sent off a number of works to Theo before leaving Pont-Aven, in
preparation for a one-man show at the Goupil Gallery which was
to open shortly.
   [2] That is, the canvas called *The Vineyard* or *Human Miseries,* now
in the Ordrupgaard Collection in Denmark; and the *Night Café* now
in Moscow.
   [3] The *Red Vineyard,* the only canvas that Vincent ever sold.
   [4] This was a portrait of his friend Mme. Ginoux.

money by when he sells, till the time (say in a year) when he has enough to risk a second voyage to Martinique.[1]

We are working hard, and our life together goes very well. I am very glad to know that you are not alone in the flat. These drawings by de Haan are *very fine,* I like them very much. Yet to do that with colour, to manage so much expression without the help of chiaroscuro in black and white, damn it all, it is not easy. And he will even arrive at *a new type of drawing* if he carries out his plan of passing through impressionism *as a school,* considering his new attempts in colour merely as studies. But in my opinion he is right over and over again to do all this.

Only there are several so-called impressionists who have not his knowledge of the figure, and it is just this knowledge of the figure which will later on come again to the surface, and which he will be all the better for. I am very anxious some day to get to know de Haan and Isaäcson. If they ever came here Gauguin would certainly say to them—go to Java for impressionist work. For Gauguin though he works hard here is still homesick for hot countries. And then it is unquestionable that if you went to Java, for instance, with the one idea of working on colour, you would see heaps of new things. Then in those brighter countries, with a stronger sun, direct shadow, as well as the cast shadow of objects and figures, becomes quite different, and is so full of colour that one is tempted simply to suppress it. That happens even here. Yet I will say no more on the importance of painting in the tropics, I am already sure de Haan and Isaäcson will feel the importance of it.

In any case, to come here some time or other would do them no harm, they would certainly find some interesting things.

Gauguin and I are going to have our dinner at home to-day, and we feel as sure and certain that it will turn out well as that it will seem to us better or cheaper.

So as not to delay this letter I will finish up for today. I

[1] The first such expedition had been undertaken the previous year.

hope to write again soon. Your arrangement about money is quite right.

I think you will like the fall of the leaves that I have done.

It is some poplar trunks in lilac cut by the frame where the leaves begin.

These tree-trunks are lined like pillars along an avenue where to right and left there are rows of old Roman tombs of a blue lilac.[1] And then the soil is covered, as with a carpet, by a thick layer of yellow and orange fallen leaves. And they are still falling like flakes of snow.

And in the avenue little black figures of lovers. The upper part of the picture is a bright green meadow, and no sky or almost none.

The second canvas is the same avenue but with an old fellow and a woman as fat and round as a ball.

But if only you had been with us on Sunday, when we saw a red vineyard, all red like red wine. In the distance it turned to yellow, and then a green sky with the sun, the earth after the rain violet, sparkling yellow here and there where it caught the reflection of the setting sun.

A handshake in thought from both of us, goodbye for the present, I will write again as soon as I can, and to our Dutchmen too.[2]

Yours,
Vincent

My dear Theo,   [Arles, second half of December 1888]
Gauguin and I went yesterday to Montpellier to see the museum there and especially the Brias room.[3] There are a lot of portraits of Brias, by Delacroix, Ricard, Courbet, Cabanel, Couture, Verdier, Tassaert, and others. Then there are pictures by Delacroix, Courbet, Giotto, Paul Potter, Botticelli, Th. Rousseau, very fine. Brias was a benefactor of artists, I shall say no more to you than that. In the portrait

---

[1] The Alyscamps at Arles.   [2] The two artists staying with Theo.
[3] Alfred Bruyas (or Brias) had left his personal collection to the Museum.

by Delacroix he is a gentleman with red beard and hair, confoundedly like you or me, and made me think of that poem
by de Musset—"*Partout ou j'ai touché la terre—un mal-
heureux vêtu de noir, auprès de nous venait s'asseoir, qui nous
regardait comme un frère.*"[1] It would have the same effect on
you, I am sure. Please do go to that bookshop where they
sell the lithographs by past and present artists, and see if you
could get, not too dear, the lithograph after Delacroix's
"Tasso in the Madhouse," since I think the figure there must
have some affinity with this fine portrait of Brias.

They have got some more Delacroixs, the study of a
"Mulatto Woman" (which Gauguin copied once),[2] the
"Odalisques," "Daniel in the Lions' Den"; and by Courbet:
first, the "Village Girls," magnificent, a woman seen from
behind, another lying on the ground in a landscape; second,
the "Woman Spinning," superb, and a whole heap more of
Courbet's. But after all you must know this collection exists,
or else know people who have seen it, and consequently be
able to talk about it. So I shan't say more about the museum
(except the Barye drawings and bronzes).

Gauguin and I talked a lot about Delacroix, Rembrandt,
etc. Our arguments are *terribly electric,* we come out of them
sometimes with our heads as exhausted as an electric battery
after it has run down. We were in the midst of magic, for
as Fromentin well says : Rembrandt is above all else a magician.

I tell you this in connection with our Dutch friends de
Haan and Isaäcson, who have so sought after and loved
Rembrandt, so as to encourage you all to pursue your
researches.

You must not be discouraged in them.

You know the strange and magnificent "Portrait of a
Man," by Rembrandt, in the Lacaze Gallery. I said to Gauguin that I myself saw in it a certain likeness in family or in

[1] "Wherever I touched the earth, a wretch clad in black came and
sat by us, scanning us like a brother."

[2] On an earlier visit to the museum, probably in 1883; this copy
has in fact recently come to light afresh.

race to Delacroix or to Gauguin himself. I do not know why, but I always call this portrait " The Traveller," or " The Man Come from Far." It is a similar and parallel idea to the one I've already spoken to you about, that I always look on the portrait of old Six, the fine portrait of the " Man with a Glove," as you in the future, and the etching by Rembrandt, " Six reading near a window in a shaft of sunlight," as you in the past and present. This is how things stand.[1] Gauguin was saying to me this morning when I asked him how he felt " that he felt his old self coming back," which gave me enormous pleasure. When I came here myself last winter, tired out and almost stunned in mind, before ever being able to begin to recover I had a strain of inward suffering too.

I do wish that some day you could see this Montpellier Museum—there are some very fine things.

Say to Degas that Gauguin and I have been to see the portrait of Brias by Delacroix at Montpellier, for we must make bold to believe that *what is is,* and the portrait of Brias by Delacroix is as like you and me as a new brother.

As for founding a way of life for artists chumming it together, you see such queer things, and I will wind up with what you are always saying—time will show. You can say all that to our friends Isaäcson and de Haan, and even boldly read them this letter. I should have written to them already if I had felt the necessary electric force.

A good hearty handshake all round from Gauguin as from me.

Yours,
Vincent

If you should be thinking that Gauguin and I have facility in our work, I assure you that work does not always come easy, and that our Dutch friends may get no more discouraged than we do in their difficulties is my wish both for them and for you.

---

[1] Gauguin had been sick in the last few weeks with some disorder of the digestive system, and had written to Theo announcing that it was necessary for him to leave Arles, since he and Vincent could not get along together.

My dear Theo,   [Arles, about December 23 1888]

Thank you very much for your letter, for the 100 fr. note enclosed and also for the 50 fr. order.

I think myself that Gauguin was a little out of sorts with the good town of Arles, the little yellow house where we work, and especially with me.[1]

As a matter of fact there are bound to be for him as for me further grave difficulties to overcome here.

But these difficulties are rather within ourselves than outside.

Altogether I think that either he will definitely go, or else definitely stay.

Before doing anything I told him to think it over and reckon things up again.

Gauguin is very powerful, strongly creative, but just because of that he must have peace.

Will he find it anywhere if he does not find it here?

I am waiting for him to make a decision with absolute serenity.

A good handshake.

                                                Vincent

[On the following day, December 24th, a telegram arrived from Gauguin that called Theo to Arles. Vincent, in a state of terrible excitement and high fever, had cut off a piece of his own ear, and brought it as a gift to a woman in a brothel. There had been a violent scene; Roulin the postman managed to get him home, but the police intervened, found Vincent bleeding and unconscious in bed, and sent him to the hospital. Theo found him there, " poor fighter and poor poor sufferer," and stayed over Christmas. Gauguin went back with Theo to Paris. By December 31st the news was better, and on the 1st, Vincent wrote this letter in pencil.]

[1] Gauguin had written to Theo that Vincent and he could not go on living together " in consequence of incompatibility of temper." The quarrel was made up, and Gauguin wrote another letter, speaking of the first as a bad dream.

My dear lad, [Arles, about January 1 1889]

I hope that Gauguin will completely reassure you, and a bit about the painting business too.

I expect to begin work again soon.

The charwoman and my friend Roulin had taken care of the house, and had put everything in order.

When I come out I shall be able to take the little old road here again, and soon the fine weather will be coming and I shall begin again on the orchards in bloom.

My dear lad, I am so terribly *distressed* at your journey. I should have wished you had been spared that, for after all no harm came to me, and there was no reason why you should put yourself to that trouble.

I cannot tell you how glad I am that you have made peace, and even more than that, with the Bongers.[1]

Say that to André from me, and give him my cordial regards.

What would I not have given for you to have seen Arles when it was fine, as it is you have seen it looking dismal.

However, keep good heart, address letters direct to me at Place Lamartine 2. I will send Gauguin's pictures that are still at the house as soon as he wishes. We owe him the money that he spent on the furniture.

A handshake, I must go back to hospital, but shall soon be out for good.

Yours,
Vincent

Write a line to Mother too for me, so that no one will be worried.[2]

---

[1] Theo was already engaged to Johanna Bonger, who had been staying with her brother, Andries, friend of Theo and Vincent in Paris. The news of the engagement seems in fact to have constituted one main cause of Vincent's breakdown, since a threat was involved that his financial backing from Theo would be cut off.

[2] On the back of this letter a short message to Gauguin was written out also.

My dear Theo,   Arles, January 23 1889

Thank you for your letter and the 50 fr. note it contained. Of course I am now safe until the arrival of your letter after the 1st. What happened about that money was entirely pure chance and misunderstanding, for which neither you nor I are responsible. By just the same mischance I could not telegraph as you said, because I did not know if you were still in Amsterdam or back in Paris. It is over now with the rest, and is one more proof of the proverb that misfortunes never come singly. Roulin left yesterday[1] (of course my wire yesterday was sent off before the arrival of your letter of this morning). It was touching to see him with his children this last day, especially with the quite tiny one, when he made her laugh and jump on his knee, and sang for her.

His voice has a strangely pure and touching quality in which there was for my ear at once a sweet and mournful cradle-song, and a kind of far-away echo of the trumpet of revolutionary France. He was not sad, however. On the contrary, he had put on his brand new uniform which he had received that very day, and everyone was making much of him.

I have just finished a new canvas which almost has what one might call a certain *chic* about it, a wicker basket with lemons and oranges, a cypress branch and a pair of blue gloves. You have already seen some of these baskets of fruit of mine.

Look here—you do know that what I am trying to do is to get back the money that my training as a painter has cost, neither more nor less.

I have a right to that, and to the earning of my daily bread.

I think it just that there should be that return, I don't say into your hands, since what we have done we have done together, and to talk of money distresses us so much.

But let it go to your wife's hands, who will join with us besides in working with the artists.

[1] He was moving to a post in Marseilles.

If I am not yet devoting much thought to direct sales, it is because my count of pictures is not yet complete, but it is getting on, and I have set to work again with a nerve like iron.

I have good and ill luck in my production, but not ill luck *only*. For instance, if our Monticelli bunch of flowers is worth 500 francs to a collector, and it is, then I dare swear to you that my sunflowers are worth 500 francs too, to one of these Scots or Americans.

Now to get up heat enough to melt that gold, those flower-tones, it isn't any old person who can do it, it needs the force and concentration of a single individual whole and entire.

When I saw my canvases again after my illness the one that seemed the best to me was the "Bedroom."

The amount we handle is a respectable enough sum, I admit, but much of it runs away, and what we'll have to watch above all is that from year's end to year's end it doesn't all slip through the net. That is why as the month goes on I keep more or less trying to balance the outlay with the output, at least in relative terms.

So many difficulties certainly do make me rather worried and timorous, but I haven't given up hope yet.

The trouble I foresee is that we shall have to be very *prudent* so as to prevent the expenses of a sale lowering the sale itself, when the time for it comes. How many times we have had occasion to see just that mischance in the lives of artists.

I have in hand the portrait of Roulin's wife, which I was working on before I was ill.[1]

In it I had ranged the reds from rose to an orange, which rose through the yellows to lemon, with light and sombre greens. If I could finish it, I should be very glad, but I am afraid she will no longer want to pose with her husband away.

You can see just what a disaster Gauguin's leaving is,

[1] The *Woman rocking a Cradle,* begun in December.

because it has thrust us down again just when we had made a
home and furnished it to take in our friends in bad times.

Only in spite of it we will keep the furniture, etc. And
though everyone will now be afraid of me, in time that may
disappear.

We are all mortal and subject to all the ailments there are,
and if the latter aren't exactly of an agreeable kind, what
can one do about it? The best thing is to try to get rid of
them.

I feel remorse too when I think of the trouble that, however involuntarily, I on my side caused Gauguin. But up to
the last days I saw one thing only, that he was working with
his mind divided between the desire to go to Paris to carry out
his plans, and the life at Arles.

What will come of all this for him?

You will doubtless be feeling that though you have a good
salary, nevertheless we lack capital, except in goods, and that
in order really to alter the unhappy position of the artists that
we know, we need to be in a stronger position. But then we
often run up against sheer distrust on their part, and the
things they are perpetually scheming among themselves,
which always end in—a *blank*. I think that at Pont-Aven
they had already formed a new group of 5 or 6, perhaps
already broken up.

They are not dishonest, it is something without a name and
one of their enfant terrible faults.

Meantime the great thing is that your marriage should not
be delayed. By getting married you will set Mother's mind
at rest and make her happy, and it is after all almost a necessity in view of your position in society and in commerce. Will
it be appreciated by the society to which you belong, perhaps
not, any more than the artists ever suspect that I have sometimes worked and suffered for the community. . . . So from
me, your brother, you will not want completely banal congratulations and assurances that you are about to be transported
straight into paradise. And with your wife you will not be
lonely any more, which I could wish for our sister as well.

That, after your own marriage, is what I should set m
heart on more than anything.

When you are married, perhaps there will be other mar
riages in the family, and in any case you will see your wa
clear and the house will not be empty any more.

Whatever I think on other points, our father and mothe
were exemplary as married people.

And I shall never forget Mother at Father's death, whe
she only said one small word : it made me begin to love dea
old Mother more than before. In fact as married people ou
parents were exemplary, like Roulin and his wife, to cit
another instance.

Well, go straight ahead along that road. During my illnes
I saw again every room of the house at Zundert, every patl
every plant in the garden, the views from the fields roun
about, the neighbours, the graveyard, the church, our kitche
garden behind—down to the magpie's nest in a tall acacia i
the graveyard.

It's because I still have earlier recollections of those firs
days than any of the rest of you.[1] There is no one left wh
remembers all this but Mother and me.

I say no more about it, since it is better that I should no
try to recall all that passed through my head then.

Only please realize that I shall be very happy when you
marriage has taken place. Look here now, if for your wife
sake it would perhaps be as well to have a picture of min
from time to time at Goupil's, then I will give up my grudg
against them, in this way :—

I said I did not want to go back to them with too naïve
picture.

But if you like you can exhibit the two pictures of sur
flowers.

Gauguin would be glad to have one, and I should ver
much like to give Gauguin a real pleasure.[2] So if he want

---

[1] Vincent was the eldest of the six children in his family.

[2] Gauguin had taken two of Vincent's *Sunflowers* away with hin
and the sunflowers of Arles bloomed again in Tahiti, when Gaugui
in 1900 nostalgically ordered sunflower seeds from París, and di

one of the two canvases, all right, I will do one of them over again, whichever he likes.

You will see that these canvases will catch the eye. But I would advise you to keep them for yourself, just for your own private pleasure and that of your wife.

It is a kind of painting that rather changes in character, and takes on a richness the longer you look at it.

Besides, you know, Gauguin likes them extraordinarily. He said to me among other things—" That . . . it's . . . the flower."

You know that the peony is Jeannin's, the hollyhock belongs to Quost, but the sunflower is somewhat my own.

And after all I should like to go on exchanging my things with Gauguin even if sometimes it would cost me also rather dear.

Did you during your hasty visit see the portrait of Mme. Ginoux in black and yellow?[1] That portrait was painted in three-quarters of an hour. I must stop for the moment.

The delay of the money was pure chance, and neither you nor I could do anything about it. A handshake.

Yours,
Vincent

My dear Theo,   [Arles, February 3 1889]
I should have preferred to reply at once to your kind letter containing 100 francs, but as I was very tired just then, and the doctor had given me strict orders to go out walking without doing any mental work, I'm in consequence only writing to you to-day. As far as work goes the month hasn't on the whole been too bad, and work distracts me, or rather keeps me in control, so that I don't deny myself it.

I have done the " Woman Rocking the Cradle " three times, and as Mme. Roulin was the model and I only the painter, I

---

still-lifes of the same subject as had decorated his room in the Yellow House.

[1] *The Arlésienne* of early November 1888.

let her choose between the three, her and her husband, but on condition that I should make another duplicate for myself of the one she chose, and I have this in hand now.

You ask me if I have read *La Mireille* by Mistral.[1] I am like you, I can only read it in fragments in the translation. But have you *heard* it yet, for you know perhaps that Gounod has set it to music, at least I think so. Naturally I do not know the music, and even if I heard it I should be watching the musicians rather than listening.

But I can tell you this, that in its words the language native to this region is extraordinarily musical in the mouth of an Arlésienne.

Perhaps in the "Woman Rocking" there's an attempt to get something of the *music* of the colouring here. It is badly painted and the chromos in the little shops are infinitely better painted technically, but all the same. . . .

By the way—this here so-called *good* town of Arles is such an odd place, that old Gauguin calls it with good reason "the dirtiest hole in the south."

And if Rivet[2] saw the population he would certainly have some bad moments, saying over and over again, "You are a sickly lot, all of you," just as he says of us; but if you catch the disease of the country, my word, you have caught it once and for all.

By which I mean that I have no illusions about myself any more. It is going very well, and I shall do everything the doctor says, but . . .

When I came out of the hospital with kind old Roulin, I thought that there had been nothing wrong with me, it was only *afterwards* that I felt I had been ill. Well, well, there are moments when I am wrung by enthusiasm or madness or prophecy, like a Greek oracle on its tripod.

And then I have great readiness of speech and speak like the Arlésiennes, but despite all this I feel so weak.

[1] Frédéric Mistral, the Provençal poet and collector of Provençal folk-lore.
[2] Doctor to the two brothers in Paris.

Once my bodily strength comes back, but also at the slightest grave symptom, I have already told Rey[1] that I would come back and put myself under the mental specialists at Aix, or under him.

Can anything come of it but trouble and suffering if we are not well, either for you or for me? So completely has our ambition foundered.

Then let us work on very quietly, let us take care of ourselves as much as we can and not exhaust ourselves in barren efforts of mutual generosity.

You will do your duty and I will do mine, since as far as that goes we have already both paid in other ways than in words, and at the end of the journey we may meet each other again with a quiet mind. But when that delirium of mine shakes up everything I dearly loved, I do not accept it as reality and I am not going to be a false prophet.

Illness or death, indeed, they have no terrors for me, but fortunately for us ambition is not compatible with the professions we follow.

But how comes it that you are thinking at this time both of the clauses of your marriage settlement and of the possibility of dying? Wouldn't it have been better quite simply to run your wife through beforehand?

After all that is the way of the north, and it is not for me to say that they have not good ways in the north.

It will all come right, indeed it will.

But I who have not a penny still say in this matter that money is one kind of coin and painting another. And I am already able to send you a consignment of the kind I spoke of in my previous letters. But it will be bigger if my strength returns.

But in case Gauguin, who has a perfect infatuation for my sunflowers, takes those two pictures from me, I should just like him to give your fiancée or you two of his own, not just average, but better than the average. And if he takes one version of the " Woman Rocking," he ought still more to give

[1] The house-surgeon at the Arles hospital.

something good in return. Without that I could not complete this series of which I was telling you,[1] which should be able to make its way into that same little window we have so often gazed at.

As for the Indépendants[2] I think that six pictures is too much by half. To my mind the " Harvest " and the " White Orchard " are enough, with the little " Provençal Girl " or the " Sower " if you like. But I don't greatly care. The one thing I have set my heart on is some day to give you a more heartening impression of this painting job of ours, by a collection of 30 or so more serious studies. That will prove again to our real friends like Gauguin, Guillaumin, Bernard, etc., that we are producing something. Well, about the little yellow house, when I paid my rent the landlord's agent was very nice, and behaved like an Arlésien by treating me as an equal. Then I told him that I had no need of a lease or a written promise of reference, and that in case of illness I should pay only as a matter of friendly agreement.

People here are sound at heart, and the spoken word is more binding than the written word. So I am keeping the house provisionally, since for the sake of my mental recovery I need to feel here that I am in my own home. Now about your removal from the Rue Lepic to the Rue Rodier, I can't offer any opinion, as I have not seen it, but the chief thing is that you too should lunch at home with your wife.

By staying in Montmartre you would the sooner be decorated and a Minister of the Arts, but as you are not keen on that, it is better to have the peace of one's own home, so I think you are quite right.

I am a little like that too. I always say to the people here who ask after my health, that I shall start like them by dying of it, and after that my illness will be dead.

This doesn't mean I shall not have long spells of respite,

[1] A decorative project for combining the *Sunflowers* and the *Women Rocking* in alternate sequence.

[2] A special " Society of Independent Artists " had been founded in Paris in 1884, for the organisation of annual exhibitions without jury interference. Vincent had first shown in this company in 1888.

but once you are ill in earnest you know quite well that you cannot contract the same illness twice, you are well, or you are ill, just as you are young or you are old. Only be sure of it, like you, I do what the doctor tells me as much as I can, and I consider that as a part of my work and the duty which I have to fulfil.

I must tell you this, that the neighbours, etc., are particularly kind to me, as everyone suffers here either from fever, or hallucinations, or madness, we understand each other like members of the same family. I went yesterday to see the girl I had gone to when I went astray in my wits.[1] They told me there that in this country things like that are not out of the ordinary. She had been upset by it and had fainted but had recovered her calm. And they spoke well of her too.

But as for considering myself as altogether sane, we must not do it. People here who are ill like me have told me the truth. You may be old or young, but there will always be moments when you lose your head. So I do not ask you to say of me that there is nothing wrong with me, or that there never will be. Only the Ricord of this is probably Raspail.[2] I have not had the fevers of this country yet, and I may still catch them. But they are well up in all this already at the hospital here, and directly you have no false shame and say frankly what you feel, you cannot go wrong.

I finish this letter for this evening. A good handshake in thought.

Yours,
Vincent

[Soon after this Vincent had his second attack, and was taken to the hospital imagining that people wanted to poison him; he recovered quickly to the point when he could resume his letters to Theo.]

[1] The girl at the brothel, Rachel, to whom Vincent had presented the detached part of his ear on December 23rd.

[2] i.e., his affliction was of a different kind from the one most common in those parts, venereal disease; Ricord in the United States had pioneered the study of the latter; while Raspail was a noted natural physician in Paris.

My dear Theo, [Arles, beginning of April 1889]

A few words to wish you and your fiancée all happiness these days.[1] It is a sort of nervous affliction with me that on festive occasions I generally find difficulty in formulating good wishes, but you must not conclude from that that I wish you happiness less earnestly than anyone else, as you well know.

I have still to thank you for your last letter, as well as for the consignment of paints from Tasset and for several numbers of *Le Fifre* with drawings by Forain. These last especially had the effect on me of making me see my own stuff as very sentimental beside them.

I waited several days before answering, not knowing which day you were leaving for Amsterdam. Besides I do not know either if you are getting married in Breda or in Amsterdam. But if as I am inclined to think it will be in Amsterdam, then I have assumed that you would find this letter there by Sunday.

By the way—only yesterday our friend Roulin came to see me. He told me to give you many greetings from him and to congratulate you. His visit gave me a lot of pleasure, he often has to carry loads you would call too heavy, but it doesn't prevent him, as he has the strong constitution of the peasant, from always looking well and even jolly. But for me, who am perpetually learning from him afresh, what a lesson for the future it is when one gathers from his talk that life does not grow any easier as one gets on in life.

I talked to him so as to have his opinion as to what I ought to do about the studio,[2] which I have to leave in any case at Easter, according to the advice of M. Salles[3] and M. Rey.

I said to Roulin that having done a good many things to put the house into a far better state than when I took it, especially as regards the gas I had put in, I considered it as a definite piece of work.

---

[1] Their marriage was about to take place.

[2] Following his third attack in March, Vincent had remained in the hospital for the time being.

[3] The Protestant clergyman who came on regular visits.

They are forcing me to leave—very well—but I should be pretty well justified in taking away the gas and making a rumpus about damages or something, only I haven't the heart to do it.

The only thing I feel I can do in this business is to tell myself that it was an attempt to make an abiding place for unknown successors. Besides, before seeing Roulin I had already been to the gas works to arrange it this way. And Roulin was of the same opinion. He expects to stay in Marseilles.

I am well just now, except for a certain undercurrent of vague sadness difficult to define—but anyway—I have rather gained than lost in physical strength, and I am working.

Just now I have on the easel an orchard of peach trees beside a road with the Alpilles in the background. It seems that there was a fine article in the *Figaro* on Monet; Roulin had read it and been struck by it, he said.

Altogether it is a rather difficult problem to decide whether to take a new flat, and even to find it, especially by the month. M. Salles has spoken to me of a house at 20 francs which is very nice, but he is not sure if I could have it.

At Easter I shall have to pay three months' rent, the removal, etc. All this is not very cheering or convenient, especially as there seems no prospect of any better luck anywhere.

Roulin said or rather hinted that he did not at all like the disquiet which has reigned here in Arles this winter, considered even quite apart from what has fallen on me.[1]

After all it is rather like that everywhere, business not too good, resources exhausted, people discouraged and . . . as you said, not content to remain spectators, and becoming nuisances from being out of work—if anybody can still make a joke or work fast, down they come on him.

And now, my dear lad, I do believe I shall soon not be ill enough to have to stay shut up. Otherwise I am beginning to get used to it, and if I had to stay for good in an asylum, I

[1] The neighbours had petitioned that Vincent should not be left at liberty.

should make up my mind to it and I think I could find subjects for painting there as well.

Write to me soon if you can find the time.

Roulin's family was still in the country and though he earns slightly more, the separate expenses are greater in proportion, and so they are not really a farthing better off, and he was not without very heavy anxieties.

Fortunately the weather is fine and the sun glorious, and people here quickly forget all their griefs for the time being and then they brim over with high spirits and illusions.

I have been re-reading Dickens' " Christmas Books " these days. There are things in them so profound that one must read them over and over, there are tremendously close connections with Carlyle.

Roulin, though he is not quite old enough to be like a father to me, has all the same a silent gravity and tenderness for me such as an old soldier might have for a young one. All the time—but without a word—a something which seems to say, we do not know what will happen to us to-morrow, but whatever it may be, think of me. And it does one good when it comes from a man who is neither embittered, nor sad, nor perfect, nor happy, nor always irreproachably right. But such a good soul and so wise and so full of feeling and so trustful. I tell you I have no right to complain of anything whatever about Arles, when I think of some things I have seen there which I shall never be able to forget.

It is getting late. Once more I wish you and Jo plenty of happiness, and a handshake in thought.

Yours,

Vincent

SAINT-REMY

My dear Theo,   [Saint-Rémy, early June 1889]

I must beg you again to send me as soon as possible some ordinary brushes, of about these sizes.[1] Half a dozen of each, please; I hope that you are well and your wife too, and that you are enjoying the fine weather a little. Here at any rate we have splendid sunshine.

As for me, my health is good, and as for my brain, that will be, let us hope, a matter of time and patience.

The director mentioned that he had had a letter from you and had written to you; he tells me nothing and I ask him nothing, which is the simplest.

He's a gouty little man—several years a widower, with very dark spectacles. As the institution is rather dead and alive, the man seems to get no great amusement out of his job, and besides he has enough to live on.

A new man has arrived, who is so worked up that he smashes everything and shouts day and night, he tears his shirts violently too, and up till now, though he is *all day long* in a bath, he gets hardly any quieter, he destroys his bed and everything else in his room, upsets his food, etc. It is very sad to see, but they are very patient here and will end by seeing him through. New things grow old so quickly—I think that if I came to Paris in my present state of mind, I should see no difference between a so-called dark picture and a light impressionist picture, between a varnished picture in oils and a mat picture done with solvent.

I mean by this that by dint of reflection, I have come by slow degrees to believe more than ever in the eternal youth of the school of Delacroix, Millet, Rousseau, Dupré and Daubigny, as much as in that of the present, or even in that of the artists to come. I hardly think that impressionism will ever do more than the romantics for instance. Between that and

[1] A sketch was enclosed.

admiring people like Léon Glaize or Perrault there is certainly a margin.

This morning I saw the country from my window a long time before sunrise, with nothing but the morning star, which looked very big. Daubigny and Rousseau have depicted just that, expressing all that it has of intimacy, all that vast peace and majesty, but adding as well a feeling so individual, so heartbreaking. I have no aversion to that sort of emotion.

I am always filled with remorse, terribly so, when I think of my work as being so little in harmony with what I should have liked to do. I hope that in the long run this will make me do better things, but we have not got to that yet.

I think that you would do well to wash the canvases which are quite, quite dry with water *and a little spirits of wine* to take away the oil and the spirit in the impasto. The same for " The Night Café " and " The Green Vineyard " and especially the landscape that was in the walnut frame. " Night " also, but that has been retouched recently and might run with the spirits of wine.

It's almost a whole month since I came here, not once has the least desire to be elsewhere come to me, only the wish to work is getting a scrap stronger.

I do not notice in the others either any very definite desire to be anywhere else, and this may well come from the feeling that we are too thoroughly shattered for life outside.

What I cannot quite understand is their absolute idleness. But that is the great fault of the South and its ruin. But what a lovely country, and what lovely blue and what a sun! And yet I have only seen the garden and what I can look at through my window.

Have you read the new book by Guy de Maupassant, " Strong as the Dead," what is the subject of it? The last thing I read in that category was Zola's " The Dream "; I thought the figure of the woman, the one who did embroidery, very very beautiful, and the description of the embroidery all in gold, just because it is as it were a question of the colour of the different yellows, whole and broken up. But the figure of the man did not seem very lifelike and the great cathedral also gave me the blues. Only that contrast of lilac and blue-black did, if you like, make the blonde figure stand out. But after all there are things like that in Lamartine.

I hope that you will destroy a lot of the things that are too bad in the batch I have sent you, or at least only show what is most passable. As for the exhibition of the Indépendants, it's all one to me, just act as if I weren't there. So as not to be indifferent, and not to exhibit anything too mad, perhaps the " Starry Night " and the landscape with yellow verdure, which was in the walnut frame. Since these are two with contrasting colours, it might give somebody else the idea of doing those night effects better than I have.

But you must absolutely set your mind at rest about me now. When I have received the new canvas and the paints, I am going off to see a little of the country.

Since it is just the season when there are plenty of flowers and consequently colour effects, it would perhaps be wise to send me five metres more of canvas.

For the flowers are short lived and will be replaced by the yellow cornfields. Those especially I hope to catch better than I did at Arles. The mistral (since there are some mountains) seems much less tiresome than at Arles, where you always got it at first hand.

When you receive the canvases that I have done in the garden, you will see that I am not too melancholy here.

Goodbye for the present, a good handshake in thought to you and Jo.

Yours,
Vincent

My dear Theo,   [Saint-Rémy, early September 1889]
I so like your letter, what you say of Rousseau and artists such as Bodmer, that they are in any case men, and such men that you would like to see the world peopled with the like of them—yes, certainly that is what I feel too.

And that J. H. Weissenbruch knows and does the muddy towpaths, the stunted willows, the foreshortening, the strange and subtle perspective of the canals as Daumier does lawyers, I think that is perfect.

Tersteeg has done well to buy some of his work; why people like that do not sell is, I think, because there are too many dealers trying to sell different stuff, with which they deceive the public and lead it astray.

Do you know that even now, if by chance I read an account of some energetic manufacturer or even more of a publisher, then I feel the same indignation, the same wrath as I used to feel when I was with Goupil and Co.

Life passes like this, time does not return, but I am dead set on my work, just for the very reason that I know the opportunities of working do not return.

Especially in my case, in which a more violent attack may destroy for ever my ability to paint.

During the attacks I feel a coward before the pain and suffering—more of a coward than I ought, and it is perhaps this very moral cowardice which, while formerly I had no desire to get better, makes me now eat like two, work hard, limit myself in my relations with the other patients for fear of a relapse—altogether I am now trying to recover like a man who has meant to commit suicide and, finding the water too cold, tries to regain the bank.

My dear brother, you know that I came to the South and threw myself into my work for a thousand reasons. Wishing to see a different light, thinking that to look at nature under a brighter sky might give us a better idea of the Japanese way of feeling and drawing. Wishing also to see this stronger sun, because one feels that without knowing it one could not understand the pictures of Delacroix from the point of view of execution and technique, and because one feels that the colours of the prism are veiled in the mist of the North.

All this is still somewhat true. Then when to this is added the natural inclination towards this South which Daudet described in *Tartarin,* and that here and there I have found besides friends and things here which I love.

Can you understand then that while finding this malady horrible, I feel that all the same I have fashioned myself links with the place that are perhaps too strong—links that may cause me later on to hanker to work here again—even though it may well be that in a comparatively short time I shall return to the North.

Yes, for I will not hide from you that in the same way that I take my food now with avidity, I have a terrible desire that comes over me to see my friends again and to revisit the northern countryside.

My work is going very well, I am finding things that I have sought in vain for years, and feeling that, I am always thinking of that saying of Delacroix's that you know, that he discovered painting when he no longer had either breath or teeth.

Well, with this mental disease I have, I think of the many other artists suffering mentally and I tell myself that this does not prevent one from exercising the painter's profession as if nothing was amiss.

When I realize that here the attacks tend to take an absurd religious turn, I should almost venture to think that this even *necessitates* a return to the North. Do not talk too much about this to the doctor when you see him—but I do not know if this does not come from living for so many months, both in the Arles hospital and here, in these old cloisters. In fact, I really must not live in such an atmosphere, one would be better off in the street. I am not indifferent, and even during the suffering religious thoughts sometimes bring me great consolation. Thus this last time during my illness a misfortune happened to me—that lithograph of Delacroix's, the " Pietà," together with some other sheets, fell into some oil and paint and was ruined.

I was distressed at this—so in between times I have occupied myself with painting it, and you will see it some day. I made a copy of it on a canvas of size 5 or 6, which I hope has feeling.

Besides having seen not long ago the " Daniel " and the " Odalisques " and the portrait of Brias and the " Mulatto Woman " at Montpellier, I still feel the impression which these created.

L.V.G.   L

That is what braces me, as with reading a fine book like Beecher Stowe's or Dickens', but what annoys me is to keep on seeing these good women who believe in the Virgin of Lourdes and make up things like that, and to think that I am a prisoner under a management of that sort, which very willingly fosters these sickly religious aberrations, when the proper thing would be to cure them. So I say again, better to go, if not into a prison, at least into the army.

I reproach myself for my cowardice, I ought rather to have defended my studio, even if it meant fighting with the police and the neighbours. Others in my place would have used a revolver, and certainly if as an artist one had killed some rotters like that, one would have been acquitted. I should have done better so, and as it is I have been cowardly and drunk.

Ill as well, yet I have not been brave. Then face to face with the suffering of these attacks I feel very frightened too, and I do not know if my zeal is anything different from what I said, it is like someone who meant to commit suicide and finding the water too cold, struggles to regain the bank.

But listen, to be confined, as I saw happen to Braat[1] in the past—fortunately that was long ago—no and again *no*. It would be different if old Pissarro or Vignon for instance would like to take me in with them. Well, I'm a painter myself, that might be arranged, and it is better that the money should go to support painters than to the excellent sisters of mercy.

Yesterday I asked M. Peyron pointblank—since you are going to Paris, what would you say if I suggested you should be kind enough to take me with you? He replied evasively—it was too sudden, he must write to you first. But he is very kind and very indulgent towards me, and while not the absolute master here—far from it—I owe many liberties to him. After all you must not only make pictures, but you must also see people, and from time to time by means of the company of others recover your balance and stock yourself with ideas. I have put aside the hope that it will not come back—on the

---

[1] A close friend of Theo's and an employee of the same firm.

contrary, we must expect that from time to time I shall have an attack. But even at those times it would be possible to go to a nursing home or even into the town prison, where there is generally a cell.

Do not fret in any case—my work goes well and look here, I can't tell you how it rekindles me to tell you sometimes how I am going to do this or that, cornfields, etc. I have done the portrait of the warder, and I have a duplicate of it for you. This makes a rather curious contrast with the self-portrait I have done, in which the look is vague and veiled, while he has something military in his small quick black eyes.

I have made him a present of it, and I shall do his wife too if she is willing to sit. She is a faded woman, an unhappy, resigned creature of small account, so insignificant that I have a great desire to paint that blade of dusty grass. I have talked to her sometimes when I was doing some olive trees behind their little house, and she told me then that she did not believe that I was ill—and indeed you would say as much yourself now if you saw me working, my brain so clear and my fingers so sure, that I have drawn that " Pietà " by Delacroix without taking a single measurement, and yet there are those four hands and arms in the foreground in it—gestures and torsions of the body not exactly easy or simple.

I beg you, send me the canvas soon if it is possible, and then I think that I shall need 10 more tubes of zinc white. All the same, I know well that healing comes—if one is brave —from within, through profound resignation to suffering and death, through the surrender of your own will and of your self-love. But that is no use to me, I love to paint, to see people and things and everything that makes our life— artificial—if you like. Yes, real life would be a different thing, but I do not think I belong to that category of souls who are ready to live and also ready at any moment to suffer.

What a queer thing *touch* is, the stroke of the brush.

In the open air, exposed to wind, to sun, to the curiosity of people, you work as you can, you fill your canvas anyhow. Then, however, you catch the real and the essential—that is the most difficult. But when after a time you take up this study again and arrange your brush strokes in the direction of the objects—certainly it is more harmonious and pleasant to look at, and you add whatever you have of serenity and cheerfulness.

Ah, I shall never be able to convey my impressions of some faces that I have seen here. Certainly this is the road on which there is something new, the road to the South, but men of the North have difficulty in penetrating it. And already I can see myself in the future, when I shall have had some success, regretting my solitude and my wretchedness here, when I saw between the iron bars of the cell the reaper in the field below. Misfortune is good for something.

To succeed, to have lasting prosperity, you must have a temperament different from mine; I shall never do what I might have done and ought to have wished and pursued.

But I cannot live, since I have this dizziness so often, except in a fourth or fifth rate condition. When I realize the worth and originality and the superiority of Delacroix and Millet, for instance, then I am bold to say—yes, I am something, I can do something. But I must have a foundation in those artists, and then produce the little which I am capable of in the same direction.

So old Pissarro is cruelly smitten by these two misfortunes at once.[1]

As soon as I read that, I thought of asking him if there would be any way of going to stay with him.

If you will pay the same as here, he will find it worth his while, for I do not need much—except to work.

Ask him straight out, and if he does not wish it, I could quite well go to Vignon's. I am a little afraid of Pont-Aven, there are so many people there, but what you say about Gauguin interests me very much. And I still tell myself that Gauguin and I will perhaps work together again.

I know that Gauguin is capable of better things than he has done, but to make that man comfortable!

I am still hoping to do his portrait.

Did you see that portrait that he did of me, painting some

[1] Pissarro had lost his mother and had trouble with his eyes.

sunflowers? Subsequently my face got much brighter, but all told it was really me, very tired and charged with electricity as I was then.

And yet to see the country, you must live with the poor people and in the little homes and public houses, etc.

And that was what I said to Bock, who was complaining of seeing nothing that tempted him or impressed him. I went for walks with him for two days and I showed him thirty pictures to be done as different from the North as Morocco would be. I am curious to know what he is doing now.

And then do you know why the pictures by Eug. Delacroix —the religious and historical pictures, the " Bark of Christ," the " Pietà," the " Crusaders," have such a hold on one? Because Eug. Delacroix when he did a " Gethsemane " had first been to observe on the spot what an olive grove was, and the same for the sea whipped by a strong mistral, and because he must have said to himself—these people of whom history tells us, doges of Venice, crusaders, apostles, holy women, were of a character and lived in a manner analogous to those of their present descendants.

And I must tell you—and you can see it in the " Woman Rocking," however much of a failure and however feeble that attempt may be—had I had the strength to continue, I should have made portraits of saints and holy women from life who would have seemed to belong to another age, and they would have been middle-class women of the present day and yet they would have had something in common with the first early Christians.

However, the emotions which that rouses are too strong, I shall stop at that, but later on, later on I do not say that I shall not return to the task.

What a great man Fromentin[1] was—for those who want to see the East—he will always remain the *guide*. He was the first to establish a link between Rembrandt and the Midi, between Potter and what he saw himself.

You are right a thousand times over—I must not think of

[1] Author of *The Masters of Past Time,* a collection of artistic essays which Vincent had read in 1884.

all that—I must create—were it only studies of cabbages and salad, to get calm, and once calm, then—whatever I might be capable of. When I see them again, I shall make duplicates of that study of the "Tarascon Diligence," of the "Vineyard," the "Harvest," and especially of the "Red Cabaret," that night café which is the most characteristic of all in its colour. But the white figure right in the middle must be done over as to colour, and better constructed. But that—I venture to say—is the real Midi, and a deliberated combination of greens with reds.

My strength has been exhausted too quickly, but I see in the distance the possibility for others of doing an infinite number of fine things. And again and again this idea remains true, that to make travel easier for others it would have been well to found a studio somewhere in this neighbourhood. To make the journey in one stage from the north to Spain, for instance, is not good, you will not see what you should see there—you must *get your eyes accustomed* first and gradually to the different light.

I have not much need to see Titian and Velasquez in the galleries, I have seen living types that have informed me better what a Midi picture is now, than before my little journey.

Good Lord, Good Lord, the good people among the artists who say that Delacroix is not of the real East. Look here, is the real East the kind of thing that Parisians like Gérôme have done?

Because you paint a bit of a sunny wall from nature and well and truly according to our way of seeing *in the North,* does that prove equally that you have seen the people of the East? Now that is what Delacroix was seeking, but it in no way hindered him from painting walls in the "Jewish Wedding" and the "Odalisques." Isn't that true?—and then Degas says that it is paying too dear for it, to drink in the cabarets while you are painting pictures, I don't deny it, but would he then like me to go into cloisters or churches, it is there that I am afraid. That is why I make an attempt to

escape in writing this letter; with many handshakes to you
and Jo.

Yours,

Vincent

I still have to congratulate you on the occasion of Mother's
birthday. I wrote to them yesterday, but the letter has not yet
gone because I have not had the presence of mind to finish it.
It is queer that already, two or three times before, I had had
the idea of going to Pissarro's; this time, after your telling me
of his recent misfortunes, I do not hesitate to ask you this.

Yes, we must finish with this place, I cannot do the two
things at once, work and take no end of pains to live with
these queer patients here—it is upsetting.

In vain I tried to force myself to go downstairs. And yet it
is nearly two months since I have been out in the open air.

In the long run I shall lose the faculty for work here, and
that is where I begin to call a halt, and I shall send them
then—if you agree—about their business.

And then to go on paying for it, no, then one or other of
the artists who is hard up will agree to keep house with me.
It is fortunate that you can write saying you are well, and
Jo too, and that her sister is with you.

I very much wish that, when your child comes,[1] I might
be back—not with you, certainly *not,* that is impossible, but in
the neighbourhood of Paris with another painter. I could
mention a third alternative, my going to the Jouves, who
have a lot of children and quite a household.

You understand that I have tried to compare the second
attack with the first, and I only tell you this, it seemed to me
to stem from some influence or other from outside, rather
than from within myself. I may be mistaken, but however it
may be, I think you will feel it quite right that I have rather
a horror of all religious exaggeration. The good M. Peyron
will tell you heaps of things, probabilities and possibilities,
and involuntary acts. Very good, but if he is more precise than
that I shall believe none of it. And we shall see then *what*

[1] Jo had announced her pregnancy.

he will be precise about, if he is precise. The treatment of patients in this hospital is certainly easy, one could follow it even while travelling, for they do absolutely *nothing*; they leave them to vegetate in idleness and feed them with stale and slightly spoiled food. And I will tell you now that from the first day I refused to take this food, and until my attack I ate only bread and a little soup, and as long as I remain here I shall continue this way. It is true that after this attack M. Peyron gave me some wine and meat, which I accepted willingly the first days, but I wouldn't want to be an exception to the rule for long, and it is right to respect the regular rules of the establishment. I must also say that M. Peyron does not give me much hope for the future, and this I think right, he makes me realize properly that *everything* is doubtful, that one can be sure of nothing beforehand. I myself expect it to return, but it is just that work takes up my mind so thoroughly, that I think that with the physique I have, things may continue for a long time in this way.

The idleness in which these poor unfortunates vegetate is a pest, but there, it is a general evil in the towns and countryside under this stronger sunshine, and having learnt a different way of life, certainly it is my duty to resist it. I finish this letter by thanking you again for yours and begging you to write to me again soon, and with many handshakes in thought.

My dear Theo, [Saint-Rémy, mid November 1889]

I have to thank you very much for a parcel of paints, which was accompanied also by an excellent woollen jacket.

How kind you are to me, and how I wish I could do something good, so as to prove to you that I would like to be less ungrateful. The paints reached me at the right moment, because those I had brought back from Arles were almost exhausted. The thing is that I have worked this month in the olive groves, because they[1] have maddened me with their Christs in the Garden, with nothing really observed. Of course with me there is no question of doing anything from

[1] Bernard and Gauguin, who had sent records of their recent work.

the Bible—and I have written to Bernard and Gauguin too
that I considered that to think, not to dream, was our duty,
so that I was astonished looking at their work that they had
let themselves go so far. For Bernard has sent me photos of
his canvases. The trouble about them is that they are a sort
of dream or nightmare—that they are erudite enough—you
can see that it is someone who is mad on the primitives—but
frankly the English Pre-Raphaelites did the thing much better,
and then Puvis and Delacroix, much more healthily than the
Pre-Raphaelites.

It is not that it leaves me cold, but it gives me a painful
feeling of collapse instead of progress. Well, to shake that
off, morning and evening these bright cold days, but with a
very fine and clear sun, I have been knocking about in the
orchards and the result has been 5 canvases of size 30,
which, with the 3 studies of olives that you have, make up at
least an attack on the problem. The olive is as mutable as
our willow or pollarded osier in the north, you know the
willows are very striking, in spite of them seeming mono-
tonous, it is the tree in character with the country. Now what
the willow is at home, that is just what the olive and the
cypress signify here. What I have done is a rather hard and
coarse realism beside their abstractions, but it will give the
feeling of the country and will smell of the soil. How I
would like to see Gauguin's and Bernard's studies from
nature, the latter talks to me of portraits—which doubtless
would please me better.

I hope to get myself used to working in the cold—in the
morning there are very interesting effects of white frost and
fog; then I still have a great desire to do for the mountains
and the cypresses what I have just done for the olives, and
have a good go at them.

The thing is that these have rarely been painted, the olive
and the cypress, and from the point of view of marketing the
pictures, they *ought* to go in England, I know well enough
what they look for there. However that may be, I am almost
sure of this, that in this way I'll do something tolerable from
time to time. It is really my opinion more and more, as I said

to Isaäcson, that if you work diligently from nature without saying to yourself beforehand—" I want to do this or that," if you work as if you were making a pair of shoes, without artistic preoccupations, you will not always do well, but the days you least anticipate it you find a subject which holds its own with the work of those who have gone before us. You learn to know a country which is fundamentally quite different from its appearance at first sight.

Contrariwise you say to yourself—" I want to finish my pictures more, I want to do them with care," lots of ideas like that, confronted by the difficulties of weather and of changing effects, are reduced to being impracticable, and I end by resigning myself and saying that it is the experience and the meagre work *of every day* which alone ripens in the long run and allows one to do things that are more complete and more true. Thus slow long work is the only way, and all ambition and resolve to make a good thing of it, false. For you must spoil quite as many canvases when you return to the onslaught every morning, as you succeed with. To paint, a regular tranquil existence would hence be absolutely necessary, and at the present time what can you do, when you see that Bernard for instance is hurried, hurried, endlessly hurried by his parents? He cannot do as he wishes, and many others are in his predicament.

You can say to yourself, I will not paint any more, but then what is one to do? Oh, we must invent a more expeditious method of painting, less costly than oil and yet lasting. A picture . . . will end by becoming as commonplace as a sermon, and a painter will become like a creature left over from last century. All the same, it is a pity it should be so. Now if the painters had understood Millet better as a man, as some like Lhermitte and Roll have grasped him, things would not be like this. We *must* work as much and with as few pretensions as a peasant, if we want to last.

And it would have been better than having grandiose exhibitions to address oneself to the people and work so that each one could have in his home some pictures or some reproductions which would be lessons, like the work of Millet.

I am quite at the end of my canvas and as soon as you can I beg you to send me 10 metres. Then I shall attack the cypresses and the mountains. I think that this will be the core of the work that I have done here and there in Provence, and then we can conclude my stay here when it is convenient. It is not urgent, for Paris after all only distracts. Yet I don't know—not being always a pessimist—I keep thinking that I have it still in my heart to paint some day a bookshop with its frontage yellow and rose, at evening, and black passers-by —it is such an essentially modern subject. Because it seems, imaginatively speaking, such a wellspring of light—I say, there would be a subject that would go well between an olive grove and a cornfield, the seed time of books and prints. I have a great longing to do it, like a light in the midst of darkness. Yes, there is a way of seeing Paris as beautiful. But after all bookshops do not run away like hares, and there is no hurry, and I am quite willing to work here for another year, which would probably be wiser.

Mother must have been a fortnight in Leyden. I have delayed sending you canvases for her, because I will include them with the canvas of the " Cornfield " for the Vingtistes.[1]

Warm regards to Jo, she is doing admirably in going on being well. Thank you again for the paints, and the woollen jacket, and a good handshake in thought.

Yours,
Vincent

[Saint-Rémy, beginning of February 1890]
My dear Theo,

I have just to-day received the good news that you are at last a father, that the most critical time is over for Jo, and lastly that the little boy is well. That does me more good and gives me more pleasure than I can put into words. Bravo —and how pleased Mother is going to be. The day before yesterday I received a fairly long and very contented letter

[1] A group of Vincent's works was going to the exhibition of this society in Brussels.

from her too. Anyhow, here it is, the thing I have for so long so much desired for you. No need to tell you that I have often thought of you these days and it touched me very much that Jo had the kindness to write to me the very night before. She was so brave and calm in her danger, it touched me profoundly. Well, it contributes much to helping me forget those last days when I was ill, I don't know in those instances where I am and my mind wanders.

I was extremely surprised at the article on my pictures which you sent me.[1] I needn't tell you that I hope to go on thinking that I do not paint like that, but I do instead see in it how I ought to paint. For the article is very right inasmuch as it indicates the gap to be filled, and I think that really the writer wrote it more to guide not only me, but the other impressionists as well, and even partly to make the breach at a good place. So he proposed an ideal collective personality to the others quite as much as to me; he simply tells me that here and there there is something good, if you like, even in my work which is at the same time so imperfect, and that is the consoling side, which I appreciate and for which I hope to be grateful. Only it must be understood that my back is not broad enough to bear such an undertaking, and in the concentration of the article on me, there's no need to tell you how steeped in flattery I feel; and in my opinion it is as exaggerated as what a certain article by Isaäcson said about you, that at present the artists had given up squabbling and that an important movement was silently getting under way in the little shop on the Boulevard Montmartre. I admit that it is difficult to speak out, to express one's ideas differently—in the same way as you cannot paint things as you see them—and so I do not mean to criticize the daring of Isaäcson or that of the other critic, but as far as we are concerned, really, we are *posing* a bit for *the model,* and indeed that is a duty and a part of one's job like any other. So if some sort

[1] Article by Albert Aurier in the *Mercure de France* of January 1890, entitled *Les Isolés.* Vincent's art was treated there in terms of its symbolist content.

of reputation comes to you and to me, the thing is to try to keep some sort of calm and, if possible, presence of mind.

Why not say what he said of my sunflowers, *with far more grounds,* of those magnificent and finished hollyhocks of Quost's, and his yellow irises, or those splendid peonies of Jeannin's? And you will foresee as I do that praise like this *must* have its opposite, the reverse of the medal. But I am glad and grateful for the article, or rather " *le cœur à l'aise* "[1] as the song in the *Revue* has it, since one may need it, as one may really need a medal. Besides, an article like that has its own merit as a critical work of art, in which light I think it is to be respected, and the writer *must* heighten the tones, syncopate his conclusions, etc. But from the beginning you must beware of bringing up your young family *too much* in an artistic ambience. Old Goupil managed his household pretty well in the Parisian briar-patch and I expect you will many a time afresh be thinking of him. Things have changed so, his cold aloofness would be shocking to-day, but his power to resist so many storms, that really was something.

Gauguin proposed, very vaguely it is true, to found a studio in his name, he, de Haan and I, but he said that first he is going through to the bitter end with his Tonkin project, and seems to have cooled off greatly, I do not exactly know why, in order to continue to paint. And he is just the sort to be off to Tonkin, he has a sort of need for expansion and he finds —and there's some justification for it—the artistic life ignoble. With his repeated experience of travel, what can one say to him?

But I hope he will feel that you and I are indeed his friends, without counting on us too much, which indeed he in no way does. He writes with much reserve, more gravely than last year. I have just written a line to Russell once more, to remind him a little of Gauguin, for I know that Russell as a man has much gravity and strength. Gauguin and Russell are countrymen at heart; not uncouth, but with a certain innate sweetness of far-off fields, more so probably than you or I, that is how they look to me.

[1] " my heart is at ease "

It is necessary—I admit—sometimes to believe in it a little in order to see it. If for my part I wanted to go on—let us call it *translating* certain sheets by Millet,[1] then to prevent anyone being able, not to criticize me, that wouldn't matter, but to make it awkward for me or hinder me by pretending that it is producing copies—then I need someone among the artists like Russell or Gauguin to carry this thing through, and to make a serious thing of it.

I have scruples of conscience about doing the things by Millet which you sent me, for instance, and which seemed to me perfectly chosen, and I took the pile of photographs and sent them without hesitation to Russell, so that I should not see them again until I have thought it over. I do not want to do it until I have heard a little of your own opinion, and a few other people's too, on the ones that will soon be reaching you.

Without that I should have scruples of conscience, a fear lest it should be plagiarizing. And not now, but in a few months' time, I shall try to get a candid opinion from Russell himself on the usefulness of the thing. In any case Russell gets roused, he grows angry, he says something true, and that is what I need sometimes. You know I find the " Virgin " so dazzling that *I have not dared* to look at her. All at once I felt a " not yet." My illness makes me very sensitive now, and I do not feel myself capable for the moment of continuing these " translations," when it concerns such masterpieces. I am calling a halt over the " Sower " which is in hand, and is not coming along as I should wish. While ill, I have thought a lot all the same about continuing this work, and how *when* I do it, I do it calmly, you will soon see when I send the five or six finished canvases.

I hope that M. Lauzet[2] will come, I have a strong desire to make his acquaintance. I have confidence in his opinion when he says it is Provence, there he touches on the difficulty, and like the other one he indicates a thing to be done rather than

---

[1] Vincent had been doing variations on some of his favourite Millet compositions.

[2] A publisher of prints.

a thing already done. Landscapes with cypresses! Ah, it
would not be easy. Aurier speaks of it too, when he says that
even black is a colour, and their flame-like appearance—I
think about it, but haven't the daring either, and I say with the
cautious Isaäcson—I do not yet feel that we can get to that.
You need a certain dash of inspiration, a ray from on high,
things not in ourselves, in order to do beautiful things. When
I had done those sunflowers, I looked for the opposite and yet
the equivalent, and I said—it is the cypress.

I will say no more—I am a little worried about a friend who
is still apparently ill, and whom I should like to go round to;
it is the one whose portrait I did in yellow and black, and
she had so altered. It is nervous attacks and the complications
of a premature change of life, altogether very painful. Last
time she was like an old grandfather. I promised to return
within a fortnight and was taken ill again myself. Anyway
the good news you have sent me and this article and heaps
of things have made me feel quite well in myself to-day. I
am sorry too that M. Salles did not find you. I thank Wil[1]
once more for her kind letter. I should have liked to answer
today, but I am putting it off until several days from now;
tell her that Mother has written me another long letter from
Amsterdam. How happy she too will be.

Meantime I remain with you in thought, though I am
finishing my letter. May Jo long remain for us what she is.
Now as for the little boy, why don't you call him Theo in
memory of our father, to me certainly it would give so much
pleasure.[2]

A handshake.

Yours,

Vincent

If you see him, start by thanking M. Aurier very much for
his article; I will send you a line for him of course and a
study.

---

[1] Their sister.
[2] In fact the boy was to be christened Vincent.

[Auvers-sur-Oise, late May 1890]

My dear Theo, my dear Jo,

Thank you for your letter which I received this morning, and for the fifty francs which were in it.

To-day I saw Dr. Gachet[1] again and I am going to paint at his house on Tuesday morning, then I shall dine with him and afterwards he will come to look at my painting. He seems very sensible, but he is as discouraged about his job as a country doctor as I am about my painting. Then I said to him that I would gladly exchange job for job. Anyway I am ready to believe that I shall end up being friends with him. He said to me besides, that if the depression or anything else became too great for me to bear, he could quite well do something to diminish its intensity, and that I must not find it awkward to be frank with him. Well, the moment when I shall need him may certainly come, however up to now all is well. And things may yet get better, I still think that it is mostly a malady of the South that I have caught, and that the return here will be enough to dissipate the whole thing. Often, very often, I think of your little one and then I start wishing he was big enough to come to the country. For it is the best system to bring them up there. How I do wish that you, Jo and the little one would take a rest in the country instead of the customary journey to Holland.

Yes, I know quite well that Mother will insist on seeing the little one, and that is certainly a reason for going, but she would surely understand if it was really better for the little one.

Here one is far enough from Paris for it to be real country, but nevertheless how changed since Daubigny. Yet not changed in an unpleasant way, there are many villas and

---

[1] The specialist to whose care Vincent had been committed; he was an art collector and had known Cézanne personally.

various modern bourgeois dwelling houses, very radiant and sunny and covered with flowers.

This in an almost lush country, just at the moment when a new society is developing in the old, is not at all unpleasing; there is much well-being in the air. I see or think I see in it a quiet like that of Puvis de Chavannes, no factories, but lovely greenery in abundance and well kept.

Please tell me sometime, which is the picture that Mlle. Bock has bought? I must write to her brother to thank them and then I shall suggest exchanging two of my studies for one of each of theirs. I have a drawing of an old vine, from which I intend to make a canvas of size 30, and a study of pink chestnuts and one of white chestnuts. But if circumstances allow it, I hope to work a little at the figure. Some pictures present themselves vaguely to my mind, which it will take time to get clear, but that will come bit by bit. If I had not been ill, I should have written to Bock and Isaäcson long ago.

My trunk has not yet arrived, which annoys me. I sent a wire this morning.

I thank you in advance for the canvas and paper. Yesterday and to-day it has been wet and stormy, but it is not unpleasant to see these effects again. The beds have not arrived either. But in spite of these annoyances, I feel happy at not being far from you two and my friends any longer. I hope you are well. It seemed to me however that you had less appetite than formerly,[1] and according to what the doctors say, constitutions like ours need very solid nourishment. So be sensible about this, especially Jo too, having her child to nurse. Really she ought to eat at least double, it would not at all be overdoing it when there are children to bring into the world and rear. Without that it is like a train going slowly where the line is straight. Time enough to reduce steam when the line is more uneven.

A handshake in thought from

Yours,
Vincent

[1] He had spent three days in Paris on his way through to Auvers.

[Auvers, early July 1890]

Dear brother and sister,

Jo's letter was really like a gospel to me, a deliverance from the agony which had been caused by the hours I had shared with you which were a bit difficult and trying for us all.[1] It was no slight thing when all of us alike felt our daily bread to be in danger, no slight thing when for other reasons than that we felt that our manner of existence was frail.

Back here, I too still felt very sad and continued to feel the storm which threatens you weighing on me as well. What is to be done—look here, I generally try to be fairly cheerful, but my life too is threatened at the very root, and my steps too are unsteady.

I feared—not altogether, but nevertheless a little—that being a burden on you, you found me forbidding, but Jo's letter proves to me clearly that you understand that for my part I am in toil and trouble as much as you are.

There—once back here I set to work again—though the brush almost slipped from my fingers, and knowing exactly what I wanted, I have since painted three big canvases already.

They are vast stretches of corn under troubled skies, and I did not need to go out of my way to try to express sadness and the extreme of loneliness. I hope you will see them soon—for I hope to bring them to you in Paris as soon as possible, since I almost think that these canvases will tell you what I cannot say in words, the health and fortifying power that I see in the country. Now the third canvas is Daubigny's garden, a picture I have been contemplating since I came here.

I hope with all my heart that the intended journey will give you a little distraction.

I often think of the little one. I think it is certainly better to bring up children than to give all your nervous energy to making pictures, but there is nothing for it, I am—at least I feel—too old to go back on my steps or to desire anything different. That desire has left me, though the mental suffering from it remains.

[1] Earlier in the month Vincent had gone on his last visit to Paris.

I am very sorry not to have seen Guillaumin again, but I am pleased that he has seen my canvases.

If I had waited, I should probably have stayed talking with him long enough to miss my train.

Wishing you luck and courage and comparative prosperity, I beg you tell Mother and our sister that I think of them very often, also I have a letter from them this morning and will reply soon.

Handshakes in thought,

> Yours,
> Vincent

My money will not last me very long this time, as on my return I had to pay the freight of the luggage from Arles. I retain very pleasant memories of that journey to Paris, for several months I had hardly dared to hope to see my friends again. I think that Dutch lady[1] has a lot of talent. Lautrec's picture, the portrait of a musician, is amazing, I was very moved by it.

My dear brother,   [Auvers, late July 1890][2]

Thanks for your kind letter and for the 50 fr. note it contained. . . . Since the thing that matters most is going well, why should I say more about things of less importance; my word, *before we have a chance of talking business more collectedly, there is likely to be a long way to go.* . . .

The other painters, whatever they think of it, instinctively keep themselves at a distance from discussions about actual trade.

Well, the truth is, we can only make our pictures speak. But still, my dear brother, there is this that I have always told you, and I repeat it once more with all the earnestness that can be imparted by an effort of a mind diligently fixed on trying to do as well as one can—I tell you again that I shall

[1] The sculptress S. de Swart.
[2] This letter, evidently his penultimate one to Theo, was found on Vincent's body after his suicide on the 27th. Several sentences dealing with the state of Theo's business are omitted.

always consider that you are something other than a simple dealer in Corot, that through my mediation you have your part in the actual production of some canvases, which even in the cataclysm retain their quietude.

For this is what we have got to, and this is all or at least the chief thing that I can have to tell you at a moment of comparative crisis. At a moment when things are very strained between dealers in pictures by dead artists, and living artists.

Well, my own work, I am risking my life for it and my reason has half-foundered owing to it—that's all right—but you are not among the dealers in men so far as I know, and you can choose your side, I think, acting with true humanity, but what's the use?

SUMMARY CHRONOLOGY
OF THE LIFE OF
VINCENT VAN GOGH

Early Years

1853   March 30th, birth of Vincent in the parsonage at Groot Zundert in North Brabant, as the eldest child of Theodorus van Gogh, pastor of the parish.

1857   May 1st, birth of his brother Theo.

1869   July 30th, enters the firm of Goupil and Co., art dealers in The Hague.

1872   August, beginning of the extant correspondence with Theo.

1873   June, is transferred by the firm to London; meanwhile in January Theo had entered the Brussels branch. The same month he is rejected by Ursula Loyer, the daughter of his London landlady.

1875   May, is sent once more to the Paris branch. Clashes with his employers. The period of his religious mysticism.

1876   April, dismissed by the firm. Goes to England in a schoolmastering post, teaching at Ramsgate and then at Isleworth. Returns to Etten in North Brabant to see his family (who have now moved there) over Christmas—and remains in Holland.

1877   Takes a position in a bookshop in Dordrecht. May 9th, moves to Amsterdam to study for the University entrance examination and so gain entry to the Theological Seminary.

1878   July, gives up his studies after fifteen months—to enter an Evangelical school in Brussels; leaves after three months only. December, undertakes to go as a preacher among the miners of the Borinage, in South Belgium, at his own expense; stays at Pâturages, preaching and working among the sick.

1879   January, obtains a temporary nomination for six

months as a lay preacher at Wasmes, in the Borinage. July, dismissed for excessive zeal. Works at his own expense at Cuesmes nearby.

1880   July/August, finds his vocation as an artist and begins to draw miners. October, goes to Brussels and takes lessons in anatomy and perspective. The payments for his support from Theo begin at this time.

Holland, 1881-1885

1881   April 12th, returns to Etten and lives with his parents. Suffers the disappointment of rejection by his cousin, Kee Vos. October, beginning of his correspondence with the artist Anthon van Rappard. December, settles in The Hague, and takes lessons with the successful painter of The Hague school, Anton Mauve.

1882   January, takes in the prostitute Clasina Maria Hoornik (Sien) and lives with her. Falls out with Mauve after only a few weeks of working with him. Starts to build a large collection of lithographs and woodcuts from English magazines. Sells twelve *Views of The Hague* commissioned by his uncle C. M. van Gogh.

1883   September, Theo comes and exerts pressure to induce him to part from Sien. Moves to Drenthe, a province in the north-east of Holland, and roams the moorland regions there for two and a half months. December, goes to stay with his family at Nuenen, a village in Brabant near Eindhoven (his father now being appointed there).

1884   At Nuenen. The period of the relationship with his neighbour Margot Begemann; family objections and the woman's attempt at suicide bring the affair to a tragic end. Does still-lifes, treatments of weavers and peasants, studies of heads. Theo finally accepts, after some hesitation, a proposal originally made by Vincent in March : namely that Theo should consider all works sent to him thereafter as his property, so that his monthly dispatches of 150 francs would become a purchase price rather than a gift or loan.

1885   At Nuenen. March 27th, death of his father. April/
       May, paints the *Potato-Eaters*. November, moves to
       Antwerp.
1886   January, enters the Academy at Antwerp. February,
       leaves for Paris.

Paris, February 1886—February 1888
1886   Welcomed by Theo and lives with him in the Rue de
       Laval. Joins the Atelier Cormon. June, moves with
       Theo to Montmartre, 54 Rue Lepic. There follows the
       period of his friendly relations with the many Parisian
       artists, and of his prolonged exposure to Japanese art.
1887   Exhibits his work informally in various places, with-
       out success. June, works at Asnières, a suburb of
       Paris, with Emile Bernard.

Arles, February 1888—May 1889
1888   February 20th, leaves for Arles in Provence. Takes a
       room there over the Restaurant Carrel. March, begins
       a regular correspondence with Bernard. May, rents a
       four-room house, 2 Place Lamartine. June, spends a
       week working at Saintes-Maries-sur-Mer. September,
       moves into the "Yellow House." October 23rd,
       arrival of Gauguin from Brittany. December, Theo
       gives advance news of his engagement to Johanna
       Bonger. December 23rd, first mental crisis; Gauguin
       leaves for Paris on the 27th, Vincent spends two weeks
       in hospital.
1889   January 7th, returns to the house and begins to paint
       again soon after. February 4th, suffers his second
       crisis; this lasts about two weeks, and is followed by a
       third attack towards the end of the month. Under
       pressure from the people of Arles, who had petitioned
       that he should remain in confinement, he stays on at
       the hospital into April. April 17th, Theo gets mar-
       ried. Vincent agrees to move to the nearby asylum of
       Saint-Paul-de-Mausole at Saint-Rémy.

Saint-Rémy, May 1889—*May* 1890

1889   May 8th, admitted to the asylum. There he has long
        periods of lucidity, interspersed by two violent attacks;
        one of these lasts from early July to around mid
        August, the other from about Christmas to about New
        Year's Day.

1890   January, an article by Albert Aurier commending Vin-
        cent's work appears in the periodical *Mercure de
        France*; late in the month occurs the sixth crisis
        (about a week in duration). January 31st, birth of a
        son to Theo (christened Vincent Willem). Mid Febru-
        ary, his seventh crisis, which lasts until mid April.
        March, sells his *Red Vineyard* in Brussels for 400
        francs. May 16th, leaves for Paris, in order to retire
        to Auvers. May 17th, visits Theo for three days in
        Paris.

Auvers-sur-Oise, May-July 1890

1890   May 21st, arrives at Auvers. Dr. Gachet takes care of
        him there. July 1st, visits Theo in Paris. July 27th,
        shoots himself, and dies on the 29th. July 30th, buried
        in the small cemetery at Auvers; Theo himself is to die
        on January 25th, 1891.

INDEX

Fontana Paperbacks

Fontana is a leading paperback publisher of fiction and non-fiction, with authors ranging from Alistair MacLean, Agatha Christie and Desmond Bagley to Solzhenitsyn and Pasternak, from Gerald Durrell and Joy Adamson to the famous Modern Masters series.

In addition to a wide-ranging collection of internationally popular writers of fiction, Fontana also has an outstanding reputation for history, natural history, military history, psychology, psychiatry, politics, economics, religion and the social sciences.

All Fontana books are available at your bookshop or newsagent; or can be ordered direct. Just fill in the form and list the titles you want.

FONTANA BOOKS, Cash Sales Department, G.P.O. Box 29, Douglas, Isle of Man, British Isles. Please send purchase price, plus 8p per book. Customers outside the U.K. send purchase price, plus 10p per book. Cheque, postal or money order. No currency.

NAME (Block letters)

_____

ADDRESS

_____

_____

_____